Liver Pathology and Alcohol

Drug and Alcohol Abuse Reviews

Edited by

Ronald R. Watson

- **Liver Pathology and Alcohol,** *1991*
- **Drug and Alcohol Abuse Prevention,** *1990*

Liver Pathology
and Alcohol

Edited by

Ronald R. Watson

University of Arizona, Tucson, Arizona

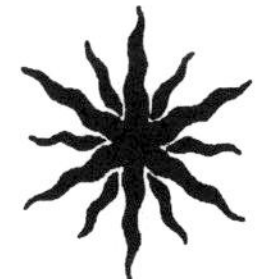

Humana Press • Totowa, New Jersey

Copyright © 1991 by The Humana Press Inc.
999 Riverview Drive
Totowa, NJ 07512 USA

Printed in the United States of America.

Library of Congress Cataloging-in-Publication Data

Liver Pathology and Alcohol/edited by Ronald R. Watson.
        p. cm. -- (Drug and alcohol abuse reviews)
    Includes bibliographical references and index.
    ISBN 0-89603-206-X
    1. Alcoholic liver diseases. I. Watson, Ronald R. (Ronald Ross)
II. Series.
    [DNLM: 1. Liver--pathology. WI 700 L78381]
RC848.A42L58 1991
616.3'62--dc20
DNLM/DLC
for Library of Congress

                                                91-20879
                                                  CIP

Contents

Preface

Alcohol and other drugs of abuse are major contributing factors to liver disease and its pathology. Alcoholic cirrhosis causes thousands of deaths each year in the United States, and encourages liver replacement. A better understanding of the mechanisms of liver pathology will significantly aid basic researchers and physicians in treating and preventing liver damage.

This book is designed especially for those researchers wishing to understand alcoholic liver disease. Therefore the role of alcohol in changing nutrition and its nutritional effects on liver disease are reviewed.

The generation of free radicals during alcohol use has been found to be an important cause of membrane changes, of cancer development, and of lipid alterations—and thus of liver pathology. In addition to alcohol, other drugs of abuse, including morphine, cocaine, marijuana, and caffeine have also been shown to be significant contributors to liver pathology.

The prevalence of drug and alcohol use and abuse today means that liver disease will continue as a major social and medical problem. The explanation of its biological origins cannot fail to help us better understand and treat the disease in the years to come.

Ronald R. Watson

Contributors

Neal L. Benowitz • *Department of Medicine, University of California, San Francisco, CA*

Puran S. Bora • *Department of Medicine, Jewish Hospital of St. Louis at the Washington University Medical Center, St. Louis, MO*

Lester M. Bornheim • *Department of Pharmacology and the Liver Center, University of California, San Francisco, CA*

Rhonda L. Boyd • *Department of Physiology and Pharmacology, Bowman Gray School of Medicine of Wake Forest University, Winston-Salem, NC*

Charles R. Breese • *Department of Physiology and Pharmacology, Bowman Gray School of Medicine of Wake Forest University, Winston-Salem, NC*

Stuart J. Chirtel • *VA Medical Center, Washington, DC and Department of Medicine, George Washington University, Washington, DC*

Anselm D'Costa • *Department of Physiology and Pharmacology, Bowman Gray School of Medicine of Wake Forest University, Winston-Salem, NC*

Charles P. Denaro • *Department of Medicine, University of California, San Francisco, CA*

Gregg Duester • *Department of Biochemistry, Colorado State University, Fort Collins, CO*

Billy W. Geer • *Department of Biology, Knox College, Galesburg, IL*

Pradeep Ghosh • *VA Medical Center, Washington, DC and Department of Medicine, George Washington University, Washington, DC*

Pieter W. H. Heinstra • *Department of Biochemistry, Leiden University, Leiden, The Netherlands*

Rolf F. Kletzien • *Department of Biological Sciences, Western Michigan University, Kalamazoo, MI*

Edward T. Knych • *Department of Pharmacology, School of Medicine, University of Minnesota, Duluth, MN*

M. R. Lakshman • *VA Medical Center, Washington DC and Department of Medicine, George Washington University, Washington, DC*

Louis G. Lange • *Department of Medicine, Jewish Hospital of St. Louis at the Washington University Medical Center, St. Louis, MO*

Renee C. Lin • *Departments of Medicine and Biochemistry, Indiana University School of Medicine, and Richard L. Roudebush VA Medical Center, Indianapolis, IN*

Lawrence Lumeng • *Departments of Medicine and Biochemistry, Indiana University School of Medicine, and Richard L. Roudebush VA Medical Center, Indianapolis, IN*

Ariane Mallat • *Department of Medicine, The Johns Hopkins University School of Medicine, Baltimore, MD*

Paul B. McCay • *Oklahoma Medical Research Foundation, Oklahoma City, OK*

Robert S. McCuskey • *Departments of Anatomy and Physiology, College of Medicine, University of Arizona, Tucson, AZ*

Robert R. Miller, Jr. • *Department of Biology, Knox College, Galesburg, IL*

Mack C. Mitchell • *Department of Medicine, The Johns Hopkins University School of Medicine, Baltimore, MD*

Siraj I. Mufti • *Department of Pharmacology and Toxicology, College of Pharmacy, University of Arizona, Tucson, AZ*

Olalekan E. Odeleye • *Department of Family and Community Medicine, University of Arizona, Tucson, AZ*

Barry J. Potter • *Division of Hepatology, Department of Medicine, Mount Sinai School of Medicine, New York, NY*

David S. Raiford • *Department of Medicine, The Johns Hopkins University School of Medicine, Baltimore, MD*

Lester A. Reinke • *Department of Pharmacology, University of Oklahoma Health Sciences Center, Oklahoma City, OK*

Edward Reyes • *Department of Pharmacology, University of New Mexico School of Medicine, Albuquerque, NM*

F. Joseph Roll • *Department of Medicine, University of California, San Francisco , CA*

Hagai Rottenberg • *Pathology Department, Hahnemann University School of Medicine, Philadelphia, PA*

Akitaka Shibuya • *Department of Internal Medicine, Kitasato University School of Medicine, Kanagawa, Japan*

Louis Shuster • *Tufts University, School of Medicine, Boston, MA*

William E. Sonntag • *Department of Physiology and Pharmacology, Bowman School of Medicine of Wake Forest University, Winston-Salem, NC*

Thomas M. Soranno • *Department of Pharmacology and Toxicology, University of Medicine and Dentistry of New Jersey, Newark, NJ*

Lester G. Sultatos • *Department of Pharmacology and Toxicology, University of Medicine and Dentistry of New Jersey, Newark, NJ*

Ralph E. Tarter • *Departments of Surgery and Medicine, University of Pittsburgh School of Medicine, Pittsburgh, PA*

David H. Van Thiel • *Department of Surgery and Medicine, University of Pittsburgh School of Medicine, Pittsburgh, PA*

Ronald R. Watson • *Department of Family and Community Medicine, University of Arizona, Tucson, AZ*

Akira Yoshida • *Department of Biochemical Genetics, Beckman Research Institute of the City of Hope, Duarte, CA*

Alcohol and Hepatic Iron Homeostasis

Barry J. Potter

Introduction

Alcoholic liver disease is associated with marked disorders of iron homeostasis. These abnormalities include changes in plasma iron turnover,[1] red cell iron incorporation,[1,2] depression of the serum levels of transferrin[3] (the major serum iron transport protein), and, in approximately one-third of chronic alcoholics, an increase in liver iron concentrations.[4] In the rat, ethanol alters the rate of synthesis and secretion of transferrin and other serum proteins by the liver.[5–7] Although these disturbances have been attributed to a variety of causes, such as a direct toxic effect of alcohol on heme synthesis,[8] negative vitamin balance,[2] altered iron absorption,[9–11] or intake of greater quantities of iron contained in some alcoholic beverages,[12,13] the mechanism(s) of these disorders remain(s) in doubt.

It becomes apparent that there is not a simplistic causal relationship between alcoholic intake and alterations to iron homeostasis when it is noted that the hematologic manifestations range from iron deficiency and anemia,[14] through megaloblastic anemia with high levels of serum iron, to hemochromatosis and siderosis.[2] Decreased levels of serum iron are frequent in alcoholics with gastrointestinal bleeding and liver disease,[2] although a normal plasma iron clearance and increased mean hepatic iron concentration

From: *Drug and Alcohol Abuse Reviews, Vol. 2: Liver Pathology and Alcohol*
Ed: R. R. Watson ©1991 The Humana Press Inc.

are associated with this decrease.[15] Increased serum iron levels are also found in some alcoholics,[2,16,17] although the diurnal variation appears to remain intact.[17] The percentage transferrin iron saturation also appears to be increased in these subjects and in male adolescent alcohol abusers.[18] Experimentally, a gradual rise in the serum iron level is seen in volunteers during alcoholic intoxication, and this falls sharply on recovery.[19]

Iron overload occurs in normal subjects if they are exposed to excessive amounts of bioavailable iron for a considerable period of time. In some areas of Ethiopia, the daily intake of iron is in the range of 100–300 mg, compared to a normal average of 15–25 mg. This extra iron is a contaminant of the food grain, however, and has a low bioavailability so that iron overload does not occur[20] in this group of people. Among the Bantu in South Africa, an excessive iron intake also occurs as a result of drinking beer fermented in iron pots. In this population, iron overload is common,[21–23] with heavy parenchymal deposits in the liver being common. Although there is still some controversy as to whether the iron overload seen in Western alcoholics is caused by the iron content of the beverage being consumed (as discussed later), at least in the Bantu, changing from home brewed beer to commercially prepared liquor has lowered the incidence of iron overload while increasing the incidence of fatty changes or alcoholic hyaline in the liver in alcoholic liver disease in this population.[24]

The predisposition to iron overloading is also genetically linked in some cases. Primary idiopathic hemochromatosis has now been shown to be an autosomal recessive disorder, with the susceptibility locus on gene 6, close to the HLA-A locus (mainly HLA-A3 and HLA-B7).[25–29] This disease has frequently been confused in the past with that of alcoholic liver disease with accompanying iron overload,[30,31] especially since approximately one-quarter of the patients presenting with idiopathic hemochromatosis also abuse alcohol,[31] but can now be better differentiated on the basis of HLA typing.[31–34]

However, although the presence of the two phenotypes — HLA-43 and HLA-B7 — is important collaborative evidence in the diagnosis of idiopathic hemochromatosis, this presence cannot be relied upon to differentiate between this and iron overload in alcoholic liver disease. Final diagnosis can usually now be made on the basis of a liver biopsy and the determination of the liver iron concentration.[4] Although liver iron levels are elevated in the alcoholics, these values are still much lower than those found in patients with idiopathic hemochromatosis. It should be noted that use of indirect methods of determining liver iron content, such as serum iron and transferrin saturation, the desferrioxamine chelation test, and serum ferritin measurement, tend to underestimate liver iron stores in idiopathic hemochromatosis and to overestimate them in alcoholic liver disease.[35]

Since the liver not only synthesizes and secretes transferrin, the major serum iron transport protein, but is also a major site of iron storage (mainly in the cytosolic iron storage protein ferritin), it is clear that any disturbances of liver function could profoundly affect iron homeostasis. Prolonged alcohol abuse leads to such marked alterations in liver function and is also associated with disturbances to iron homeostasis, as has been mentioned earlier. Although considerable, but fragmented, evidence is available, what still remains to be elucidated is exactly how these various disturbances occur and their relationship to the liver in acute and chronic alcohol intoxication. This review will therefore attempt to remedy this situation and to present a cohesive picture of the effects of alcohol on liver iron homeostasis, based on the current understanding of normal iron metabolism. To aid our understanding of the abnormalities occurring as a result of alcohol intoxication, a brief review of normal iron metabolism will be given prior to discussing the effects in detail.

Normal Iron Homeostasis

Iron-containing compounds are vital to life. The body of an average 75-kg man contains between 3.5–4 g of iron (approx 45–50 mg/kg). Of this, 2–2.5 g are to be found in the hemoglobin molecule in erythrocytes, and up to 1 g in the body iron stores (principally in ferritin in the liver). Of the rest, 300 mg are present in myoglobin, 80 mg in heme enzymes, and a further 100 mg in nonheme enzymes. Only 3 mg are present in the serum, mostly complexed to transferrin, although approx 20 mg are turned over per day, principally from the recycling of iron from senescent red cells. Iron balance in the body is exquisitely balanced. Less than 1 mg/d is lost from the body of normal males, postmenopausal females, and prepubertal females. About 65% of this loss occurs via the gastrointestinal tract and most of the rest through the skin, with only small quantities being lost in the urine. In women, the menstrual losses are an additional 0.4–0.5 mg/d, although the range varies widely.[36,37] To balance these losses, an equal amount of iron in a bioavailable form needs to be acquired from the diet.

Iron Absorption

Iron absorption from the food is a complex process, dependent on its form and the composition of the rest of the diet. In a normal diet, approx 15 mg of iron are taken in daily. Of this, less than 8 mg can be solubilized in the digestive tract and only 3 mg taken up by the mucosa. From this, 1 mg of iron enters the plasma in the portal vein. For practical purposes, dietary iron can be divided into two types: heme- and nonheme-bound. Heme iron absorption is unaffected by the composition of the diet and is therefore generally considered to be in the most bioavailable form. Nonheme iron absorption is, however, markedly influenced by the constituents of the diet and is poorly bioavailable unless some enhancing substance, such as ascorbic acid or meat, is taken up along with it. For example, only 1% of the iron from some vegetables is absorbed, whereas up to 25% may be absorbed from red meats.[38] When meat is taken with maize, however, this value is reduced by half.

Nonheme iron must be in an ionized form before it can be absorbed. The valency of this ionized iron is also important for its uptake. Ferric iron is poorly soluble above pH 3, and at pH 8 (the pH of the duodenum) the solubility is of the order of $10^{-18}M$, compared to $1.6 \times 10^{-2}M$ for ferrous iron.[39] The counter ion is also important; ferric chloride is much more soluble than ferric phosphate, which is an important constituent of many vegetables.[39] In aqueous solution, ferric ions are bound to each other through water bridges and at alkaline pH, precipitation of the metallic hydroxide will occur, making the iron totally unavailable to the mucosal cells. Absorption of ferrous iron correlates well with the dose administered, up to 0.5 g,[40] and there appears to be no defined upper limit as may be seen in iron poisoning.

It thus appears that the ferric nonheme iron released by digestion of food must be both ionized and complexed in some form for mucosal absorption to occur. It has been suggested that the iron released following peptic digestion in the stomach is stabilized by mucopolysaccharides if other constituents of the diet, such as ascorbate, citrate, or amino acids, do not perform this task.[41] This process does not appear to be altered in diseases such as idiopathic hemochromatosis or iron deficiency anemia, where iron uptake is known to be modified.[42–44]

Although there is some evidence that bile may affect iron absorption, this work is still the subject of controversy. Ferrous salts are taken up more readily in the presence of bile in the iron deficient dog[45] and bile duct ligation lowers ferric iron absorption in rats.[46] This effect, however, is not seen in vivo in humans.[47]

Uptake of nonheme iron by the mucosa is extremely rapid and, at least in rats, iron may be detected in the portal circulation in less than 26 s after its entry into the gut lumen.[48] Maximal absorption of iron occurs in the duodenum and jejunum, where the efficiency increases from the distal to the proximal region.[49] This effect is less pronounced in iron deficiency, because of an enhanced absorptive capacity of the distal portion of the jejunum.[50] However, in mice, iron deficiency has been shown to result in a doubling of iron uptake by the proximal region, but no change in uptake by the distal portion of the small intestine.[51] The enhanced uptake has been shown to be the result of an increase in V_{max}, and is also seen in hypoxia and pregnancy in mice.[52]

Iron transport by the intestinal mucosa consists of at least three sequential steps:

1. Uptake of iron from the gut lumen by the intestinal brush borders;
2. Intracellular transport or storage; and
3. Iron release into the portal circulation.[53]

Iron binding to microvillous membranes appears to be specific, saturable, and significantly higher for the ferrous form,[54] suggesting the presence of high affinity binding sites on the membranes and an active transport system for iron across this barrier. Studies using membrane vesicles indicate that both active transport and simple diffusion are involved in the microvillous uptake of ferrous iron.[55] Uptake studies with ferric iron have also shown that membrane transport of iron is the rate-limiting step[56] and that uptake from distal ileum vesicles represents predominantly transport and is higher than that in vesicles from duodenum.[57] Following hypoxia, there appears to be an increase in ferric iron uptake only in duodenal vesicles[57] and no effect on ferrous iron uptake.[58] Further analysis has shown the presence of a relatively low affinity transport site (K_m ca. 83 1M) in proximal intestine brush borders[59] and a single high capacity, high affinity binding site (K_d < 5 1M) in duodenal microvillous membranes.[60] This latter binding component appears to be principally lipid in nature, since it can be extracted into chloroform/methanol solution and is both heat and protease resistant. There is now some evidence that free fatty acids may also act as mediators for the transport of Fe^{2+} across intestinal brush border membranes.[61] Furthermore, rats fed high fat diets tend to have higher liver iron contents than those fed low fat diets.[62] Other groups, however, have suggested that the membrane transport component may be a 100-kDa glycoprotein.[63]

Once iron is taken up by microvillous membrane, it appears to become bound to specific carriers and is either rapidly transported to the serosal side of the mucosal cell or stored in cytosolic ferritin. The nature of the carrier(s) has still not been clearly determined. Several groups have suggested that transferrin-like proteins are involved,[64–68] although it is possible that there may be transferrin contamination of the various preparations.[69] There is also some evidence that the iron is chelated to lower mol wt ligands, such as amino acids, although it is not clear whether these play a part in iron transport.[70,71] Iron not immediately transported to the serosal side of the mucosal cell becomes sequestered in ferritin within 2–6 h in the rat and is accompanied by a burst of ferritin synthesis.[72] The current consensus is that this ferritin is purely a storage vehicle for excess iron and is not directly involved in the transfer of iron to the plasma.[50,71] However, mucosal iron stores in ferritin correlate inversely with iron absorption and directly with body iron stores.[73]

Little is known about the delivery of iron from the mucosal cell to serum transferrin. There has been no conclusive isolation of a receptor mechanism for apotransferrin. Huebers and coworkers have suggested that transferrin is involved in the *luminal* uptake of iron and then acts as a shuttle for mucosal iron transport.[74] As has been mentioned earlier, transferrin-like immunoreactive proteins have been observed in the mucosa and the concentration appears to increase in iron deficiency.[75] If this transferrin is not a contamination artifact, then either transferrin is actively synthesized by the mucosal cells, or a recycling mechanism is present that is similar to that seen for other cells — except that iron would be donated to transferrin. Transfer of iron to transferrin does, however, appear to require an intact cytoskeleton.[76]

Heme iron does not appear to be taken up by a receptor-mediated mechanism. Degradation of heme by xanthine oxidase occurs inside the mucosal cell and the iron released into the intracellular pool.[77] Xanthine oxidase has also been shown to be involved in the incorporation of iron into transferrin directly in the intestine,[78] but the significance of this has not been thoroughly investigated.

Plasma to Cell Cycle

More than 95% of the iron in the plasma circulates bound to transferrin, the principal iron transport protein, and the remainder (nontransferrin-bound iron) is either complexed to low mol wt chelators, sequestered in serum ferritin, or is attached to heme-containing breakdown products. The transferrin molecule consists of a single polypeptide chain with a mol wt of approx 78 kDa. There are two iron binding sites on the molecule, designated N- and C-terminal binding sites, respectively. Ferric iron is bound, complexed through bicarbonate ions, and the stability of the iron–bicarbonate–transferrin complex is pH-dependent, iron only being easily removed below pH 6. Whether these two binding sites are identical in their iron binding and donating properties has been a source of controversy for over 20 years since the proposal by Fletcher and Huehns that these sites differed in their ability to donate iron to reticulocytes for hemoglobin synthesis.[79,80] It now appears that the transferrin–reticulocyte interaction is extremely sensitive to environmental variables, which may account for the earlier discrepancies in the relative iron donating properties of the two sites. Since the normal range of transferrin saturation in humans is of the order of 45–55%, controversy has also arisen over the occupancy of these iron binding sites.[81–83] Although there is a considerable range in the occupancy ratio, it seems that the N-terminal site is predominantly occupied in most human subjects.[83] This is in accord with the finding that the N-terminal site has an affinity for iron 1.38 times greater than that for the C-terminal site.[84] It should be noted that the rate of clearance of iron from transferrin is proportionally greater for diferric transferrin than for either monoferric form.[85]

Transferrin-bound iron circulates in the plasma and is downloaded at either sites of utilization, such as the erythroid marrow, or storage, such as the liver. Since the principal use of iron in the body is in the production of hemoglobin, the reticulocyte has been the cell most frequently chosen to study iron–transferrin–cell interactions. Reticulocyte receptors for transferrin have now been isolated and characterized by several groups (*see* Seligman[86] or May and Cuatrecasas[87] for reviews of these data). More recently, investigations using K562 and Hep G2 cell lines have now helped clarify much of the mechanism of iron uptake by the cell. The transferrin receptor has been shown to have an observed mol wt of approx 180 kDa and is composed of two 90–94 kDa identical subunits attached through a single disulfide bridge.[88,89] Posttranslational modification of the receptor occurs, following synthesis in the endoplasmic reticulum, and the mature 760 amino acid monomer is a transmembrane phosphoglycoprotein with covalently attached fatty acids.[90,91] Each monomeric subunit can bind a molecule of transferrin, implying an accumulation of a maximum of 4 atoms of iron per receptor at any one time on the cell surface! Thus, this system has the potential to deliver the huge quantities of iron required by reticulocytes actively synthesizing hemoglobin (a rate that could, theoretically, run at greater than a million iron atoms/min for each cell[92]).

The transferrin receptor is intimately involved in the rapid delivery of iron from the plasma to cells that are actively synthesizing iron containing proteins. It has been shown that diferric or monoferric transferrin bind to these specific receptors on the cell surface in a temperature and energy dependent process.[93,94] Coated pit formation occurs followed by internalization of the receptor–transferrin–iron complex into endocytic vesicles.[95–97] Acidification ensues (probably as a result of proton pumping by the Na^+/H^+ transport system), lowering the pH of the veqicle to $\leq$pH 5.5. This leads to the release of the iron from the receptor-bound transferrin.[98] In other receptor systems, such as the asialoglycoprotein receptor system, this lowering of the pH causes the receptor to dissociate from the membrane receptor and this is thought to trigger the steps leading to the fusion with a secondary lysosome and subsequent degradation of the ligand. However, iron-free (apo)transferrin has a very high affinity for its receptor at this acidic pH[99] and therefore does not separate from it. The steps leading to fusion with secondary lysosomes do not occur and the apotransferrin is then recycled back to the cell surface still attached to the transferrin receptor. At physiological pH, the receptor has a much higher affinity for iron-loaded transferrin than for apotransferrin, and the apotransferrin is therefore released back into the plasma, undegraded, to bind more iron.[100] This cycle is shown in Fig. 1.

Recycling of transferrin in Hep G2 cells normally takes about 16 min: 4 min for binding, 5 min for internalization of the complex, 7 min for its return to the cell surface, and 15 s for the release of apotransferrin back into the medium.[101] At the present time, it is not known how the iron released from transferrin enters the cytosol from the endosome (which occurs 6–10 min after vesicle formation). It is thought that the iron must be chelated to a small molecule for transport into the cell, such as pyrophos-

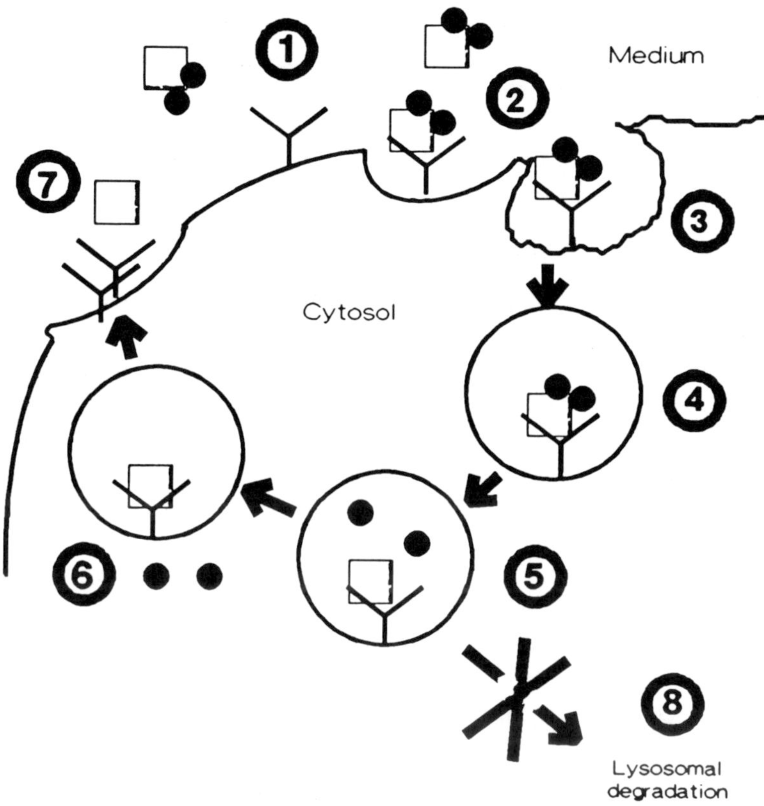

Fig. 1. The cellular uptake of transferrin-bound iron by receptor-mediated recycling. (1) Empty transferrin receptors are expressed on the cell surface. Binding of iron-loaded transferrin to these receptors (2) leads to the formation of clathrin-coated pits (3). These pits are then pinched off and form an endosome in the cell cytosol (4). The pH inside the endosome drops to approximately pH 5.5, causing release of the iron, which is then transported into the cytoplasm by an unknown mechanism (6). At this lowered pH, apotransferrin has a high affinity for the transferrin receptor and is therefore transported back to the cell surface (7) where, at physiological pH, it has a much lower affinity for the receptor and is released into the medium, freeing the receptor to bind more iron-loaded transferrin. Because transferrin does not dissociate from its receptor in the cell, the normal signal to fuse with a secondary lysosome is not given and lysosomal degradation (8) of transferrin does not occur.

phate, ATP, or ADP,[102] since uncomplexed iron is toxic to the cell (as discussed later). The expression of transferrin receptors in most proliferating or metabolizing cells appears now to be regulated by iron availability. Chelation of intracellular iron by desferrioxamine leads to an increase in the receptor mRNA,[103] and it seems that there are at least two genetic elements present for regulation of the transferrin receptor gene,[104] which is thought to be located on chromosome 3.[105]

Hepatic Iron Storage

As the liver is not only a major storage site for iron, but also synthesizes transferrin, interactions of iron-loaded transferrin with the various cells of the liver probably represents one of the critical factors in iron homeostasis. Less evidence is available on the mode of action of liver transferrin receptors than for those on reticulocytes. The author's laboratory has isolated a putative 90-kDa transferrin receptor from rat liver by affinity chromatography and has also shown that the OKT9 monoclonal antibody (an antibody to the human transferrin receptor) inhibits iron uptake by the isolated rat hepatocyte.[106] Isolated hepatocytes have now been shown to exhibit all the characteristics of a specific receptor-mediated mechanism for transferrin binding and iron uptake.[106–110] The controversy centered around the suggestion that the major liver transferrin receptors resided on endothelial cells, rather on the hepatocytes,[112,113] has now been resolved and shown to be mainly caused by the collagenase perfusion technique employed.[114] However, accumulated data now suggest that there are (at least) two mechanisms operating in the hepatocyte: specific transferrin receptors at low transferrin concentrations and a nonspecific bulk endocytosis mechanism at higher levels.[115–118] In the light of the finding that transferrin receptors recycle in the absence of bound transferrin,[119] this is clearly an area that still needs to be evaluated for its influence on iron uptake by the liver.

Not only is the mechanism for iron uptake across the liver plasma membrane unclear, but that for transport of iron in the cell to sites of utilization and/or storage within ferritin molecules has also not been well defined. Once across the plasma membrane barrier, iron enters a transitory "labile" iron pool, from which it can be readily chelated and mobilized. If it is not required for the synthesis of heme proteins, from this pool it enters the ferritin molecule. Ferritin is a ubiquitous iron-storage protein consisting of complexes of two subunits of mol wt 21 kDa (H) and 19 kDa (L) that form a protein shell within which iron is stored in a semicrystalline form. Synthesis of this protein shell is induced by iron administration,[120] resulting from the shift of ferritin mRNA from messenger ribonucleoproteins to polysomes and subsequent active translation.[121] Chelation studies have shown that removal of the intracellular iron pool results in an increase in free ferritin mRNA and a reduction in that associated with polysomes.[120] Induction of ferritin mRNA synthesis with sodium butyrate increases the synthesis of ferritin proportionately, but the capacity for modulation of ferritin synthesis in response to iron is preserved,[122] suggesting that ferritin synthesis depends on both regulatory signals and transcription rates. As with the transferrin receptor, there is now known to be a specific iron responsive element in the H chain mRNA (in the 5' untranslated region), although this represses the regulation of ferritin translation by iron.[123]

As iron loading increases, the pattern of ferritin deposition changes from predominantly cytosolic arrays associated with lysosomes (but not inside them[124]) to condensed aggregates within the lysosomes, which represent hemosiderin (a condensed semicrystalline degradation product of ferritin). These lysosomes are much more fragile than normal, possibly as a result of free radical formation by the stored hemosideral iron.[125] There is some evidence that this hemosideral iron is not readily accessible initially to chelation therapy, but gradually becomes so with treatment,[126] probably liberated through lysosomal digestion or cell death. These iron "compartments" exist in both the hepatocytes and Kupffer cells of the liver, as well as the reticuloendothelial (RE) cells of the spleen and bone marrow. In vitamin C deficient guinea pigs, the relative proportion of iron stored as ferritin is decreased in favor of hemosiderin, and the release of iron from the RE system is reduced. This suggests that vitamin C may increase the mobility of iron between the various "compartments," especially facilitating the mobilization of RE iron.[127] However, there is little evidence as to how iron is mobilized back to the serum from these "compartments." It is unlikely to be located on the freshly synthesized transferrin since Baker and coworkers[128] have shown that iron efflux from the hepatocyte is virtually zero in transferrin-free medium (in spite of normal transferrin synthesis by these cells) and increases markedly in the presence of apotransferrin. The problem has yet to be solved as to whether transferrin acts solely as a serum iron transporter, or has a more specific role in the control of iron mobilization and apotransferrin synthesis through membrane interaction.

Although transferrin-bound iron is the major source of iron in the hepatocyte, it is not the only one. Other iron sources include hemoglobin (complexed to haptoglobin), heme (bound to hemopexin), and plasma ferritin. These sources are not significant in normal healthy individuals. Although it has been suggested that there are receptor-mediated mechanisms for the uptake of iron in these various forms, to date only one receptor system has been conclusively isolated and partially characterized. Mack and coworkers have isolated a hepatic membrane receptor for ferritin[129] and partially purified it by affinity chromatography. The isolated receptor is fairly insoluble and so no reliable mol wt has been obtained, but these workers have been able to determine the number of receptors (approx 30,000) per hepatocyte.

The Reticuloendothelial System

The RE system, which includes the Kupffer cells in the liver, acquires virtually all of its iron by phagocytosis of senescent red cells or their fragments, and as such may be regarded as an extension of the erythron, i.e., once iron is taken up by the erythroid marrow, the majority remains intracellular until released by the RE cells. After phagocytosis, the iron is released from heme by heme oxygenase and then either released to plasma transferrin or stored in ferritin for subsequent release at a later interval. As with the mucosal cells, the exact mechanism of iron donation to plasma transferrin has not been elucidated. Like almost every cell in the body, the RE cells express transferrin receptors on their cell surface. These receptors may be downregulated following functional activation in vivo[130] with a concomitant increase in intracellular ferritin.[131]

Ethanol and Dietary Iron

As has been said earlier, alcohol has profound effects on iron homeostasis. It is also associated with the development of a number of hematological abnormalities that include megaloblastic anemia, transient hemolysis with hyperlipidemia, reversible sideroblastic erythropoiesis, thrombocytopenia, siderosis, and hemochromatosis.[132] Whether these changes are caused solely by alcohol or by changes in the diet is often difficult to elucidate because many of the early studies were performed either on laboratory volunteers, skid-row alcoholics, or on patients with late-term alcoholic cirrhosis. At least one study has been performed, however, on noncirrhotic alcoholics under controlled conditions and has shown that many of the hematological aberrations, including alterations to serum iron, still occur in the absence of liver damage and in the face of normal nutrition.[133] Considerable controversy has also arisen as to the effects of the quantities of iron in the beverage of choice for intoxication, fueled by the findings of siderosis among the Bantu drinking Kaffir beer and the early confusion over alcoholic siderosis and idiopathic hemochromatotics who drank heavily.

Experimentally, there is no doubt that alcoholic beverages influence iron absorption. Whether this is because of the alcohol itself, or other constituents of the drink is also controversial. Absorption of ferric chloride in humans, as measured by its incorporation into red cells, appears to be enhanced in the presence of ethanol from a test dose of either whiskey or brandy.[134] Since this does not occur in achlorhydric subjects, and is not seen with either ferrous salts or hemoglobin iron, this enhancement was considered by these workers to be caused by the stimulation of gastric acid production by alcohol (and thus the maintenance of more iron in a bioavailable form). Other workers, however, using whole body counting techniques, have found that a single dose of whiskey appears to reduce iron absorption and that removing the alcohol from the whiskey does not alter this observation.[135]

Experiments in animals have been equally confusing. MacDonald and Pechet, using radioiron-labeled wine, failed to observe any increase in absorption in rats.[136] Tapper et al. observed a marked decrease in iron absorption in rats in the presence of a large dose of whiskey.[137] They also saw no change in iron absorption in rats given a liquid alcohol diet, or ip injections of ethanol, for up to 4 wk. Mazzanti and coworkers have shown that chronically alcoholic rats retain a larger percentage of a test dose of radioiron and suggest that a reduction in enterocyte turnover may be contributing to this effect.[138] An interesting study by Fairweather-Tait and colleagues has recently shown that consumption of wine, whiskey, and ethanol by male Wistar rats resulted in higher liver iron concentrations, whereas beer and cider had no effect.[139] Since ethanol alone had the greatest effect and cider the least, the hypothesis that the effects of ethanol are moderated by other components of the beverage is again in favor. These effects could still be secondary, however, to the long-term effects of ethanol on the metabolism of a variety of compounds. For example, folic acid metabolism is well known to be altered in chronic alcoholism[140] and it has been shown that in alcoholic, folate deficient rabbits, iron uptake increases significantly.[141] Administration of folic acid to these rabbits returns the iron-absorption values to normal. Other factors, such as endotoxin, have been shown to not only reduce iron uptake, but also to shunt the iron taken up by the mucosa to ferritin.[142] In idiopathic hemochromatosis, there is a decrease in mucosal ferritin, presumably leading to decreased storage of iron in the mucosal cells by these patients.[143]

Changes in iron distribution to mucosal proteins in experimental animals are often seen in response to dietary iron and/or body iron stores. Shunting of iron to mucosal ferritin is decreased when animals are placed on a low iron diet and increased when the iron content of the diet is returned to normal.[144] Similarly, the number of transferrin receptors found on the basolateral membranes from intestinal cells are inversely proportional to the body iron stores.[145] However, these receptors do not appear to be directly involved in iron absorption since, following the induction of hemolysis with phenylhydrazine, iron absorption increased almost threefold without a concomitant change in the receptor number or affinity. As yet, no investigation has been made into the effects of ethanol on these receptors.

Because of these experimental findings in animals, it is not surprising that the increased intake of iron in alcoholics has often been considered to be associated with greater quantities of iron found in the beverages themselves. Wine (especially red wine) contains large amounts of iron and many French investigators have long considered this to be a prime cause of siderosis in alcoholics.[146–148] At least one English group of workers has found hepatic siderosis to be unusual among British alcoholics, and has attributed this to the low intake of wine by these patients.[149] The average iron and alcohol content of the different types of alcoholic beverages may be seen in Table 1. A more recent study by Jakobovits et al., however, showed that the incidence of siderosis in British alcoholics (as estimated by stainable parenchymal iron) to be as high as 57%,[150] although the occurrence of significant hepatic iron deposition was low. Approximately 7% of these patients had grades III and IV siderosis and there was no significant difference between the sexes. In the female alcoholics studied by these workers, there was a significant inverse degree of correlation between age and the degree of siderosis, which was not seen in males. The male alcoholics showed, however, an inverse correlation between the quantity of alcohol consumed and the degree of siderosis, as well as a correlation between the TIBC and the degree of siderosis. In this group of alcoholic patients, the average daily intake of iron was approx 1.5 mg, compared to 7.2 mg from other sources,

Table 1
Average Iron and Alcohol Content of Common Potables*

Beverage	Iron, mg/L	Alcohol, g/L
Beers	0.1–0.5	22–66
Alcoholic ciders	3.0–5.0	38–105
White wines	5.0–12.0	88–102
Red wines	6.5–13.0	89–101
Port and sherry	3.0–5.0	156–161
Spirits (70% proof)	Trace	315

*Adapted from Jakobovits et al., 1979.[150]

and there appeared to be no relationship between the amount of iron ingested and the degree of siderosis observed.

The lack of correlation between the degree of hepatic siderosis and the quantity of iron taken up in alcoholic beverages (apart from that seen in the South African Bantu) has also been seen in red wine drinkers. Miralles Garcia and de Castro del Pozo have shown that there is no correlation between iron ingestion from red wine (up to 23 mg/d) and hepatic iron deposition.[151] This is in contrast to the findings of a postmortem study by Powell, who found a significant correlation between both the quantities of iron and alcohol ingested and hepatic siderosis in alcoholics and their close relatives.[152] Other groups, however, have found no correlation between hepatic siderosis and the length of drinking history.[79,150,153] Although the presence of hepatic siderosis has often been considered to be abnormal, several groups have nonetheless found stainable iron in many of their hematologically normal control subjects.[153–156] Whether this is normal, or reflects hitherto undetected abnormalities in iron homeostasis, is not clear. In most cases this stainable liver iron is only grade I or II, and biopsies from these "control" subjects do not show grades III and IV siderosis. These latter grades invariably denote significantly increased hepatic iron deposition and this may be seen in a small, but significant, number of alcoholics.

The presence of liver disease in alcoholics may also affect hepatic iron deposition. Overall, most groups have found that the severity of the liver disease does not appear to be the determining factor; the percentage of precirrhotic patients with siderosis being of the order of 50–65% of those examined, and this value does not change significantly in the presence of cirrhosis.[144,150,153,157] Lundvall and Weinfeld, using a desferrioxamine chelation test on alcoholics with precirrhotic liver disease, showed an increase in excreted chelated iron in the first test, followed by lowered iron excretion in subsequent ones.[158] Since this change was sometimes accompanied by a decline in the SGOT levels in these patients, these authors concluded that the initial excess desferrioxamine-induced iron excretion was probably a result of increased liver cell injury. However, it is also possible that this increased initial excretion of iron reflects removal of iron from the hepatic labile iron pool where it is not only readily available for chelation, but also for the generation of free radicals, leading to lipid peroxidation and subsequent cell damage (and hence increased SGOT levels ...).

Cirrhosis of the liver also affects iron absorption, although the effect appears to be different in humans from that observed in experimental animals. In patients with cirrhosis, administration of a test dose of oral iron in the presence of ethanol results in a significant elevation in the serum iron curve, which is not seen in control subjects.[159] Since the ethanol did not affect either the level of endogenous serum iron or the serum clearance of exogenous iron, this elevation of the curve has been ascribed to increased absorption in cirrhosis. Since this curve could be normalized by the oral administration of pancreatin, it has been suggested that the abnormal iron absorption seen in alcoholic cirrhosis could occur as a result of diminished pancreatic activity in these patients. This diminished activity could result from hypoproduction, delayed transport, or increased inactivation of pancreatic enzymes caused by portal hypertension, intestinal venostasis, or collateral circulation. However, in the latter case, no correlation has been found between the extent of the bypass and changes in iron uptake in either humans[160] or experimental animals.[161]

Several groups have attributed the increased iron absorption to concomitant liver damage, or to other factors, such as anemia or inflammation,[162,163] rather than diminished pancreatic activity. It should be noted, however, that iron absorption is normal in acute viral hepatitis.[164] Other candidates for this effect include xanthine oxidase deficiency,[165,166] hypoxia,[167,168] or even hyperhemolysis.[169,170] In the rat, however, increased deposition of hepatic iron is associated with nutritional cirrhosis and tends to be lowered by the administration of ethanol to these experimental animals.[171] Since this effect is also seen in control animals, it has been suggested that this may be a result of a redistribution of storage iron produced by chronic ethanol ingestion and not from diminished iron absorption or total body iron.

Whether iron absorption is increased in response to experimental chronic alcohol administration seems to depend on the technique used to measure adsorption and the time-frame involved. In experiments using isolated intestinal loops and everted gut sacs, a single bolus of ethanol resulted in decreased ferrous iron uptake over 30 min in control animals.[137] The same experiments on animals fed a liquid alcohol diet for up to 4 wk, however, elicited no change in uptake when compared to animals on the control diet. The use of whole body counting 9 d after the administration of ferric iron to animals on this same liquid alcohol diet showed increased iron absorption, but no apparent increase in hepatic iron deposition.[138] A comparable study in human alcoholics, also using whole body counting 14 d after a test meal containing 2 mg ferrous sulfate and radiolabeled ferric citrate, showed no differences between the alcoholics and control subjects in radioiron absorption, although patients with iron deficiency anemia took up significantly more of the test dose.[172] The addition of ethanol (0.5 g/kg body wt) to the test meal tended to increase absorption, but not markedly so, in both controls and alcoholic patients. In the light of these conflicting studies, many workers now consider that the increased liver iron concentrations seen in many alcoholics are unlikely to be caused by increased iron absorption occurring as a result of chronic alcohol ingestion. Since iron absorption is increased in response to changes in iron homeostasis, it is probable that any increase in iron absorption occurs secondarily to changes caused by ethanol intoxication.

Effects of Ethanol
on Liver Iron Homeostasis

The liver is often erroneously considered to be a single, homogeneous system of cells. This is probably because the major cell type — the hepatocyte — comprises 85% of the organ. However, the nonparenchymal cells of the liver also have separate discrete functions that may or may not interact with those of the hepatocytes. In particular, the Kupffer cells are part of the reticuloendothelial system (RES) and as such are involved in the removal of senescent red blood cells from the circulation. Since the hepatocyte is a major site of (nonheme) iron deposition, it is clearly possible to differentiate at least two types of iron overload. Thus, transfusional iron overload, as can occur following treatment of β-thalassemia, results in an initial iron loading of the Kupffer cells, which subsequently spills over into the parenchymal cells. Primary idiopathic hemochromatosis, on the other hand, results in an initial iron loading of the hepatocytes. The hepatocyte population of the liver is itself not homogeneous. It is now well known that the liver acinus can be divided into three zones, relative to the portal vein, and that hepatocytes from each of these zones have slightly different metabolic activities. Because there are metabolic gradients across the acinus, it is also possible to observe different types of liver damage and iron loading, depending on whether the material originates from the gut or other parts of the body. Thus, low alcohol concentrations will affect primarily the periportal cells, but heavy intoxication will affect all parts of the acinus. Once liver damage intervenes, however, the picture becomes more complicated. Besides fatty liver and fibrosis, inflammatory infiltrates can also occur and these, together with the contents of dying cells, can cause radical changes in hepatic iron homeostasis.

Perhaps because of these intricacies, there have been very few attempts to elucidate what effect alcohol has on iron uptake by the liver. As part of the author's ongoing investigation into the effects of ethanol on iron homeostasis, the effects of ethanol on transferrin-bound iron uptake by freshly isolated rat hepatocytes have been closely studied. Initial studies appeared to show that hepatocytic uptake of transferrin-bound iron was depressed by approx 25–30% in the presence of 10 m*M* ethanol.[173] Total transferrin binding appeared to be unchanged from that of control cells, but the mol ratio of iron to transferrin on cell membranes isolated after 90 min incubation was also markedly reduced in the presence of ethanol, suggesting increased retention of apotransferrin. Further studies with these cells, using both weakly and strongly buffered media, have provided further insight into the acute effects of ethanol on transferrin-bound iron uptake by the hepatocyte.[110] The depression of iron uptake was found to persist with hepatocytes that had been preincubated with 10 m*M* ethanol in weakly buffered medium for 90 min prior to the addition of diferric transferrin. Increasing the buffering capacity of the system, or the addition of a metabolic inhibitor of alcohol dehydrogenase (4-methylpyrazole), returned iron uptake to control values. Products of alcohol metabolism, such as acetaldehyde, acetate and lactate, and 3-butanol (an alcohol not metabolized by alcohol dehydrogenase) all had no influence on iron uptake. Investigation of transferrin-bound iron uptake over the pH range 6–8.5 revealed a marked

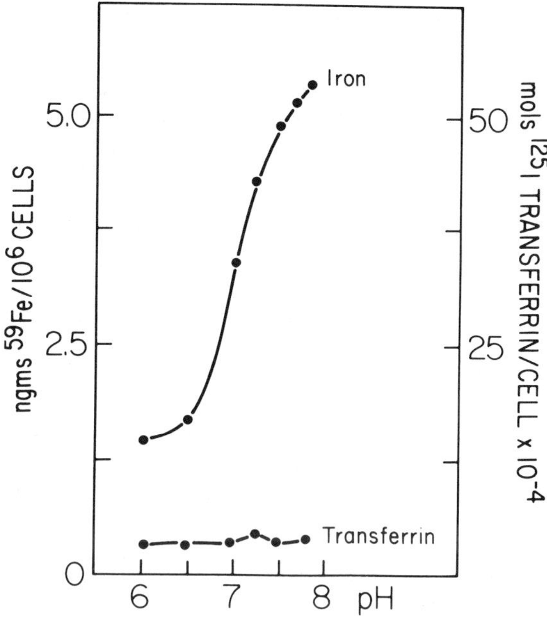

Fig. 2. The effect of pH on the uptake of transferrin-bound iron and transferrin binding by freshly isolated suspensions of rat hepatocytes. (From Beloqui et al.,[110] with permission of the publisher.)

dependency on pH of iron uptake, but not transferrin binding, as can be seen in Fig. 2. In the light of modern theory on transferrin receptor recycling, it can be seen that the lowered iron uptake at lower pH values is almost certainly a result of an increased affinity of apotransferrin for the receptor and a slower release of it back into the medium prior to the binding of iron-loaded transferrin.

Whether this effect observed in vitro is operative in vivo is not clear. A mild acidosis has been observed in humans following ethanol ingestion,[174] which has been related to an increase in serum lactic acid levels,[175] although acetate production may also be a contributory factor.[176,177] In contrast, a combined metabolic/respiratory alkalosis has been seen in alcoholics during ethanol withdrawal.[178,179] Although the pH effects seen in vivo are small, over a long time-frame these changes could disrupt normal liver iron homeostasis. Within the microenvironment of the hepatic sinusoid, these pH changes could be more severe than those measured in peripheral blood, resulting in more dramatic changes in iron uptake, mobilization, and storage.

Chronic alcohol intake in the rat, however, does have a more marked effect on hepatic iron uptake. Transferrin-bound iron uptake rates by isolated hepatocytes are less than 40% of those found with the pair-fed animals, and the presence of 50 m*M* ethanol in the medium lowers uptake still further to only 27% of control values.[180] Although the total number of transferrin receptors remains unchanged, many more are expressed on the cell surface at 4°C (85% vs 44% for control hepatocytes). Assuming that the iron uptake is all receptor-mediated, this would imply that, at least in the rat, chronic alcoholism leads to a reduced receptor recycling rate. This has also been seen with the asialoglycoprotein receptor.[181] Since use of this alcohol diet leads to the development of fatty liver in the rat, it is not unreasonable to assume that this lowered rate of receptor recycling is caused by changes in the hepatocyte membrane fluidity. However, iron loading of these animals during the development of chronic alcoholism leads to a dramatic increase in the rates of iron uptake to supra-control values,[182] an effect also seen in response to endotoxin (*vide infra*).

Although comparable studies have not been performed with human hepatocytes, transferrin-bound iron uptake has been studied in human alcoholics, utilizing ^{52}Fe (produced in a cyclotron) to minimize the long-term radiation hazard that would ensue from using iron isotopes with longer half-lives.[183] In this study, hepatic uptake and plasma clearance of transferrin-bound iron were measured and compared to the liver iron and serum iron in patients with alcoholic liver disease, as well as patients with primary biliary cirrhosis or polycythemia rubra vera (who served as controls for this study). Over a 4-h period, less than 2.5% of the transferrin-bound iron was taken up by the livers of the controls. A significantly higher quantity was taken up by patients with alcoholic fatty liver (11.8 ± 0.8%) or alcoholic cirrhosis (7.7 ± 1.3%), but the greatest quantity of transferrin-bound iron was taken up by the livers of the patients with primary biliary cirrhosis (13.3 ± 1.3%). The mean serum iron concentrations in the alcoholics were significantly greater than the other two groups and these values correlated well with the observed hepatic iron uptake rates in these alcoholic patients. No such correlation was seen with the patients with either PBC or polycythemia rubra vera and there were no correlations between liver iron or serum ferritin and hepatic uptake in any of the groups studied.

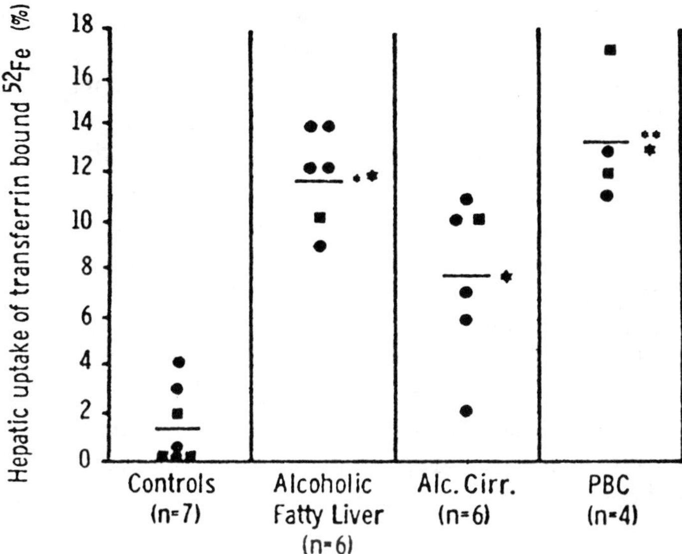

Fig. 3. Uptake of transferrin-bound iron in patients with alcoholic liver disease and primary biliary cirrhosis. (From Chapman et al.,[183] with permission of the authors and publisher.)

The hepatic uptake values for transferrin-bound iron in these patients is shown in Fig. 3.

Since all of the alcoholic patients studied here had some form of liver disease, these data tend to support the suggestion made earlier that iron uptake is increased in patients with liver damage.[184] Whether it is also related to liver iron deposition is less clear. The alcoholic patients in this study had significantly higher liver iron concentrations than the patients with PBC. In an earlier study, Pollycove et al. observed that transferrin-bound iron uptake in 3 patients with alcoholic cirrhosis was relatively normal, and significantly lower than for patients with idiopathic hemochromatosis.[185] All of the alcoholic patients in this study, however, were iron deficient. In other studies, patients with cirrhosis have been shown to have hepatic iron uptake values comparable to those seen in idiopathic hemochromatosis[186] and the alcoholic cirrhotics in the study of Chapman and colleagues.[183] Since the transferrin receptor and liver iron stores appear to have a reciprocal relationship in idiopathic hemochromatosis,[187] it is not readily apparent just what cellular mechanism is causing the increased hepatic iron uptake. It may be a primary phenomenon, or occurring secondarily to liver damage.[183–187] Since, in the study by Chapman et al.,[183] iron uptake was lower in patients with alcoholic cirrhosis than in those with fatty liver, the increased hepatic iron uptake may be considerably modulated by a decrease in the number of viable hepatocytes. This could also explain the variations seen between the various studies reviewed here, and implies that overall liver function must also be taken into consideration.

The apparent relationship between serum iron and hepatic iron uptake in alcoholics is interesting. As has been said earlier, the hepatic transferrin receptors have a higher affinity for iron loaded transferrin, and it has been shown that the hepatic uptake of transferrin-bound iron correlates significantly with the percentage transferrin iron saturation.[188,189] It has long been known that alcohol abuse can cause significant increases in the serum iron concentration and related parameters and that this occurs independently of liver damage.[4,14,35,190–192] The increased serum iron concentrations could therefore increase the uptake of transferrin-bound iron by the liver. Since the serum transferrin concentration may be low in patients with cirrhosis, resulting from decreased hepatic synthesis (*vide infra*), this will also tend to result in the increased liver uptake of circulating iron.

In normal individuals, more than 95% of the iron circulates in the serum bound to transferrin. There is now considerable evidence that a portion of the remaining fraction, designated nontransferrin bound (NTB) iron, is bound to a protein, whereas the larger fraction is present as some form of low mol wt complex.[193–196] This NTB iron can be extremely efficiently cleared from the plasma by the liver[197] by a passive, saturable process that is not regulated by liver iron stores.[198] NTB iron concentrations can reach up to 30% of the total serum iron in iron storage disorders[199] and could clearly have marked effects both on hepatic iron deposition and tissue damage. Although sera from both treated[186] and untreated[200] hemochromatosis patients result in a higher than normal hepatic iron uptake in test systems, this NTB fraction appears to be normal in patients with alcoholic liver disease ($3.3 \pm 0.7\%$ vs $3.2 \pm 0.3\%$ for controls[199]) and thus would not be expected to show this effect. However, the turnover of this NTB iron fraction has not yet been examined in patients with alcoholic liver disease.

Two other mechanisms for the changes seen in liver iron in alcoholics should also be considered, although as yet they have not been thoroughly investigated. The first is that this iron arises from ineffective erythropoiesis following prolonged alcohol ingestion.[8] In human alcoholics, serum iron values tend to decrease for up to 3 d after alcohol withdrawal, accompanied by a reversion of the abnormal accumulation of erythroblastic hemosiderin to normal. The suggestion that these findings indicate a direct interference in heme synthesis[8,14] is only part of the story. Plasma erythropoietin levels have been shown to be elevated in alcoholic mice, but the number of "erythropoietin-responsive cells" appear to be reduced, leading to an impaired response.[201] In addition, hyperferremia may be observed, occurring as a result of interference in the utilization of iron by the red cells, and this also leads to excess mitochondrial iron accumulation.[202,203] The occurrence of ineffective erythropoiesis, besides changing serum iron parameters, also results in the excess production of both heme and hemoglobin, both of which may be taken up by the liver parenchymal cells. Although this pathway is not normally of much importance, if the reticuloendothelial system is overwhelmed (or blocked), uptake of these compounds by the liver could have some effect on liver iron homeostasis.

Although serum ferritin levels have been measured in alcoholic patients, there have been no studies on its uptake, at the cellular level, in alcoholism. There is now some evidence that ferritin functions as a carrier protein, as well as a cellular iron storage vehicle,[204,205] and hepatic membrane receptors have been isolated from the livers of several species, including humans.[206–208] Unlike the transferrin receptor, ferritin uptake does not appear to be downregulated by iron overload and as such appears to be independent of hepatic iron status.[209] There is now evidence that the NTB iron levels seen in thalassemia and idiopathic hemochromatosis may in fact be caused by circulating ferritin,[210] but, since this fraction is insignificant in alcoholics, it is unlikely that it plays a major role in the elevation of hepatic iron stores. However, ferritin liberated through tissue destruction in alcoholic liver disease will clearly be rapidly cleared by other viable cells within the liver.

Whatever pathway is used to bring iron to the hepatocyte membrane, the mechanism for its entry into the cell has not yet been elucidated with any certainty. It is also not known in what (complexed) form it enters the labile cytosolic iron pool, prior to being shunted either to the mitochondria for the production of heme proteins or into the storage in cytosolic ferritin. It is assumed that under normal circumstances the iron is complexed to reduce its cellular toxicity, since otherwise it would contribute to lipid peroxidation by the production of deleterious free radicals. Under normal circumstances, biosynthesis of ferritin is regulated by iron in the absence of alterations in mRNA levels, there being an iron-responsive *cis*-acting element in the 5' leader region of ferritin mRNA.[211] It has also been shown that hemin and protoporphyrin IX derepress ferritin synthesis in vitro[212] and may in fact induce it, as well as destabilizing transferrin receptor mRNA. However, as in the case of iron absorption, contradictory results have been reported for the effects of ethanol on ferritin synthesis. Nadkarni and Deshpande observed that ferritin synthesis in rats in vivo was reduced in response to chronic alcohol administration.[213] Brissot et al., however, using a human hepatoma cell line (Hep G2), showed that alcohol could induce ferritin synthesis,[214] although the ethanol concentration used for induction was rather high (>250 mM). It is possible that the reduction in ferritin synthesis seen in the animal studies may be a result of a nutritional deficiency, since ascorbic acid deficiency in guinea pigs has been shown to lower both tissue[215] and serum[216] ferritin levels. It is interesting to note that recent work by Roeser's group has shown that two types of tissue ferritin have now been identified: cytosolic and lipid-associated ferritin.[217] Only the cytosolic ferritin appears to be affected by ascorbic acid deficiency. These workers consider that lipid-associated ferritin represents ferritin recruited from the cytosol and sequestered to lipid membranes, where it acts as a metabolic sink for iron. This should, in turn, decrease the risk of membrane damage through iron associated lipid peroxidation. What effect ethanol has on lipid-associated ferritin has not yet been determined.

Although the degree of hepatic iron loading seen in alcoholics is much less than that seen in idiopathic hemochromatosis, there is an increased incidence of siderosis. At least one group of investigators has considered that, in patients with hepatic cirrhosis, the iron accumulation occurs secondarily to the development of cirrhosis.[218] Powell and Kerr have shown that, in patients with idiopathic hemochromatosis, iron deposition in the liver was the same for both alcoholic and nonalcoholic subjects, with only 25% of the alcoholics showing the morphologic changes associated with alcoholic liver disease superimposed on those caused by hemochromatosis.[219] Subjects who are heterozygous for the hemochromatosis allele and are alcoholics rarely develop overt iron storage disease.[220,221] In several studies of alcoholics, however, there has been a definite lack of correlation between hepatic siderosis and drinking history.[4,150,153]

One of the problems of diagnosing and treating iron overload is that true quantitation of the iron deposition in the liver can only be made from a liver biopsy,[222] which is not always feasible. There is now some evidence that the serum ferritin concentration correlates linearly with body iron stores, each mg of storage iron equating to approx 0.1 µg/L of serum ferritin.[223–227] However, there are some disease states in which the plasma ferritin values are abnormally raised, such as liver disease, some forms of cancer, and infections.[228,229] In the case of liver disease, the increased serum ferritin concentrations are thought to result from the release of cytosolic ferritin from damaged liver cells.[230,231] (It has also been suggested that serum ferritin concentrations more accurately represent reticuloendothelial iron stores, since they fall dramatically following treatment of megaloblastic anemia.)[232] Values for serum ferritin in a variety of disease states, besides alcoholic liver disease, may be seen in Fig. 4.[233] In one study, over two-thirds of a population of heavy drinkers had raised serum ferritin levels.[234] However, these elevated values were associated with raised serum γ-glutamyl transferase concentrations, suggesting that the liver was the source of the serum ferritin. The elevated ferritin levels in alcoholics have also been shown to be unrelated to erythropoietic activity.[235] It is now generally agreed that a serum ferritin level greater than 300 µg/L is very unlikely to be the result of alcohol-induced liver damage if the γ-glutamyl transferase values are below 50 U/L.[236]

Most of the evidence for cellular injury and fibrosis resulting from excess liver iron deposition is based mainly on clinical observations and is largely circumstantial.[237] Iron overload in infants with thalassemia major tends to result in collagen deposition prior to any other evidence of liver injury, and this deposition may lead to cirrhosis, rather than cellular necrosis.[238] In idiopathic hemochromatosis, there is an age-related rise in hepatic iron accumulation and a threshold of hepatic iron deposition for the development of fibrosis and cirrhosis (22 mg/g dry wt of liver).[239] In patients with concomitant alcoholism, the development of fibrosis occurred earlier, suggesting some form of synergism between the effects of iron and alcohol. Several mechanisms have been proposed to account for the development of fibrosis and cirrhosis following iron overload. Iron overload itself may directly stimulate collagen synthesis, independently of the development of liver damage.[240] Cellular damage can also occur as a result of iron catalyzed lipid peroxidation, leading to increased organelle and membrane

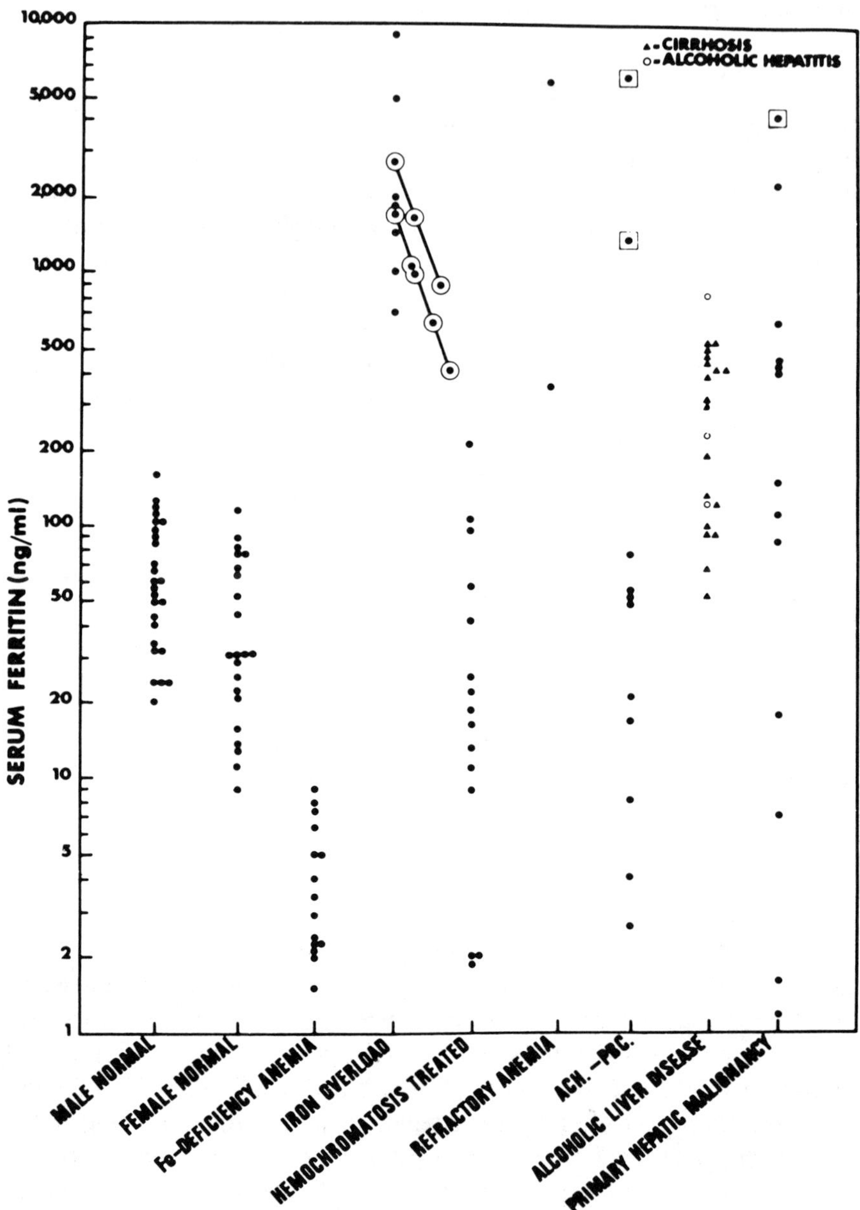

Fig. 4. Serum ferritin concentration as measured by radioimmunassay in normal subjects and various diseases. ACH = active chronic hepatitis; PBC = primary biliary cirrhosis; ▣ = patients with massive or submassive hepatic necrosis; ⊙ = repeated venesections; ▲ = cirrhosis; ○ = alcohol hepatitis. (From Powell et al.,[233] with permission of the authors and publisher.)

26

fragility.[241–243] Although ethanol has been shown to increase lipid peroxidation both in vivo[244–247] and in vitro,[248–253] the role of lipid peroxidation in the generation of alcoholic liver disease is still unclear. This is, however, beyond the scope of this chapter and the reader is referred either to Irving et al.,[254] or elsewhere in this volume for a more detailed treatise on the effects of ethanol on lipid peroxidation.

The Reticuloendothelial System

Although the reticuloendothelial system is intimately involved in the recycling of red cell iron from hemoglobin, it has not been studied as thoroughly in terms of this processing in alcoholic liver disease. There appears to be no direct evidence that ethanol *per se* alters red cell survival rates,[255] and it is often considered that the hemolytic syndromes resulting from alcohol intoxication are probably secondary to other alcohol-induced events.[132] However, there is an impaired release of reticuloendothelial iron in response to alcohol administration in experimental animals.[256] This is mirrored by reduced plasma iron turnover and an increase in marrow transit time. There also tends to be an increase in iron retained in the spleen, as well as the liver. It is interesting to note that female rats tend to show a greater increase in hepatic iron storage under the influence of ethanol. Whereas females tend to store more iron (in ferritin) than males under normal conditions,[257] the increased hepatic iron concentration resulting from ethanol administration appears to be restricted to the nonferritin fraction.[256]

Although iron overloaded spleens in other diseases have been shown to result in increased lipid peroxidation,[258] no such conclusive studies have been performed in alcoholic liver disease. Indeed, some studies on alcoholics have suggested that the reticuloendothelial system may be iron deficient.[259] This is more likely to be caused by increased hemolysis following heavy drinking leading to increased heme turnover.[260] It is debatable whether the increase in hemolysis occurs as a result of increased lipid peroxidation since only minor changes in susceptibility have been seen in red cells from alcoholic patients and this is markedly decreased in the presence of cirrhosis.[261] This latter abnormality appears to be related to liver protein synthesis rather than to a decreased red cell membrane content of polyunsaturated fatty acids. Although ineffective erythropoiesis can be observed in alcoholics, alcohol-induced bone marrow damage appears to be reversible and the toxic effect appears to be peripheral to the marrow.[262]

It should be remembered that the Kupffer cells are both part of the reticuloendothelial system and reside in the liver. Like monocytes and macrophages, they have membrane receptors for transferrin.[263–265] Although not yet studied in alcoholic liver disease, iron uptake from transferrin by these cells has been shown to be reduced in patients with untreated hemochromatosis[266] and the cells found to contain significant quantities of hemosiderin.[267] However, peripheral blood monocytes from patients with idiopathic hemochromatosis do not appear to synthesize ferritin more rapidly than those from control subjects,[268] although earlier reports suggested that there was an abnormal release of reticuloendothelial iron from labeled erythrocytes in these patients.[269] This could, of course, reflect the type of iron overload occurring. In transfusional siderosis, most of the excess iron is presented as hemoglobin in red cells and therefore the iron would be deposited in the reticuloendothelial system. In idiopathic hemochromatosis, the iron is thought to enter by a more physiological route and is therefore directed primarily to the parenchymal cells. Since anemia, red cell hemolysis, and siderosis have all been observed in alcoholic liver disease, it is probable that the aforementioned mechanisms will be operative at some time during the course of chronic alcohol intoxication. It is unlikely, however, that reticuloendothelial transport of iron plays a primary role in the abnormalities of iron homeostasis that occur during alcoholism.

Serum Transferrin

Since the liver is not only a major site of iron storage, but also synthesizes transferrin, ethanol intoxication may lead to changes in the turnover of this protein. The relationship between alcohol abuse and disturbances to protein metabolism is well-known.[250] Although chronic ethanol abuse is known to cause hepatomegaly and an accumulation of protein in the liver,[270] the effects on individual proteins have been less well-established, and may even depend on the system used to examine protein metabolism. Furthermore, ethanol (or its metabolic products, such as acetaldehyde) may also have an effect on the secretory mechanism involved in the movement of proteins into the plasma.[271–273] Alterations to pH brought about by alcohol metabolism have also been shown to alter hepatic synthesis of transferrin and albumin, as well as other plasma proteins.[110,274] Studies on the acute effects of ethanol have shown that it depresses the fractional synthesis of transferrin in vitro, but this effect can be reversed by the simultaneous administration of an amino acid mixture.[275] Other effects, such as fasting and changes in atmospheric pressure, have also been shown to alter transferrin synthesis in vivo.[276] Differences in protein synthesis between chronic and acute alcohol intoxication in rats, however, have been seen if the radiolabeled amino acids are infused continuously, rather than injected as a bolus;[277] the rates tend to be elevated in acute treatment and depressed in chronic alcoholism in the rat.

Transferrin synthesis is also regulated by both serum and hepatic storage iron. In iron deficiency, there is an increased hepatic transferrin release, which can be equated with enhanced *de novo* synthesis, and this enhancement can be reduced back to normal by refeeding with iron.[278] There is a similar relationship between the rate of iron uptake and transferrin synthesis.[279] However, inflammation, which is also associated with a fall in serum iron and iron-binding capacity, does not appear to result in increased serum transferrin concentration[280] — at least in the short term. [^{14}C]Leucine incorporation into transferrin and ceruloplasmin has been shown to be increased over fourfold in turpentine-treated mice,[1] whereas the transferrin levels rise to 160% of control values after 72 h (with a concomitant rise in the serum unsaturated iron-binding capacity).

The metabolism of transferrin in patients with alcoholic liver disease has been studied in the author's laboratory.[281] Highly purified radiolabeled human transferrin was injected into six patients with alcoholic fatty liver and five with alcoholic cirrhosis. Six healthy individuals, with a daily alcohol intake of less than 40 g, were also studied. The plasma disappearance curves for these patients may be seen in Fig. 5. Although there were no significant differences in the mean fractional catabolic rate and plasma volume in the patients with alcoholic cirrhosis, when compared to the control subjects, the calculated synthesis rates for transferrin were significantly different, as may be seen in Fig. 6. The diminished synthesis seen in alcoholic cirrhosis (0.44 ± 0.05 mg/kg/h vs 0.84 ± 0.03 mg/kg/h for the controls) resulted in a markedly lower serum transferrin concentration (1.8 ± 0.3 g/L vs a control value of 3.1 ± 0.2 g/L). The serum transferrin levels for patients with alcoholic fatty liver were within the normal range (2.8 + 0.2 g/L), which implied that the elevated synthesis seen in this group (0.99 ± 0.08 mg/kg body wt/h) was owing to an elevated fractional turnover rate of transferrin in their plasma.

Although the lowered synthesis rates for transferrin in the patients with cirrhosis may be explained in terms of the liver's diminished synthetic

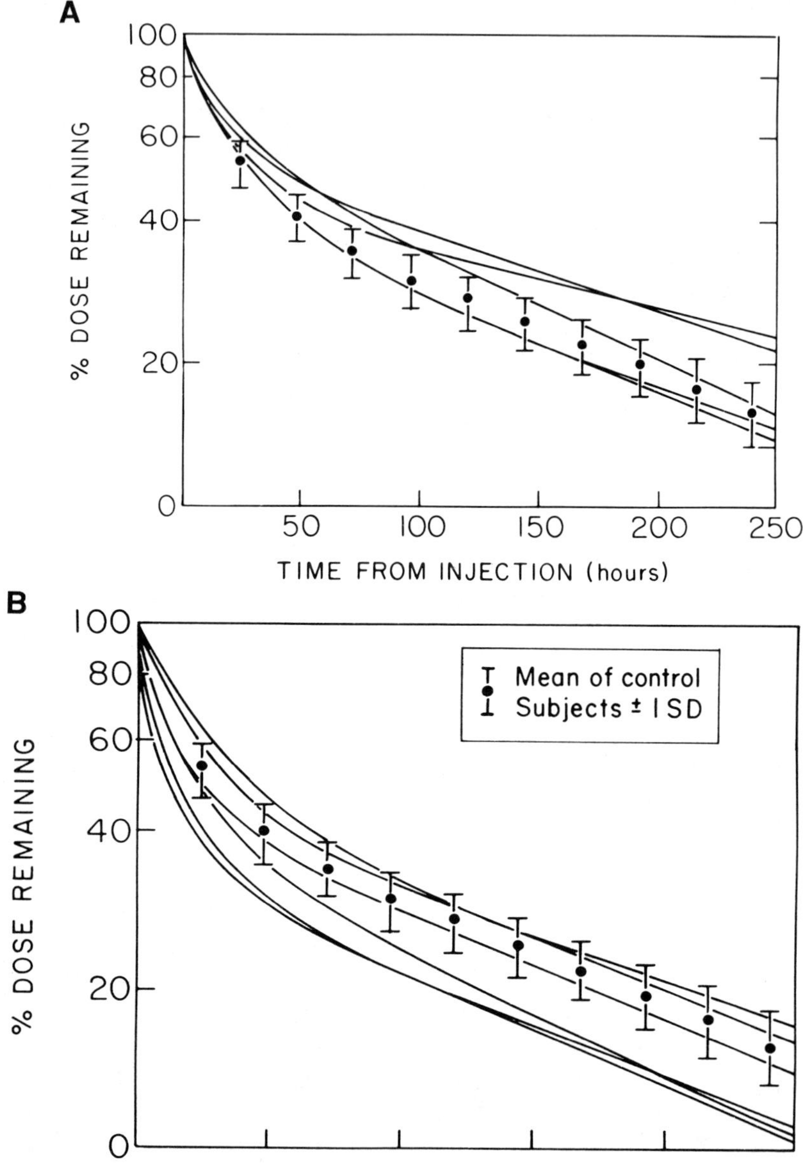

Fig. 5. Plasma disappearance curves of plasma-bound radioactivity after the intravenous injection of ^{125}I-transferrin into patients with alcoholic liver disease. **(A)** Individual disappearance curves for transferrin in six patients with alcoholic fatty liver. **(B)** The corresponding individual plasma disappearance curves for five patients with alcoholic cirrhosis. The "average" curve for the six control subjects (± the standard deviation) is also shown (●). (Reproduced with permission of the publisher from Potter et al.[281])

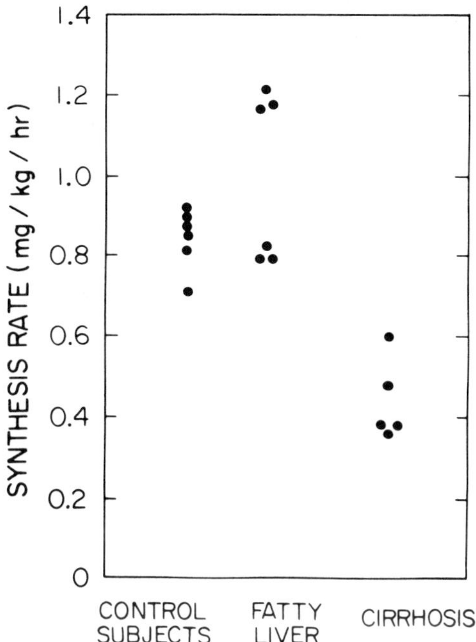

Fig. 6. Intravenous synthesis rates for transferrin in alcoholic liver disease. Values are derived from the integrated rate equations of Nosslin.[322] (Reproduced from Potter et al.,[281] with permission of the publisher.)

capacity, the elevation of these rates in those subjects with fatty liver is somewhat unexpected since, as has been mentioned previously, acute alcohol administration in the rat often results in decreased transferrin synthesis. It is possible that, in the noncirrhotic alcoholic patient, transferrin is acting as an acute phase reactant and the elevated synthesis may correspond to that seen by Beaumier et al.[1] in experimental inflammation. Another explanation is that the increased turnover may be attributable to these patients ceasing drinking just prior to the study, leading to the stimulation of erythropoiesis. None of these patients had any evidence of hemolysis, which could also increase transferrin metabolism.[282] Since none of these patients had significant hepatic iron deposition (i.e., greater than grade 1 siderosis), it is unlikely that their hepatic iron stores had any influence on the observed synthetic rate. However, as is shown in Fig. 7, the serum total iron binding capacity correlates well with the IV transferrin synthesis rate. This is not seen in the control subjects.

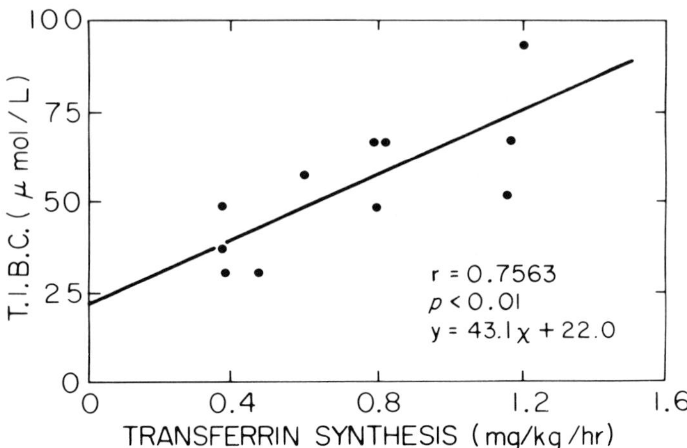

Fig. 7. The correlation between Total Iron Binding Capacity (TIBC) and transferrin synthesis in alcoholic liver disease. $r = 0.7563$; $p = < 0.01$; $y = 43.1_x + 22.0$. (Reproduced with permission of the publisher from Potter et al.[281])

Precise information about the site(s) of transferrin catabolism is unavailable at the present time. Although earlier work in rats, using in vitro liver perfusion,[283] suggested that the liver could account for approx 10% of the catabolism in the intact animal, it has subsequently been shown that endocytic degradation by the liver cells only occurs with artificially denatured transferrin.[284] This finding is in agreement with the work of Regoeczi et al., who suggested that desialylated transferrin is cleared by the bone marrow in rabbits.[285] Furthermore, evidence of clearance by the asialoglycoprotein receptor on the hepatocyte[286] of desialylated transferrin is controversial.[287,288] In addition, the hepatocyte receptors are specific for the native iron-transporting molecule and binding of denatured transferrin or apotransferrin is greatly reduced.[107,109] This indirect evidence would suggest, therefore, that as the liver is also the site of transferrin synthesis, the effects of transferrin metabolism would be on synthesis *per se*, rather than on catabolism.

Alcohol does not only affect the rate of synthesis. Considerable evidence has now accumulated to suggest that it also alters the structure of transferrin. Several groups have now confirmed that there is an abnormal microheterogeneity of transferrin that can be observed in the serum of many alcoholics.[288–292] The abnormality appears as a transferrin component with an isoelectric point of pH 5.7 and it has been suggested that this is related to changes in the structure and composition of the carbohydrate moiety of this glycoprotein.[293–295] More recent work, however, has shown that the defect is more complex and involves galactose and *N*-acetylglucosamine, as well as sialic acid.[296] Detection of this carbohydrate-deficient transferrin has now been refined into a potentially useful test for the detection of alcohol abuse.[297,298] These elevated values for carbohydrate-deficient transferrin in alcoholics gradually decrease in most subjects after cessation of drinking ($t_{1/2} = 16 \pm 5$ d).[299] Lieber and coworkers consider that, for the assessment of treatment outcome, the combination of carbohydrate-deficient transferrin and the γ-glutamyl transferase levels as markers yield a sensitivity of 95%.[299]

Why this change in transferrin sialic acid content occurs following alcohol abuse is not known. It could be owing to either a degradative process, or incomplete glycosylation occurring during synthesis. Acetaldehyde is known to alter the incorporation of glucosamine into glycoproteins,[300] but this does not explain the change in terminal glycosylation. It appears that some resialylation of asialotransferrin can occur[301] and the addition of microtubule inhibitors can increase the proportion of asialoglycoproteins undergoing resialylation.[302] Microtubule inhibition is paralleled by a corresponding reduction in intracellular transport and secretion of proteins. As a result proteins accumulate in Golgi-derived vesicles, which are rich in sialyltransferase,[303] and these vesicles have a tendency to fuse with lysosomes.[304] Thus it is possible that resialylation may occur in stalled, Golgi-derived vesicles, or similar organelles.[305] Since sialyltransferase is a membrane-bound enzyme in Golgi bodies, some alcohol-related perturbation of this organelle may be a factor in these alterations, especially as alcohol has been shown to alter the density distribution of these bodies.[287,306] Ethanol has been shown to alter ectosialyltransferase activity, but not that of neuraminidase, in the developing rat brain.[307] More recent work in human alcoholics suggests that the altered transferrin found in these patients is probably caused by an impaired uptake of sialic acid-deficient transferrin by the hepatocyte owing to membrane dysfunction, rather than a defect in sialylation.[308]

Experimental work on hepatic iron uptake from asialotransferrins, however, has not shown the expected result. Normal liver cells take up iron more rapidly from asialotransferrin than native transferrin.[287,309] It has been suggested that asialotransferrin could be taken up by either the transferrin or the asialoglycoprotein receptor,[310] but Regoeczi and Koj consider that asialotransferrin binds to each of these sequentially and switches from the asialoglycoprotein receptor to the transferrin receptor at an acidified subcellular site.[311] However, in alcohol-fed rats, iron uptake by freshly isolated hepatocytes from rat asialotransferrin is less than 55 of control values and, in the presence of 50 mM ethanol, this value drops to 67% of controls.[180] Binding of asialotransferrin to these cells was threefold higher than for native transferrin, suggesting that binding was occurring with receptors other than the transferrin receptor, and was the same in control and alcohol-fed rats. Casey and coworkers have shown that alcohol impairs the recycling of asialoglycoprotein receptors, so that, if the asialotransferrin is recycling via this receptor, iron uptake from this macromolecule would inevitably be reduced. If this occurs in humans, then it is unlikely that the altered transferrins contribute to the hemosiderosis seen in some alcoholics.

Endotoxins

Endotoxins are toxic cell-wall components of gram-negative bacteria and are usually lipopolysaccharides. They are present in large quantities in the gut as a result of the death of the normal gut flora, such as *Escherichia coli*. Normally only small quantities of these pass into the portal circulation, where they are rapidly detoxified by the liver reticuloendothelial cells. The increased antibody production and hypergammaglobulinemia frequently seen in liver disease are now considered to be partly a result of the failure of the liver to clear absorbed antigens. As a result of decreased Kupffer cell activity in patients with alcoholic hepatitis,[312] serum titers of antibodies to *E. coli* O antigens tend to be much higher and more frequent in patients with alcoholic liver disease.[313,314] The levels are also greater in patients with cirrhosis than in those with fatty liver, and the presence of alcoholic hepatitis elevates these values further.[315] Endotoxins themselves have been quantitated in peripheral venous blood and found to occur more often in patients with alcoholic cirrhosis than in those with nonalcoholic cirrhosis.[316] Experimentally, the administration of endotoxin to rats on an alcoholic diet induces hepatic necrosis.[317]

It is now well known that bacterial infection leads to a hypoferremic response, involving a marked reduction in transferrin-bound iron. A similar effect can be seen following the administration of endotoxins to rats and mice.[318,319] Although the reticuloendothelial system has been considered to be responsible for the production of this hypoferremic state, the exact mechanism of this iron removal from the plasma has not been elucidated. The author's laboratory has now established that hepatocytic uptake of transferrin-bound iron is involved in the generation of experimental hypoferremia by endotoxins.[320] Transferrin-bound iron uptake by hepatocytes from endotoxin treated rats is not increased until 24 h after treatment, as may be seen in Fig. 8. A similar effect is seen with nontransferrin-bound iron (Fig. 9), although the rate of uptake of this material is much greater. Transferrin synthesis by these cells, however, is significantly reduced at 1 h (Fig. 10), and returns to normal values by 24 h. The number of transferrin receptors involved in iron uptake is also reduced by endotoxin (Fig. 11), both in terms of the total available (as determined by transferrin binding at 37°C) and those expressed on the cell surface (binding at 4°C). However, the percentage internalized, i.e., involved in transferrin recycling, is increased from about 20% in controls to ca. 40% following endotoxin treatment. The rate of recycling of the receptor is also increased, as may be seen in Fig. 12, from 18 ± 2 min to 11 ± 1 min 24 h after treatment.

Extrapolation of this elevated iron uptake to humans would indicate significant effects of endotoxins on iron homeostasis. Normally, between 30 and 35 mg of iron are recycled through the blood each day, of which 2.5–4.5 mg are handled by the parenchymal cells and the rest by the reticuloendothelial system. Because the blood only contains about 5 mg of iron unassociated with heme at any one moment, elevation of hepatocytic uptake by two to three times, in conjunction with the observed reduction in iron release, could by itself account for the hypoferremia seen after infection or endotoxin administration. The increased uptake of nontransferrin-bound iron (one to two orders of magnitude greater than that seen for transferrin-bound iron) ensures that little nonheme iron remains in the plasma. The reduced transferrin binding also observed, which is more than offset by faster endocytic recycling, implies more apotransferrin in the serum available to chelate iron and make it unavailable to invading pathogenic bacteria. However, in vivo, it is less likely that this is the sole, or even necessarily the major, contributor to the observed hypoferremia. It would nevertheless act as an efficient secondary or alternative system to the reticuloendothelial system to ensure that little or no iron was made readily available to invading bacteria.

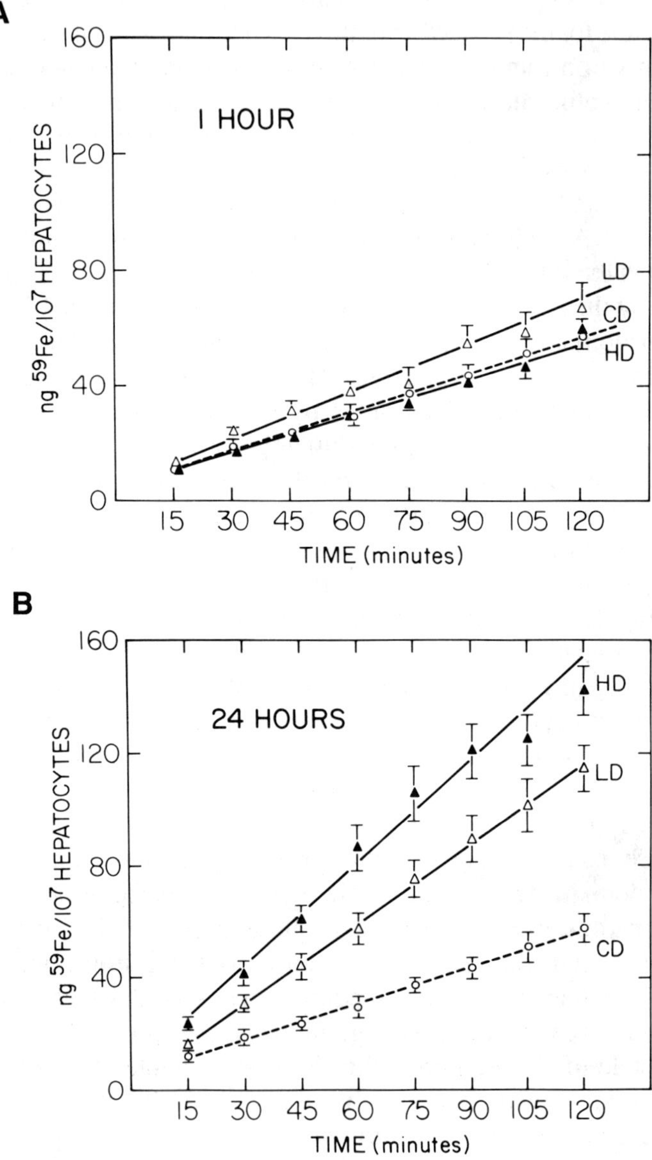

Fig. 8. Uptake of transferrin bound iron by suspensions of hepatocytes
isolated either 1 h **(A)** or 24 h **(B)** after endotoxin administration. Hepatocytes, at
a final concentration of $2.5 \pm 0.5 \times 10^6$ cells/mL were incubated at 37°C in Leibovitz
L-15 medium containing 50 mM HEPES and 2% bovine serum albumin in the

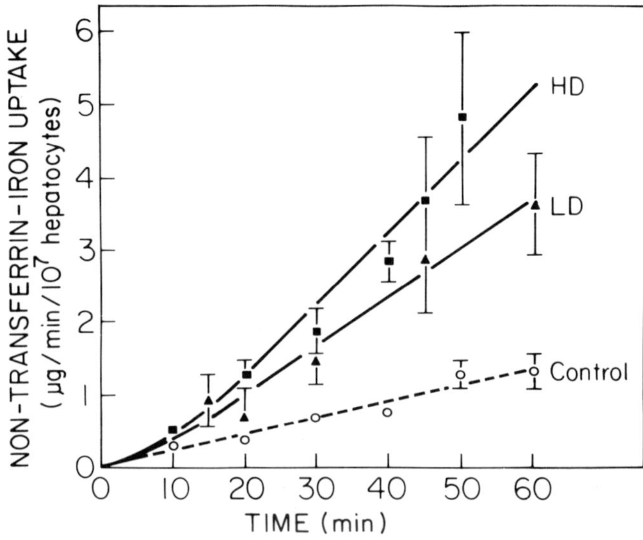

Fig. 9. Uptake of nontransferrin-bound iron by suspensions of rat hepatocytes isolated 24 h after endotoxin administration. The cells were incubated in the presence of 5 μM nontransferrin-bound [59]Fe. Other conditions are the same as in Fig. 8. (Reproduced with permission of the publisher from Potter et al.[320])

These data may also explain some of the anomalies seen in patients with alcoholic liver disease. As has been mentioned previously, these patients have significantly increased titers to *E. coli* O antigens (and presumably to antigens from other gram-negative bacteria), suggesting large fluxes of endotoxins owing to increased gastrointestinal permeability to these antigens as a result of alcohol abuse. Although ethanol administration to rats results in the impairment of transferrin endocytosis and iron uptake, endotoxins dramatically alter the iron homeostatic mechanism and indeed not only reverse this inhibition caused by ethanol abuse but increase uptake to values greater than those seen in nonalcoholic rats treated with endotoxin.[321] It can be seen from these experiments that endotoxins have several signifi-

---

presence of 100 μg/mL diferric ^{59}Fe-labeled transferrin. HD = hepatocytes isolated from rats injected ip with 25 mg/kg lipopolysaccharide from *E. coli* 026:B6; LD = hepatocytes from rats treated with 2.5 mg/kg lipopolysaccharide; CD = hepatocytes from control rats (injected with an equivalent volume of saline). (Reproduced from Potter et al.,[320] with permission of the publisher.)

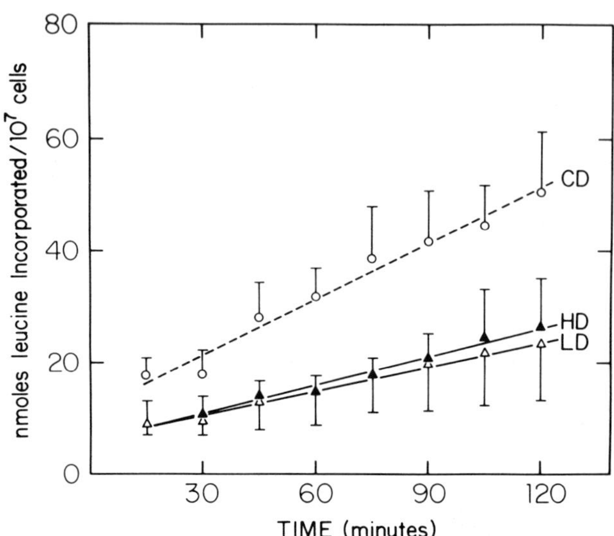

Fig. 10. Incorporation of [³H]leucine into transferrin by suspensions of hepatocytes isolated 1 h after endotoxin administration. Incorporation of leucine into immunoprecipitable transferrin was determined by the method of Yeoh et al.[323] Other conditions were as in Fig. 8. (Reproduced with permission of the publisher from Potter et al.[320])

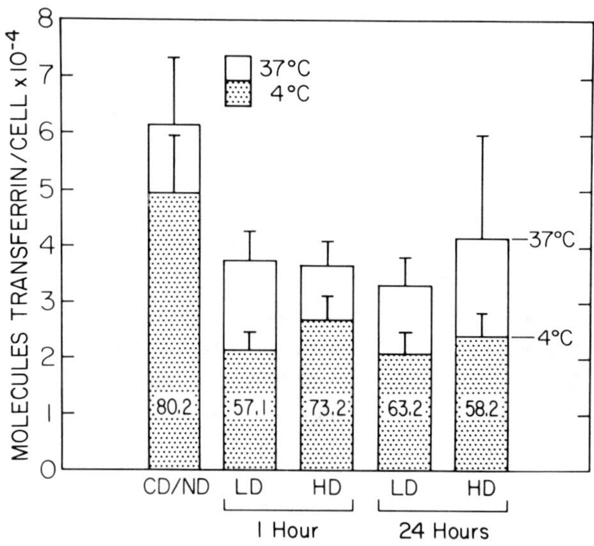

Fig. 11. Transferrin binding to isolated hepatocytes. Histogram values are given for 4 and 37°C. Values within the stippled areas represent the percentage of (surface) binding at 4°C to that at 37°C (total number of receptor sites). □ = 37°C; ▓ = 4°C. (Reproduced with permission of the publisher from Potter et al.[320])

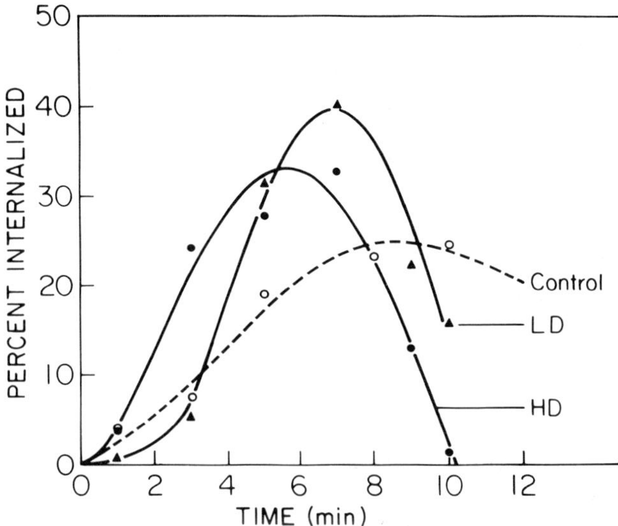

Fig. 12. Transferrin receptor recycling by hepatocytes isolated 24 h after endotoxin administration. After cell surface labeling with ^{125}I, suspensions of hepatocytes were incubated at 37°C in the presence of limited quantities of diferric transferrin. At preset intervals, aliquots were taken, chilled and subjected to proteolysis of the surface receptors with trypsin. The cells were then lysed, the membranes dissolved, and the internalized transferrin receptors quantitated by measurement of the radioactivity after immunoprecipitation. Other conditions are as in Fig. 8. (Reproduced with permission of the publisher from Potter et al.[320])

cant and distinct effects on iron metabolism by the hepatocyte. However, only the long-term direct action of endotoxin or its modulated effect, possibly through products secreted by the reticuloendothelial system, such as interleukin 1 or tissue necrosis factor, alters iron homeostasis within the parenchyma.

Conclusions

From this brief review of the literature, it can be seen that ethanol has the potential for disrupting almost every aspect of hepatic iron homeostasis. However, there still seems to be considerable disagreement as to exactly what its mode of action is, as the observed effects tend to depend on the experimental design or the model used. To date, insufficient attention has been paid to the metabolites of ethanol, particularly acetaldehyde, which may play a far greater role in the pathogenesis of alcoholic liver disease. It is possible that all, some, or none of the mechanisms described in this review actually result in the disturbed hepatic iron homeostasis seen in alcoholic liver disease. Considerably more research is required to elucidate the overall mode of action of ethanol on hepatic iron homeostasis.

References

[1] D. L. Beaumier, M. A. Caldwell, and B. E. Holdbein (1984) Inflammation triggers hypoferremia and ceruloplasmin in mice. *Infect. Immun.* **46,** 489–494.

[2] E. R. Eichner and R. S. Hillman (1971) The evolution of anemia in alcoholic patients. *Am. J. Med.* **50,** 218–232.

[3] L. S. Valberg, C. N. Ghent, D. A. Lloyd, J. V. Frei, and M. J. Chamberlain (1978) Diagnostic efficacy of tests for the detection of iron overload. *Canad. Med. Assoc. J.* **119,** 229–236.

[4] R. W. Chapman, M. Y. Morgan, M. Laulicht, A. V. Hoffbrand, and S. Sherlock (1982) Hepatic iron stores and markers of iron overload in alcoholics and patients with idiopathic hemochromatosis. *Dig. Dis. Sci.* **27,** 909–916.

[5] E. Baraona, P. Pikkarainen, M. Salaspuro, F. Finkelman, and C. S. Lieber (1980) Acute effects of ethanol in hepatic protein synthesis and secretion in the rat. *Gastroenterology* **79,** 104–111.

[6] K. N. Jeejeebhoy, M. J. Phillips, A. Bruce-Robertson, J. Ho, and V. Sodtke (1972) The effect of cortisol on the synthesis of rat plasma albumin, fibrinogen and transferrin. *Biochem. J.* **130,** 533–538.

[7] S. Mookerjea and A. Chow (1969) Impairment of glycoprotein synthesis in acute ethanol. *Biochim. Biophys. Acta* **184,** 83–92.

[8] D. O. B. Hourihane and D. G. Weir (1970) Suppression of erythropoiesis by alcohol. *Br. Med. J.* **i,** 86–89.

[9] A. E. Davis and J. Badendock (1962) Iron absorption in pancreatic disease. *Lancet* **ii,** 5–8.

[10] R. W. Charlton, P. Jacobs, M. Seftel, and T. M. Bothwell (1964) Effects of alcohol on iron absorption. *Br. Med. J.* **2,** 1427–1429.

[11] E. W. Sorensen (1966) Studies on iron absorption. *Acta Med. Scand.* **180,** 241–244.

[12] E. B. Flink (1971) Mineral metabolism in alcoholism, in *The Biology of Alcoholism,* vol. 1. B. Kissin and M. Begleiter, eds. Plenum, London, pp. 377–395.

[13] J. P. von Wartburg and J. Papenberg (1970) Biochemical and enzymatic changes induced by chronic ethanol intake, in *International Encyclopedia of Pharmacology and Therapeutics,* vol 22. J. Tremolieres, ed. Pergamon, Oxford, pp. 301–343.

[14] M. E. Conrad and J. E. Barton (1980) Anemia and iron kinetics in alcoholism. *Semin. Hematol.* **17,** 149–163.

[15] C. Kimber, D. J. Deller, R. N. Ibbotson, and H. Lander (1965) The mechanism of anemia in chronic liver disease. *Q. J. Med.* **34,** 33–64.

[16] N. Krasner, K. M. Cochran, R. I. Russel, H. A. Carmichael, and G. C. Thompson (1976) Alcohol and absorption from the small intestine. 1. Impairment of absorption from the small intestine in alcoholics. *Gut* **17,** 245–248.

[17] B. Speck (1970) Die tagesschwankungen des serumeisens und der latenten eisenbindungskapazitat dei hepatitis, leberzirrhose, alkoholismus, hamcchromatose und aplastischer anamie. *Schweiz Med. Wochenshr.* **100,** 303–305.

[18] I. M. Friedman, H. C. Kraemer, F. S. Mendoza, and L. D. Hammer (1988) Elevated serum iron concentration in adolescent alcohol users. *Am. J. Dis. Children* **142,** 156–159.

[19] J. Linderbaum and C. S. Lieber (1969) Hematologic effects of alcohol in man in the absence of nutritional deficiency. *N. Engl. J. Med.* **281,** 333–338.

[20] Y. Hofvander (1968) Haematological investigations in Ethiopia with special reference to a high iron intake. *Acta Med. Scand. Suppl.* **494,** 1–74.

[21] A. R. P. Walker and V. B. Arvidsson (1953) Iron overload in the South African Bantu. *Trans. Roy. Soc. Trop. Med. Hyg.* **47,** 536–548.

[22] T. H. Bothwell, R. W. Charlton, and H. C. Seftel (1965) Oral iron overload. *S. Afr. Med. J.* **39,** 892–900.

[23] L. D. Baker (1986) Alcohol consumption among South African blacks and its relationship to iron overload. *S. Afr. Med. J.* **70,** 160–62.

[24] C. Isaacson (1978) The changing pattern of liver disease in South African Blacks. *S. Afr. Med. J.* **53,** 365–368.

[25] M. Simon, M. Bourci, B. Genetet, and R. Fauchet (1977) Idiopathic hemochromatosis: Demonstration of recessive transmission and early detection by family HLA typing. *N. Engl. J. Med.* **297,** 1017–1021.

[26] A. Bomford, A. J. Eddleston, L. A. Kennedy, J. R. Batchelor, and R. Williams (1977) Histocompatability antigens as markers of abnormal iron metabolism in patients with idiopathic haemochromatosis and their relatives. *Lancet* **i,** 327–329.

[27] G. E. Cartwright, C. Q. Edwards, K. Kravitz, M. Skolknick, D. B. Amos, A. Johnson, and L. Buskgaer (1979) Hereditary hemochromatosis: Phenotypic expression of the disease. *N. Engl. J. Med.* **301,** 175–179.

[28] T. H. Bothwell and R. W. Charlton (1982) A general approach to the problems of iron deficiency and iron overload in the population at large. *Semin. Hematol.* **19,** 54–67.

[29] T. E. Meyer, D. Ballot, T. H. Bothwell, A. Green, D. P. Derman, R. D. Baynes, T. Jenkins, P. L. Jooste, E. D. Du Toits, and P. Jacobs (1987) The HLA linked iron loading gene in an Afrikaner population. *J. Med. Genet.* **24,** 48–353.

[30] R. A. MacDonald (1961) Idiopathic hemochromatosis, a variant of portal

cirrhosis and idiopathic hemosiderosis. *Arch. Intern. Med.* **107,** 606–616.

[31] L. W. Powell (1975) The role of alcoholism in hepatic iron storage disease. *Ann. NY Acad. Sci.* **252,** 124–134.

[32] M. Simon, M. Bourel, B. Genetet, R. Fauchet, G. Edan, and P. Brissot (1977) Idiopathic hemochromatosis and iron overload in alcoholic liver disease: Differentiation by HLA phenotype. *Gastroenterology* **73,** 655–658.

[33] M. Simon, J.-L. Alexandre, M. Bourel, B. Le Marec, and C. Scordia (1977) Heredity of idiopathic haemochromatosis: A study of 106 families. *Clin. Genet.* **11,** 327–341.

[34] D. Conte, A. Piperno, C. Mandeli, S. Fargion, M. Cesana, L. Brunelli, L. Ferrario, P. Velio, M. G. Zaramella, C. Tiribelli, G. Fiorelli, and P. A. Bianchi (1986) Clinical, biochemical and histological features of primary haemochromatosis: A report of 67 cases. *Liver* **6,** 310–315.

[35] P. Brissot, M. Bourel, D. Herry, J.-P. Verger, M. Messner, C. Beaumont, F. Regnouard, B. Ferrand, and M. Simon (1981) Assessment of liver iron content in 271 patients: A reevaluation of direct and indirect methods. *Gastroenterology* **80,** 557–565.

[36] L. Hallberg, A.-M. Hogdahl, L. Nilsson, and G. Rybo (1966) Menstrual blood loss and iron deficiency. *Acta Med. Scand.* **180,** 639–650.

[37] S. K. Cole, W. Z. Billewicz, and A. M. Thomson (1971) Source of variation in menstrual blood loss. *J. Obstet. Gynaecol. Br. Commonwealth* **78,** 933–939.

[38] M. Layrisse and C. Martinez-Torres (1971) Food iron absorption: Iron supplementation of food, in *Progress in Hematology,* vol VI. E. B. Brown and C. V. Moore, eds. Grune and Stratton, New York, pp. 137–160.

[39] W. Forth and W. Rummel (1973) Iron absorption. *Physiol. Rev.* **53,** 724–792.

[40] T. H. Bothwell, G. Pirzio-Biroli, and C. A. Finch (1958) Iron absorption. I. Factors influencing absorption. *J. Lab. Clin. Med.* **51,** 24–36.

[41] A. Jacobs and P. M. Miles (1969) Intraluminal transport of iron from stomach to small intestinal mucosa. *Br. Med. J.* **iv,** 778–781.

[42] P. M. Smith, F. Studley, and R. Williams (1969) Postulated gastric factor enhancing iron absorption in haemochromatosis. *Br. J. Haematol.* **16,** 443–449.

[43] L. W. Powell and E. Wilson (1970) *In vivo* intestinal mucosal uptake of iron, body iron absorption and gastric juice iron-binding in idiopathic haemochromatosis. *Austral. Ann. Med.* **19,** 226–231.

[44] A. Jacobs and P. M. Miles (1968) The iron-binding properties of gastric juice. *Clin. Chim. Acta.* **24,** 87–92.

[45] M. S. Wheby, M. E. Conrad, S. E. Hedberg, and W. H. Crosby (1962) The role of bile in the control of iron absorption. *Gastroenterology* **42,** 319–324.

[46] D. A. Webling and E. S. Holdsworth (1966) Bile and the absorption of strontium and iron. *Biochem. J.* **100,** 661–663.

[47] H. Brise (1962) Effect of surface-active agents on iron absorption. *Acta Med. Scand.* **171 (Suppl. 376),** 47–50.

[48] M. S. Wheby, L. G. Jones, and W. H. Crosby (1964) Studies on iron absorption. Intestinal regulatory mechanisms. *J. Clin. Invest.* **43,** 1433–1442.

[49] M. S. Wheby (1970) Site of iron absorption in man. *Scand. J. Haematol.* **7,** 56–62.

[50] B. S. Narasinga Rao (1981) Physiology of iron absorption and supplementation. *Br. Med. Bull.* **37,** 25–30.

[51] A. Muir and U. Hopfer (1985) Regional specificity of iron uptake by small intestinal brush-border membranes from normal and iron deficient mice. *Am. J. Physiol.* **248,** G376–G379.

[52] K. B. Raja, I. Bjarnason, R. J. Simpson, and T. J. Peters (1987) In vitro measurement and adaptive response of Fe^{3+} uptake by mouse intestine. *Cell. Biochem. Function.* **5,** 69–76.

[53] M. A. Savin and J. D. Cook (1978) Iron transport by isolated rat intestinal mucosal cells. *Gastroenterology* **75,** 688–694.

[54] T. M. Cox and M. W. O'Donnell (1981) Studies on the binding of iron by rabbit intestinal microvillous membranes. *Biochem. J.* **194,** 753–759.

[55] J. J. M. Marx and P. Aisen (1981) Iron uptake by rabbit intestinal mucosal membrane vesicles. *Biochim. Biophys. Acta* **649,** 297–304.

[56] R. J. Simpson and T. J. Peters (1984) Studies of Fe^{3+} transport across isolated intestinal brush-border membrane of the mouse. *Biochim. Biophys. Acta* **772,** 220–226.

[57] R. J. Simpson, K. B. Raja, and T. J. Peters (1985) Fe^{3+} transport by brush-border membrane vesicles isolated from normal and hypoxic mouse duodenum and ileum. *Biochim. Biophys. Acta* **814,** 8–12.

[58] R. J. Simpson and T. J. Peters (1985) Fe^{2+} uptake by intestinal brush-border membrane vesicles from normal and hypoxic mice. *Biochim. Biophys. Acta* **814,** 381–388.

[59] R. J. Simpson and T. J. Peters (1986) pH-sensitive transport of Fe^{2+} across purified brush-border membrane from mouse intestine. *Biochim. Biophys. Acta* **856,** 109–114.

[60] R. J. Simpson and T. J. Peters (1986) Cholate-soluble and -insoluble iron binding components of rabbit duodenal brush-border membrane. Relevance to Fe^{2+} uptake by brush border membrane vesicles. *Biochim. Biophys. Acta* **859,** 227–236.

[61] R. J. Simpson and T. J. Peters (1987) Transport of Fe^{2+} across lipid bilayers: Possible role of free fatty acids. *Biochim. Biophys. Acta* **898,** 187–195.

[62] P. E. Johnson, H. C. Lukaski, and T. D. Bowman (1987) Effects of level and saturation of fat and iron level and type in the diet on iron absorption and utilization by the rat. *J. Nutr.* **117,** 501–507.

[63] M. W. O'Donnell and T. M. Cox (1982) Microvillar iron-binding glycoproteins isolated from the rabbit small intestine. *Biochem. J.* **202,** 107–115.

[64] W. N. Pearson and M. Reich (1969) Studies of ferritin and a new iron-binding protein found in the intestinal mucosa of the rat. *J. Nutr.* **99,** 137–140.

[65] M. Worwood and A. Jacobs (1971) Absorption of ^{59}Fe in the rat: Iron binding substances in the soluble fraction of intestinal mucosa. *Life Sci.* **10,** 1363–1373.

[66] S. Pollack and F. D. Lasky (1976) A new iron-binding protein isolated from intestinal mucosa. *J. Lab. Clin. Med.* **87,** 670–679.

[67] H. Huebers, E. Huebers, W. Rummel, and R. C. Crichton (1976) Isolation and characterization of iron-binding proteins from rat intestinal mucosa. *Eur. J. Biochem.* **66,** 447–455.

[68] J. W. Halliday, L. W. Powell, and U. Mack (1976) Iron absorption in the rat: The search for possible intestinal mucosal carriers. *Br. J. Haematol.* **34,** 237–250.

[69] G. Johnson, P. Jacobs, and L. R. Purves (1983) Iron binding proteins of iron-absorbing rat intestinal mucosa. *J. Clin. Invest.* **71,** 1467–1476.

[70] R. G. Sheehan and E. P. Frenkel (1972) The control of iron absorption by the gastrointestinal mucosal cell. *J. Clin. Invest.* **51,** 224–231.

[71] M. C. Linder, V. Dunn, E. Isaacs, D. Jones, M. Van Volkom, and H. N. Munro (1975) Ferritin and intestinal iron absorption: Pancreatic enzymes and free iron. *Am. J. Physiol.* **228,** 196–201.

[72] J. A. Smith, J. W. Drysdale, A. Goldberg, and H. N. Munro (1968) The effect of enteral and parenteral iron on ferritin synthesis in the intestinal mucosa of the rat. *Br. J. Haematol.* **14,** 79–86.

[73] M. A. Savin and J. D. Cook (1980) Mucosal iron transport by rat intestine. *Blood* **56,** 1029–1035.

[74] H. A. Huebers, E. Huebers, E. Csiba, W. Rummel, and C. A. Finch (1983) The significance of transferrin for intestinal iron absorption. *Blood* **61,** 283–290.

[75] K. Osterloh, K. Schuman, C. Ehtechami, and W. Forth (1985) Transferrin in isolated cells from rat duodenum and jejunum. *Blut* **51,** 41–47.

[76] G. Johnson, P. Jacobs, and L. R. Purves (1985) The effects of cytoskeletal inhibitors on intestinal iron absorption in the rat. *Biochim. Biophys. Acta* **843,** 83–91.

[77] R. B. Dawson, S. Rafal, and L. R. Weintraub (1970) Absorption of hemoglobin iron: The role of xanthine oxidase in the intestinal, heme-splitting reaction. *Blood* **35,** 94–103.

[78] R. W. Topham, J. H. Woodruff, and M. C. Walker (1981) Purification and characterization of the intestinal promoter of Fe^{3+}-transferrin formation. *Biochemistry* **20,** 319–324.

[79] J. Fletcher and E. R. Huehns (1968) Function of transferrin. *Nature* **218,** 1211–1214.

[80] O. Zak and P. Aisen (1990) Evidence for functional differences between the

two sites of rabbit transferrin: Effects of serum and carbon dioxide. *Biochim. Biophys. Acta* **1052,** 24–28.

[81] J. J. Marx, J. A. G. K. Gebbink, T. Nishisato, and P. Aisen (1982) Molecular aspects of the binding of absorbed iron to transferrin. *Br. J. Haematol.* **52,** 105–110.

[82] H. A. Huebers, B. Josephson, E. Huebers, E. Csiba, and C. A. Finch (1984) Occupancy of the iron binding sites of transferrin. *Proc. Natl. Acad. Sci. USA* **81,** 4326–4330.

[83] O. Zak and P. Aisen (1986) Nonrandom distribution of iron in circulating transferrin. *Blood* **68,** 157–161.

[84] J. Williams and K. Moreton (1980) The distribution of iron between the metal-binding sites of transferrin in human serum. *Biochem. J.* **185,** 483–488.

[85] M. Cazzola, H. A. Huebers, M. H. Sayers, A. P. MacPhail, M. Eng, and C. A. Finch (1985) Transferrin saturation, plasma iron turnover, and transferrin uptake in normal humans. *Blood* **66,** 935–939.

[86] P. A. Seligman (1983) Structure and function of the transferrin receptor, in *Progress in Hematology,* vol XIII. E. B. Browm, ed. Grune and Stratton, New York, pp. 131–146.

[87] W. S. May, Jr and P. Cuatrecasas (1985) Transferrin receptor: Its biological significance. *J. Membrane Biol.* **88,** 205–215.

[88] I. S. Trowbridge and M. B. Omary (1981) Human cell surface glycoprotein related to cell proliferation is the receptor for transferrin. *Proc. Natl. Acad. Sci. USA* **78,** 3039–3043.

[89] C. A. Enns and H. H. Sussman (1981) Physical characterization of the transferrin receptor in human placentae. *J. Biol. Chem.* **256,** 9820–9823.

[90] M. B. Omary and I. S. Trowbridge (1981) Covalent binding of fatty acid to the transferrin receptor in cultured human cells. *J. Biol. Chem.* **256,** 4715–4718.

[91] C. Schneider, R. Sutherland, R. Newman, and M. Greaves (1982) Structural features of the cell surface receptor for transferrin that is recognized by the monoclonal antibody OKT9. *J. Biol. Chem.* **257,** 8516–8522.

[92] F. M. van Bockxmeer and E. H. Morgan (1979) Transferrin receptors during rabbit reticulocyte maturation. *Biochim. Biophys. Acta* **584,** 76–83.

[93] J. H. Jandl and J. H. Katz (1963) The plasma-to-cell cycle of transferrin. *J. Clin. Invest.* **42,** 314–326.

[94] Z. Zaman, M. Heynen, and R. L. Verwilgen (1980) Studies on the mechanism of transferrin iron uptake by reticulocytes. *Biochim. Biophys. Acta* **632,** 553–561.

[95] C. Harding, J. Meuser, and P. Stahl (1983) Receptor-mediated endocytosis of transferrin and recycling of the transferrin receptor in rat reticulocytes. *J. Cell Biol.* **97,** 329–339.

[96] C. R. Hopkins and I. S. Trowbridge (1983) Internalization and processing of

transferrin and the transferrin receptor in human carcinoma A431 cells. *J. Cell Biol.* **97,** 508–521.

[97] J. A. Hanover, M. C. Willingham, and I. Paston (1984) Kinetics of transit of transferrin and epidermal growth factor through clathrin-coated membranes. *Cell* **39,** 283–293.

[98] P. Aisen and L. Listowsky (1980) Iron transport and storage proteins. *Ann. Rev. Biochem.* **49,** 357–393.

[99] A. Dautry-Varsat, A. Ciechanover, and H. F. Lodish (1983) pH and the recycling of transferrin during receptor-mediated endocytosis. *Proc. Natl. Acad. Sci. USA* **80,** 2258–2262.

[100] R. D. Klausner, G. Ashwell, J. van Renswoude, J. B. Harford, and K. R. Bridges (1983) Binding of apotransferrin to K562 cells: Explanation of the transferrin cycle. *Proc. Natl. Acad. Sci. USA* **80,** 2263–2266.

[101] A. Ciechanover, A. L. Schwartz, A. Dautry-Varsat, and H. F. Lodish (1983) Kinetics of internalization and recycling of transferrin and the transferrin receptor in a human hepatoma cell line. *J. Biol. Chem.* **258,** 9681–9689.

[102] K. Konopka and I. Romslo (1980) Uptake of iron from transferrin by isolated rat mitochondria mediated by phosphate compounds. *Eur. J. Biochem.* **107,** 433–439.

[103] K. K. Rao, J. B. Harford, T. Rouault, A. McClelland, F. H. Ruddle, and R. D. Klausner (1986) Transcriptional regulation by iron of the gene for the transferrin receptor. *Mol. Cell. Biol.* **6,** 236–240.

[104] J. L. Casey, B. Di Jeso, K. Rao, R. D. Klausner, and J. B. Harford (1988) Two genetic loci participate in the regulation by iron of the gene for the human transferrin receptor. *Proc. Natl. Acad. Sci. USA* **85,** 1787–1791.

[105] C. A. Enns, H. A. Suomalainen, J. E. Gebhardt, J. Scroder, and H. H. Sussman (1982) Human transferrin receptor: Expression of the receptor is assigned to chromosome 3. *Proc. Natl. Acad. Sci. USA* **79,** 3241–3245.

[106] R. M. Nunes, O. Beloqui, B. J. Potter, and P. D. Berk (1986) Evidence for receptor mediated uptake of transferrin iron by rat hepatocytes. *Ann. NY Acad. Sci.* **463,** 327–329.

[107] S. P. Young and P. Aisen (1981) Transferrin receptors and the uptake and release of iron by isolated hepatocytes. *Hepatology* **1,** 114–119.

[108] S. P. Young and P. Aisen (1980) The interaction of transferrin with isolated hepatocytes. *Biochim. Biophys. Acta* **633,** 145–153.

[109] R. M. Nunes, J. M. Prieto, and B. J. Potter (1982) Mediation of a receptor mechanism in the uptake of iron from transferrin by the hepatocyte. *Protides Biol. Fluids* **29,** 455–458.

[110] O. Beloqui, R. M. Nunes, B. Blades, P. D. Berk, and B. J. Potter (1986) Depression of iron uptake from transferrin by isolated hepatocytes in the presence of ethanol is a pH-dependent consequence of ethanol metabolism. *Alcohol. Clin. Exp. Res.* **10,** 463–470.

[111] E. H. Morgan and E. Baker (1986) Iron uptake and metabolism by hepatocytes. *Fed. Proc.* **45,** 2810–2816.

[112] R. Soda and M. Tavassoli (1984) Liver endothelium and not hepatocytes or Kupffer cells have transferrin receptors. *Blood* **63,** 270–276.

[113] W. Vogel, A. Bomford, S. Young, and R. Williams (1987) Heterogeneous distribution of transferrin receptors on parenchymal and nonparenchymal liver cells: Biochemical and morphological evidence. *Blood* **69,** 264–270.

[114] T. Kishimoto and M. Tavassoli (1986) Recovery of transferrin receptors on hepatocytes membranes after collagenase perfusion. *Biochem. Biophys. Res. Commun.* **134,** 711–715.

[115] J.-C. Sibille, J.-N. Octave, Y.-J. Schneider, A. Trouet, and R. R. Crichton (1982) Transferrin protein and iron uptake by cultured hepatocytes. *FEBS Lett.* **150,** 365–369.

[116] C. G. D. Morley and A. Bezkorovainy (1983) The behavior of transferrin receptors in rat hepatocyte plasma membranes. *Clin. Physiol. Biochem.* **1,** 318–328.

[117] M. A. Page, E. Baker, and E. H. Morgan (1984) Transferrin and iron uptake by rat hepatocytes in culture. *Am. J. Physiol.* **246,** G26–G33.

[118] C. G. D. Morley and A. Bezkorovainy (1985) Cellular iron uptake from transferrin: Is endocytosis the only mechanism? *Int. J. Biochem.* **17,** 553–564.

[119] C. Watts (1985) Rapid endocytosis of the transferrin receptor in the absence of bound transferrin. *J. Cell Biol.* **100,** 633–637.

[120] J. W. Drysdale and H. N. Munro (1966) Regulation of synthesis and turnover of ferritin in rat liver. *J. Biol. Chem.* **241,** 3630–3637.

[121] J. Rogers and H. N. Munro (1987) Translation of ferritin light and heavy subunit mRNA's is regulated by intracellular chelatable iron levels in rat hepatoma cells. *Proc. Natl. Acad. Sci. USA* **84,** 2277–2281.

[122] A. Rouault, M. W. Hentze, A. Danas, W. Caughman, J. B. Harford, and R. D. Klausner (1987) Influence of altered transcription on the translational control of human ferritin expression. *Proc. Natl. Acad. Sci. USA* **84,** 6335–6339.

[123] T. A. Rouault, M. W. Hentze, S. W. Caughman, J. B. Harford, and R. D. Klausner (1988) Binding of a cytosolic protein to the iron-responsive element of human ferritin messenger RNA. *Science* **241,** 1207–1210.

[124] T. C. Iancu and H. B. Neustein (1977) Ferritin in human liver cells of homozygous beta-thalassemia: Ultrastructural observations. *Br. J. Haematol.* **37,** 527–535.

[125] C. A. Seymor and T. J. Peters (1978) Organelle pathology in primary and secondary haemochromatosis with special reference to lysosomal changes. *Br. J. Haematol.* **40,** 239–253.

[126] B. Model (1979) Advances in the use or iron-chelating agents for the treatment of iron overload, in *Progress in Hematology,* vol XI. E. B. Brown, ed. Grune and Stratton, New York, pp. 267–312.

[127] D. A. Lipschitz, T. H. Bothwell, H. C. Seftel, A. C. Wapnick, and R. W. Charlton (1971) The role of ascorbic acid in the metabolism of storage iron. *Br. J. Haematol.* **20,** 155–163.

[128] E. Baker, A. G. Morton, and A. S. Tavill (1980) The regulation of iron release from the perfused liver. *Br. J. Haematol.* **45,** 607–620.

[129] U. Mack, L. W. Powell, and J. W. Halliday (1983) Detection and isolation of a hepatic membrane receptor for ferritin. *J. Biol. Chem.* **258,** 4672–4675.

[130] T. A. Hamilton, P. W. Gray, and D. O. Adams (1984) Expression of the transferrin receptor on murine peritoneal macrophages is modulated by in vitro treatment with interferon gamma. *Cell. Immunol.* **89,** 478–488.

[131] R. Andreesen, J. Osterholz, H. Bodemann, K. J. Bross, U. Costabel, and G. W. Lohr (1984) Expression of transferrin receptors and intracellular ferritin during terminal differentiation of human monocytes. *Blut* **49,** 195–202.

[132] N. Colman and V. Herbert (1980) Hematologic complications of alcoholism: Overview. *Semin. Hematol.* **17,** 164–176.

[133] M. Myrhed, L. Berglund, and L. E. Bottiger (1977) Alcohol consumption and hematology. *Acta Med. Scand.* **202,** 11–15.

[134] R. W. Charlton, P. Jacobs, H. Seftel, and T. H. Bothwell (1964) Effects of alcohol on iron absorption. *Br. Med. J.* **2,** 1427–1429.

[135] A. Celada, H. Rudolf, and A. Donath (1978) Effect of a single ingestion of alcohol on iron absorption. *Am. J. Hematol.* **5,** 225–237.

[136] R. A. MacDonald and G. S. Pechet (1964) Absorption by rats of iron in wine. *Proc. Soc. Exp. Biol. Med.* **117,** 54–56.

[137] E. J. Tapper, S. Bushi, R. D. Ruppert, and N. J. Greenberger (1968) Effect of acute and chronic ethanol treatment on the absorption of iron in rats. *Am. J. Med. Sci.* **255,** 46–52.

[138] R. Mazzanti, K. S. Srai, E. S. Debnam, A. M. Boss, and P. Gentilini (1987) The effect of chronic ethanol consumption on iron absorption in rats. *Alcohol Alcohol.* **22,** 47–52.

[139] S. J. Fairweather-Tait, S. Southon, and Z. Piper (1988) The effect of alcoholic beverages on iron and zinc metabolism in the rat. *Br. J. Nutr.* **60,** 2Q-215.

[140] J. Lindenbaum (1980) Folate and vitamin B_{12} deficiencies in alcoholism. *Semin. Hematol.* **17,** 113–118.

[141] A. Celada, H. Rudolf, and A. Donath (1979) Effects of experimental chronic alcohol ingestion and folic acid deficiency on iron absorption. *Blood* **54,** 906–915.

[142] F. El-Shobaki and W. Rummel (1985) Mucosal iron binding proteins aand the inhibition of iron absorption by endotoxin. *Blut* **50,** 95–101.

[143] P. Whittaker, B. S. Skikne, A. M. Covell, C. Flowers, A. Cooke, S. R. Lynch, and J. D. Cook (1989) Duodenal iron proteins in idiopathic hemochromatosis. *J. Clin. Invest.* **83,** 261–267.

[144] R. W. Topham, S. A. Joslin, and J. S. Prince, Jr (1985) The effect of short-

term exposure to low iron diets on the mucosal processing of ionic iron. *Biochem. Biophys. Res. Commun.* **133**, 1092–1G57.

[145] G. J. Anderson, L. W. Powell, and J. W. Halliday (1990) Transferrin receptor distribution and regulation in the rat small intestine. Effect of iron stores and erythropoiesis. *Gastroenterology* **98**, 576–585.

[146] A. Gilbert and A. Gernet (1896) Cirrhose alcoolique hypertrophique pigmentaire. *Com. Rend. Acad. Sci.* (Paris) **3**, 1078–1081.

[147] J. Lereboullet, R. Levillain, and B. Debesse (1956) L'hepatosiderose. Sa frequence chez les alcooliques, etudes statistique de 350 examens anatomique. *Bull. Mem. Soc. Med. Hop. Paris* **72**, 684–689.

[148] J. Andre (1961) Le demembrement des hemachromatosis. *Rev. Int. Hepatol.* **11**, 113–174.

[149] M. Barry (1973) Iron and chronic liver disease. *J. Royal Coll. Physicians* **8**, 52–62.

[150] A. W. Jakobovits, M. Y. Morgan, and S. Sherlock (1979) Hepatic siderosis in alcoholics. *Dig. Dis. Sci.* **24**, 305–310.

[151] J. M. Miralles Garcia and S. de Castro del Pozo (1976) Iron deposits in chronic alcoholics. Special studies in relation to the iron contained in red wine. *Acta Hepatogastroenterol.* **23**, 10–19.

[152] L. W. Powell (1966) Normal human iron storage and its relation to etnanol consumption. *Australas Ann. Med.* **15**, 110–115.

[153] O. Lundvall, A. Weinfeld, and P. Lundin (1969) Iron stores in alcohol abusers. I. Liver iron. *Acta Med. Scand.* **185**, 259–269.

[154] G. S. Pechet, S. W. French, J. Levy, and R. A. MacDonald (1965) Histologic and chemical tissue iron. *Arch. Pathol.* **79**, 452–461.

[155] A. Weinfeld, P. Lundin, and O. Lundvall (1968) Significance for the diagnosis of iron overload of histochemical and chemical iron in the livers of control subjects. *J. Clin. Pathol.* **21**, 35–40.

[156] C. Q. Edwards, M. Carroll, P. Bray, and G. E. Cartwright (1977) Hereditary haemochromatosis. Diagnosis in siblings and children. *N. Engl. J. Med.* **297**, 7–13.

[157] P. Scheuer, R. Williams, and A. R. Muir (1962) Hepatic pathology in relatives of patients with idiopathic haemochromatosis. *J. Pathol. Bacteriol.* **84**, 53–64.

[158] O. Lundvall and A. Weinfeld (1969) Iron stores in alcohol abusers. II. As measured with the desferrioxamine test. *Acta Med. Scand.* **185**, 271–277.

[159] V. Hoenig, M. Brodanova, and C. Kordac (1968) Effect of ethanol on iron tolerance and endogenous serum iron in liver cirrhosis. *Scand. J. Gastroenterol.* **3**, 334–338.

[160] R. Williams, H. S. Williams, P. J. Scheuer, C. S. Pitcher, E. Loiseau, and S. Sherlock (1967) Iron absorption and siderosis in chronic liver disease. *Q. J. Med.* **36**, 151–166.

[161] R. C. Doberneck, D. B. Nunn, D. G. Johnson, and B. K. Chun (1963) Iron

metabolism after portacaval shunt in dogs. *Arch. Surg.* **87,** 751–756.

[162] S. P. Balcerzak, W. W. Peternel, and E. W. Heinle (1967) Iron absorption in chronic pancreatitis. *Gastroenterology* **53,** 257–264.

[163] J. Murray and N. Stein (1967) Effect of ligation of the pancreatic duct on the absorption of radio iron by rats. *Gastroenterology* **53,** 38–41.

[164] E. Klein and W. Schmitt (1956) Eisenresorption und serum-transferrin bei leberkrankheiten. *Klin. Wschr.* **34,** 297–300.

[165] L. W. Powell and B. T. Emmerson (1966) Haemosiderosis associated with xanthine oxidase inhibition. *Lancet* **i,** 239–240.

[166] V. Hoenig, A. M. Brodanova, J. Strejceck, and V. Kordac (1967) Allopurinol and iron metabolism. *Lancet* **i,** 387.

[167] G. A. Mendel (1963) Studies on iron absorption. I. The relationship between the rat of erythropoiesis, hypoxia and iron absorption. *Blood* **18,** 727–736.

[168] L. R. Weintraub, W. H. Conrad, and W. Crosby (1965) Regulation of the intestinal absorption of iron by the rate or erythropoiesis. *Br. J. Haematol.* **11,** 432–438.

[169] C. S. Pitcher and R. Williams (1963) Reduced red cell survival in jaundice and its relation to abnormal glutathione metabolism. *Clin. Sci.* **24,** 239–252.

[170] P. G. Frick and J. F. Schmid (1965) Das hamolytische syndrom bei der akuten und chronischen hepatitis. *Klin. Wschr.* **43,** 305–309.

[171] L. W. Powell (1967) The effect of cirrhosis and ethanol ingestion on hepatic iron deposition in the rat. *J. Pathol. Bacteriol.* **93,** 157–166.

[172] R. W. Chapman, M. Y. Morgan, A. M. Boss, and S. Sherlock (1983) Acute and chronic effects of alcohol on iron absorption. *Dig. Dis. Sci.* **28,** 321–327.

[173] R. M. Nunes, O. Beloqui, B. J. Potter, and P. D. Berk (1984) Iron uptake from transferrin by isolated hepatocytes: Effect of ethanol. *Biochem. Biophys. Res. Commun.* **125,** 824–830.

[174] M. E. Rubini, C. R. Kleeman, and E. Lamdin (1955) Studies on alcohol diuresis. I. The effect of ethyl alcohol ingestion on water, electrolyte and acid-base metabolism. *J. Clin. Invest.* **34,** 439–455.

[175] P. B. Oliva (1970) Lactic acidosis. *Am. J. Med.* **48,** 209–255

[176] F. Lundquist, N. Tygstrup, K. Winkler, K. Mellengaard, and S. Munk-Peterson (1962) Ethanol metabolism and production of free acetate in the human liver. *J. Clin. Invest.* **41,** 955–96i.

[177] H. M. Redetski, T. A. Koener, J. R. Hughes, and A. G. Smith (1972) Osmometry in the evaluation of alcohol intoxication. *Clin. Toxicol.* **5,** 343–363.

[178] J. D. Beard and D. H. Knott (1968) Fluid and electrolyte balance during acute withdrawal in chronic alcoholic patients. *J. Am. Med. Assoc.* **204,** 133–139.

[179] S. M. Wolfe and M. Victor (1976) The relationship of hypomagnesemia and alkylosis to alcohol withdrawal symptoms. *Ann. NY Acad. Sci.* **162,** 973–984.

[180] B. J. Potter and T. A. McHugh (1988) Iron uptake from transferrin (Tf) and asialotransferrin (ATf) by hepatocytes from alcohol-fed rats. *Alcohol. Clin. Exp. Res.* **12,** 320 (Abstract).

[181] C. A. Casey, S. L. Kragskow, M. F. Sorrell, and D. J. Tuma (1990) Effect of chronic ethanol administration on total asialoglycoprotein receptor content and intracellular processing of asialoorosomucoid in isolated rat hepatocytes. *Biochim. Biophys. Acta* **1052,** 1–8.

[182] B. J. Potter and T. A. McHugh (1989) Effects of iron loading on iron uptake from transferrin by hepatocytes from alcohol-fed rats. *Gastroenterology* **96,** A646 (Abstract).

[183] R. W. Chapman, M. Y. Morgan, R. Bell, and S. Sherlock (1983) Hepatic iron uptake in alcoholic liver disease. *Gastroenterology* **84,** 143–147.

[184] L. Heilmeyer (1967) Pathogenesis of hemochromatosis. *Medicine* (Baltimore) **46,** 209–215.

[185] M. Pollycove, R. A. Fawwaz, and H. S. Winchell (1971) Transient hepatic deposition of iron in primary haemochromatosis with iron deficiency following venesection. *J. Nucl. Med.* **12,** 28–30.

[186] R. G. Batey, J. E. Pettit, A. W. Nicholas, S. Sherlock, and A. V. Hoffbrand (1978) Hepatic iron clearance from serum in treated hemochromatosis. *Gastroenterology* **75,** 856–859.

[187] M. Lombard, A. Bomford, M. Hynes, N. V. Naoumov, S. Roberts, J. Crowe, and R. Williams (1989) Regulation of the hepatic transferrin receptor in hereditary hemochromatosis. *Hepatology* **9,** 1–5.

[188] A. G. Morton and A. S. Tavill (1978) The control of hepatic iron uptake: Correlation with transferrin synthesis. *Br. J. Haematol.* **39,** 497–507.

[189] M. S. Wheby and G. Umpiere (1964) Effect of transferrin saturation on iron absorption in man. *N. Engl. J. Med.* **271,** 1391–1395.

[190] L. W. Sullivan and V. Herbert (1964) Suppression of hematopoiesis by ethanol. *J. Clin. Invest.* **43,** 2048–2062.

[191] J. Lindenbaum and C. S. Lieber (1969) Hematologic effects of alcohol in man in the absence of nutritional deficiency. *N. Engl. J. Med.* **281,** 333–338.

[192] L. S. Valberg, C. N. Ghent, D. A. Lloyd, J. V. Frei, and M. J. Chamberlain (1978) Diagnostic efficiency of tests for the detection of iron overload in chronic liver disease. *Can. Med. Assoc. J.* **119,** 229–236.

[193] R. J. Dern, A. Monti, and M. F. Glynn (1963) Studies with doubly labelled iron, IV. Evidence for a second iron binding system in plasma. *J. Lab. Clin. Med.* **61,** 2Q-291.

[194] F. Hosain and C. A. Finch (1964) Ferrokinetics: A study of transport iron in plasma. *J. Lab. Clin. Med.* **64,** 905–914.

[195] B. Sarkar (1970) State of iron (III) in normal human serum: Low molecular

weight of protein ligands besides transferrin. *Can. J. Biochem.* **48,** 1339–1350.

[196] R. G. Batey, S. Shamir, and J. Wilms (1981) Properties and hepatic metabolism of non-transferrin-bound iron. *Dig. Dis. Sci.* **26,** 1084–1088.

[197] P. Brissot, T. L. Wright, W.-L. Ma, and R. A. Weisiger (1985) Efficient clearance of non-transferrin-bound iron by rat liver. Implications for hepatic iron loading in iron overload states. *J. Clin. Invest.* **76,** 1463–1470.

[198] T. L. Wright, P. Brissot, W.-L. Ma, and R. A. Weisiger (1986) Characterization of non-transferrin-bound iron clearance by rat liver. *J. Biol. Chem.* **261,** 10909–10914.

[199] R. G. Batey, P. Lai Chun Fong, S. Shamir, and S. Sherlock (1980) A non-transferrin-bound serum iron in idiopathic hemochromatossis. *Dig. Dis. Sci.* **25,** 340–346.

[200] R. A. Fawwaz, H. S. Winchell, M. Pollycove, and T. Sargent (1967) Hepatic iron deposition in humans. *Blood* **30,** 417–421.

[201] M. J. Giglio, R. C. Santoro, and E. Bozzini (1984) Effect of chronic ethanol administration on production and response to erythropoietin in the mouse. *Alcohol. Clin. Exp. Res.* **8,** 323–325.

[202] L. W. Sullivan and V. Herbert (1964) Suppression of hematopoiesis by ethanol. *J. Clin. Invest.* **43,** 2048–2062.

[203] J. D. Hines (1969) Reversible megaloblastic and sideroblastic marrow abnormalities in alcoholic patients. *Br. J. Haematol.* **16,** 87–101.

[204] H. Kondo, K. Saito, P. Grasso, and P. Aisen (1988) Iron metabolism in the erythrophagocytosing Kupffer cell. *Hepatology* **8,** 32–38.

[205] J.-C. Sibille, H. Kondo, and P. Aisen (1988) Interactions between isolated hepatocytes and Kupffer cells in iron metabolism: A possible role for ferritin as an iron carrier protein. *Hepatology* **8,** 296–301.

[206] U. Mack, L. W. Powell, and J. W. Halliday (1983) Detection and isolation of a hepatic membrane receptor for ferritin. *J. Biol. Chem.* **248,** 4672–4675.

[207] P. C. Adams, L. W. Powell, and J. W. Halliday (1988) Isolation of a human hepatic ferritin receptor. *Hepatology* **9,** 719–721

[208] P. C. Adams, U. Mack, L. W. Powell, and J. W. Halliday (1988) Isolation of a porcine hepatic ferritin receptor. *Comp. Biochem. Physiol.* (B) **90,** 837–841.

[209] P. C. Adams and L. A. Chau (1990) Hepatic ferritin uptake and hepatic iron. *Hepatology* **1,** 805–808.

[210] P. Pootrakul, B. Josephson, H. A. Huebers, and C. A. Finch (1988) Quantitation of ferritin iron in plasma, an explanation for non-transferrin iron. *Blood* **71,** 1120–1123.

[211] M. W. Hentze, S. W. Caughman, T. A. Rouault, J. G. Barriocanal, A. Dancis, J. B. Harford, and R. D. Klausner (1987) Identification of the iron-responsive element for the translational regulation of human ferritin mRNA. *Science* **238,** 1570–1573.

[212] J.-J. Lin, M. M. Daniels-McQueen Patino, L. Gaffield, W. E. Walden, and R. E. Thach (1990) Derepression of ferritin messenger RNA translation by hemin in vitro. *Science* **247,** 74–77.

[213] G. D. Nadkarni and U. R. Deshpande (1982) Liver ferritin synthesis following chronic alcohol administration to rats: Modulation by propythiouracil. *Experientia* **38,** 372–373.

[214] R. Moirand, G. Lescoat, N. Hubert, J. F. Dezier, and N. Pasdeloup (1989) Ethanol induction of ferritin in a human hepatoblastoma cell line (HepG$_2$). *Hepatology* **10,** 573 (Abstract).

[215] H. P. Roeser, D. J. Sizemore, A. Nikles, and B. E. Cham (1983) Tissue ferritin in scorbutic guinea pigs. *Br. J. Haematol.* **55,** 325–333.

[216] H. P. Roeser, J. W. Halliday, D. J. Sizemore, A. Nikles, and D. Willgos (1980) Serum ferritin in ascorbic acid deficiency. *Br. J. Haematol.* **45,** 459–466.

[217] B. E. Cham, H. P. Roeser, and A. C. Nickles (1990) Ascorbic acid deficiency affects the metabolism of cytosolic ferritin but not lipid-associated ferritin in livers of guinea pigs. *Biochem. J.* **267,** 535–537.

[218] S. M. Sabesin and L. B. Thomas (1964) Parenchymal siderosis in patients with pre-existing portal cirrhosis. A pathologic entity simulating idiopathic and transfusional hemochromatosis. *Gastroenterology* **46,** 447–485.

[219] L. W. Powell and J. F. R. Kerr (1975) The pathology of the liver in hemochromatosis, in *Pathobiology Annual,* H. Joacim, ed. Academic, New York, pp. 317–337.

[220] M. L. Bassett, J. W. Halliday, and L. W. Powell (1981) HLA typing in idiopathic haemochromatosis: Distinction between homozygotes and heterozygotes with biochemical expression. *Hepatology* **1,** 120–126.

[221] M. L. Bassett, J. W. Halliday, R. A. Ferris, and L. W. Powell (1904) Hemochromatosis: Predictive accuracy of biochemical screening tests. *Gastroenterology* **87,** 628–633.

[222] D. J. Pounder (1984) Problems in the necropsy diagnosis of alcoholic liver disease. *Am. J. Forensic Med. Pathol.* **5,** 103–108.

[223] G. H. Addison, M. R. Beamish, C. N. Hales, M. Hodgkins, A. Jacobs, and P. Llewellin (1972) An immunoradiometric assay for ferritin in the serum of normal subjects and patients with iron deficiency and iron overload. *J. Clin. Pathol.* **25,** 326–329.

[224] G. O. Walters, F. M. Miller, and M. Worwood (1973) Serum ferritin concnetration and iron stores in normal subjects. *J. Clin. Pathol.* **26,** 770–772.

[225] D. A. Lipschitz, J. D. Cook, and C. A. Finch (1974) A clinical evaluation of serum ferritin. *N. Engl. J. Med.* **290,** 1213–1216.

[226] W. R. Bezwoda, T. H. Bothwell, J. D. Torrance, A. P. MacPhail, R. W. Charlton, G. Kay, and J. Levin (1979) The relationship between marrow iron stores, plasma ferritin concentrations and iron absorption. *Scand. J. Haematol.* **22,** 113–120.

[227] T. H. Bothwell, R. W. Charlton, J. D. Cook, and C. A. Finch (1979) *Iron metabolism in man.* Blackwell, Oxford, pp. 90–103.

[228] M. Worwood (1979) Serum ferritin. *CRC Crit. Rev. Clin. Lab. Sci.* **10,** 171–204.

[229] S. Nakano, T. Kumada, K. Sugiyama, H. Watahili, and I. Takeda (1984) Clinical significance of serum ferritin for hepatocellular carcinoma. *Am. J. Gastroenterol.* **79,** 623–627.

[230] C. W. Aungst (1968) Ferritin in body fluids. *J. Lab. Clin. Med.* **71,** 517–522.

[231] J. Prieto, M. Barry, and S. Sherlock (1975) Serum ferritin in patients with iron overload and with acute and chronic liver diseases. *Gastroenterology* **68,** 525–533.

[232] S. Hussein, M. Laulicht, and A. V. Hoffbrand (1978) Serum ferritin in megaloblastic anaemia. *Scand. J. Haematol.* **20,** 241–245.

[233] L. W. Powell, J. W. Halliday, and L. V. McKeering (1975) Studies of serum ferritin with emphasis on its importance in clinical medicine, in *Proteins of Iron Storage and Transport in Biochemistry and Medicine,* R. R. Crichton, ed. North Holland, Amsterdam, pp. 215–221.

[234] H. Kristenson, G. Fex, and E. Trell (1981) Serum ferritin, gammaglutamyl-transferase and alcohol consumption in healthy middle-aged men. *Drug Alcohol Depend.* **8,** 43–50.

[235] L. Lundin, R. Hallgren, G. Birgegard, and L. Wide (1981) Serum ferritin in alcoholics and relation to liver damage, iron state and erythropoietic activity. *Acta Med. Scand.* **209,** 327–331.

[236] T. E. Meyer, C. Kassianides, T. H. Bothwell, and A. Green (1984) Effects of heavy alcohol consumption on serum ferritin concentrations. *S. Afr. Med. J.* **6,** 573–575.

[237] L. W. Powell and H. M. Lloyd (1975) Haemochromatosis. *Arch. Int. Med.* **135,** 1269.

[238] T. C. Iancu, H. B. Neustein, and B. H. Landing (1977) The liver in thalassaemia major: Ultrastructural observations, in *Iron Metabolism,* Ciba Foundation Symposium #51, Elsevier, Amsterdam, pp. 293–316.

[239] M. L. Bassett, J. W. Halliday, and L. W. Powell (1986) Value of hepatic iron measurements in early hemochromatosis and determination of the critical iron level associated with fibrosis. *Hepatology* **6,** 24–29.

[240] L. R. Weintraub, A. Goral, J. Grasso, C. Franzblau, A. Sullivan, and S. Sullivan (1985) Pathogenesis of hepatic fibrosis in experimental iron overload. *Br. J. Haematol.* **59,** 321–331.

[241] B. F. Trump, J. M. Valigorsky, A. A. Arstila, W. J. Mergner, and T. D. Kinney (1973) The relationship of intracellular pathways of iron metabolism to cellular iron overload and iron storage diseases. *Am. J. Pathol.* **72,** 295–324.

[242] H. L. Bonkowsky, J. F. Healy, P. R. Sinclair, J. F. Sinclair, and J. S. Pomeroy (1981) Iron and the liver: Acute and long-term effects of iron loading on hepatic haem metabolism. *Biochem. J.* **196**, 57–64.

[243] B. R. Bacon, A. S. Tavill, G. M. Brittenham, C. H. Park, and R. O. Recknagel (1983) Hepatic lipid peroxidation in vivo in rats with chronic iron overload. *J. Clin. Invest.* **71**, 429–439.

[244] N. R. DiLuzio (1966) A mechanism of acute ethanol-induced fatty liver and the modification of liver injury by antioxidants. *Lab. Invest.* **15**, 50–63.

[245] R. C. Reitz (1975) A possible mechanism for the peroxidation of lipids due to chronic ethanol consumption. *Biochim. Biophys. Acta* **380**, 145–154.

[246] A. Boveris, C. G. Fragga, A. I. Varsavsky, and O. R. Koch (1983) Increased chemiluminescence and superoxide production in the livers of chronically ethanol-treated rats. *Arch. Biochem. Biophys.* **227**, 534–541.

[247] G. Krikun and A. I. Cederbaum (1986) Effect of chronic ethanol consumption on microsomal lipid peroxidation: Role of iron and comparison between controls. *FEBS Lett.* **208**, 292–296.

[248] U. Koster, D. Albrecht, and H. Kappus (1977) Evidence for carbon tetrachloride and ethanol-induced lipid peroxidation in vivo demonstrated by ethane production in mice and rats. *Toxicol. Appl. Pharmacol.* **41**, 639–648.

[249] R. E. Litov, D. H. Irving, J. E. Downey, and A. L. Tappel (1978) Lipid peroxidation: A mechanism involved in acute ethanol toxicity as demonstrated by in vivo pentane production in the rat. *Lipids* **13**, 305–307.

[250] C. S. Lieber (1980) Alcohol, protein metabolism and liver injury. *Gastroenterology* **79**, 373–390.

[251] S. Shaw, E. Jayatilleke, and C. S. Lieber (1988) Lipid peroxidation as a mechanism of alcoholic liver injury: Role of iron mobilization and microsomal induction. *Alcohol* **5**, 135–140.

[252] A. I. Cederbaum (1989) Oxygen radical generation by microsomes: Role of iron and implications for alcohol metabolism and toxicity. *Free Rad. Biol. Med.* **7**, 559–567.

[253] V. D. Antonenkov, S. V. Pirozhkov, S. V. Popova, and L. F. Pachenko (1989) Effect of chronic ethanol treatment on lipid peroxidation in rat liver homogenate and subcellular fractions. *Int. J. Biochem.* **21**, 1191–1195.

[254] M. G. Irving, J. W. Halliday, and L. W. Powell (1988) Association between alcoholism and increased hepatic iron stores. *Alcohol. Clin. Exp. Res.* **12**, 7–13.

[255] R. A. Cooper (1980) Hemolytic syndromes and red cell membrane abnormalities in liver disease. *Semin. Hematol.* **17**, 103–112.

[256] J. Sanchez, M. Casas, and R. Rama (1988) Effect of chronic ethanol administration on iron metabolism in the rat. *Eur. J. Haematol.* **41**, 321–325.

[257] M. C. Linder, J. R. Moor, L. E. Scott, and H. N. Munro (1973) Mechanism of

sex difference in rat tissue iron stores. *Biochim. Biophys. Acta* **297,** 70–80.

[258] A. D. Heys and T. L. Dormandy (1981) Lipid peroxidation in iron-overloaded spleens. *Clin. Sci.* **60,** 295–301.

[259] D. Savage and J. Lindenbaum (1986) Anemia in alcoholics. *Medicine* **65,** 322–338.

[260] A. Kristensson-Aas, S. Wallerstedt, C. Alling, G. Cederblad, and B. Magnusson (1986) Haematological findings in chronic alcoholics after heavy drinking with special reference to haemolysis. *Eur. J. Clin. Invest.* **16,** 178–183.

[261] M. R. Clemens, H. Einsele, H. Remmer, and H. D. Waller (1985) Decreased susceptibility of red blood cells to lipid peroxidation in patients with alcoholic liver cirrhosis. *Clin. Chim. Acta* **145,** 283–288.

[262] F. Michot and J. Gut (1987) Alcohol-induced bone marrow damage: A bone marrow study in alcohol-dependent individuals. *Acta Haematol.* **78,** 252–257.

[263] M. Kumazawa, M. Misaki, M. Baba, T. Shima, and S. Suzuki (1986) Transferrin receptor on rat Kupffer cells in primary culture. *Liver* **6,** 138–144.

[264] R. Andreesen, J. Osterholz, H. Bodemann, K. J. Bross, U. Costabel, and G. W. Lohr (1984) Expression of transferrin receptors and intracellular ferritin during terminal differentiation of human monocytes. *Blut* **49,** 195–202.

[265] T. Nishisato and P. Aisen (1982) Uptake of transferrin by rat peritoneal macrophages. *Br. J. Haematol.* **52,** 631–640.

[266] D. J. Sizemore and M. L. Bassett (1984) Monocyte transferrin-iron uptake in hereditary hemochromatosis. *Am. J. Hematol.* **16,** 347–354.

[267] L T. Yam, H. E. Finkel, L. R. Weintraub, and W. H. Crosby (1968) Circulating iron-containing macrophages in hemochromatosis. *N. Engl. J. Med.* **275,** 512–514.

[268] M. L. Bassett, J. W. Halliday, and L. W. Powell (1982) Ferritin synthesis in peripheral blood monocytes in idiopathic hemochromatosis. *J. Lab. Clin. Med.* **100,** 137–145.

[269] G. Fillet and G. Marsaglia (1975) Idiopathic hemochromatosis: Abnormality in RBC transport of iron by the reticuloendothelial system. *Blood* **46,** 1007.

[270] E. Baraona, M. T. Leo, S. A. Borowsky, and C. S. Lieber (1975) Alcoholic hepatomegaly: Accumulation of protein in the liver. *Science* **190,** 794–795.

[271] M. A. Rothschild, M. Oratz, J. Morland, S. S. Schreiber, A. Burks, and B. Martin (1980) Effects of ethanol on protein synthesis and secretion. *Pharmacol. Biochem. Behav.* **13 (Suppl. 1),** 31–36.

[272] G. D. Volentine, D. J. Tuma, and M. F. Sorrell (1984) Acute effects of ethanol on hepatic glycoprotein secretion in the rat. *Gastroenterology* **86,** 225–229.

[273] M. F. Sorrell, J. M. Nauss, T. M. Donahue, Jr, and D. J. Tuma (1983) Effect of chronic ethanol administration on hepatic glycoprotein secretion in the rat. *Gastroenterology* **84,** 580–586.

[274] B. Wallin, J. Morland, and A.-M. Fikke (1981) Combined effects of ethanol and pH-change on protein synthesis in isolated rat hepatocytes. *Acta Pharmacol. Toxicol.* **49**, 134–140.

[275] K. N. Jeejeebhoy, M. J. Phillips, A. Bruce-Robertson, J. Ho, and U. Sodtke (1972) The acute effects of ethanol on albumin, fibrinogen and transferrin synthesis in the rat. *Biochem. J.* **126**, 1111–1126.

[276] M. E. Gardiner and E. H. Morgan (1981) Effect of reduced atmospheric pressure and fasting on transferrin synthesis in the rat. *Life Sci.* **29**, 1641–1648.

[277] A. Smith-Keilland and J. Morland (1981) Reduced hepatic protein synthesis after long term ethanol treatment in fasted rats. Dependence on animal handling before measurement. *Biochem. Pharmacol.* **30**, 2377–2379.

[278] A. G. Morton and A. S. Tavill (1977) The role of iron in the regulation of hepatic transferrin synthesis. *Br. J. Haematol.* **36**, 383–394.

[279] A. G. Morton and A. S. Tavill (1978) The control of hepatic iron uptake: Correlation with transferrin synthesis. *Br. J. Haematol.* **39**, 4497–507.

[280] M. J. O'Shea, D. Kershnobich, and A. S. Tavill (1973) Effects of inflammation on iron and transferrin metabolism. *Br. J. Haematol.* **25**, 707–714.

[281] B. J. Potter, R. W. G. Chapman, R. M. Nunes, D. Sorrentino, and S. Sherlock (1985) Transferrin metabolism in alcoholic liver disease. *Hepatology* **5**, 714–721.

[282] S. Jarnum and N. A. Lassen (1961) Albumin and transferrin metabolism in infectious and toxic diseases. *Scand. J. Clin. Lab. invest.* **40**, 2143–2152.

[283] R. Hoffenberg, A. H. Gordon, E. G. Blake, and L. N. Louis (1970) Plasma protein catabolism in the rat. The effect of alterations of albumin concentration and dietary protein depletion. *Biochem. J.* **118**, 401–404.

[284] J. P. Milsom and R. G. Batey (1979) The mechanism of hepatic iron uptake from native and denatured transferrin and its subcellular metabolism in the liver cell. *Biochem. J.* **182**, 117–125.

[285] E. Regoeczi, P. A. Chindemi, M. W. C. Hatton, and L. R. Berry (1980) Galactose-specific elimination of human asialotransferrin by the bone marrow in the rabbit. *Arch. Biochem. Biophys.* **205**, 76–84.

[286] G. Ashwell and A. G. Morell (1974) The role of surface carbohydrates in the hepatic recognition and transport of circulating glycoproteins, in *Advances in Enzymology,* vol 41. A. Meister, ed. Wiley, New York, pp. 99–128.

[287] E. Regoeczi, P. A. Chindemi, and M. T. Debanne (1984) Transferrin glycans: A possible link between alcoholism and hepatic siderosis. *Alcohol. Clin. Exp. Res.* **8**, 287–292.

[288] S. P. Young, A. Bomford, and R. Williams (1983) Dual pathways for the uptake of rat asialotransferrin by rat hepatocytes. *J. Biol. Chem.* **258**, 4972–4976.

[289] H. Stibler, C. Allgulander, S. Borg, and K. G. Kjellin (1978) Abnormal microheterogeneity of transferrin in serum and cerebrospinal fluid in alcoholism. *Acta Med. Scand.* **204,** 49–56.

[290] H. Stibler, S. Borg, and C. Allgulander (1979) Clinical significance of abnormal heterogeneity of transferrin in relation to alcohol consumption. *Acta Med. Scand.* **206,** 275–281.

[291] O. Vesterberg, S. Petren, and D. Schmidt (1984) Increased concentrations of a transferrin variant after alcohol abuse. *Clin. Chim. Acta* **141,** 33–39.

[292] E. L. Storey, U. Mack, L. W. Powell, and J. W. Halliday (1985) Use of chromatofocusing to detect a transferrin variant in serum of alcoholic subjects. *Clin. Chem.* **31,** 1543–1545.

[293] H. Stibler, O. Sydow, and S. Borg (1980) Quantitative estimation of abnormal microheterogeneity of serum transferrin in alcoholics. *Pharmacol. Biochem. Behav.* **13 (Suppl. 1),** 47–51.

[294] H. Stibler and S. Borg (1981) Evidence of a reduced sialic acid content in serum transferrin in male alcoholics. *Alcohol. Clin. Exp. Res.* **5,** 545–549.

[295] C. J. Dekker, M. J. Kroos, C. Van der Heul, and H. G. Van Eijk (1984) Iron uptake from sialotransferrins by rat reticulocytes. *Int J. Biochem.* **16,** 787–792.

[296] H. Stibler and S. Borg (1986) Carbohydrate composition of serum transferrin in alcoholic patients. *Alcohol. Clin. Exp. Res.* **10,** 61–64.

[297] H. Stibler, S. Borg, and M. Joustra (1986) Micro anion exchange chromatography or carbohydrate-deficient transferrin in relation to alcohol consumption (Swedish patent 8400587–5). *Alcohol. Clin. Exp. Res.* **10,** 535–544.

[298] U. J. Behrens, T. M. Worner, L. F. Braly, F. Schaffner, and C. S. Lieber (1988) Carbohydrate-deficient transferrin, a marker for chronic alcohol consumption in different ethnic populations. *Alcohol. Clin. Exp. Res.* **12,** 427–432.

[299] U. Behrens, T. M. Worner, and C. S. Lieber (1988) Changes in carbohydrate-deficient transferrin levels after alcohol withdrawal. *Alcohol. Clin. Exp. Res.* **12,** 539–544.

[300] M. F. Sorrell and D. J. Tuma (1978) Selective impairment of glycoprotein metabolism by ethanol and acetaldehyde in rat liver slices. *Gastroenterology* **75,** 200–208.

[301] E. Regoeczi, P. A. Chindemi, M. T. Debanne, and P. A. Charlwood (1982) Partial resialylation of human asialotransferrin type 3 in the rat. *Proc. Natl. Acad. Sci. USA* **79,** 2226–2230.

[302] E. Regoeczi, P. A. Charlwood, and P. A. Chindemi (1985) The effects of cytotropic compounds on the resialylation of human asialotransferrin type 3 in the rat. *Exp. Cell. Res.* **157,** 495–503.

[303] M. T. Debanne and E. Regoeczi (1981) Subcellular distribution of human asialotransferrin type 3 in the rat liver. *J. Biol. Chem.* **256,** 11266–11272.

[304] L. Marzella and H. Glaumann (1980) Increased degradation in rat liver induced by vinblastine: I. Biochemical characterization. *Lab. Invest.* **42,** 8–17.

[305] M. D. Snider and O. C. Rogers (1985) Intracellular movement of cell surface receptors after endocytosis: Resialylation of asialo-transferrin receptor in human erythroleukemia cells. *J. Cell Biol.* **100,** 826–834.

[306] J. J. M. Bergeron, J. H. Ehrenreich, P. Siekevitz, and G. E. Palade (1973) Golgi fractions prepared from rat liver homogenates. I. Isolation procedure and morphological characterization. *J. Cell Biol.* **59,** 45–72.

[307] H. Stibler, E. Burns, T. Kruckeberg. P. Gaetano, E. Cerven, S. Borg, and B. Tabakoff (1983) Effect of ethanol on synaptosomal sialic acid metabolism in the developing rat brain. *J. Neurosci.* **59,** 21–35.

[308] S. Petren and O. Vesterberg (1988) Concentration differences in isoforms of transferrin in blood from alcoholics during abuse and abstinence. *Clin. Chim. Acta.* **175,** 183–188.

[309] C. J. Dekker, M. J. Kroos, C. Van der Heul, and H. G. Van Eijk (1985) Uptake of sialo and asialo transferrins by isolated rat hepatocytes. Comparison of a heterologous and a homologous sytem. *Int. J. Biochem.* **17,** 701–706.

[310] S. P. Young, A. Bomford, and R. Williams (1983) Dual pathways for the uptake of rat asialotransferrin by rat hepatocytes. *J. Biol. Chem.* **258,** 4972–4976.

[311] E. Regoeczi and A. Koj (1985) Diacytosis of human asialotransferrin type 3 in the rat liver is due to the sequential engagement of two receptors. *Exp. Cell. Res.* **160,** 1–8.

[312] S. P. Wilkinson, J. Canalese, and R. Williams (1980) Consequences of kupffer cell failure in fulminant hepatic failure and cirrhosis with particular reference to endotoxaemia, in *The Reticuloendothelial System and the Pathogenesis of Liver Disease.* H. Liehr and M. Grun, eds. Elsevier/North Holland Biomedical Press, Amsterdam, pp. 337–340.

[313] H. Prytz, M. Bjorneboe, F. Orskov, and M. Hilden (1973) Antibodies to Escherichia coli in alcoholic and non-alcoholic patients with cirrhosis of the liver. *Scand. J. Gastroenterol.* **8,** 433–438.

[314] A. Simjee, J. Hamilton-Miller, H. Thomas, W. Brumfitt, and S. Sherlock (1975) Antibodies to Escherichia coli in chronic liver diseases. *Gut* **16,** 871–875.

[315] P. Staun-Olsen, M. Bjorneboe, H. Prytz, A. C. Thomsen, and F. Orskov (1983) *Escherichia coli* antibodies in alcoholic liver disease. Correlation to alcohol consumption, alcoholic hepatitis and serum IgA. *Scand. J. Gastroenterol.* **18,** 889–896.

[316] C. Bode, V. Kugler, and J. C. Bode (1987) Endotoxemia in patients with alcoholic and non-alcoholic cirrhosis and in subjects with no evidence of chronic liver disease following acute alcohol excess. *J. Hepatol.* **4,** 8–14.

[317] B. S. Bhagwandeen, M. Apte, L. Manwarring, and J. Dickeson (1987) Endotoxin induced hepatic necrosis in rats on an alcohol diet. *J. Pathol.* **151,** 47–53.

[318] R. J. Elin and S. M. Wolf (1974) The role of iron in non-specific resistance to infection induced by endotoxin. *J. Immunol.* **112,** 737–745.

[319] R. F. Kampschmidt and G. A. Schultz (1961) Hypoferremia in rats following injection of bacterial endotoxin. *Proc. Soc. Exp. Biol. Med.* **106,** 870–871.

[320] B. J. Potter, B. Blades, T. A. McHugh, R. M. Nunes, O. Beloqui, P. A. Slott, and J. H. Rand (1989) Effects of endotoxin on iron uptake by the hepatocyte. *Am. J. Physiol.* **257,** G524–G531.

[321] B. J. Potter, T. A. McHugh, and J. H. Rand (1988) The effects of endotoxins on iron uptake by hepatocytes from chronically alcohol-fed rats. *Hepatology* **8,** 1240 (Abstract).

[322] B. Nosslin (1973) Analysis of disappearance time curves after single injection of labeled proteins, in *Protein Turnover,* Ciba Foundation Symposium 9 (New Series). G. E. W. Wolsteinholm and M. O'Connor, eds. Assoc. Sci. Publ., Amsterdam, pp. 113–130.

[323] G. C. T. Yeoh, J. A. Wassenberg, E. Edkins, and I. T. Oliver (1979) Synthesis and secretion of albumin and transferrin by foetal rat hepatocyte cultures. *Biochim. Biophys. Acta* **565,** 347–355.

The Pathogenesis
of Inflammation
in Alcoholic Liver Disease

F. Joseph Roll

Introduction

In the US and many other Western countries, alcohol-related* liver injury is responsible for the majority of deaths caused by liver disease.[1] We have no specific therapy except abstinence from alcohol, which in many patients fails to prevent progression of the disease. This has given strong impetus to attempts to understand the pathogenesis of the disease and develop treatments to supplement abstinence.

In the early part of this century, alcohol-related liver disease was thought to be primarily a result of the malnutrition that usually accompanies alcoholism, but the response of patients with alcoholic liver disease to nutritional therapy in randomized, controlled trials has been disappointing. More recently, investigators surveying this field have stressed the toxic effects of alcohol itself and have assigned to malnutrition, at most, a contributory role.[2] A multitude of effects of alcohol or its metabolite acetalde-

*Alcohol and ethanol are used synonymously in this chapter.

From: *Drug and Alcohol Abuse Reviews, Vol. 2: Liver Pathology and Alcohol*
Ed: R. R. Watson ©1991 The Humana Press Inc.

hyde on such cellular functions as protein secretion, mitochondrial energy production, membrane fluidity, redox state, and cytoskeletal function have been documented;[3] in vitro studies have suggested that acetaldehyde can increase transcription rates for collagen in cultured fibroblasts,[4] raising the possibility that cirrhosis might result directly from alcohol metabolism. However, even high concentrations of alcohol do not damage liver cells in vitro,[5] and it has been difficult to explain the full spectrum of human alcohol-related liver injury on the basis of any of the effects of alcohol described to date.

With the current interest in the toxic effects of alcohol it is often assumed that the inflammation that is such a striking feature of alcoholic hepatitis clinically and pathologically (*see below*) is a nonspecific response to alcohol-induced liver-cell injury. According to this view, leukocytes are attracted by dying liver cells, cell components such as condensed intermediate filaments ["alcoholic hyaline"], or fragments of the extracellular matrix and accumulate in the liver to remove the dead cells and debris in a "house-keeping" role. This assumption has to be reexamined in the light of recent studies that suggest a mechanism by which viable liver cells may elicit an inflammatory response, such as that seen in alcoholic hepatitis. These studies have shown that:

1. Alcohol metabolism by the liver is associated with an increased rate of lipid peroxidation in vivo.
2. Liver cells metabolizing alcohol generate, via a lipid peroxide intermediate, a substance that is a chemoattractant for polymorphonuclear leukocytes.
3. In vitro, activated polymorphonuclear leukocytes are themselves cytotoxic to liver cells and destructive of extracellular matrix.

These observations suggest the hypothesis that inflammation is a primary problem in alcohol-related liver disease and that, like certain arthritides and autoimmune disorders, alcoholic liver disease may be a process in which the inflammatory response is misdirected and becomes predominantly destructive rather than protective of the organism. This chapter will begin by describing the spectrum of alcohol-related liver disease and will then summarize the evidence for a primary role of inflammation in its genesis, focusing on studies from our laboratory of a chemoattractant generated by liver cells metabolizing ethanol.

The Spectrum
of Alcohol-Related Liver Disease

Alcoholic Fatty Liver

Alcoholic fatty liver is characterized histologically by the deposition of large droplets of fat in liver cells. This may involve only a few, or nearly all, of the cells. Similar deposits may be seen in livers of obese individuals, in normal volunteers given ethanol for several weeks and rarely in nonobese, normal individuals.[6,7] The fat appears to be primarily in the form of triacylglycerol. The predominant reason for the fat accumulation associated with alcohol ingestion is not known,[8] but evidence has been gathered in experimental animals and in humans for several potential mechanisms which may act in concert, including an increase in fatty acid uptake by the liver,[9] inhibition of hepatic fatty acid oxidation,[10] and increased synthesis of fatty acids.[11] Whether fatty liver has any ill effects in humans is controversial. It has been reported that some patients with simple fatty liver have a subtle increase in fibrous tissue around hepatic central veins, called perivenular fibrosis, which presages the development of cirrhosis,[12] but this has not been found in all studies[13] and prior episodes of frank inflammation cannot be excluded in these patients. It has also been claimed that fatty liver progresses directly to cirrhosis in the baboon model of alcoholic liver disease; however, published reports of serial liver biopsies in these animals describe mononuclear cell infiltrates that temporally precede or accompany the fibrosis.[14] In summary, alcoholic fatty liver has not been conclusively shown to cause frank liver-cell injury or fibrosis.

Alcoholic Hepatitis

Alcoholic hepatitis and cirrhosis are more serious forms of liver disease that occur in only 15% of alcoholics. Clinically, alcoholic hepatitis is characterized by jaundice, gastrointestinal symptoms, prolonged fever, leukocytosis, an elevated erythrocyte sedimentation rate, and an enlarged, tender liver. In many ways it mimics an acute inflammatory process, such as a bacterial infection. Histologically there is a characteristic inflammatory cell infiltrate composed predominantly of polymorphonuclear leukocytes, but including macrophages and lymphocytes, swelling and degeneration of liver cells around central veins, and condensation of liver-cell intermediate filaments giving rise to hepatocyte inclusions known as "alcoholic hyaline" or "Mallory bodies."[15] By contrast, in some other types of hepatitis, such as viral hepatitis, neutrophils are not prominent, although there may be a comparable degree of liver-cell necrosis. This observation suggests that liver-cell damage itself does not always cause an influx of polymorphonuclear leukocytes. There may also be fat accumulation in liver cells and a spidery fibrosis in the vicinity of central veins, perhaps reflecting overlap of alcoholic hepatitis with the other two manifestations of alcohol-related liver disease. Alcoholic hepatitis has a high mortality; approximately one-third of the patients in control groups in clinical treatment trials die within the first 4 wk after hospitalization.[16]

Alcoholic Cirrhosis

At least half of the patients with the lesion of alcoholic hepatitis who continue to consume alcohol (and many who do not) go on to develop cirrhosis within 2–3 yr.[17] Cirrhosis is characterized histologically by the appearance of abundant extracellular matrix, consisting primarily of collagen bundles that disrupt the normal architecture of the liver and distort blood vessels.[15] Smooth muscle-like cells, so-called myofibroblasts, populate the scar tissue and are likely responsible for formation and contraction of the bundles of collagen.[18–20] Clinically, the cirrhotic phase is dominated by complications stemming from the obstruction to blood flow through the liver by the proliferating scar: portal hypertension with shunting of blood through esophageal varices, hepatic encephalopathy, and impaired liver cell function. Mortality during the first year after presentation is 25%.[21]

The Role of Inflammation

In trying to understand the pathogenesis of alcohol-related liver disease, a fundamental question is whether the inflammation seen in alcoholic hepatitis is necessary for liver-cell injury and/or subsequent fibrosis. The evidence at present is primarily clinical and is indirect. A role in injury is suggested by the observations that the illness often persists for months after withdrawal from alcohol and that improvement in serum transaminases and other measures of liver injury parallels resolution of histologic inflammation.[22,23] There is also an excellent correlation between the histologic findings of inflammation and liver-cell injury in coded liver biopsies of patients with alcoholic hepatitis.[23] Moreover, antiinflammatory drugs, such as corticosteroids, have been shown to reduce mortality in a subset of patients with severe disease.[24]

What is the evidence that alcoholic hepatitis is a precursor of cirrhosis? Again the clinical evidence is indirect and is based on two observations:

1. As previously noted, when patients with alcoholic hepatitis are studied by means of serial liver biopsies a high proportion are found to develop cirrhosis during a followup period of several years,[17,25] and
2. In large groups of alcoholic individuals, those with inflammation (i.e., alcoholic hepatitis) gave a history of an average of 10.3 yr of alcoholism, whereas those with cirrhosis had a 17.1-yr history of alcoholism.[26]

These data are in accord with clinical experience in the US and Europe: With the exception of studies of perivenular fibrosis described earlier, there is no evidence that patients progress to cirrhosis without inflammation. The experience of certain Asian patients who have progressive fibrosis without hepatitis is often cited as evidence that alcoholic hepatitis may not always precede cirrhosis, but we now know that sporadic hepatitis C infection is common in this population and frequently leads to chronic hepatitis and cirrhosis.[27] Hence, chronic viral infection cannot be excluded as the cause of fibrosis in these patients.

In summary, clinical data suggests that alcoholic hepatitis almost always *precedes* cirrhosis. This is entirely consistent with evidence that the liver, like other organs, responds differently to acute than to chronic injury and inflammation. Like a sutured surgical wound, a self-limited injury to the liver, no matter how severe, usually heals without scarring and fibrosis. This is most clearly demonstrated by studies of hepatotoxins in animals. A single dose of carbon tetrachloride adminstered to a rat causes extensive liver necrosis, but this is followed by complete restoration of normal structure. If the toxin is given for several weeks, fibrosis develops but is fully reversible when the carbon tetrachloride is stopped.[28] The clinical counterpart of this is a patient who survives *acute* virus- or drug-induced fulminant hepatic failure. Even though most of the liver of such a patient is destroyed, the organ will frequently regenerate with a normal structure.[29] In contrast, if the injury is subacute or *chronic,* then fibrosis may dominate the repair process and cirrhosis can result. Thus, 10% of patients with chronic hepatitis B infection and 40–50% of those with chronic hepatitis C go on to cirrhosis,[30,31] and, in the example of carbon tetrachloride experimental injury, if administration of the toxin is continued beyond several weeks, then an irreversible cirrhosis results.[28]

There are in medicine many other examples of pathologic fibrosis associated with chronic inflammation, including sclerosis of renal glomeruli in glomerulonephritis, scarring of heart valves in rheumatic fever, pulmonary fibrosis of the idiopathic variety, and hepatic fibrosis from chronic active hepatitis or schistosomiasis. What is the evidence that it is the inflammatory response itself that is causing the fibrosis? The best-studied example is schistosomiasis, for which good animal models are available: Here T-cells activated by antigen from the egg of the worm have been shown to be responsible for release of factors that stimulate hepatic fibroblasts to proliferate and increase their collagen synthesis.[32] Another well-studied example is the liver fibrosis induced in rats by injection of streptococcal cell-wall material. Wahl et al. have shown that, in contrast to controls, nude rats lacking only T-lymphocytes do not develop hepatic fibrosis when the bacterial cell-wall material is administered.[33] In other cases the evidence is largely indirect: For example, in pulmonary fibrosis inflammatory cells from the affected tissue can be shown in vitro to release cytokines (e.g., platelet-derived growth factor) that are known to be capable of stimulating mesenchymal cell proliferation, migration, and extracellular matrix synthesis.[34] In the inflammatory infiltrate of alcoholic hepatitis, macrophages and lymphocytes are abundant. These mononuclear inflammatory cells may be responsible for the cirrhotic phase of the disease.

These observations suggest, then, that the lesion of alcoholic hepatitis is pivotal in the development of significant complications and that the inflammatory response seen in alcoholic hepatitis is closely linked to the mechanism by which alcohol injures the human liver.

Neutrophils and Liver Injury

The Role of Neutrophils in Cell and Tissue Injury

The primary role of neutrophils is in defense against foreign organisms, but, as mentioned previously, it is becoming clear that neutrophils can also be destructive agents in a number of diseases, including ischemia–reperfusion injury to the heart and other organs, rheumatoid arthritis, psoriasis, ulcerative coliitis, and Arthus reactions.[35] Before discussing the evidence for neutrophil-mediated liver injury, I will mention some of the

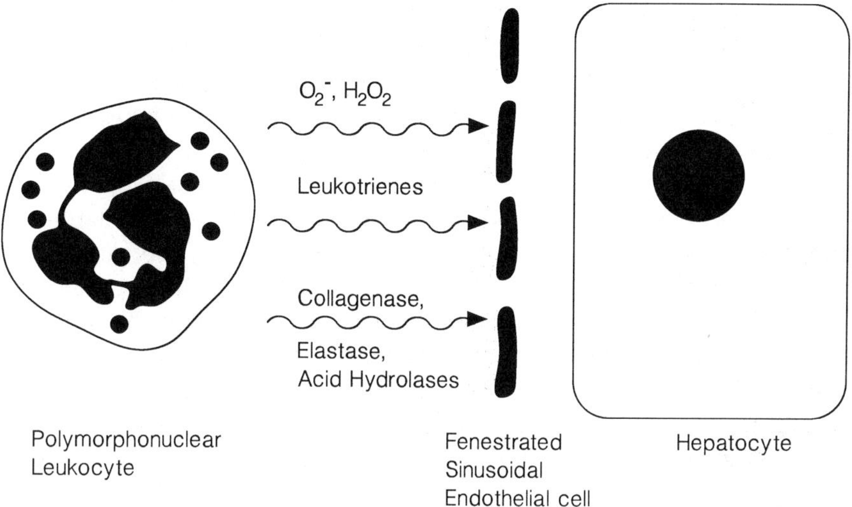

Fig. 1. Neutrophil products that are potentially cytotoxic to liver-derived cells.

mechanisms by which these cells exert toxicity. Becker distinguishes oxidative from nonoxidative mechanisms of neutrophil cytotoxicity.[36] Oxidant mechanisms include the production of O_2^-, H_2O_2, and, possibly, $\cdot OH$ by the neutrophil membrane-associated NADPH oxidase system (Fig. 1). The relative importance of these oxidants is still debated and may depend in part on the system being studied. Under most circumstances, O_2^- is not as reactive as $\cdot OH$ and is readily consumed by dismutation to H_2O_2, but there is some doubt whether neutrophils can generate $\cdot OH$ under physiologic conditions.[37] Neutrophil oxidative toxicity is at present thought to be attributable to the oxidizing ability of either H_2O_2 or hypochlorous acid, an enzyme secreted by neutrophils during degranulation. The mechanisms by which these oxidants damage target cells are still hypothetical, but include

1. "Oxidative stress," a shift in the redox state of the cell that ultimately leads to a rise in cytosolic calcium and cell injury, and
2. Direct oxidative attack on key proteins, membrane phospholipids, or DNA, causing cell death.[38]

Support for the oxidative mechanisms of target-cell injury comes from studies showing a protective effect of exogenous scavengers, such as superoxide dismutase, and of endogenous antioxidant defense mechansims, such as glutathione and glutathione peroxidase. Of particular relevance to liver toxicity is the observation that neutrophils can be stimulated to release increased quantities of oxidants by exposure to bacterial lipopolysaccharide,[39] which has been reported to be present in splanchnic blood of patients with liver disease.[40]

Nonoxidative mechansims of injury include the numerous proteases secreted by neutrophils during activation: elastase, collagenase, gelatinase, cathepsin, and acid hydrolases. These are known to be capable of degrading the extracellular matrix, and, given the importance of matrix for cell viability and function,[41] enzymes could mediate toxicity by this means. Alternatively, they may cause injury by attacking carbohydrates or proteins on the surface of target cells. The metabolism of H_2O_2 to HOCl by the granule enzyme myeloperoxidase and the oxidative inactivation of α-1-proteinase inhibitor by HOCl illustrate the possibility of cooperative effects of oxidative and nonoxidative mechanisms.[37] Neutrophils also produce another major group of mediators, termed eicosanoids, such as prostaglandins, leukotrienes, lipoxins, and thromboxanes (Fig. 1). Some of these are cytoprotective, but others may potentiate tissue injury by causing vasodilatation or by recruiting other inflammatory cells. Hepatocytes can convert some of these compounds to vasoactive glutathione derivatives, and this may play a role in certain types of liver injury.[42] It was recently reported that neutrophils activated by endotoxin can synthesize and secrete biologically active tumor necrosis factor α.[43] The cytotoxic effects of this cytokine are well described, and it may prove to be an important mediator of neutrophil-induced cell injury.

There are now several published studies implicating macrophages in liver injury in experimental models,[44,45] but to date there have been only a limited number of studies of the participation of neutrophils in liver injury. Cytotoxicity of neutrophils for a variety of endothelial cells or cell lines was described previously.[46] Morphologic studies of in vivo models of liver injury, such as that of endotoxin administration, have suggested that neutrophil adherence to the endothelium is an early event;[47] however, the effect of neutrophil depletion has not been tested.

A series of in vitro experiments demonstration cytotoxicity of neutrophils for hepatocytes has been reported by Mavier et al.[48,49] In these experiments, rat hepatocytes were incubated with stimulated human neutrophils, and toxicity was assessed by measuring release of the hepatocyte enzyme alanine amintransferase and by looking for ultrastructural changes. Mavier et al. demonstrated that incubation of liver cells with unstimulated neutrophils for up to 16 h was not associated with any significant toxicity. In contrast, incubation with neutrophils treated with opsonized zymosan particles — a standard activating stimulus — provoked significant release of hepatocyte aminotransferase activity.[48] Supernatants of neutrophils stimulated for 2 h with zymosan could be substituted for the neutrophils themselves, and, by the use of inhibitors, the cytotoxicity was shown to be attributable to proteases, such as cathepsin G and elastase, rather than to an oxidative mechanism.[49] In preliminary work, these authors showed that stimulation of the acute-phase response in the liver cells protected against cytotoxicity, probably by increasing the concentration of protease inhibitors in the medium and/or the hepatocytes.[50] It is not clear whether the cytotoxicity is a direct effect of the proteases on hepatocytes or an indirect effect of the enzymes via matrix degradation with subsequent loss of cell adhesion and viability. As with all such in vitro studies, the effect of isolating the liver cells from their normal matrix and from plasma factors is unknown, and in vivo studies in animal models of neutrophil-mediated liver injury are needed.

Neutrophil Chemotaxis and Chemoattractants

In a strict sense, chemotactic factors are substances that cause directed movement of cells (e.g., neutrophils) along a concentration gradient, but most chemotactic factors also have other effects on the cells they stimulate. For example, in vivo, in response to a chemotactic stimulus, circulating neutrophils adhere to endothelium locally, penetrate the endothelial lining (i.e., undergo diapedesis), migrate in a directed fashion along a concentration gradient, and secrete a number of potentially toxic products, including reduced oxygen intermediates ($\cdot$OH, H_2O_2, and HOCl), enzymes (such as elastase and collagenase), and arachidonic acid derivatives (such as leukotrienes, lipoxins, thromboxanes, and prostaglandins).[51] The release of these arachidonic acid derivatives, which are themselves mediators of inflammation, may serve to amplify or modulate the inflammatory response by recruiting either other neutrophils or the second wave of defenders, monocytes and macrophages. In general, chemotactic factors are not cell-specific, and the same factors usually are chemotactic for both neutrophils and macrophages. Nor do these factors act only on leukocytes: The chemotactic lipid leukotriene B_4 exerts a chemotactic effect on fibroblasts as well as neutrophils[52] and macrophages and it increases the ability of endothelial cells to adhere to neutrophils.[53] Both peptide chemotactic factors, such as C5a, and lipid chemotactic factors, such as leukotriene B_4, have been identified, and binding studies show that these ligands bind unique receptors. After ligand binding, the intracellular cascade of activation seems to follow a common path involving activation of a guanine nucleotide binding protein, activation of phospholipase C, increased phosphoinositide metabolism, and intracellular calcium.[54] Certain agonists, such as phorbol myristate acetate, are capable of directly activating the intracellular signal transduction pathway.

Although the complex biochemical events that take place in the target cell after exposure to a chemotactic stimulus are being unraveled, there is to date no convenient way to measure chemotactic activity except by bioassay. One of the methods most commonly used is the Boyden chamber assay.[55] In this assay, the chemoattractant substance is placed in the lower compartment of a two-compartment Plexiglas™ chamber. A filter with pores just large enough to admit a migrating cell separates the lower chamber from the upper chamber, into which is placed a suspension of freshly isolated neutrophils. After a suitable incubation period, the filter is removed, fixed, stained, and examined under a microscope. In one commonly used assay, the "leading front" assay, the distance that the leading front of neutrophils has moved through the filter in a given period of time (total migration) is recorded. The distance moved by cells in response to buffer alone is also measured (stimulated random motility). Chemotaxis (net migration) is calculated by subtracting stimulated random motility from total migration. By varying the location and concentration of stimulus above and below the filter, a truly chemotactic stimulus can be distinguished from one that merely stimulates random migration. In support of the physiologic significance of these in vitro assays, it has been found that substances that are chemotactic for leukocytes in the Boyden chamber also cause local accumulations of neutrophils when injected into the skin.[56]

The chemotactic response may be blocked by stimulus-specific inhibitors, such as chemotactic-factor inactivator (which blocks the response to C5a), by agents that act on microtubules, such as colchicine, and also by high concentrations of a chemotactic factor itself.[57] The latter effect is referred to as "deactivation." The mechanism is not known, but the effect may be a result of saturation of receptors so that the cell can no longer recognize a chemotactic gradient. It has been suggested that deactivation plays a role in retaining recruited neutrophils at the site of inflammation.

Neutrophil Function
in Alcoholic Liver Disease

In studies of the increased susceptibility to infection manifested by patients with alcoholic liver disease, DeMeo et al. reported defective in vitro neutrophil chemotaxis in response to complement components generated from serum of the majority of patients with alcoholic cirrhosis.[58] These investigators were able to determine that the problem was an inhibition of chemotaxis by the patients' serum, rather than a deficiency in the patients' neutrophils. Subsequently other investigators showed that such patients have elevated levels of a protein (chemotactic-factor inactivator) that blocks C5a-stimulated chemotaxis.[59,60] Defective neutrophil phagocytosis and intracellular killing of bacteria have also been described in alcoholic liver disease.[61] MacGregor has confirmed that neutrophils from patients with alcoholic cirrhosis exhibit decreased directed migration in response to complement components, but he also found normal chemotactic response to f-met-leu-phe in vitro;[62] moreover, the delivery of neutrophils in vivo in skin window trauma in these patients was normal. It was suggested that skin window trauma releases a number of different chemotactic mediators and that, because the previously described inhibitor is specific for C5a-induced chemotaxis, the neutrophils of these patients may be quite capable of responding to other stimuli. Investigators have also looked at the effect of alcohol itself on neutrophil function. In one of these studies, the investigators isolated neutrophils from healthy volunteers who had ingested moderate amounts of alcohol (blood alcohol levels approx 100 mg%) and examined 11 different neutrophil functions in vitro.[63] They found that alcohol exposure significantly affected only one function: bacterial phagocytosis. Higher concentrations of alcohol, such as those found in many chronic alcoholic patients, may impair a wider range of functions in vitro and probably play a role in the increased incidence of infection in these patients. Given that neutrophil infiltration of the liver is prominent in alcoholic hepatitis, it appears that directed migration is not abolished in these patients despite the effects of chemotactic-factor inactivator and alcohol itself.

Alcohol Metabolism
and the Formation of Chemoattractants

Lipid Peroxidation
and Chemoattractants

What is the evidence that lipid peroxidation is involved in formation of some chemoattractants? Certain polar lipids are among the most potent chemotactic substances known, and many of these are generated by enzymatic or nonenzymatic oxidation of free fatty acids. A good example is the generation of leukotriene B_4 (5S-12R-dihydroxy-6,14-*cis*-8,10-*trans*-eicosatetraenoic acid) from the abundant membrane lipid arachidonic acid. Arachidonic acid itself has no chemotactic activity, but it can be oxidized by an enzyme in neutrophils via a hydroperoxide intermediate, 5-hydroperoxyeicosatetraenoic acid, to the dihydroxy acid, which is chemotactic at nanomolar concentrations. Structure–function studies of LTB_4 analogs lacking one or the other hydroxyl group and of isomers of the dihydroxy acid reveal that the two hydroxyl groups in their appropriate positions are critical for chemotactic activity.[64] In vivo, in neutrophils, a specific enzyme (5-lipoxygenase) is responsible for the formation of the hydroperoxide intermediate, but nonenzymatic formation of the intermediate by halothane free radicals in vitro has also been described.[65]

Nonenzymatic, free-radical-mediated formation of a chemoattractant from arachidonic acid has been described by Perez et al., who exposed arachidonic acid to a superoxide-generating system consisting of acetaldehyde and xanthine oxidase in the presence and absence of a variety of radical scavengers.[66] In the absence of scavengers, a polar lipid was formed from arachidonic acid that had chemotactic activity. Scavengers of singlet oxygen virtually completely blocked generation of the activity and scavengers of other oxygen-derived free radicals, superoxide and hydroxyl radical, were partially inhibitory. In addition, Petrone et al. incubated human plasma with a superoxide-generating system consisting of xanthine oxidase and xanthine, and showed superoxide dismutase inhibitable production of a lipid chemoattractant.[67] Injection of this material into the skin of rats induced neutrophil accumulation. Neither of these compounds has yet been chemically characterized.

Another example of chemoattractants arising from lipid peroxidation in vivo is the formation of aldehydes, principally 4-hydroxynonenal, which has been extensively studied by Esterbauer et al. and Comporti.[68,69] The hydroxyalkenals are short-chain aldehydes that appear to be derived from scission of lipid peroxides formed enzymatically and nonenzymatically from phospholipid-bound long-chain fatty acids, such as arachidonic and linoleic acids.[68] Lipid peroxidation and production of these aldehydic products are found in association with many types of cell injury. For example, 4-hydroxynonenal can be isolated from pleural exudates in rats or generated in isolated liver cells or in microsomal preparations stimulated by carbon tetrachloride or ADP–iron. These aldehydes are substrates for glutathione transferase and aldehyde dehydrogenase, and it has been suggested that the enzymes are involved in their detoxification.[70] However, it is not yet clear whether lipid peroxides or aldehydes are causing injury or are merely byproducts of injured cells.[68,71] Recently Curzio et al. reported that 4-hydroxynonenal at micromolar concentrations is chemotactic for human neutrophils.[72] Homologs of chain length from 8 to 15 carbon atoms have been shown to stimulate chemotaxis of human neutrophils at concentrations ranging from 10^{-6} (4-hydroxyundecanal) to as low as $10^{-12}M$ (4-hydroxyoctenal),[72] and some of these are also produced during peroxidation of liver microsomal lipids.[68]

A chemotactic aldehyde with a structure somewhat different from either LTB_4 or 4-hydroxynonenal is reportedly produced by the metabolism of exogenous arachidonic acid by porcine leukocytes.[73] This compound has been identified as 12-oxododeca-5,8,10-trienoic acid, a 12-carbon carboxylic acid with a carbonyl group at the C-12 position and lacking any hydroxyl groups. It is postulated to arise by cleavage of arachidonic acid by 12-lipoxygenase. This compound apparently does not stimulate superoxide production or neutrophil aggregation, but is chemotactic for human neutrophils.

These examples illustrate that peroxidation reactions, both enzymatic and nonenzymatic, can convert ubiquitous, inactive precursors to biologically active products. Although the direct toxicity of lipid peroxides is still controversial, some of their derivatives clearly have chemotactic activity and may in part explain the accumulation of inflammatory cells at sites of lipid peroxidation as a result of drug toxicity.

Alcohol Metabolism:
A Source of Lipid Peroxidation

DiLuzio, more than 20 years ago, proposed that ethanol metabolism by the liver induces lipid peroxidation in that organ.[74] This has been confirmed by some,[75] but other investigators have failed to find evidence for lipid peroxidation following exposure to alcohol.[76] Some of the discrepancies may well be attributable to methodologic differences[77] or difficulties in measuring lipid peroxidation.[71] Recently the proposal has gained more attention, with evidence for ethanol-induced lipid peroxidation coming from several different lines of investigation. First, free radicals and oxygen, in the presence of catalytic iron, are known to react with polyunsaturated fatty acids to yield lipid hydroperoxides.[78] These can form alkoxy and peroxy radicals that propagate and undergo cyclization to form internal endoperoxides that are detected (as the breakdown product, maldonaldehyde) by the thiobarbituric acid assay for lipid peroxidation. Alkoxy and peroxy radicals may fragment or be reduced to fatty acid aldehydes, ketones, and alcohols as described previously. A number of studies have linked ethanol metabolism to free-radical generation in vitro and in vivo.[77] Microsomal generation of free radicals is the system studied most intensively. Several groups have reported that in vitro microsomes from rats fed ethanol produce oxygen-derived radicals at an accelerated rate.[79] The source is believed to be NADPH-cytochrome P-450 reductase, which is induced by ethanol. Reinke et al. have reported detecting by electron paramagnetic resonance spectrometry carbon-centered radicals formed in vivo and ethanol-derived (1-hydroxyethyl) radicals formed in vitro by liver microsomes from rats fed ethanol.[80] Finally, acute ethanol administration has also been shown to increase superoxide anion formation by rat liver mitochondria.[81]

Another potential source of radicals is the cytosolic enzyme xanthine oxidase, which can use either acetaldehyde or xanthine as a substrate to produce superoxide.[82] Because the K_m of the enzyme for acetaldehyde is in the low millimolar range, whereas acetaldehyde concentrations in the liver are thought to be maintained in the 10–50 μM range by the lower-K_m mitochondrial enzyme acetaldehyde dehydrogenase, it has been suggested that acetaldehyde is not a physiologic substrate for the enzyme.[83] However, the situation is made more complex by evidence that acetaldehyde binds rapidly and reversibly to proteins close to the site of its formation and so may not freely diffuse to the mitochondrial enzyme,[83] but may reach high concentrations locally and be oxidized to a significant extent by cytosolic mechanisms. In this regard it may be significant that Weiner has reported that approx 20% of acetaldehyde metabolism by rat liver could not be accounted for by acetaldehyde dehydrogenase.[84] In addition there is evidence that the interaction between acetaldehyde and xanthine oxidase may also produce longer-lived acetaldehyde radicals[85] that could contribute to lipid peroxidation.

Evidence against a role for acetaldehyde in alcohol-mediated lipid peroxidation has been presented by Kato et al.[86] These investigators reported that acute administration of ethanol to rats was associated with increased hepatic lipid peroxidation that could be blocked by administration of the xanthine oxidase inhibitor allopurinol. They then performed experiments to determine the most likely substrate for xanthine oxidase under these conditions. When ethanol was given in conjunction with an acetaldehyde dehydrogenase inhibitor to raise hepatic acetaldehyde, no further increase in lipid peroxidation occurred. The authors interpreted these results as showing that acetaldehyde was probably not serving as a substrate for the enzyme and generating the lipid peroxidation. They noted that purine substrates for xanthine oxidase (i.e., xanthine/hypoxanthine) were increased under the experimental conditions and suggest that these are giving rise to the lipid peroxides.

Aldehyde oxidase, like xanthine oxidase, is a molybdenum flavohemoprotein, found in human liver cytosol, that can use acetaldehyde as an electron donor in the reduction of oxygen.[86] The primary substrates of this enzyme are thought to be xenobiotics having a quinoline or pyridine ring rather than aldehydes. The reported K_m for aldehydes is relatively high (1.0–3.5 mM)[87,88] but, as is the case for xanthine oxidase, aldehyde compartmentation might make these compounds more significant substrates in vivo. Indeed, a recent study suggested that aldehyde oxidase is an important source of free radicals and lipid peroxidation in rat liver cells metabolizing alcohol.[88]

Thus, there is now a fairly convincing body of evidence that in experimental animals ethanol metabolism is associated with increased lipid peroxidation. Unfortunately, there are important differences between the responses of humans and all other species to alcohol. Even within the human species there may be inherited differences in susceptibility to alcoholic liver disease.[89] For this reason, it is critical to carry out human studies also. Several groups studying human subjects have found evidence for increased lipid peroxidation. Suematsu et al. reported that alcoholic subjects have higher hepatic and plasma levels of lipid peroxides.[90] More recently, Vendemiale et al. administered acute doses of alcohol or an isocaloric carbohydrate solution to normal, healthy subjects and measured plasma ethanol levels and malondialdehyde by high-performance liquid chromatography hourly for up to 6 h afterward.[91] Plasma ethanol levels reached a peak of approx 140 mg% 3 h after ethanol was started, and malondialdehyde was significantly increased after 4 h in the group given ethanol.

A number of defense mechanisms exist in cells and plasma to handle the ongoing flux of both free radicals and lipid peroxides.[92] These compounds include vitamin E, glutathione, glutathione peroxidase, metallothionein, superoxide dismutase, and others. Any reduction of these defense mechanisms at a time when oxidant stress is increased, for example, during alcohol metabolism, could potentiate the risk of radical-mediated injury. Glutathione is an important and well-studied example. This compound acts as a substrate for glutathione peroxidase in the detoxification of hydrogen peroxide within cell cytosol, and there is good evidence for alcohol-induced perturbations in glutathione metabolism, which may contribute to liver injury (*see* the chapter by Mitchell, this volume). Vitamin E and glutathione peroxidase are both depleted by ethanol administration.[93] Superoxide dismutase may be induced by chronic ethanol administration.[94]

In summary, evidence is accumulating from studies in both experimental animals and humans that acute and chronic ethanol metabolism by the liver lead to increased free-radical generation and lipid peroxidation. Postulated mechanisms include increased activity of the electron-transport chains of microsomes or mitochondria, metabolism of ethanol or acetaldehyde to radicals and increased substrates (e.g., acetaldehyde or purines) for cytosolic oxidases. However, the relative importance of these mechanisms is unknown, and the contribution of defects in antioxidant mechanisms also remains to be defined.

Generation of a Chemoattractant by Liver Cells Metabolizing Alcohol

Several years ago, seeking an explanation for the neutrophilic infiltrates seen in alcoholic hepatitis, we found that, when primary cultures of rat hepatocytes were incubated with modest concentrations of ethanol (2–20 mM), they generated a polar lipid with chemotactic activity for human neutrophils (Fig. 2).[95] The activity was released into the medium in a time- and concentration-dependent manner, and maximal chemotactic activity was generated after 6 h of incubation with 10 mM ethanol (Fig. 2). The appearance of the activity was not attributable to loss of cell viability

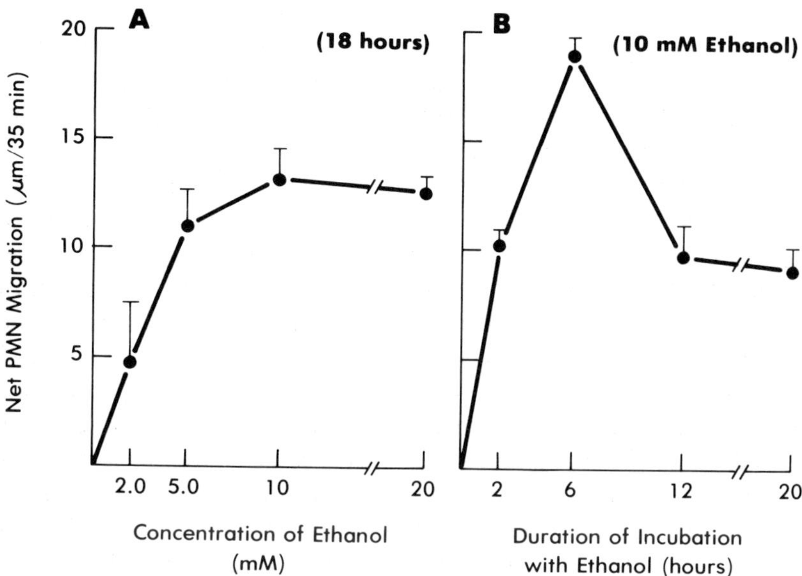

Fig. 2. Migration of human neutrophils in response to medium of rat hepatocytes incubated with ethanol: **(A)** response to medium incubated with increasing concentrations of ethanol for 18 h; **(B)** response to medium of cells incubated with 10 m*M* ethanol for various periods of time. Reprinted from the *Journal of Clinical Investigation*, 1984, vol. 74, pp. 1350–1357 by copyright permission of the American Society for Clinical Investigation.

as judged by exclusion of trypan blue or release of intracellular enzymes. It did depend on metabolism of ethanol to acetaldehyde, and the latter could substitute for ethanol in stimulating formation of activity. Subsequently we found that human hepatocytes produce an apparently identical activity and that rat neutrophils do not respond to the chemotactic factor.[96] Although the reason for this is not known it is interesting in this regard that Kreisle et al. have shown that rat neutrophils do not have high-affinity receptors for leukotriene B_4, another lipid chemoattractant.[97] The lack of response to the ethanol-induced chemotactic factor may explain why rats do not develop significant inflammation in response to ethanol exposure.[98] Since we described this lipid chemotactic activity, there have been preliminary reports of other chemotactic factors, which appear to be proteins, released by hepatocytes exposed to ethanol.[99]

Because of previous reports of free-radical generation and lipid peroxidation resulting from alcohol metabolism, we looked for a role for these processes in production of the chemotactic lipid by hepatocytes. We attempted to inhibit chemotactic-activity production by adding the radical scavengers superoxide dismutase and catalase to intact cells exposed to alcohol. However, we were unable to demonstrate any effect.[95] To exclude the possibility that these radical scavengers did not gain access to an intracellular site of radical production, we repeated the experiments in a cell-free alcohol-metabolizing system consisting of rat liver cytosol. In this system, oxygen-radical scavengers blocked generation of the activity completely.[100] Figure 3 shows a hypothetical pathway, based on studies in the cell-free system, for generation of the chemotactic factor from acetaldehyde in hepatocytes. Complete inhibition by superoxide dismutase or catalase implies that both O_2^- and H_2O_2 are necessary. Dependence on both of these oxygen intermediates may be explained by their interaction in the iron-catalyzed Haber-Weiss reaction (Eq. 3) to form the reactive $\cdot OH$ radical that can attack polyunsaturated fatty acids to produce lipid peroxides.[71] In this reaction, the role of O_2^- is thought to be reduction of ferric iron (Eq. 1), which then catalyzes the reduction of H_2O_2 to the hydroxyl radical ($\cdot OH$) (Eq. 2).

$$Fe^{3+} + O_2^- \longrightarrow Fe^{2+} + O_2 \tag{1}$$

$$Fe^{2+} + H_2O_2 \longrightarrow Fe^{3+} + \cdot OH + OH^- \tag{2}$$

$$\text{catalytic Fe}$$
$$\text{Net: } O_2^- + H_2O_2 \longrightarrow O_2 + \cdot OH + OH^- \tag{3}$$

In support of this sequence, we found that scavengers of the hydroxyl radical, as well as the iron chelator desferrioxamine, inhibited generation of the chemotactic activity.[100] Hultcrantz et al. have further explored the requirement for iron in production of chemotactic activity in studies of rat dietary models of iron deficiency and iron overload.[101] Hepatocytes isolated from iron-deficient, iron-loaded and control rats were incubated with ethanol (10 mM), and the generation of chemotactic activity was assayed. Control and iron-loaded cells produced chemotactic activity as expected, but iron-deficient cells failed to produce any activity. Addition of ferric citrate to the iron-deficient cells restored chemotactic-activity production, and addition of desferrioxamine to the iron-loaded cells blocked their ability to generate

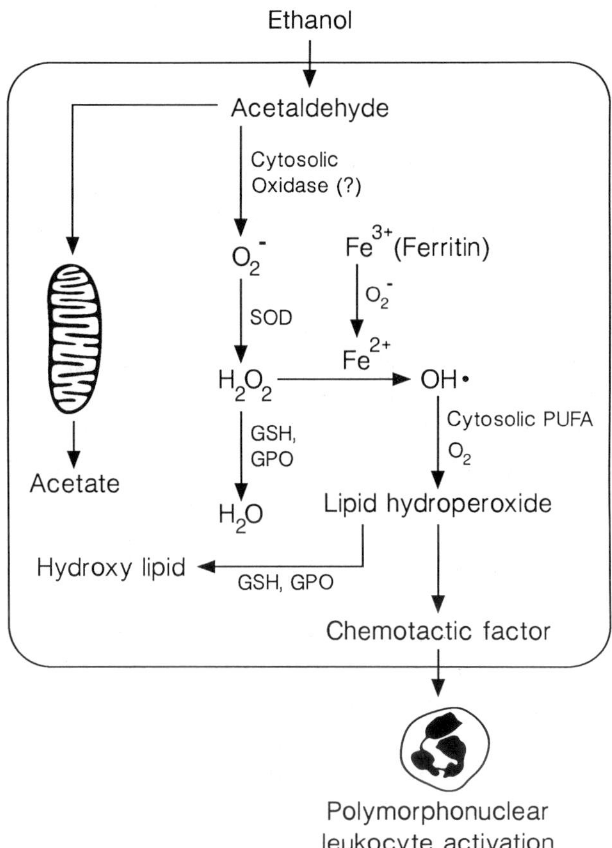

Fig. 3. Hypothetical pathway of generation of chemotactic factor in a hepatocyte metabolizing ethanol. The cytosolic polyunsaturated fatty acid (PUFA) that acts as a precursor is thought to be arachidonic acid.

the factor. The intracellular source of the iron that is responsible is not known, but, based on measurements of the changes in total cellular iron in these experiments, Hultcrantz et al. concluded that a small intracellular pool of "free" iron was probably involved in production of the factor. In normal hepatocytes, most iron is sequestered as Fe^{3+} in the storage proteins ferritin and hemosiderin, but a small fraction, perhaps 2–10% of total cellular iron, probably exists bound to low-mol-wt compounds.[102] Britton et al. have recently shown that this low-mol-wt cytosolic iron is catalytically active in stimulating lipid peroxidation by liver microsomes.[103] They also showed that the activity was inhibited by desferrioxamine and enhanced by iron loading. The size of the free pool may be controlled by variables other than the extent of iron loading, and this may be relevant to the observations of Hultcrantz et al. For example, iron can be released as Fe^{2+} from ferritin by biological reductants such as superoxide, xanthine, NADH, or NADPH.[104] Because some of these reductants are produced during alcohol metabolism they may play a role in providing reduced iron for generation of chemotactic factor.

The involvement of oxygen-derived radicals and iron in production of a polar lipid chemoattractant suggest that the factor may be a lipid peroxide or have a lipid peroxide intermediate. Selenium-dependent glutathione peroxidase is the principal hydrogen peroxide-scavenging enzyme in liver cytosol. It requires reduced glutathione as a hydrogen donor and can reduce both H_2O_2 and lipid hydroperoxides. If a lipid peroxide or H_2O_2 are intermediates in the formation of the chemotactic activity (Fig. 3) then depleting cytosol of glutathione and glutathione peroxidase should result in greater amounts of activity being produced. To test this hypothesis, Neuschwander-Tetri raised rats from weaning on a selenium-deficient diet to deplete their livers of glutathione peroxidase (to <5% of control), and then gave them an acute dose of L-buthionine sulfoximine to deplete them of glutathione (to <15% of control). He found that liver cytosol from glutathione- and glutathione peroxidase-deficient rats, when incubated with ethanol, appeared to generate 500-fold as much chemotactic activity as control cytosol.[105] When exogenous glutathione and glutathione peroxidase were added back to the depleted cytosol, the amount of chemotactic activity reverted to that found in normal cells. These results are strongly suggestive of a peroxide intermediate(s) at some point in the pathogenetic sequence (Fig. 3) and emphasizes the importance of endogenous antioxidant mechanisms in limiting production of this activity. The precursor of the chemotactic factor from hepatocytes is unknown, but is postulated to be a polyunsaturated fatty acid, such as arachidonic acid (Fig. 3). Arachidonic and other long-chain fatty acids are not confined to cell membrane compartments, but are known to be present in liver cytosol associated with the carrier protein, fatty acid binding protein.[106] Support, but not proof, of its derivation from arachidonic acid is the observation that, on reverse-phase high-performance liquid chromatography, it comigrates with a previously described chemotactic activity produced by the cooxidation of arachidonic acid and acetaldehyde by xanthine oxidase.[66] Current efforts are directed at identification of the chemical structure of the lipid by gas chromatography/mass spectroscopy.

Is this factor produced in vivo? In preliminary experiments to approach this question, we have administered ethanol by gavage to rats and assayed their serum, pre- and post-ethanol administration, for chemotactic activity. No activity was found in the pre-ethanol serum, but chemotactic activity with the same properties as the factor was detectable in the post-ethanol serum diluted up to 1:20, suggesting that the factor is produced in vivo and escapes intrahepatic degradation.

Thus, liver cells metabolizing ethanol in vitro generate a polar lipid with chemotactic activity for human neutrophils. An identical factor is produced in vivo in rats given intragastric ethanol. The structure of this compound(s) is not yet identified, but there is evidence that it is formed in liver cytosol by the action of oxygen-derived free radicals and iron on an unsaturated fatty acid, such as arachidonic acid.

Summary

The pathogenesis of alcoholic liver disease is still unknown. There is a strong association of both alcoholic hepatitis and subsequent cirrhosis with an inflammatory response, which could explain the damage seen in these phases of the disease. There is now evidence that liver cells metabolizing alcohol cause the lipid peroxidation leading to formation of one or more chemotactic factors, which may explain the neutrophil influx in alcoholic hepatitis. Further studies are needed to obtain chemical identification of this factor and to determine both whether it is present in the plasma of human subjects ingesting alcohol and how it is correlated with the presence of alcoholic hepatitis.

References

[1] National Center for Health Statistics (1987) Monthly Vital Statistics Report. Advance Report of Final Mortality Standards, **vol. 38,** No.5. Supplement, (1989).

[2] C. S. Lieber (1988) Biochemical and molecular basis of alcohol-induced injury to liver and other tissues. *N. Engl. J. Med.* **319,** 1639–1650.

[3] C. S. Lieber (1988) Metabolic effects of ethanol and its interaction with other drugs, hepatotoxic agents, vitamins, and carcinogens: A 1988 update. *Semin. Liver Dis.* **8,** 47–68.

[4] D. A. Brenner and M. Chojkier (1987) Acetaldehyde increases collagen gene transcription in cultured human fibroblasts. *J. Biol. Chem.* **262,** 17690–17695.

[5] P. J. Syapin and E. P. Noble (1979) Studies on ethanol's effects on cells in culture, in *Biochemistry and Pharmacology of Ethanol,* vol. I. E. Majchrowicz and E. P. Noble, eds. Plenum, New York, pp. 521–540.

[6] E. Rubin and C. S. Lieber (1968) Alcohol-induced hepatic injury in nonalcoholic volunteers. *N. Engl. J. Med.* **278,** 869–905.

[7] R. N. M. MacSween, P. P. Anthony, and P. J. Scheuer, eds. (1979) *Pathology of the Liver.* Churchill Livingstone, London.

[8] D. Zakim and T. D. Boyer (1990) Alcoholic Liver Disease, in *Hepatology: A Textbook of Liver Disease,* vol. II. D. Zakim and T. D. Boyer, eds. W.B. Saunders, Philadelphia, pp. 821–869.

[9] E. B. Feigelson, W. W. Pfaff, A. Karmen, and D. Steinberg (1961) The role of plasma free fatty acids in development of fatty liver. *J. Clin. Invest.* **40,** 2171–2179.

[10] D. Zakim and J. Green (1968) Relation of ethanol inhibition of hepatic fatty acid oxidation to ethanol-induced fatty liver. *Proc. Soc. Exp. Bio. Med.* **127,** 138–142.

[11] C. S. Lieber and R. Schmid (1961) The effect of ethanol on fatty acid metabolism: Stimulation of hepatic fatty acid synthesis in vitro. *J. Clin. Invest.* **40,** 394–399.

[12] C. S. Lieber, M. Nakano, and T. M. Worner (1981) Ultrastructure of the initial stages of hepatic perivenular fibrosis after alcohol. *Trans. Assoc. Am. Physicians* **94,** 292–300.

[13] A. Burt and R. N. M. MacSween (1986) Hepatic vein lesions in alcoholic liver disease: Retrospective biopsy and necropsy study. *J. Clin. Pathol.* **39,** 63–67.

[14] H. Popper and C. S. Lieber (1980) Histogenesis of alcoholic fibrosis and cirrhosis in the baboon. *Am. J. Pathol.* **98,** 695–716.

[15] A. Baptista, L. Bianchi, J. de Groote, V. J. Desmet, P. Gedigk, G. Korb, R. N. M. MacSween, H. Popper, P. J. Scheuer, M. Schmid, H. Theeler, and W. Wepler (1981) Alcoholic liver disease: Morphological manifestations. *Lancet* **i,** 707–711.

[16] T. F. Imperiale and A. J. McCullough (1990) Do corticosteroids reduce mortality from alcoholic hepatitis? *Ann. Intern. Med.* **113,** 299–307.

[17] A. Pares, J. Caballeria, M. Bruguera, M. Torres, and J. Rodes (1986) Histological course of alcoholic hepatitis: Influence of abstinence, sex and extent of hepatic damage. *J. Hepatol.* **2,** 33–42.

[18] R. Rudolph, W. J. McClure, and M. Woodward (1979) Contractile fibroblasts in chronic alcoholic cirrhosis. *Gastroenterology* **76,** 704–709.

[19] J. J. Maher (1990) Hepatic fibrosis caused by alcohol. *Semin. Liver Dis.* **10,** 66–73.

[20] S. L. Friedman (1990) Cellular sources of collagen and regulation of collagen production in liver. *Semin. Liver Dis.* **10,** 20–29.

[21] W. J. Powell and G. Klatskin (1968) Duration of survival in patients with Laennec's cirrhosis. *Am. J. Med.* **44,** 406–420.

[22] W. C. Maddrey, J. K. Boitnott, M. S. Bedine, F. L. Weber, E. Mezey, and R. I. White (1978) Corticosteroid therapy of alcoholic hepatitis. *Gastroenterology* **75,** 193–199.

[23] J. K. Boitnott and W. C. Maddrey (1981) Alcoholic liver disease: I. Interrelationships among histologic features and the histologic effects of prednisolone therapy. *Hepatology* **1,** 599–612.

[24] R. L. Carithers, H. F. Herlong, A. M. Diehl, E. W. Shaw, B. Combes, H. J. Fallon, and W. C. Maddrey (1989) Methylprednisolone therapy in patients with severe alcoholic hepatitis. *Ann. Intern. Med.* **110,** 685–690.

[25] T. I. A. Sorensen, K. D. Bentsen, M. Orholm, G. Hoybye, K. Eghoje, and P. Christoffersen (1984) Prospective evaluation of alcohol abuse and alcoholic liver injury in men as predictors of development of cirrhosis. *Lancet* **ii,** 241–244.

[26] W. K. Lelbach (1974) Organic pathology related to volume and pattern of alcohol use, in *Research Advances in Alcohol and Drug Problems.* R. J. Gibbins, Y. Israel, H. Kalant, R. E. Popham, W. Schmidt and R. G. Smart, eds. Wiley, New York, pp. 93–198.

[27] I. Saito, T. Miyamura, A. Ohbayashi, H. Harada, T. Katayama, S. Kikuchi, Y. Watanabe, S. Koi, M. Onji, Y. Okta, Q.-L. Choo, M. Houghton, and G. Kuo (1990) Hepatitis C virus infection is associated with the development of hepatocellular carcinoma. *Proc. Natl. Acad. Sci. USA* **87,** 6547–6549.

[28] G. R. Cameron and W. A. E. Karunaratne (1936) Carbon tetrachloride cirrhosis in relation to liver regeneration. *J. Pathol. Bacteriol.* **42,** 1–21.

[29] G. G. Karvountzis, A. G. Redeker, and R. L. Peters (1974) Long term follow-up studies of patients surviving fulminant viral hepatitis. *Gastroenterology* **67,** 870–877.

[30] J. H. Hoofnagle, D. A. Shafritz, and H. Popper (1987) Chronic type B hepatitis and the "healthy" HBsAg carrier state. *Hepatology* **7,** 758– 763.

[31] J. L. Dienstag and H. J. Alter (1986) Non-A, non-B hepatitis: Evolving epidemiologic and clinical perspective. *Semin. Liver Dis.* **6,** 67–81.

[32] D. J. Wyler and L. J. Rosenwasser (1982) Fibroblast stimulation in schistosomiasis. *J. Immunol.* **129,** 1706–1710.

[33] S. M. Wahl, D. A. Hunt, J. B. Allen, R. L. Wilder, L. Paglia, and A. R. Hand (1986) Bacterial cell wall-induced hepatic granulomas. *J. Exp. Med.* **163,** 884–902.

[34] Y. Martinet, W. N. Rom, G. R. Grotendorst, G. R. Martin, and R. G. Crystal (1987) Exaggerated spontaneous release of platelet-derived growth factor by alveolar

macrophages from patients with idiopathic pulmonary fibrosis. *N. Engl. J. Med.* **317,** 202–209.

[35] H. L. Malech and J. I. Gallin (1987) Current concepts: Immunology: Neutrophils in human diseases. *N. Engl. J. Med.* **317,** 687–694.

[36] E. L. Becker (1988) the cytoxic action of neutrophils on mammalian cells in vitro. *Prog. Allergy* **40,** 183–208.

[37] S. J. Weiss (1989) Tissue destruction by neutrophils. *N. Engl. J. Med.* **320,** 365–376.

[38] J. L. Farber, M. E. Kyle, and J. B. Coleman (1990) Biology of disease: Mechanisms of cell injury by activated oxygen species. *Lab. Invest.* **62,** 670–679.

[39] L. A. Guthrie, L. C. McPhail, P. M. Henson, and R. B. Johnston (1984) Priming of neutrophils for enhanced release of oxygen metabolites by bacterial lipopolysaccharide. *J. Exp. Med.* **160,** 1656–1671.

[40] J. P. Nolan and D. S. Camara (1982) Endotoxin, sinusoidal cells and liver injury, in *Progress in Liver Disease,* vol. 7. H. Popper and F. Schaffner, eds. Grune and Stratton, New York, pp. 361–376.

[41] D. M. Bissell, D. M. Arenson, J. J. Maher, and F. J. Roll (1987) Support of cultured hepatocytes by a laminin-rich gel. *J. Clin. Invest* **79,** 801–812.

[42] D. Keppler, W. Hagmann, S. Rapp, C. Denzlinger, and H. K. Koch (1985) The relation of leukotrienes to liver injury. *Hepatology* **5,** 883–891.

[43] D. B. Dubravec, D. R. Spriggs, J. A. Mannick, and M. L. Rodrick (1990) Circulating human peripheral blood granulocytes synthesize and secrete tumor necrosis factor α. *Proc. Natl. Acad. Sci. USA* **87,** 6758–6761.

[44] M. J. P. Arthur, P. Kowalski-Saunders, and R. Wright (1986) Corynebacterium parvum-elicited hepatic macrophages demonstrate enhanced respiratory burst activity compared with resident Kupffer cells in the rat. *Gastroenterology* **91,** 174–181.

[45] M. Chojkier and J. Fierer (1985) D-Galactosamine hepatotoxicity is associated with endotoxin sensitivity and mediated by lymphoreticular cells in mice. *Gastroenterology* **88,** 115–121.

[46] D. E. Gannon, J. Varani, S. H. Phan, J. H. Ward, J. Kaplan, G. O. Till, R. H. Simon, U. S. Ryan, and P. A. Ward (1987) Source of iron in neutrophil-mediated killing of endothelial cells. *Lab. Invest.* **57,** 37–44.

[47] H. J. Schlayer, H. Laaf, T. Peters, H. E. Schaefer, and K. Decker (1989) Tumor necrosis factor (TNF) mediates lipopolysaccharide (LPS)-elicited neutrophil sticking to sinusoidal endothelial cells in vivo, in *Cells of the Hepatic Sinusoid,* vol. 2. E. Wisse, D. L. Knook, and K. Decker, eds. Kupffer Cell Foundation, Rijswijk, The Netherlands, pp. 319–324.

[48] B. Guigui, J. Rosenbaum, A. M. Preaux, N. Martin, E. S. Zafrani, D. Dhumeaux, and P. Mavier (1988) Toxicity of phorbol myristate acetate-stimulated polymorphonuclear neutrophils against rat hepatocytes. *Lab. Invest.* **59,** 831–837.

[49] P. Mavier, A. M. Preaux, B. Guigui, M. C. Lescs, E. S. Zafrani, and D. Dhumeaux (1988) In vitro toxicity of polymorphonuclear neutrophils to rat hepatocytes; evidence for a proteinase-mediated mechanism. *Hepatology* **8,** 254–258.

[50] P. Mavier, A. M. Preaux, J. Rosenbaum, A. Mallat, and D. Dhumeaux (1989) Acute inflammatory reaction reduces toxicity of polymorphonuclear cells to hepatocytes. *Hepatology* **10,** 611 (abstract).

[51] R. A. Lewis, K. F. Austen, and R. J. Soberman (1990) Leukotrienes and other products of the 5–1ipoxygenase pathway. *N. Engl. J. Med.* **323,** 645–655.

[52] H. Mensing and B. M. Czarnetzki (1984) Leukotriene B_4 induces in vitro fibroblast chemotaxis. *J. Invest. Dermatol.* **82,** 9–12.

[53] R. L. Hoover, M. J. Karnovsky, K. F. Austen, E. J. Corey, and R. A. Lewis (1984) Leukotriene B_4 action on endothelium mediates augmented neutrophil/ endothelial adhesion. *Proc. Natl. Acad. Sci. USA* **81,** 2191–2193.

[54] P. N. Devreotes and S. H. Zigmond (1988) Chemotaxis in eukaryotic cells: A focus on leukocytes and dictyostelium. *Annu. Rev. Cell. Biol.* **4,** 649–86.

[55] P. C. Wilkinson (1988) Micropore filter methods for leukocyte chemotaxis. *Methods Enzymol.* **162,** 38–50.

[56] R. A. Lewis and K. F. Austen (1984) The biologically active leukotrienes:biosynthesis, metabolism, receptors, functions, and pharmacology. *J. Clin. Invest* **73,** 889–897.

[57] J. M. Shields and W. S. Haston (1985) Behaviour of neutrophil leucocytes in uniform concentrations of chemotactic factors: Contraction waves, cell polarity and persistence. *J. Cell. Sci.* **74,** 75–93.

[58] A. N. DeMeo and B. R. Andersen (1972) Defective chemotaxis associated with a serum inhibitor in cirrhotic patients. *N. Engl. J. Med.* **286,** 735–740.

[59] D. E. Van Epps, R. G. Strickland, and R. C. Williams (1975) Inhibitors of leukocyte chemotaxis in alcoholic liver disease. *Am. J. Med.* **59,** 200–207.

[60] R. A. Robbins, R. K. Zetterman, T. J. Kendall, G. L. Gossman, H. P. Monsour, and S. I. Rennard (1987) Elevation of chemotactic factor inactivator in alcoholic liver disease. *Hepatology* **7,** 872–877.

[61] I. A. Rajkovic and R. Williams (1986) Abnormalities of neutrophil phagocytosis, intracellular killing and metabolic activity in alcoholic cirrhosis and hepatitis. *Hepatology* **6,** 252–262.

[62] R. R. MacGregor (1990) in vivo neutrophil delivery in men with alcoholic cirrhosis is normal despite depressed in vitro chemotaxis. *Alcohol. Clin. Exp. Res.* **14,** 195–199.

[63] J. X. Corberand, P. F. Laharrague, and G. Fillola (1989) Human neutrophils are not severly injured in conditions mimicking social drinking. *Alcohol. Clin. Exp. Res.* **13,** 542–546.

[64] C. A. Dahinden, R. M. Clancy, and T. E. Hugli (1984) Stereospecificity of

leukotriene B_4 and structure–function relationships for chemotaxis of human neutrophils. *J. Immunol.* **133,** 1477–1482.

[65] B. Bosterling and J. R. Trudell (1984) Production of 5- and 15-hydro-peroxyeicosatetraenoic acid from arachidonic acid by halothane-free radicals generated by UV-irradiation. *Anesthesiology* **60,** 209–213.

[66] H. D. Perez, B. B. Weksler, and I. M. Goldstein (1980) Generation of a chemotactic lipid from arachidonic acid by exposure to a superoxide-generating system. *Inflammation* **4,** 313–327.

[67] W. F. Petrone, D. K. English, K. Wong, and J. M. McCord (1980) Free radicals and inflammation: Superoxide-dependent activation of a neutrophil chemotactic factor in plasma. *Proc. Natl. Acad. Sci. USA* **77,** 1159–1163.

[68] H. Esterbauer, H. Zollner, and R. J. Schaur (1990) Aldehydes formed by lipid peroxidation: Mechanisms of formation, occurrence, and determination, in *Membrane Lipid Oxidation.* C. Vigo-Palfrey, ed. CRC Press, Boca Raton, pp. 239–268.

[69] M. Comporti (1985) Biology of disease; lipid peroxidation and cellular damage in toxic liver injury. *Lab. Invest.* **53,** 599–623.

[70] U. H. Danielson, H. Esterbauer, and B. Mannervik (1987) Structure-activity relationships of 4–hydroxyalkenals in the conjugation catalysed by mammalian glutathione transferases. *Biochem. J.* **247,** 707–713.

[71] J. M. C. Gutteridge (1988) Lipid peroxidation: Some problems and concepts, in *Oxygen Radicals and Tissue Injury: Proceedings of a Brook Lodge Symposium,* Augusta, MI, April 1987, pp. 9–19.

[72] M. Curzio, H. Esterbauer, C. DiMauro, G. Cecchini, and M. U. Dianzani (1986) Chemotactic activity of the lipid peroxidation product 4–hydroxynonenal and homologous hydroxyalkenals. *Biol. Chem. Hoppe-Seyler* **367,** 321–329.

[73] W. C. Glasgow, T. M. Harris, and A. R. Brash (1986) A short-chain aldehyde is a major lipoxygenase product in arachidonic acid-stimulated porcine leukocytes. *J. Biol. Chem.* **261,** 200–204.

[74] N. R. DiLuzio (1963) Prevention of the acute ethanol-induced fatty liver by antioxidants. *The Physiologist* **6,** 169.

[75] H. Rouach, M. Clement, M. T. Orfanelli, B. Janvier, J. Nordmann, and R. Nordmann (1983) Hepatic lipid peroxidation and mitochondrial susceptibility to peroxidative attacks during ethanol inhalation and withdrawal. *Biochim. Biophys. Acta* **753,** 439–444.

[76] S. Hashimoto and R. O. Recknagel (1968) No chemical evidence of hepatic lipid peroxidation in acute ethanol toxicity. *Exp. Mol. Pathol.* **8,** 225–242.

[77] A. I. Cederbaum (1989) Introduction: Role of lipid peroxidation and oxidative stress in alcohol toxicity. *Free Rad. Biol. Med.* **7,** 537–539.

[78] S. D. Aust and B. A. Svingen (1982) The role of iron in enzymatic lipid peroxidation, in *Free Radicals in Biology,* V. W. A. Pryor, ed. Academic, NY, pp. 1–28.

[79] A. I. Cederbaum (1987) Microsomal generation of hydroxyl radicals: Its role in microsomal ethanol oxidizing system (MEOS) activity and requirement for iron. *Ann. NY Acad. Sci.* **492,** 35–49.

[80] L. A. Reinke, E. K. Lai, C. M. DuBose, and P. B. McCay (1987) Reactive free radical generation in vivo in heart and liver of ethanol-fed rats: Correlation with radical formation in vitro. *Proc. Natl. Acad. Sci. USA* **84,** 9223–9227.

[81] J. Sinaceur, C. Ribiere, D. Sabourault, and R. Nordmann (1985) Superoxide formation in liver mitochondria during ethanol intoxication: Possible role in alcohol hepatotoxicity, in *Free Radicals in Liver Injury.* G. Poli, K. H. Cheeseman, M. U. Dianzani, and T. F. Slater, eds. IRL, Oxford, pp. 175–177.

[82] I. Fridovich (1989) Oxygen radicals from acetaldehyde. *Free Rad. Biol. Med.* **7,** 557,558.

[83] M. G. Irving, S. J. Simpson, W. M. Brooks, R. S. Holmes, and D. M. Doddrell (1985) Application of the reverse DEPT polarization-transfer pulse sequence to monitor in vitro and in vivo metabolism of ^{13}C-ethanol by ^{1}H-NMR spectroscopy. *Int. J. Biochem.* **17,** 471–478.

[84] H. Weiner (1987) Subcellular localization of acetaldehyde oxidation in liver. *Ann. NY Acad. Sci.* **492,** 25–34.

[85] S. Puntarulo and A. I. Cederbaum (1989) Chemiluminescence from acetaldehyde oxidation by xanthine oxidase involves generation of and interactions with hydroxyl radicals. *Alcohol. Clin. Exp. Res.* **13,** 84–90.

[86] S. Kato, T. Kawase, J. Alderman, N. Inatomi, and C. S. Lieber (1990) Role of xanthine oxidase in ethanol-induced lipid peroxidation in rats. *Gastroenterology* **98,** 203–210.

[87] K. V. Rajagopsalan and P. Handler (1964) Hepatic aldehyde oxidase. *J. Biol. Chem.* **239,** 2027–2038.

[88] S. Shaw and E. Jayatilleke (1990) The role of aldehyde oxidase in ethanol-induced hepatic lipid peroxidation in the rat. *Biochem. J.* **268,** 579–583.

[89] Z. Hrubec and G. S. Omenn (1981) Evidence of genetic predisposition to alcoholic cirrhosis and psychosis: Twin concordances for alcoholism and its biological end points by zygosity among male veterans. *Alcohol. Clin. Exp. Res.* **5,** 207–215.

[90] T. Suematsu, T. Matsumura, N. Sato, T. Miyamoto, T. Ooko, T. Kamada, and H. Abe (1981) Lipid peroxidation in alcoholic liver disease in humans. *Alcohol. Clin. Exp. Res.* **5,** 427–430.

[91] G. Vandemiale, E. Altomare, I. Grattagliano, and O. Albano (1989) Increased plasma levels of glutathione and malondialdehyde after acute ethanol ingestion in humans. *J. Hepatol* **9,** 359–365.

[92] B. Halliwell (1987) Oxygen radicals and metal ions:potential antioxidant intervention strategies, pp. 526–30, in Cross CE, moderator. Oxygen radicals and human disease. *Ann. Intern. Med.* **107,** 526–545.

[93] A. R. Tanner, I. Bantock, L. Hinks, B. Lloyd, N. R. Turner, and R. Wright (1986) Depressed selenium and vitamin E levels in an alcoholic population. *Dig. Dis. Sci.* **31,** 1307–1312.

[94] I. E. Dreosti, S. J. Manuel, and R. A. Buckley (1982) Superoxide dismutase (EC 1.15.1.1), manganese and the effect of ethanol in adult and foetal rats. *Br. J. Nutr.* **48,** 205–210.

[95] H. D. Perez, F. J. Roll, D. M. Bissell, S. Shak, and I. M. Goldstein (1984) Production of chemotactic activity for polymorphonuclear leukocytes by cultured rat hepatocytes exposed to ethanol. *J. Clin. Invest.* **74,** 1350–1357.

[96] F. J. Roll, D. M. Bissell, and H. D. Perez (1986) Human hepatocytes metabolizing ethanol generate a non-polar chemotactic factor for human neutrophils. *Biochem. Biophys. Res. Commun.* **137,** 688–694.

[97] R. A. Kreisle, C. W. Parker, G. L. Griffin, R. M. Senior, and W. F. Stenson (1985) Studies of leukotriene B_4–specific binding and function in rat polymorphonuclear leukocytes: Absence of a chemotactic response. *J. Immunol.* **134,** 3356–3363.

[98] E. Mezey, J. J. Potter, R. J. Slusser, and W. Abdi (1977) Changes in hepatic collagen metabolism in rats produced by chronic ethanol feeding. *Lab. Invest.* **36,** 206–214.

[99] Y. Shiratori, H. Takada, K. Hai, K. Matsumoto, K. Kamii, K. Okano, and M. Tanaka (1989) A mechanism of accumulation and activation of neutrophils and monocytes in alcoholic liver injury; roles of chemotactic factors produced by hepatocytes. *Hepatology* **10,** 704 (abstract).

[100] F. J. Roll, M. A. Alexander, and H. D. Perez (1987) Generation of chemotactic activity by hepatic ethanol metabolism involves hydroxyl (OH) radical. *Hepatology* **7,** 1040 (abstr).

[101] R. Hultcrantz, D. M. Bissell, and F. J. Roll (1991) Iron mediates production of a neutrophil chemoattractant by rat hepatocytes metabolizing ethanol. *J. Clin. Invest.* **87,** 45–49.

[102] J. D. Gower, G. Healing, and C. J. Green (1989) Determination of desferrioxamine-available iron in biological tissues by high-pressure liquid chromatography. *Anal. Biochem..* **180,** 126–130.

[103] R. S. Britton, M. Ferrali, C. J. Magiera, R. O. Recknagel, and B. R. Bacon (1990) Increased prooxidant action of hepatic cytosolic low-molecular-weight iron in experimental iron overload. *Hepatology* **11,** 1038–1043.

[104] R. Topham, M. Goger, K. Pearce, and P. Schultz (1989) The mobilization of ferritin iron by liver cytosol: A comparison of xanthine and NADH as reducing substrates. *Biochem. J.* **261,** 137–143.

[105] B. A. Neuschwander-Tetri and F. J. Roll (1990) Chemotactic activity for human PMN generated during ethanol metabolism by rat hepatocytes: Role of glutathione and glutathione peroxidase. *Biochem. Biophys. Res. Commun.* **167,** 1170–1176.

[106] N. M. Bass (1985) Function and regulation of hepatic and intestinal fatty acid binding proteins. *Chem. Phys. Lipids* **38,** 95–114.

Liver Cell Membrane Adaptation to Chronic Alcohol Consumption

Hagai Rottenberg

Introduction

Ethanol, which is a weak anesthetic, affects the physical properties and modulates the function of all biological membranes. Whereas it is evident that the acute intoxicating effects of ethanol result from its interaction with the membranes of the central nervous system (CNS), similar effects, which may modulate cell metabolism, probably occur in liver cells as well. Chronic alcohol ingestion leads to profound changes in many organs. Although many of these changes, particularly those associated with long-term alcohol use, are pathological, there are also adaptive changes, particularly at the level of cell membranes, which ameliorate the effects of ethanol, at least for the short term. Whether these adaptive changes of membrane composition, structure, and function delay or accelerate the onset of the pathological changes in human alcoholics is still an open question. In the following, I shall review the evidence for the adaptation of cell membranes to chronic alcohol ingestion, with special emphasis on liver cell membranes.

From: *Drug and Alcohol Abuse Reviews, Vol. 2: Liver Pathology and Alcohol*
Ed: R. R. Watson ©1991 The Humana Press Inc.

Adaptation to Chronic Alcohol Consumption: Tolerance and Dependence

Organisms respond to chronic alcohol intake, as to many other environmental stresses, by a variety of defense mechanisms on several different levels. These mechanisms can be classified into two distinct classes: tolerance and dependence. Tolerance can be defined as an attenuation of the biological response to a given dose of alcohol. Dependence involves adjustment of optimal biological activity to the continuous presence of ethanol. Dependence expresses itself adversely when alcohol is withdrawn abruptly, resulting in a severe "withdrawal syndrome." Both tolerance and dependence are widely observed in human alcoholics.[1] Although these biological responses of adaptation are protective, and hence, beneficial for the short term, there are reasons to believe that they are harmful to humans in the long term. Tolerance may lead to increased alcohol consumption as the individual attempts to reach a desired response. Since most of the pathological effects of alcohol depend on high concentrations of ethanol, tolerance may increase the probability of pathological complications for alcoholics. Dependence results in a severe withdrawal syndrome, and its frequent occurrence may contribute to the damaging effect of alcohol consumption on various organs. An understanding of the biological processes that lead to tolerance and dependence may lead to the development of therapies that ameliorate the harmful effects of these processes.

Mechanisms of Tolerance

Some aspects of tolerance involve the response of the organism as a whole. Thus, a significant component of tolerance is behavioral and depends on learning.[2] Another mechanism affecting the entire organism is metabolic and depends on the development of alternative metabolic pathways for alcohol clearance.[3] The learning processes that lead to tolerance involve brain membranes, neurotransmitters, receptors, and membrane transport systems, such as channels and carriers. Of these, the most thoroughly documented effects are those of the neuropeptide arginine vasopressin, which appears to maintain learned tolerance through its interaction with a particular class of brain receptors.[4] Another neurotransmitter that appears to play a role in the development of tolerance is norepinephrine, which acts through its effect on adenylate cyclase and, presumably, cAMP levels.[5] A calcium channel that is induced by cAMP has also been implicated in the development of tolerance. When the voltage-dependent dihydropyridine (DHP)-sensitive calcium channel is blocked the development of tolerance is delayed.[6]

These systems may all be part of the process of acquisition of tolerance by learning. However, tolerance to ethanol is exhibited, not only by the whole animal, but also on a cellular level and even by individual membrane systems when assayed in vitro. For instance, the stimulating effect of alcohol on the muscimol enhancement of the chloride flux of the $GABA_A$ receptor complex is not observed in membranes from ethanol-fed animals.[7] Many other membrane enzymes and transport systems, which are inhibited or stimulated by ethanol, exhibit attenuated responses to ethanol in membranes from ethanol-fed animals (*see later discussion*). Moreover, the effect of ethanol on the physical properties of membranes is also greatly attenuated in membranes from ethanol-fed animals.[8] Thus, the question arises: Do the various membrane systems develop tolerance to ethanol independently, or is there a common mechanism, as has been suggested,[9] that results in general attenuation of the effect of ethanol on membrane enzymes, receptors, and transport systems? After reviewing these studies in more detail, I shall attempt to answer this question.

Mechanisms of Dependence

Unlike the case of tolerance that operates, in part, on the level of the whole animal and involves learned behavioral response, it appears that dependence results from the cumulative response of several individual systems on the level of receptors, channels, and enzymes. Two interacting systems that may be responsible for the occurrence of seizures after withdrawal are the NMDA-receptor Ca^{2+} channel and the GABA-receptor Cl^- channel. Acute ethanol administration stimulates the Cl^- flux through the GABA receptor[10] and may lead to downregulation of the system in ethanol-fed animals, whereas acute alcohol inhibits Ca^{2+} flux through the NMDA receptor channel[11] and thus, leads to upregulation of this system in ethanol-fed animals. Since increased NMDA-sensitivity reduces GABAergic activity in itself, these adaptations appear to be interconnected and are thought to be responsible for alcohol withdrawal seizures.[12] Benzodiazepines, which enhance GABAergic activity, are the drugs of choice for controlled alcohol withdrawal; NMDA-receptor inhibitors can also prevent seizures.[13]

Another Ca[+] channel, which is inhibited by acute ethanol and appears to be upregulated in ethanol-fed animals, as well as in cells cultured in the presence of ethanol, is the DHP-sensitive voltage dependent Ca^{2+} channel.[14,15] This channel may also contribute to dependence and withdrawal syndrome.[16] In contrast, adenylate cyclase, which is stimulated by ethanol, leading to increased cAMP levels after acute administration of alcohol to neural cells, is downregulated in cells cultured in the presence of ethanol.[17] The chronic alcohol-induced impairment of the activity of adenylate cyclase appears to result from alteration of the properties of the α subunit of the G_s protein that mediates the agonist-induced activation of adenylate cyclase.[18] Although these changes in the CNS appear to be largely responsible for the neurological manifestations of the withdrawal syndrome, similar changes in membrane enzyme activity probably occur in cells of various other organs, and may contribute to organ damage when alcohol is withdrawn. Thus, lymphocytes from chronic-alcoholic patients show reduced levels of receptor stimulated cAMP and resistance to the stimulating effects of alcohol.[19] Similar abnormalities in adenylate cyclase were observed in platelets from alcoholics.[20]

Alcohol Effects on Biological Membranes

Partition of Ethanol in Biological Membranes

The effects of ethanol on membrane structure and function depend on the solubility of ethanol in the membrane. Ethanol is a weak ampiphilic molecule. In longer chain alcohols the additive hydrophobic interactions of the methylene groups are dominant and these alcohols partition preferentially into the membrane.[21] However, in ethanol the hydrophobic and hydrophilic forces are almost equal and, hence, the partition coefficients are very low. Because of the low partition coefficients of ethanol in buffer:membrane systems, it is technically very difficult to measure directly ethanol partition by binding assays. The value most frequently used in the literature (e.g., $K_p = 0.1$, where K_p is the ratio of ethanol concentration in the membrane to ethanol concentration in the medium) was obtained from an extrapolation of the partition coefficients of the homologous series of n-alkanols.[21] However, it is doubtful whether such extrapolation can be justified to very short alcohols (e.g., ethanol and methanol). As indicated earlier, in short alcohols the hydrophobic interaction of the methylene groups are weak compared to the hydrophilic interactions. The interaction of the alcohols with the membrane could be dominated by hydrogen bonding and polar interactions with the phospholipid polar head group and glycerol backbone. Thus, the extrapolation from longer chain alcohols, which essentially considers only the hydrophobic interactions, could not be expected to be very accurate. Only a few attempts have been made to determine ethanol partition coefficients in biological membranes and phospholipid vesicles directly from the distribution of radiolabeled ethanol. These studies yielded values that are considerably higher than those extrapolated from long chain alcohols.[22–25] In mitochondria and SR vesicles, K_p values in the range 1–4 were obtained; in synaptosomes, values in the range 0.3–1.0 were determined. However, in the red blood cell membrane, K_p was below 0.4, which is closer to the extrapolated values. Another direct determination of ethanol binding to DMPC liposomes by ^{2}H-NMR has yielded K_p values that are considerably higher (15–45) than the value obtained by radiolabeled distribution.[26] Since the lipid composition, lipid phase structures, and the fatty acid composition of phospholipid acyl-chain all affect the partition of ethanol,[27] direct determinations of binding are necessary for the evaluation of the effect of ethanol on biological membranes.

Ethanol partition and its dependence on membrane properties can also be estimated indirectly by a variety of techniques. Artificial phospholipid membranes, when composed of one or two phospholipid species, exhibit prominent, sharp phase transitions from gel to liquid crystalline. These are shifted when solvents (such as ethanol) are incorporated into the membrane. The concentration dependence of such shifts allows the calculation of partition coefficients.[27] Unfortunately, these methods cannot be used with most biological membranes because those do not show simple sharp transitions. Measurements of ethanol partition in PC and PE liposomes have yielded very low values (0.03–0.1) compared to the direct measurement of binding in biological membranes and liposomes.[22–26] It should be emphasized that the absolute values determined by this method are dependent on the validity of the theory of ideal solutions and the assumption that ethanol does not bind to the gel phase, both of which may not be appropriate to these systems.

We have used the well-known observation that anesthetics protect red blood cells from hypotonic hemolysis[21] to obtain the relative partition of alcohols and anesthetics in plasma membranes of red blood cells from control- and ethanol-fed rats.[28] The absolute values of ethanol partition coefficient can be estimated from these measurements as follows: To obtain 60%

protection from hemolysis by halothane, 5 mM anesthetic was added to the suspension. The same protection was obtained by 175 mM ethanol. Hence, the ratio of partition coefficients, halothane/ethanol, is 35. We have found previously, by direct binding assay, that the halothane partition coefficient in rat RBC is 16.[29] Hence, ethanol partition in plasma membrane from RBC can be estimated to be 0.46.

More recently, we have developed other indirect methods that are highly sensitive. These methods are based on the effect of alcohols (and anesthetics) on the membrane dielectric constant and yield K_p values that are comparable to the values obtained by direct binding assays (Rottenberg, in preparation).

One way to attenuate the effect of ethanol on biological membranes is to reduce the partition coefficients of ethanol. We have shown that in ethanol-fed rats the partition coefficients of ethanol in membranes from liver mitochondria and synaptosomes are greatly reduced.[22] This observation was confirmed later by another laboratory.[24] Thus, it appears that on prolonged administration of ethanol an adaptive change occurs in the membrane lipid composition that reduces the partition of ethanol into the membrane and may fully account for the observed tolerance. The reduction of partition coefficients is not specific to ethanol. The partition coefficients of local anesthetics, inhalation anesthetics, long-chain alcohols, and hydrophobic alkanes are also reduced.[22,28,29] Moreover, this adaptation was observed in every membrane that was tested: synaptic plasma membrane, red blood cell plasma membranes, and liver mitochondrial and microsomal membranes.[22,28–30] The fact that this change is associated with changes in lipid composition (as shown later) and is retained by liposomes made from purified phospholipid from ethanol-fed rats (Rottenberg, in preparation, and ref. *30*) indicates that it is the change in phospholipid composition that leads to the observed reduction of the partition coefficients.

In warm-blooded animals the first response to ethanol is hypothermia. It is generally observed that lowering the temperature, which increases membrane order, reduces the partition coefficients of amphiphilic molecules.[31] Although it was not demonstrated experimentally yet that alcohol partition is reduced at lower temperatures, it is very likely that this is indeed the case. The sensitivity of membranes to the effects of alcohol on both structure and function is greatly diminished at low temperature, most probably because of reduced partition.[31,32] The hypothermic response develops within minutes of administration of alcohol. However, when alcohol is administered chronically, tolerance is induced slowly and the hypothermic effect is attenuated.

Based on physicochemical considerations, it can be expected that in phospholipid bilayers ethanol would be localized near the membrane surface with the hydroxyl group located near the polar head-groups in the glycerol backbone region, whereas the alkane moiety is buried in the more hydrophobic region of the fatty acid acyl-chains. For long-chain alcohols and sterols there is ample experimental evidence that supports this expectation (cf refs. 33,34). The evidence that exists concerning the location of ethanol is not as extensive, but appears to confirm this prediction as well.[35] However, various experimental findings have raised the question whether there is more than one binding site for ethanol in phospholipid membranes. The unusual concentration dependence of the partition coefficients of ethanol as measured by NMR and radiolabeled ethanol binding[25,26] have led to the suggestion of two binding sites, a polar surface site and hydrophobic core site. However, the effect of high concentration of ethanol on its partition simply indicates that as the membrane composition is altered by incorporation of ethanol, its bulk properties are modulated. Thus, ethanol not only affects its own partition but also the partition of other amphiphilic molecules.[22] This suggests that the system does not behave like an ideal solution (which is hardly expected), but does not necessarily mean that more than one distinct binding site is involved. Moreover, although the NMR data suggest increased binding of ethanol at high concentration,[26] the radiolabeled binding indicates decreased binding.[25] Unless this discrepancy is resolved, no conclusion can be derived from these observations. Nevertheless, it is possible that specific binding sites (not necessarily glycerophospholipids) exist in biological membranes. The most compelling evidence in this regard comes from studies of the effect of gangliosides, which enhanced the sensitivity of lipid vesicles to the effects of ethanol and anesthetics on fluidity[36] and were reported to introduce a new binding site for alcohols at the lipid/water interface.[37] It has also been shown that synaptosomal plasma membranes from ethanol sensitive mice (LS) contain three times as much GM_1 gangliosides as ethanol resistant mice (SS).[38] This is compatible with the reported finding of enhanced binding of ethanol to liposomes containing GM_1[37] and may account for the difference in alcohol sensitivity between SS and LS mice. However, the reports that gangliosides (including GM_1) antagonize ethanol intoxication[39,40] appear to contradict these findings.

Although it has been suggested frequently that membrane proteins or protein-lipid interfaces may provide distinct binding sites for ethanol, no convincing evidence exists to support these suggestions. However, it is well known that most biological membranes are asymmetric. The distribution of membrane components, such as phospholipids, cholesterol, proteins, gangliosides, and so forth, between the two leaflets of the membranes is highly asymmetric. Moreover, in many cells, segregated domains of different compositions often exist on the same face of the membrane.[41] Since membrane composition determines the ethanol partition coefficients, it can be predicted that alcohol would partition unequally between different domains of the membranes. Although there are no direct measurements of partition that can discriminate between membrane domains, it is possible to assess the effects of ethanol on the two membrane leaflets separately by using fluorescent probes that can be quenched selectively on one side of the membrane. By this method it was demonstrated that the ethanol effect on membrane fluidity is greater on the outer leaflet of synaptosomes.[42] Whether this is because of different partition coefficients or different susceptibility to fluidization has not been established yet. However, we believe that as a first approximation the sensitivity to the alcohol effect on fluidity depends on partition (as discussed later) and, hence, suggest that these results indicate differences in the partition coefficient of ethanol between the two leaflets. Indeed, the outer face of synaptic plasma membrane is enriched with gangliosides. The finding that gangliosides increase the partition of ethanol[37] supports the interpretation that the increased sensitivity of the outer leaflet is caused by a higher partition coefficient of ethanol. It has also been shown that the synaptosomal membrane resistance to ethanol, which is observed in ethanol-fed mice, is mostly owing to a reduction in the ethanol sensitivity of the exofacial leaflet, thus resulting in a more symmetric membrane.[43] It was suggested that this is the result of reduced asymmetry of cholesterol distribution. It is thus possible that the reduction of the partition coefficient observed in synaptosomes is specific to the exofacial leaflet. Although these results are intriguing, it should be pointed out that resistance to the fluidizing effect of ethanol is exhibited by membranes that contain no cholesterol (e.g., mitochondria) and is retained by symmetric phospholipid vesicles extracted from ethanol-fed animals.[44] Thus, membrane asymmetry in itself should not be considered necessary for the resistance to ethanol observed in membranes from ethanol-fed animals.

Ethanol Effects on Membrane Structure

General anesthetics and amphiphilics, including ethanol, affect the structure and physical properties of membranes. The hypothesis that ethanol (and anesthetics) modulate membrane functions through their effects on the physical properties of membrane lipids led to intensive study of these effects. Particular attention has been focused on the effects of ethanol on membrane fluidity (reviewed in refs. *8,41,45*). As has been pointed out frequently, there is no precise physical definition of "membrane fluidity," a concept that incorporates both static parameters, such as order, and dynamic parameters, such as viscosity. Although, in general, increased order is associated with increased viscosity, these are two different parameters that can vary independently.

In principle, it should be possible to determine these two parameters separately. However, in most types of measurements, particularly as applied to biological membranes, these effects are not sufficiently separated, so that the ambiguous characterization of these measurements, as related to membrane "fluidity" is probably a justified compromise. Most studies of the effects of ethanol on the fluidity of biological membranes utilize either spin-labeled fatty acids or hydrophobic fluorescence polarization probes. In general, both techniques show that ethanol (like other anesthetics) increases membrane fluidity. The results of the spin-probe studies are usually expressed as decreased order parameter (S), whereas the results of the fluorescence polarization are expressed as decreased polarization (P), anisotropy (A), or microviscosity (η). However, both methods, particularly as applied to biological membranes, incorporate static and dynamic parameters, although the mix might be different with different probes. It is, therefore, no surprise that there is a considerable lack of quantitative agreement between the effects of ethanol on membrane fluidity, as estimated by different probes and when different methods of data analysis are employed. These studies have been reviewed frequently[8,41,45] and it is sufficient to summarize these studies here very briefly: There is excellent correlation between the biological effects of ethanol and anesthetics, both in vivo and in vitro, and their effect on membrane fluidity. However, the concentration of ethanol (and anesthetics), which produces significant intoxication or even narcotic effects, is associated with relatively small changes in fluidity. Moreover, it is possible to produce changes of similar magnitude by other means (e.g., increased temperature) without producing the intoxication effect. The correlation between the biological effects of alcohols and anesthetics and membrane fluidity is no better than the correlation between the biological effect of alcohols and their partition coefficients. Thus, at present there is really no evidence to refute the notion that the correlation between fluidity modulation by alcohol and anesthetics and the biological activity is simply the result of a strong correlation between fluidity modulation and partition. In other words, it is quite possible that membrane fluidization by ethanol is simply another quantitative indication of the partition of ethanol into the membrane and is totally irrelevant to the mechanism of action of these agents. In fact, it is possible to use fluidity probes for estimation of partition coefficients of alcohol and anesthetics.[46]

Perhaps the most important finding related to the alcohol effects on membrane fluidity is the observation first reported by Chin and Goldstein[47] that synaptic membranes and red blood cells from ethanol-treated mice are resistant to the fluidizing effects of ethanol. This observation was confirmed and extended by many laboratories. It was found that liver organelle membranes, such as mitochondria[44] and microsomes,[48] as well as liver plasma membranes,[49] isolated from ethanol-fed rats are also resistant to the fluidizing effects of ethanol. Moreover, these membranes are also resistant to fluidization by anesthetics.[22,29] In addition, membranes from a strain of mice that are resistant to the narcotic effects of ethanol (SS) are also more resistant to the fluidizing effects of ethanol than ethanol-sensitive mice (LS).[50] The resistance to ethanol fluidization was also detected in blood cells from alcoholic patients.[51,52] All these and similar findings[8] were thought to confirm the role of the fluidizing effect of ethanol in producing the pharmacological effects of ethanol. However, as we pointed out earlier, these changes, to the extent that they were specifically examined, appear to correlate with the changes in the partition coefficients of ethanol and anesthetics in membranes from ethanol-fed animals. Thus, we are justified in concluding that the resistance to fluidization by alcohol is just another indication for the reduction of the partition coefficient and probably has no biological significance in itself.

This conclusion does not imply that ethanol effects on membrane lipids are irrelevant to its biological action. There are other effects on membrane properties that have not received much attention, but may be of greater relevance. For instance, ethanol and anesthetics affect the cooperative properties of membrane lipid. Thus, the various transitions in phospholipid membranes between gel to liquid crystalline, interdigitated layers, and hexagonal arrays are all sensitive to ethanol.[53,54] In biological membranes, at physiological temperatures, the major phase transitions are largely suppressed. However, subtle transitions that affect lipid segregation, protein aggregation, fusion, and other important membrane processes probably do occur. Moreover, lipid–protein interactions may depend on lipid-phase structure, which thus modulates protein function. In mitochondria, which exhibit subtle temperature-dependent lipid transitions that affect respiratory enzyme activity at the physiological range, acute alcohol lowers the transition temperatures, whereas chronic ethanol consumption leads to an increase in the transition temperature and to a resistance to the effects of ethanol on respiration.[31,32,55] Another physical property that is affected by ethanol and anesthetics is the dielectric constant, which may be important in modulating ion transport, channel activation, and other processes that depend on electrostatic interactions.[56]

Alcohol Effects
on Membrane Lipid Composition

It is evident that the changes that occur in membranes of chronic alcoholics that result in reduced partition coefficients of ethanol and its consequent tolerance (e.g., resistance to fluidization, tolerance of enzymes, receptors, and channels) are the result of modification of lipid composition. However, despite enormous effort by many groups, it is still not possible to characterize these changes precisely and to relate them to the observed modulation of the membrane response. Because of the use of different animal models, different diets and ethanol feeding protocols, and different procedures of membrane preparation and lipid analysis, there is little consensus about these changes. However, significant differences between control and ethanol-fed are almost universally observed.[57] The most consistent changes that were reported are in the acyl-chain composition of the phospholipids and can be characterized generally as a decrease of the degree of saturation.[58] There is indeed direct evidence for the reduction of the activity of the enzyme desaturase.[59] Other changes are more controversial. Cholesterol was reported to be elevated in plasma membranes by one group,[60] but unchanged[28,61] or even lowered[62] by other groups. Anionic phospholipids were reported to be elevated in brain membranes by one group,[57] but no other group has found similar changes in brain membranes or other tissues. It is also not clear what property of the modified lipids leads to reduced partition (or resistance). It was suggested that the modified membranes from ethanol-fed animals are more "ordered" than those of controls.[8] Since partition of amphiphilic molecules strongly depends on lipid packing and membrane "order," such a change would be sufficient to explain the reduced partition and the resulting resistance to ethanol's effect. However, the reported data on the difference in "order" between membranes from ethanol-fed and control animals are also controversial. It should be emphasized again, that in part, these conflicting results are related to differences in animal species, feeding protocols, membrane preparation, and so on. However, in this case, even more important is the use of different probes to estimate membrane order and the ambiguity inherent in the interpretation of these measurements. For instance, the partition probe 5-doxyl-decane always shows large, significant increased "order" in membranes from ethanol-fed rats (cf refs. *22,28,29,31,63*). It is, of course, highly significant that this is a partition probe and that the change in membrane "order" is indicated by the change in partition. Other probes sense this increased "order" to a lesser extent. The order parameter of 5-doxyl-stearate is often found to be higher in ethanol-fed rats (cf ref. *22*), but 12-doxyl-stearate did not show this difference in the same preparation.[31] Similarly, time resolved fluorescence measurements of DPH do not show different order.[29,30] These findings are consistent with the interpretation that the structural changes occur close to the surface (where ethanol resides), but is not detected in the core of the membrane. Moreover, since the partition probe 5-doxyl-decane is the most sensitive indicator of this change, it is likely that this is precisely the change in membrane structure that results in reduced partition of ethanol and other anesthetics.

It has been claimed that the change in the phospholipid's property that produces resistance to the fluidizing effects of ethanol is contributed by a very small fraction of the total phospholipids. Taraschi et al. have claimed that phospholipid vesicles of any composition can be made resistant to the fluidizing effects of ethanol when a very small amount (less than 2.5%) of the PI obtained from liver microsomes of ethanol-fed rats is incorporated.[64] However, we have recently conducted a study, essentially identical to that of Taraschi et al., that does not support their finding. We have found that the resistance to ethanol disordering in phospholipids from liver microsomes from ethanol-fed rats is not restricted to PI, but instead is shared equally by all classes of phospholipids. Moreover, the degree of resistance to fluidization in vesicles of mixed lipids is strictly proportional to the fraction of phospholipids from ethanol-fed animals, regardless of the class of lipids (Rottenberg, Bittman, and Lee, in preparation). Thus, our results are compatible with the hypothesis that the bulk properties of the phospholipid membrane are modified in ethanol-fed animals in a manner that changes the packing of the polar residues near the surface, and thus reduces the partition of both ethanol and anesthetics.

Effects of Ethanol on Membrane Enzymes, Receptors, and Channels

High concentrations of ethanol and other anesthetics affect the activity of numerous membrane enzymes, receptors, and channels (cf refs. *45,56,65*). Many, but not all, of these effects can be related to the effects of anesthetics on the physical properties of the membranes and show little specificity when the activity is related to the membrane concentration of these agents. It is interesting to note, however, that although some enzymes, transporters, and channels are stimulated by high concentrations of ethanol, others are inhibited. If the only relevant effect of ethanol on membrane structure is the increase of membrane fluidity, one would expect ethanol addition to be equivalent to increased temperature, which is generally associated with increased activity. Thus, the fact that many enzymes and channels are inhibited by high concentrations of ethanol suggests that even at high concentration of ethanol its nonspecific effects do not always result from increased fluidity. As discussed earlier, ethanol can inhibit the activity of enzymes and channels through its effects on lipid–protein interactions, which determine the protein conformation, or on protein–protein interactions. The effect on the membrane dielectric constant could also be important in many processes. There are several reports that indicate that the effects of ethanol on enzymes and channels are considerably attenuated in membranes from ethanol-fed animals. For example, Ca^{2+}-uptake by rat liver microsomes is inhibited by ethanol, in vitro, and the extent of this inhibition is greatly reduced in liver microsomes from ethanol-fed rats.[48] Similarly, mitochondrial ATPase and electron transport is stimulated by ethanol, but this stimulation is greatly attenuated in mitochondria isolated from ethanol-fed rats.[32] Similar effects were observed with the Na^+-K^+ ATPase and phospholipase A_2.[8] It is hard to conceive separate specific ethanol-induced changes in these and other enzymes that lead to the observed tolerance, particularly since the effect of ethanol is significant only at high ethanol concentrations, well above the in vivo concentration obtained during ethanol-feeding. It is reasonable to assume that a change in the physical properties of the membrane is the basis of the apparent tolerance of several diverse membrane enzymes. However, as discussed earlier, this change does not appear to be related specifically to resistance to membrane fluidization since the inhibitory effect of alcohol on ion transport cannot be attributed to membrane fluidization. However, a reduction of the partition coefficient of ethanol would result in tolerance to any effect of alcohol on membrane enzymes, regardless of its mechanism, provided that the effect is mediated by the membrane lipids. The magnitude of the observed reductions in ethanol partition coefficients is sufficient to account for the observed degree of tolerance to the nonspecific effect of ethanol on membrane enzymes and channels.

It is still an open question whether ethanol can interact directly with specific membrane proteins in a manner that is completely independent of its interaction with lipids. There is one example of a soluble protein (luciferase) that is inhibited by alcohols and other anesthetics, which appear to bind to a hydrophobic site and hence their potency correlates with their lipid/water partition coefficients. This sole example has been postulated to be the prototype for the action of alcohol and anesthetics on membrane enzyme.[66] To date, there is little evidence to support this hypothesis. Studies of specific effects of anesthetics on various channels and receptors suggest specific saturable sites of interaction for local anesthetics. However, even though the effects of ethanol and general anesthetics can often be described in considerable molecular detail, no evidence for specific saturable protein binding sites for ethanol exists.[56,67]

Nevertheless, in recent years a growing number of channels have been identified that exhibit extremely high sensitivity to ethanol. From the pharmacological point of view, these are the systems that are expected to be most affected, in vivo, both in acute and chronic alcohol ingestion. Prominent among these are the NMDA Ca^{2+} channel, which is inhibited[11] and the $GABA_A$ Cl^- channel, which is stimulated.[10] Voltage dependent Ca^{2+} channels are also significantly inhibited by pharmacologically relevant concentration of ethanol (i.e., 20–100 mM).[15] The effect of ethanol on cAMP is also observed at pharmacological concentrations in some cells and appears to depend mostly on stimulation of adenylate cyclase.[17] The mechanisms of the effects of ethanol on these ethanol-sensitive channels and enzymes have not been determined as yet. However, it is very unlikely that the effects can be attributed to membrane fluidization since pharmacological concentrations of ethanol have little effect on membrane fluidity.[8]

Adaptation to Alcohol
of Liver Cell Membranes

The majority of the studies on alcohol's effects on membranes were conducted with CNS membranes. This is understandable since the CNS is the site of the acute pharmacological effects of ethanol intoxication and also plays prominently in the pathological effects associated with chronic alcoholism. However, other organs are also damaged by long-term use of alcohol and it is possible that the effects of alcohol on the membranes of these organs contribute to the pathology of chronic alcoholism. The liver is, however, unique in that most of the metabolism of ethanol occurs in the liver and the effects of chronic alcohol use on liver membranes could be partially owing to its metabolism. Nevertheless, most of the direct effects of ethanol on membranes, as discussed in the preceding section, were also observed in liver membranes and some of the effects of long-term use of alcohol can be described as adaptation to the continuous presence of ethanol.

Mitochondria

The effects of chronic-alcoholism on liver mitochondria have been studied extensively. In ethanol-fed animals, as well as in humans, chronic alcoholism results in gross changes in mitochondrial morphology.[68] In addition, there is a significant decrease in the activities of several key enzymes of oxidative phosphorylation.[69,70] However, it is doubtful whether the latter changes could be considered to be an adaptation to the presence of ethanol. The reduced activities of respiratory enzymes of rat liver mitochondria, which develops over a period of 4–5 wk, are not observed in rat brain mitochondria (Thayer and Rottenberg, in preparation) or in rat heart mitochondria after a comparable period.[71] It is thus probable that these changes are associated with alcohol metabolism, which occurs in part in the mitochondria and is not caused by direct effect of ethanol on mitochondrial membranes. However, as discussed earlier, the stimulating effect of ethanol on the ATPase and respiration is attenuated in ethanol-fed rats[32] and this change is associated with resistance to the fluidizing effect of ethanol and anesthetics.[22,31,44] Moreover, as has been reported by several groups, there are significant changes in the acyl-chain composition of mitochondrial phospholipids,[22,72] and the partition coefficients of ethanol and other amphiphilics are significantly reduced.[22] In addition, the mitochondrial-lipid phase-transitions are shifted to higher temperatures and the membrane becomes resistant to the effects of alcohol on these transitions.[31,32] All these facts suggest that similar to other membranes the mitochondrial membranes in ethanol-fed rats are adapted to the presence of ethanol by change in the phospholipid composition, which reduces the partition coefficients of ethanol. These observations are, however, hard to reconcile with the fact that no known system of the mitochondrial membrane is sufficiently sensitive to the pharmacological effects of ethanol. If pharmacological concentrations of ethanol do not significantly affect any of the important mitochondrial functions, why should the membrane adapt to the in vitro effects of high concentrations of ethanol? Perhaps an answer to this intriguing question could be found when the mechanism of adaptation is fully elucidated. As discussed in the next main section, it appears that the mechanism of adaptation is general and not specific to a particular membrane. Moreover, the adaptation may be driven by a product of alcohol ingestion and not directly by the effects of ethanol on membrane enzymes (*see* the next main section).

Microsomes

Liver microsomes are vesicles formed from the membranes of the endoplasmatic reticulum. As mentioned earlier, Ca^{2+} uptake, which is inhibited by ethanol, is enhanced in membranes from ethanol-fed rats and is partially resistant to the inhibitory effect of ethanol.[48] These changes are also associated with a change in the acyl-chain composition of the microsomal phospholipids[72] with shifts in lipid transition temperatures, and with a resistance to the fluidizing effects of ethanol.[48] Moreover, these changes are also accompanied by a reduction of the partition coefficients of amphiphilic compounds, which are exhibited by the isolated phospholipids.[30] Ca^{2+} transport in microsomes is more sensitive to the pharmacological range of ethanol than the mitochondrial enzymes but still probably not significant, in vivo. The fact that both mitochondria and microsomes adapt in a similar way suggests a generalized mechanism of adaptation (*see* the next main section).

Plasma Membranes

The effects of ethanol ingestion on liver plasma membrane are more controversial than the effects on liver organelle membranes. In part, this may be owing to the fact that it is much more difficult to obtain purified plasma membrane preparation from liver cells. Particularly in liver from ethanol-fed animals, the increased triglyceride content and the changes in the properties (and densities) of all particulate fractions make it extremely difficult to obtain purified plasma membranes by differential centrifugation. It has been reported that plasma membranes from liver of ethanol-fed animals contain less cholesterol and are more fluid than control.[62] However, others reported that these membranes are more ordered than control[73] and contain more cholesterol.[74] Again, these contradictions may be owing to procedures and methods, as discussed above. Nevertheless, it appears that these membranes too are more resistant to the fluidizing effects of ethanol.[49] Thus, although there is not sufficient evidence to substantiate this conclusion, it appears likely that these membranes also undergo the same adaptation process reported for red blood cell plasma membrane, synaptic plasma membrane, and liver mitochondria and microsomes as described earlier. The strong effect of pharmacological concentration of ethanol on various ion channels of the CNS has not been observed with liver cells. Long-term incubation of isolated liver cells with pharmacological concentration of ethanol inhibits insulin-induced amino acid uptake.[75] However, it is doubtful whether this effect occurs in vivo. Ethanol, in vitro, also appears to stimulate phospholipase C. However, this effect is very transient and is only significant at high concentration of ethanol.[76]

Mechanism of Adaptation to Ethanol and Its Reversal After Withdrawal

Little is known about the sequence of events that leads to the adaptation of membranes to chronic-ethanol ingestion or about the reversal of this process that is observed after withdrawal from ethanol. However, the time course of these events has been studied in some detail. Behavioral tolerance and dependence can be demonstrated within an hour of ethanol administration.[77] This does not mean that the membrane changes described earlier take place in this period. Initially, short-term tolerance most probably depends on different mechanisms. In mice exposed to ethanol by inhalation, the development of behavioral tolerance over a few day period paralleled the increased resistance to synaptic membrane fluidization by ethanol. Tolerance disappeared within 30 h of withdrawal, and the same time was required for the disappearance of the resistance of the synaptic membrane to fluidization by ethanol.[77] We have correlated the reduction in partition coefficient of ethanol in rat red blood cells with ethanol feeding and its withdrawal. About 2 wk of high-ethanol diet is required for the maximal reduction of the partition coefficient of ethanol (and other alcohols). The partition coefficient returns to normal value within 24 h after withdrawal. When alcohol was readministered 4 d after withdrawal, it took, again, 2 wk to obtain maximal reduction in partition coefficient.[28] A very similar time course was observed in the development and disappearance of the resistance to fluidization by ethanol of the microsomal membranes.[78] These studies demonstrate again the strong correlations between tolerance, resistance to fluidization of membranes by ethanol, and reduction in partition coefficients. These findings strengthen the argument that the reduction of the partition coefficients is the molecular basis of tolerance, at least as observed, in vitro, on membrane preparations.

What is the signal that initiates and terminates these changes, and why does the change develop relatively slowly and disappear quickly? One significant clue to this puzzle may be found in the observation that the time course of the changes in membrane properties is exactly the same as the time course of changes in serum cholesterol.[28] It is well known that chronic alcoholism, both in animal models and in humans, is associated with elevation of the serum cholesterol, which is mostly accounted for by increased HDL cholesterol.[3] As was discussed earlier, it has been suggested that increased cholesterol/phospholipid ratio in the membrane results in resistance to the effects of ethanol.[60] However, since such an increase is not universally observed, and moreover since the resistance to ethanol is exhibited by isolated phospholipids free of cholesterol, this could not be the explanation. We have suggested an alternative explanation, which postulates that the changes in phospholipid composition are in direct response to the elevation of serum cholesterol and are intended to maintain a constant cholesterol/phospholipid ratio in cell membranes.[28,63] It is well known that the cholesterol/phospholipid ratio of different membranes is carefully regulated.[79] Thus, the mechanism for this precise regulation already exists and need not be induced specifically by ethanol. The effect on ethanol partition, which is not specific, is suggested to be a beneficial side effect of this regulation. Indeed, cholesterol is an alcohol and probably shares with ethanol the same binding area close to the membrane surface.[35] Hence, reduction of cholesterol binding should be associated with reduction of binding of other amphiphilic compounds, including ethanol.

This hypothesis also fully explains the unusual time course of development and disappearance of membrane tolerance. Simply, membrane phospholipid changes follow closely the change in serum cholesterol levels. It is also compatible with the fact that ethanol induces a specific increase in the level of HDL, since HDL is responsible for the removal of cholesterol. We have recently measured the kinetics of cholesterol transfer between RBC membranes and lipoprotein in control and ethanol-fed rats. The rate of cholesterol transfer from RBC to lipoprotein is considerably enhanced in blood from ethanol-fed rats, which is compatible with our hypothesis (Rottenberg, to be published).

Conclusions and Outlook

Liver cell membranes undergo adaptation to chronic ethanol ingestion, which is similar to the adaptation of CNS and blood cell membranes, and is probably common to all tissues. This adaptation is manifested by a resistance to the effects of ethanol on membrane enzymes, receptors, and channels, as well as by changes in the activities of these systems and by resistance to the membrane fluidizing effect of ethanol and anesthetics. Many, if not all, of these changes are attributed to a reduction in the partition coefficient of ethanol and other amphiphilic drugs, which is the result of changes in the lipid composition of the membrane. The generality of these phenomena, which include membranes that are not sensitive to the pharmacological effects of ethanol, suggests a general, whole body, mechanism of adaptation. We have suggested that the elevation of serum cholesterol, which appears to result from the metabolism of ethanol, leads to changes in phospholipid composition, which reduce the partition of cholesterol and other amphiphilic molecules, including ethanol.

More specific membrane effects of low concentration of ethanol have been described recently in CNS membranes. However, to date the existence of membrane processes sensitive to low pharmacological concentration of ethanol in the liver has not been detected. It would be of great interest if such processes can be identified. The role, if any, of the adaptation of liver cell membranes in liver pathology induced by chronic alcoholism has not been elucidated. Significant adaptive changes in liver calcium metabolism may result in excess calcium loading during withdrawal and thus contribute to liver injury. However, these changes have not been fully characterized as yet.

References

[1] B. Tabakoff and J. D. Rothstein (1983) Biology of tolerance and dependence, in *Medical and Social Aspects of Alcohol Abuse*. B. Tabakoff, P. B. Sutker, and C. L. Randall, eds. Plenum, New York, p. 187.

[2] R. L. Alkana, D. A. Finn, and R. D. Malcolm (1983) The importance of experience in the development of tolerance to ethanol hypothermia. *Life Sci.* **32,** 2685–2692.

[3] C. S. Lieber (1990) Mechanism of ethanol induced hepatic injury. *Pharmacol. Ther.* **46,** 1–41.

[4] P. L. Hoffman (1987) Central nervous system effects of neurohypopyseal peptides, in *The Peptides*. vol. 8. S. Udenfriend and J. Meienhofer, eds. Academic, New York, pp. 239–295.

[5] G. Szabo, P. L. Hoffman, and B. Tabakoff (1988) Forskolin promotes the development of ethanol tolerance in 6-hydroxy-dopamine-treated mice. *Life Sci.* **42,** 615–621.

[6] P. H. Wu, T. Pham, and C. A. Narango (1987) Nifedipine delays the acquisition of tolerance to ethanol. *Eur. J. Pharmacol.* **139,** 233–236.

[7] A. M. Allen and R. A. Harris (1989) Acute and chronic ethanol treatment alter GABA receptor-operated chloride channels. *Pharmacol. Biochem. Behav.* **27,** 665–670.

[8] D. B. Goldstein (1984) The effects of drugs on membrane fluidity. *Ann. Rev. Pharmacol. Toxicol.* **24,** 43–64.

[9] M. W. Hill and A. D. Bangham (1975) General depressant drug dependence: A biophysical hypothesis. *Adv. Exp. Med. Biol.* **59,** 1–9.

[10] P. D. Suzdak, R. D. Schwartz, P. Skolnick, and S. M. Paul (1986) Ethanol stimulates GABA receptor-mediated chloride transport in rat brain synaptoneurosomes. *Proc. Natl. Acad. Sci. USA* **83,** 4071–4075.

[11] D. M. Lovinger, G. White, and F. F. Weight (1989) Ethanol inhibits NMDA-activated ion current in hypocampal neuros. *Science* **243,** 1721–1724.

[12] K. A. Grant, P. Valverius, M. Hudspith, and B. Tabakoff (1990) Ethanol withdrawal seizures and the NMDA receptor complex. *Eur. J. Pharmacol.* **176,** 289–296.

[13] R. A. Morrisett, A. H. Rezvani, D. Overstreet, D. S. Janowsky, W. A. Wilson, and H. S. Swartzwelder (1990) MK-801 potently inhibits alcohol withdrawal seizures in rats. *Eur. J. Pharmacol.* **176,** 103–105.

[14] R. O. Messing, C. L. Carpenter, I. Diamond, and D. A. Greenberg (1986) Ethanol regulates calcium channels in clonal neural cells. *Proc. Natl. Acad. Sci. USA* **83**, 6213–6215.

[15] S. Dollin, H. Little, M. Hudspith, C. Pagonis, and J. Littleton (1987) Increased dihydropyridine-sensitive calcium channels in rat brain may underlie ethanol physical dependence. *Neuropharmacology* **26**, 275–279.

[16] J. M. Littleton, H. J. Little, and M. A. Whitington (1990) Effect of dihydropyridine calcium channel antagonists in ethanol withdrawal: doses required, sterospecificity and action of Bay K 8644. *Psychopharmacology* **100**, 387–392.

[17] A. S. Gordon, K. Collier, and I. Diamond (1986) Ethanol regulation of adenosine receptor-stimulated cAMP levels in clonal neural cell line: An in vitro model of cellular tolerance to ethanol. *Proc. Natl. Acad. Sci. USA* **83**, 2105–2108.

[18] P. T. Nhamburo, P. L. Hoffman, and B. Tabakoff (1988) Cholera toxin-induced ADP-ribosylation of 46 Kda protein is decreased in brains of ethanol-fed mice. *Adv. Alcohol Subst. Abuse.* **7**, 103–105.

[19] L. E. Nagy, I. Diamond, and A. Gordon (1988) Cultured lymphocytes from alcoholic subjects have altered cAMP signal transduction. *Proc. Natl. Acad. Sci. USA* **85**, 6973–6976.

[20] B. Tabakoff, P. L. Hoffman, J. M. Lee, T. Saito, B. Willard, and F. DeLeon-Jones (1988) Differences in platelet enzyme activity between alcoholics and nonalcoholics. *N. Engl. J. Med.* **318**, 134–139.

[21] P. Seeman (1972) The membrane actions of anesthetics and tranquilizers. *Pharmacol. Rev.* **24**, 583–655.

[22] H. Rottenberg, A. Waring, and E. Rubin (1981) Tolerance and cross-tolerance in chronic alcoholics. Reduced membrane binding of ethanol and other drugs. *Science* **213**, 583–585.

[23] L. Herbette, F. C. Messino, and A. M. Katz (1982) The interaction of drugs with the sarcoplasmatic reticulum. *Ann. Rev. Pharmacol. Toxicol.* **22**, 413–434.

[24] A. Leguicher, F. Beague, and R. Nordmann (1987) Concomitant changes of ethanol partitioning and disordering capacities in rat synaptic membranes. *Biochem. Pharmacol.* **36**, 2045–2048.

[25] M. M. Sarasua, K. R. Faught, S. L. Steedman, M. D. Gordin, and M. K. Washington (1989) A comparison of ethanol partitioning in biological and model membranes: Nonideal partitioning is enhanced in synaptosomal membranes. *Alcohol. Clin. Exp. Res.* **13**, 698–705.

[26] G. P. Kreishman, C. Graham-Brittain, and R. Hitzemann (1985) Determination of the ethanol partition coefficients to the interior and the surface of DMPC liposomes using ^{2}H-NMR spectroscopy. *Biochem. Biophys. Res. Commun.* **130**, 301–305.

[27] E. S. Rowe (1983) Lipid chain length and temperature dependence of ethanol-phosphatidylcholine interactions. *Biochemistry* **22**, 3299–3305.

[28] H. Rottenberg (1986) Membrane solubility of ethanol in chronic alcoholism. *Biochim. Biophys. Acta* **855,** 211–222.

[29] S. Kelly-Murphy, A. J. Waring, H. Rottenberg, and E. Rubin (1984) Effects of chronic ethanol consumption on the partition of lipophilic compounds into erythrocyte membranes. *Lab. Invest.* **50,** 174–183.

[30] Y. Nie, C. D. Stubbs, B. W. Williams, and E. Rubin (1989) Ethanol causes decreased partitioning into biological membranes without changes in lipid order. *Arch. Biochem. Biophys.* **268,** 349–359.

[31] A. J. Waring, H. Rottenberg, T. Ohnishi, and E. Rubin (1982) The effect of chronic ethanol consumption on temperature-dependent physical properties of liver mitochondrial membranes. *Arch. Biochem. Biophys.* **216,** 51–61.

[32] H. Rottenberg, D. E. Robertson, and E. Rubin (1980) The effect of ethanol on the temperature dependence of respiration and ATPase activities of rat liver mitochondria. *Lab. Invest.* **42,** 318–326.

[33] J. M. Pope and D. W. Dubro (1986) The interaction of n-alkanes and n-alcohols with lipid bilayer membranes: A ^{2}H-NMR study. *Biochim. Biophys. Acta* **858,** 243–253.

[34] E. S. Rowe, A. Fernandes, and R. G. Khalifah (1987) Alcohol interactions with lipid: A ^{13}C-NMR study using butanol labeled at C-1. *Biochim. Biophys. Acta* **905,** 151–161.

[35] L. G. Herbette (1985) X-ray and neutron diffraction for probing the interactions of small molecules with membrane structure. *Curr. Top. Bioen.* **14,** 21–52.

[36] R. A. Harris, G. I. Groh, D. M. Baxter, and R. J. Hitzemann (1984) Gangliosides enhance the membrane actions of ethanol and pentobarbitol. *Mol. Pharmacol.* **25,** 410–417.

[37] C. Graham-Brittain, R. J. Hitzemann, and G. P. Kreishman (1989) Detection of a novel binding site for butanol in DPPC/GM_1 liposomes by ^{2}H-NMR spectroscopy. *Prog. Clin. Biol. Res.* **292,** 23–31.

[38] D. Ullman, R. C. Baker, and R. A. Deitrich (1987) Gangliosides of LS and SS mouse cerebellar and whole brain synaptosomal plasma membranes. *Alcohol. Clin. Exp. Res.* **11,** 158–162.

[39] W. R. Klemm, R. Boyles, J. Matthew, and L. Cherlan (1988) Gangliosides, or sialic acid antagonize ethanol intoxication. *Life Sci.* **43,** 1837–1843.

[40] B. L. Hungund, M. V. Reddy, V. A. Bharucha, and S. P. Mahadik (1990) Monosialogangliosides (GM_1 and AGF_2) reduce acute ethanol intoxication. *Drug. Devel. Res.* **19,** 443–451.

[41] W. G. Wood and F. Schroeder (1988) Membrane effects of ethanol: Bulk lipid versus lipid domain. *Life Sci.* **43,** 467–475.

[42] F. Schroeder, W. J. Morrison, C. Gorka, and W. G. Wood (1988) Transbilayer effects of ethanol on fluidity of brain membrane leaflets. *Biochim. Biophys. Acta* **946,** 85–94.

[43] W. G. Wood, C. Gorka, and F. Schroeder (1989) Acute and chronic effect of ethanol on chronic membrane domains. *J. Neurochem.* **52,** 1925–1930.

[44] A. J. Waring, H. Rottenberg, T. Ohinshi, and E. Rubin (1981) Membranes and phospholipids of liver mitochondria from chronic alcoholic rats are resistant to membrane disordering by alcohol. *Proc. Natl. Sci. USA* **78,** 2582–2586.

[45] R. A. Deitrich, T. V. Dunwiddie, R. A. Harris, and V. G. Erwin (1989) Mechanism of action of ethanol: Initial central nervous system actions. *Pharmacol. Rev.* **41,** 489–537.

[46] E. Lissi, M. C. Bianconi, A. T. Amaral, E. Paula, L. E. B. Blanch, and S. Schriers (1990) Methods for the determination of partition coefficients based on the effect of solutes upon membrane structure. *Biochim. Biophys. Acta* **1021,** 46–50.

[47] J. H. Chin and D. B. Goldstein (1977) Drug tolerance in biomembranes. A spin label study of the effects of ethanol. *Science* **196,** 684,685.

[48] B. Ponnappa, A. J. Waring, J. B. Hoek, H. Rottenberg, and E. Rubin (1982) Chronic ethanol ingestion increases calcium uptake and resistance to molecular disordering by ethanol in liver microsomes. *J. Biol. Chem.* **257,** 10,141–10,146.

[49] A. Schuler, J. Muscat, E. Diez, C. Fernandez-Checa, F. G. Ganlones, and A. M. Municio (1984) The fluidity of plasma membrane from ethanol-treated rat liver. *Mol. Cell. Biochem.* **64,** 89–95.

[50] D. B. Goldstein, J. H. Chin, and R. C. Lyon (1988) Ethanol disordering of spin-labeled mouse brain membranes: Correlation with genetically determined ethanol sensitivity of mice. *Proc. Natl. Acad. Sci. USA* **79,** 4231–4233.

[51] F. Beauge, H. Stibler, and S. Bork (1985) Abnormal fluidity and surface carbohydrates content of erythrocyte membrane in alcoholic patients. *Alcoholism* **9,** 322–326.

[52] W. G. Wood, S. Lahiri, C. Gorka, H. J. Armbrecht, and R. Strong (1987) In vivo effects of ethanol on erythrocyte membrane fluidity of alcoholic patients: An electron spin resonance study. *Alcohol. Clin. Exp. Res.* **11,** 332–335.

[53] E. S. Rowe (1987) Induction of lateral phase separations in binary lipid mixture by alcohol. *Biochemistry* **26,** 46–51.

[54] C. P. S. Tilcock and P. R. Cullis (1987) Lipid polymorphism. *Ann. NY Acad. Sci.* **42,** 88–102.

[55] H. Rottenberg, D. E. Robertson, and E. Rubin (1985) The effect of temperature and chronic ethanol feeding on the proton electrochemical potential and phosphate potential in rat liver mitochondria. *Biochim. Biophys. Acta* **809,** 1–10.

[56] J. R. Elliot and D. A. Haydon (1989) The action of neutral anesthetics on ion conductance of nerve membrane. *Biochim. Biophys. Acta* **988,** 257–280.

[57] G. Y. Sun and A. Y. Sun (1985) Ethanol and membrane lipids. *Alcohol. Clin. Exp. Res.* **9,** 164–180.

[58] J. M. Littleton and G. John (1977) Synaptosomal membrane lipids of mice

during continuous exposure to ethanol. *J. Pharm. Pharmacol.* **29,** 579–580.

[59] S. Umeki, H. Shiojiri, and Y. Nozawa (1984) Chronic ethanol administration decreases fatty acyl-CoA desaturase activities in rat liver microsomes. *FEBS Lett.* **169,** 274–278.

[60] J. H. Chin, L. M. Parson, and D. B. Goldstein (1978) Increased cholesterol content of erythrocytes and brain membranes in ethanol-tolerant mice. *Biochim. Biophys. Acta* **513,** 358–363.

[61] D. R. Wing, D. J. Harvey, J. Hughes, P. G. Dunbar, K. A. McPherson, and W. D. N. Paton (1982) Effect of chronic ethanol administration on the composition of membrane lipid in the mouse. *Biochem. Pharmacol.* **31,** 3431–3439.

[62] S. Yamada and C. S. Lieber (1984) Decrease in micoviscosity and cholesterol content of rat liver plasma membranes after chronic ethanol feeding. *J. Clin. Invest.* **74,** 2285–2289.

[63] H. Rottenberg (1987) Partition of ethanol and other amphiphilic compounds modulated by chronic alcoholism. *Ann. NY Acad. Sci.* **492,** 112–124.

[64] T. F. Taraschi, J. S. Ellingson, A. Wu, R. Zimmerman, and E. Rubin (1986) Phosphatidylinositol from ethanol-fed rats confers membrane tolerance to ethanol. *Proc. Natl. Acad. Sci. USA* **83,** 9398–9402.

[65] W. A. Hunt (1985) *Alcohol and Biological Membranes.* Guilford, New York.

[66] N. P. Frank and W. R. Lieb (1987) What is the molecular nature of general anesthetic target sites? *Trends Pharmacol.* **8,** 169–174.

[67] S. A. Forman and K. W. Miller (1989) Molecular sites of anesthetic action in postsyroptic nicotinic membranes. *Trends Pharmacol.* **10,** 447–452.

[68] D. J. Svoboda and R. T. Manning (1964) Chronic alcoholism with fatty methamorphosis of the liver: Mitochondrial alteration in hepatic cells. *Am. J. Pathol.* **44,** 645–654

[69] A. I. Cederbaum, C. S. Lieber, and E. Rubin (1974) Effects of chronic ethanol treatment on mitochondrial function: Damage to coupling site I. *Arch. Biochem. Biophys.* **165,** 560–569.

[70] W. S. Thayer (1987) Effect of ethanol on proteins of mitochondrial membranes. *Ann. NY Acad. Sci.* **492,** 193–206.

[71] C. C. Cunningham, D. L. Kouri, K. R. Beeker, and P. I. Spach (1989) Comparison of effects of long-term ethanol consumption on the heart and liver of the rat. *Alcohol. Clin. Exp. Res.* **13,** 58–65.

[72] C. Cunningham, C. S. Filus, R. E. Bottenus, and P. I. Spach (1982) The effect of ethanol consumption on the phospholipid composition of rat liver microsomes and mitochondria. *Biochim. Biophys. Acta* **72,** 225–233.

[73] E. N. Lewis, I. W. Levin, and C. J. Steer (1989) Infrared spectroscopic study of ethanol-induced changes in rat liver plasma membranes. *Biochim. Biophys. Acta* **986,** 161–166.

[74] B. Rovinski and E. A. Hosein (1983) Adaptive changes in lipid composition of rat liver plasma membranes during postnatal development following maternal ethanol ingestion. *Biochim. Biophys. Acta* **735,** 407–417.

[75] J. Rosa and E. Rubin (1980) Effects of ethanol on amino acid uptake by rat liver cells. *Lab. Invest.* **43,** 366–372.

[76] J. B. Hoek, A. P. Thomas, R. Rubin, and E. Rubin (1987) Ethanol-induced mobilization of calcium by activation of phosphoinositide-specific phospholipase C in intact hepatocytes. *J. Biol. Chem.* **262,** 682–691.

[77] D. B. Goldstein (1987) Ethanol induced adaptation in biological membranes. *Ann. NY Acad. Sci.* **492,** 103–111.

[78] T. F. Taraschi, J. S. Elingson, A. Wu, R. Zimmerman, and E. Rubin (1986) Membrane tolerance to ethanol is rapidly lost after withdrawal: A model for studies of membrane adaptation. *Proc. Natl. Acad. Sci. USA* **83,** 3669–3673.

[79] R. A. Cooper and J. F. Strauss III (1984) Regulation of cell membrane cholesterol, in *Physiology of Membrane Fluidity,* vol. 1. M. Shinitzky, ed. CRC, Boca Raton, FL, pp. 73–98.

The Effect of Prenatal Alcohol Exposure on γ-Glutamyl Transpeptidase

Edward Reyes

Introduction

Although the adverse effects of the maternal consumption of alcohol have been recognized for thousands of years, it is only since 1973 that attempts to study the effects of alcohol on the developing fetus have been undertaken. The term Fetal Alcohol Syndrome (FAS) was used by Jones et al. to describe the pattern of abnormalities occurring in children born to alcoholic mothers.[1-3] The percentage of offspring with FAS born to alcoholic women varies from 32 to 76%, depending on the population studied.[4] The incidence of FAS worldwide is 0.19% of live births.[5] It is evident that the problems associated with the maternal consumption of alcohol are of economic concern.

Clinical Manifestations of FAS

The clinical manifestations of FAS include facial dysmorphosis, overall growth deficiencies, a variety of neurologic dysfunctions, microcephaly, and mild to moderate mental retardation.[1-3] Mental retardation is one of the most common and most serious problems associated with alcohol teratogenicity.[5,6] Alcohol consumption during pregnancy is the greatest known

From: *Drug and Alcohol Abuse Reviews, Vol. 2: Liver Pathology and Alcohol*
Ed: R. R. Watson ©1991 The Humana Press Inc.

health hazard to the unborn and is considered one of the most common causes of mental retardation with a known etiology. The prenatal exposure to alcohol produces morphological, biochemical, behavioral, and physiological abnormalities.

Physiological and Pathophysiological Functions of γ-Glutamyl Transpeptidase

γ-Glutamyl transpeptidase (EC 2.3.2.2) is widely distributed in plants and animals and exists both as a soluble and membrane bound enzyme.[7,8] The enzyme has been studied and, at least partially, characterized in kidney, brain, and liver.[9-16] Although the enzyme has been extensively purified and studied in kidney, the present chapter will be concerned only with the enzyme in brain and liver. Evidence suggests that multiple forms of the enzyme may exist in brain[11,12,17] and liver.[18] Early kinetic studies using a partially purified preparation of enzyme from sheep brain provided nonlinear double reciprocal plots suggesting that more than one form of the enzyme was present in brain.[17] Later studies on rat brain revealed multiple forms of the enzyme that were isolated by concanavalin A fractionation.[12,19]

Kottgen et al.[18] showed that in rat liver two forms of the enzyme were present. In adult liver, γ-GTP exists in an asialo form, whereas in fetal liver it is sialylated.[18] The fetal form of the enzyme has more sialic acid than the adult form.[10,15,20-22]

Physiological Function of γ-GTP

The major function of γ-GTP is related to the metabolism of glutathione.[23-25] The enzyme catalyzes the hydrolysis of the γ-glutamyl-cysteine bond in glutathione. γ-GTP is the only enzyme capable of hydrolyzing glutathione. The enzyme is also an integral part of the γ-glutamyl cycle and will transfer the γ-glutamyl group from glutathione to an amino acid or peptide. Additionally, it may utilize glutamine as substrate, but glutathione is the preferred substrate. Evidence suggests that γ-GTP may also convert leukotriene C to leukotriene D by removal of a glutamyl residue.[26]

The pattern of development of the enzyme may provide a clue as to its physiological function. High γ-GTP activity has been demonstrated in fetal liver of both rat and humans, with much lower levels in adult tissue than in fetal tissue.[27–29] In liver, γ-GTP activity reaches a peak just prior to birth and then enzyme activity begins to fall toward adult levels.[28] A marked increase in γ-GTP activity was also found in tissues of chick embryo, between embryonic day 11 and hatching.[30,31] In mouse brain capillaries, γ-GTP specific activity continues to increase after birth until approx 12 mo of age.[32] γ-GTP activity in amniotic fluid showed a gradual decrease with advancing pregnancy.[33] Activity of γ-GTP in human fetal membranes was found to increase to week 30.[34] The higher activities of the enzyme during development suggest that it may be involved in the transport of vital nutrients or in the regulation of glutathione at a critical period in the development of the organism.

Pathophysiological Function of γ-GTP

Several clinical cases have been reported in which inborn errors of metabolism result in deficiencies in enzymes of the γ-glutamyl cycle and glutathione synthesis.[35] Patients with deficiencies of enzymes of the γ-glutamyl cycle have some degree of mental retardation.[36] Drugs, such as phenytoin and phenobarbital, which have been shown to produce an increase in γ-GTP activity, have also been shown to produce teratogenic effects as evidenced by the hydantoin and barbital syndromes.[37–39] Enzyme inducing drugs have also been shown to produce an elevation of γ-GTP activity in sera.[37–43] The rise of γ-GTP activity is inhibited in the presence of protein synthesis inhibitors, such as cycloheximide. The activity of the enzyme is also shown to be increased by treatment with drugs that induce hepatocarcinogenesis.[44]

γ-GTP as a Diagnostic Aid

The measurement of serum γ-GTP activity has been utilized as a diagnostic aid in liver disease and neurological disorders. Serum γ-GTP has been fractionated by using polyacrylamide gradient gel electrophoresis.[45] The appearance of specific isoenzyme forms of γ-GTP *in sera* have been examined for use as a diagnostic index for hepatoma. Elevated urinary γ-GTP levels following treatment with the aminoglycoside antibiotics have suggested that measurement of urinary γ-GTP can be used as an indicator of acute nephrotoxicity.[46] Hexachlorobenzene increases γ-GTP activity in liver and serum, and thus it appears to be a sensitive marker of hexachlorobenzene intoxication.[47] γ-GTP activity in serum has also been used to aid in the diagnosis of problems associated with high alcohol consumption.

Effects of Alcohol
on γ-Glutamyl Transpeptidase

An early in vitro study in our laboratory has provided evidence that alcohol produces an increase in γ-GTP activity. In this study, a purified fraction of an isoenzyme of γ-GTP from brain was shown to be activated when it was incubated with varying amounts of alcohol.[48,49] Alcohol increased the affinity of the enzyme for the substrate, γ-glutamyl-*p*-nitroanilide, in a dose dependent manner.

Human Studies

Several investigators have shown that alcoholics as well as problem drinkers have higher than normal serum γ-GTP levels.[50–55] In some instances, the enzyme activity is approx 20 times the normal value. It has also been shown that in a normal population there is a positive correlation between serum γ-GTP activity and the drinking habits of an individual. In a study of problem drinkers, it was shown that there is a positive correlation between serum γ-GTP activity and the amount of alcohol consumed by the individual.[53,54] In patients who manifested an elevated γ-GTP level and who had a history of alcohol abuse, the fetal form of the enzyme was more active than it was in controls.[51,56] It was observed that in patients who consumed large amounts of alcohol, not only was the enzyme activity increased, but a second form of the enzyme was present in the serum.[53] This observation agrees with that of Sawabu et al.[45] and Kok et al.[57] Chronic alcohol consumption appears to alter the ratio of fetal to adult forms of the enzyme.[55] Mean serum and hepatic γ-GTP activity in alcoholics is significantly increased compared to that in control patients.[58] In this study, the activity in the liver correlated well with that in the serum, indicating that ethanol-induced increases in serum γ-GTP activity are attributable, in part, to its rise in the liver of alcoholics. Teschke et al. demonstrated the same relationship between serum and liver γ-GTP activity.[59] Because of the relationship between elevated γ-GTP activities and alcohol consumption, serum γ-GTP was measured in pregnant women in an effort to identify pregnancies at risk for the fetal alcohol syndrome.[60] The sensitivity of the serum γ-GTP test in identifying those women who consumed more than 30 g of alcohol per day was 25%. It was the author's conclusion therefore that γ-GTP screening should not be used as a mass screening test during pregnancy to identify women who consume excessive amounts of alcohol and are at risk of bearing children with FAS.

Animal Studies

The administration of alcohol via the inhalational route and the administration by liquid diets have been used as means of administering alcohol to rats for prolonged periods of time. Animal studies using rats have also shown that γ-GTP activity in serum, liver, and brain is elevated following the chronic administration of alcohol.[52,56,61–64] Liquid diets have been utilized as the method of choice to administer alcohol to rats, particularly in pregnant animals. The administration of alcohol via a liquid diet has produced increases in γ-GTP activity in brain and liver. Morland et al. attribute the increase in γ-GTP activity in the alcohol treated animals to a decrease in enzyme activity in the pair-fed controls.[56] Yamada et al. obtained the same results, and attributed the increased γ-GTP activity in rats fed pelleted diets to impurities in the diet.[64] In another study, the administration of an alcohol diet to rats for a period of 6 wk resulted in an increase in γ-GTP activity with no control diet or aging effects.[65] Following an 11-wk period of alcohol consumption, no difference in the turnover rates in γ-GTP was observed, although an increase in γ-GTP activity was seen.[62]

In a recent study it was shown that rats maintained on a liquid diet containing 35% of its caloric content as alcohol for 5–6 wk had an increase in liver γ-GTP activity.[66] Furthermore, the increase in γ-GTP activity is associated with an enhanced removal of glutathione from the circulation. Studies to elucidate the mechanism by which alcohol induces γ-GTP in liver are under way by Barouki et al.[67] and others.

Effects of *In Utero* Exposure to Alcohol on γ-GTP

Although several studies have shown that alcohol produces an elevation in γ-GTP activity in the adult, little is known regarding the effects of the *in utero* administration of alcohol on γ-GTP. Leiuyer et al. have measured γ-GTP activity in childred born to alcoholic mothers[68] γ-GTP activity was found to be increased in infants born to alcoholic mothers.[68]

Effects in Animal Models

Animal models have been utilized to gather what information is available regarding the effects of alcohol on the developing fetus. Because alcohol passes freely from the maternal circulation to the fetus and through breast milk to the neonate, we conducted a series of experiments to determine if consumption of alcohol during gestation and lactation would cause alterations in brain γ-GTP activity similar to that seen in adults.[69–73] To our knowledge our laboratory is the only one where the effects of the *in utero* administration of alcohol on γ-GTP have been studied in the rat model. Our laboratory has utilized a liquid diet to produce an animal model of FAS.[72]

Our model agrees well with the effects reported for FAS in the human. Offspring of mothers that have received 35% of their calories in the form of alcohol come from smaller litters, are smaller, have a higher mortality rate, and exhibit learning deficits as adults.[72,74] We have also shown that the activity of γ-GTP in brain and liver is elevated at birth in the offspring of mothers that have received alcohol during gestation. Litter size does not have an effect on γ-GTP activity.[75] Determination of γ-GTP activity in 30-d-old pups in various regions of brain indicates that the *in utero* administration of alcohol produces an increase in enzyme activity and that this effect is long lasting. Serum γ-GTP activity in the pups is also elevated.

Effects on Ontogenesis

A series of experiments were conducted in our laboratory to ascertain the effects of the *in utero* exposure of alcohol on liver γ-GTP. We examined the effects of alcohol on total enzyme activity, on ontogenic development, and on the ratio of adult to fetal forms of γ-GTP. The experiments evaluating the effects of the *in utero* administration of alcohol on the ontogenic development of γ-GTP in brain and liver are described in the remainder of this chapter and in a previous research report.[70]

Feeding Paradigm. Sprague-Dawley rats were maintained on a 12-h light/dark cycle with lights on between 0700 and 1900 h. Mature female rats were placed with healthy mature males overnight. Vaginal smears were taken each morning to establish evidence of copulation.[72,76] When spermatozoa were identified on the vaginal smear the female was placed in an individual hanging, wire bottomed cage and started on one of five experimental diets as described by Reyes et al.[70,72,73] Three of the groups were placed on a liquid BioServ diet (Bioserv Inc., Frenchtown, NJ) containing either 2.0% v/v alcohol (10% ethanol derived calories; 10% EDC), 4.0%

v/v alcohol (20% EDC), or 6.7% v/v alcohol (35% EDC). Another liquid diet group was pair-fed (PF) to the 35% EDC group. All groups (PF, 10% EDC, 20% EDC) received the same volume of isocalorically equivalent food as the 35% EDC group. The diets were made isocalorically equivalent with a maltose-dextrin mixture. On the day before the mothers were due, they were given *ad libitum* chow and water. A fifth group of pregnant females (LC) were maintained on lab chow and water *ad libitum* to control for the effects of paired feeding. In addition, another separate set of pregnant females maintained on the LC diet was used to provide the untreated surrogate mothers. On the day following parturition, litters were culled to six pups and cross-fostered onto surrogate mothers. For determinations of enzyme activity before birth, the pups were taken by cesarean section following anesthesia of the mothers with sodium pentobarbital.

The livers were removed and placed in ice-cold *tris*-buffered saline, homogenized, and centrifuged. The supernatant (soluble fraction) was assayed for γ-GTP activity and protein content. The pellet was resuspended in *tris*-buffered saline containing 1% deoxycholic acid, let stand over night at 4°C, and centrifuged. The supernatant (membrane bound fraction) was then assayed for γ-GTP activity and protein.

γ-GTP Assay. γ-GTP activity was determined by a modification of the procedure described by Rosalki and Tarlow[77] with a Beckman U40 series spectrophotometer. A typical reaction mixture was as follows: protein (25–100 mg); γ-glutamyl-*p*-nitroanilide (5.4 mM); glycylglycine (110.5 mM); and Tris-HCl (92 mM) in a total volume of 2.0 mL. The reaction pH was 8.5. Following a 20-min incubation period at 37°C the increase in absorbance at 410 nm was determined. The reaction was stopped by the addition of trichloroacetic acid to the incubation mixture. One unit of γ-GTP is that amount of enzyme activity that will liberate 1 μmol of *p*-nitroaniline/min/mg protein. Protein was assayed by the method described by Lowry et al.[78]

Table 1 shows the effects of the *in utero* administration of various doses of alcohol on γ-GTP in liver and brain of newborn rats (day 0). Also shown in Table 1 is the effect of alcohol on body, brain, and liver weights. The higher the dose of alcohol a mother is given during pregnancy, the smaller the birth weights of her offspring. The weights of the pups from the mothers receiving the lower doses of alcohol were not significantly smaller than the pair-fed control. There is also a negative correlation between alcohol dose and brain and liver weights of the offspring. The *in utero* administra-

Table 1

The Effects of *In Utero* Exposure to Alcohol
on γ-Glutamyl Transpeptidase in Brain and Liver in Rats at Birth

Treatment	N	Body weight, g	Brain weight, mg	Brain[c] γ-GTP, U ($\times 10^{-2}$)	Liver weight, mg	Liver γ-GTP, U ($\times 10^{-2}$)
LC	15	$6.66 \pm .22$[b]	268 ± 5	$0.425 \pm .017$	285 ± 12	7.046 ± 1.021
0% EDC	22	$6.03 \pm .12$	256 ± 3	$0.347 \pm .035$	280 ± 9	$5.178 \pm .443$
11% EDC	17	$5.66 \pm .20$	263 ± 7	$0.346 \pm .031$	256 ± 12	$4.559 \pm .453$
21% EDC	12	$5.44 \pm .19$	253 ± 8	$0.460 \pm .065$	248 ± 12	$8.634 \pm .671$*[#]
35% EDC	24	$4.67 \pm .16$*	234 ± 5*	$1.165 \pm .515$	217 ± 9[#]	$5.188 \pm .448$
		$F_{(3,71)} = 10.6$[a]	$F_{(3,71)} = 4.8$[a]	$F_{(3,71)} = 1.3$	$F_{(3,71)} = 5.4$[a]	$F_{(3,71)} = 13$[a]

[a] Significance at $p < 0.05$. Statistical analysis by one way analysis of variance. Significance of group comparisons used Newman-Keuls post hoc test.

[#] Significantly different relative to 0% EDC control.

*Significantly different relative to all groups.

[b] Values are presented as mean $\pm$ SEM.

[c] A maximum of two pups from a single litter were used for γ-GTP determinations. One unit of γ-GTP is that amount of enzyme that will liberate 1 μmol of *p*-nitroaniline/min/mg protein.

tion of the 21% EDC diet increased γ-GTP activity in the liver in the offspring, whereas the 35% EDC did not seem to have an effect. A previous study, however, had shown γ-GTP to be elevated in 1-d-old pups.[72] We therefore examined the effects of the *in utero* administration of alcohol on the ontogenic development of γ-GTP. The effects of the *in utero* administration of alcohol on the ontogenesis of liver γ-GTP from gestational age 18–120 d after birth were determined.

Figure 1 shows the effects of the *in utero* administration of alcohol on the ontogenic development of the soluble form of γ-GTP in rat liver from birth to day 120. γ-GTP activity in liver of LC and 0% EDC rats appears to reach a maximum at birth and then decreases toward the adult level. Adult levels are approx one-tenth that of the newborn. This pattern is similar to that observed by Igarashi et al., who have shown that in liver γ-GTP activity increases until birth and then immediately following birth enzyme activity decreases toward adult levels.[28] Also seen in Fig. 1 are the effects of various doses of alcohol on the ontogenesis of γ-GTP. Treatment of the mothers with 21% EDC and 35% EDC diets produces a transitory elevation in γ-GTP activity, which then decreases toward the control levels.

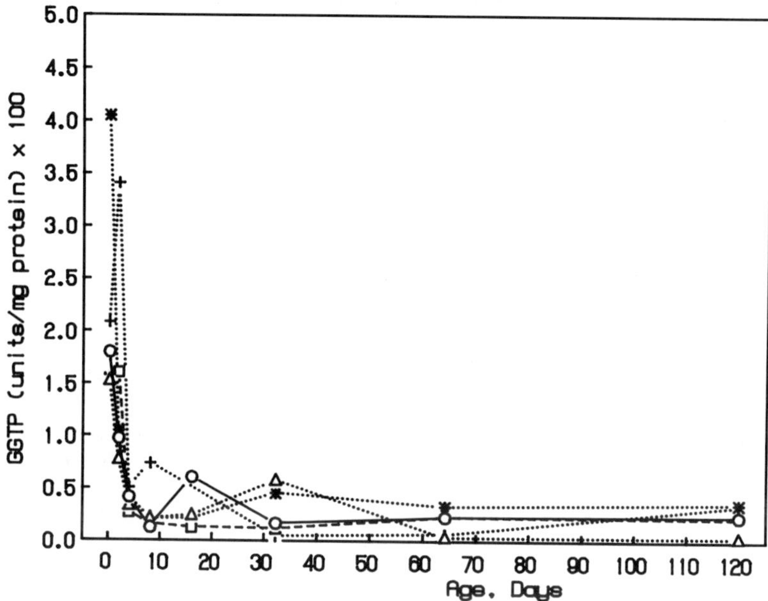

Fig. 1. The effects of *in utero* administration of alcohol on ontogenesis of soluble liver γ-GTP from birth to day 120. γ-GTP activity was determined by the method described by Rosalki and Tarlow.[77] Mothers were treated with various doses of alcohol in liquid diets as described in text. Δ = 0% EDC; + = 35% EDC; ○ = LC; □ = 11% EDC; ✱ = 21% EDC.

The effects of the *in utero* administration of alcohol on the deoxycholic acid soluble (membrane bound) fraction of γ-GTP from g18 to day 8 are illustrated in Fig. 2. By and large the same pattern is seen as that of the soluble enzyme in Fig. 1. The 35% EDC diet produces an increase in γ-GTP activity in the pups at g18 and at 1 d of age. We believe that two explanations of the data are possible at this time. The higher doses of alcohol may increase GTP activity as early as g18. An alternative explanation may be that the higher doses of alcohol produce a delay in development of the enzyme. That is, the peak that is normally seen at birth is not seen until day 1. It may be that both phenomena are occurring simultaneously, an increase in γ-GTP activity and a delay in its development. Alcohol may also interfere with the conversion of the fetal form of the enzyme to the adult form of the enzyme.

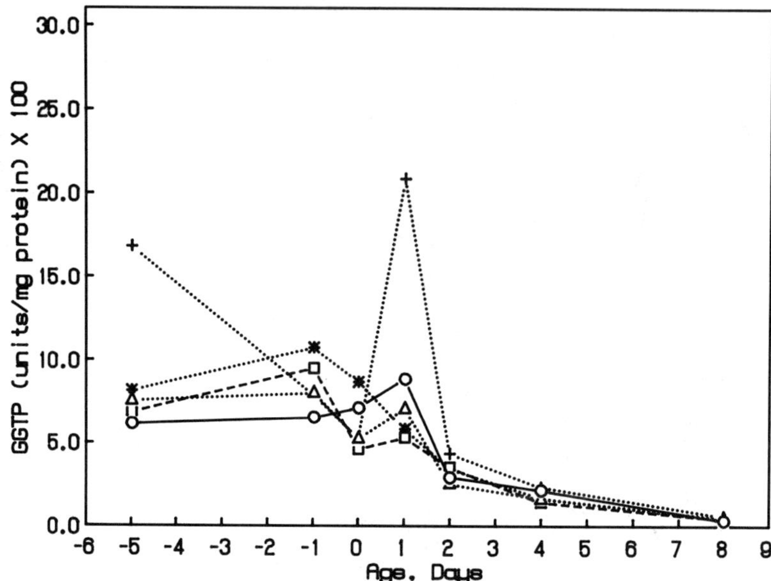

Fig. 2. The effects of *in utero* administration of alcohol on ontogenesis of membrane bound liver γ-GTP from gestational age 18 to day 8. γ-GTP activity was determined by the method described by Rosalki and Tarlow.[77] Mothers were treated with various doses of alcohol in liquid diets as described in text. Pups were taken by cesarean section following anesthesia of mothers with sodium pentobarbital. Δ = 0% EDC; + = 35% EDC; □ = 11% EDC; ○ = LC; ✳ = 21% EDC.

Effects on Isoenzyme Makeup

Electrophoretic examination for γ-GTP isoenzyme forms was performed on serum from neonatal rats (1 d old) that were exposed to alcohol *in utero*.[71] The zymograms of serum from the alcohol exposed neonates were found to have a peak of activity unique to this group.[71]

In an effort to determine if the *in utero* administration of alcohol altered the ratio of fetal to adult forms of the enzyme, the effects of *in utero* administration of alcohol on the isoenzyme makeup at birth and at 4 d of age were determined. An aliquot of the membrane bound enzyme was incubated with a slurry of concanavalin A and then centrifuged. The supernatant was assayed for γ-GTP activity to determine the amount of the adult form of the enzyme. The pellet that contained γ-GTP bound to the concanavalin A was then incubated with a solution of 50 mg/mL of glucopyranoside and centrifuged. The supernatant was assayed to determine the amount of the fetal form of the enzyme. In the LC group, the fetal form of the γ-GTP represented 65% of the total liver enzyme activity at birth. The *in utero* exposure of the pups to the 35% EDC diet did not alter the isoenzyme makeup of the liver. At 4 d of age the percentage of fetal form decreased to 58% in both the control and in the alcohol-treated animals.

More studies must be conducted to better understand the effects of the *in utero* administration of alcohol on γ-GTP. Certainly the question of what is γ-GTP doing is the fetus has to be addressed as well as how does the presence of alcohol alter this function.

Acknowledgments

Work cited from the author's laboratory was supported in part by NIH grant AA06759 and MBRS program grant RR08139.

References

[1] K. L. Jones and D. W. Smith (1973) Recognition of the fetal alcohol syndrome in early infancy. *Lancet* **ii,** 999–1001.

[2] K. L. Jones, D. W. Smith, A. P. Streissguth, and N. C. Myrianthopoulos (1974) Outcome in offspring of chronic alcoholic women. *Lancet* **1,** 1076–1078.

[3] K. L. Jones, D. W. Smith, C. N. Ulleland, and A. P. Streissguth (1973) Pattern of malformation in offspring of chronic alcoholic mothers. *Lancet* **i,** 1268–1271.

[4] J. W. Hanson, A. P. Streissguth, and D. W. Smith (1978) The Effects of moderate alcohol consumption during pregnancy on fetal growth and morphogenesis. *J. Pediatrics* **92,** 457–460.

[5] E. L. Abel, and R. J. Sokol (1986) Incidence of fetal alcohol syndrome and economic impact of FAS-related anomalies. *Drug Alcohol Depend.* **19,** 51–70.

[6] A. P. Streissguth, C. S. Herman, and D. W. Smith (1978) Intelligence, behavior, and dysmorphogenesis in the fetal alcohol syndrome: A report on 20 patients. *J. Pediatrics* **92,** 363–367.

[7] P. Selvaraj and K. A. Balasubramanian (1983) Soluble forms of γ-glutamyl-transferase in human adult liver, fetal liver, and primary hepatoma compared. *Clin. Chem.* **29,** 90–95.

[8] S. J. Sulakhe, and W. W. Lautt (1985) The activity of hepatic γ-glutamyl-transpeptidase in various animal species. *Comp. Biochem. Physiol. [C]* **82B,** 263,264.

[9] Z. O. Echetebu and D. W. Moss (1982) Multiple forms of human γ-glutamyl-transferase. *Enzyme* **27,** 1–8.

[10] E. Kottgen, W. Reutter, and W. Gerok (1978) Induction and superinduction of sialylation of membrane bound γ-glutamyltransferase during liver regeneration. *Eur. J. Biochem.* **82,** 279–284.

[11] L. Lisy, F. Stastny, and Z. Lodin (1979) Regional distribution of membrane-bound γ-glutamyl transpeptidase activity in mouse brain: Comparison with rabbit brain. *Neurochem. Res.* **4,** 747–753.

[12] E. Reyes and D. T. Barela (1980) Isolation and purification of multiple forms of γ-glutamyl transpeptidase from rat brain. *Neurochem. Res.* **5,** 159–170.

[13] E. Reyes and G. C. Palmer (1976) Biochemical localization of γ-glutamyl transpeptidase within cellular elements of the rat cerebral cortex. *Res. Comm. Chem. Pathol. Pharmacol.* **14,** 759–762.

[14] P. Selvaraj and K. A. Balasubramanian (1983) Comparison of electrophoretic and immunological properties of gamma-glutamyl transpeptidase from human adult liver, fetal liver and primary hepatoma. *Enzyme* **30,** 21–28.

[15] P. Selvaraj and K. A. Balasubramanian (1985) Comparative structural and lectin-binding studies on γ-glutamyltransferase from human adult liver, fetal liver and primary hepatoma. *Eur. J. Biochem.* **153,** 485–490.

[16] A. Szewczuk (1966) A soluble form of γ-glutamyl transpeptidase in human tissues. *Clin. Chim. Acta* **14,** 608–614.

[17] E. Reyes and E. E. Prather (1976) Subcellular and regional localization of γ-glutamyl transpeptidase in sheep brain. *Neurochem. Res.* **1,** 251–259.

[18] E. Kottgen, W. Reutter, and W. Gerok (1976) Two different gamma-glutamyltransferases during development of liver and small intestine: A fetal (sialo-) and an adult (asialo-) glycoprotein. *Biochem. Biophys. Res. Commun.* **72,** 61–66.

[19] E. Reyes, L. Lewis, and L. Saland (1980) Isolation of γ-glutamyl transpeptidase from glial cells. *Proc. West. Pharmacol. Soc.* **23,** 381–383.

[20] D. Menard, C. Malo, and R. Calvert (1981) Development of γ-glutamyl-transpeptidase activity in mouse small intestine: Influence of cortisone and thyroxine. *Biol. Neonate* **40,** 70–77.

[21] N. Tateishi, T. Higashi, K. Nakashima, and Y. Sakamoto (1980) Nutritional significance of increase in γ-glutamyltransferase in mouse liver before birth. *J. Nutr.* **110,** 409–415.

[22] A. Zorzano, L. Ruiz Del Arbol, and E. Herrera (1989) Effect of liver disorders on ethanol elimination and alcohol and aldehyde dehydrogenase activities in liver and erythrocytes. *Clin. Sci.* **76,** 51–57.

[23] A. Meister (1983) Metabolism and transport of glutathione and other γ-glutamyl compounds, in *Functions of Glutathione Biochemical, Physiological, Toxicological & Clinical Aspects.* A. Larsson, S. Orrenius, A. Holmgren, and B. Mannervik, eds. Raven, New York, pp. 1–11.

[24] A. Meister (1985) The fall and rise of cellular glutathione levels: Enzyme-based approaches. *Curr. Topics Cell Reg.* **26,** 383–394.

[25] U. Stenius, K. Rubin, D. Gullberg, and J. Hogberg (1990) γ-Glutamyl-transpeptidase-positive rat hepatocytes are protected from GSH depletion, oxidative stress and reversible alterations of collagen receptors. *Carcinogenesis* **11**, 69–73.

[26] L. Orning and S. Hammarstrom (1982) Kinetics of the conversion of leukotriene C by γ-glutamyl transpeptidase. *Biochem. Biophys. Res. Commun.* **4**, 1304–1309.

[27] P. M. Iannaccone and J. Koizum (1983) Pattern and rate of disappearance of gamma-glutamyl transpeptidase activity in fetal and neonatal rat liver. *J. Histochem. Cytochem.* **31**, 1312–1316.

[28] T. Igarashi, T. Satoh, K. Ueno, and H. Kitagaua (1981) Changes of gamma-glutamyltranspeptidase activity in the rat during development and comparison of the fetal liver, placental and adult liver enzymes. *Life Sci.* **29**, 483–491.

[29] H. Ishii, S. Yasuraoka, Y. Shigeta, S. Takagi, and T. Kamiya (1978) Hepatic and intestinal gamma-glutamyl transpeptidase activity: Its activation by chronic ethanol administration. *Life Sci.* **23**, 1393–1398.

[30] V. Lisy, F. Stastny, and J. Sedlacek (1981) Developmental formation and cortisol regulation of gamma-glutamyl transpeptidase in brain and spinal cord of chick embryo. *Dev. Neurosci.* **4**, 401–407.

[31] F. Stastny and V. Lisy (1981) Cortisol regulation of gamma-glutamyl transpeptidase in liver, choroid plexus, blood plasma and cerebrospinal fluid of developing chick embryo. *Dev. Neurosci.* **4**, 408–415.

[32] V. Lisy, F. Stastny, and Z. Lodin (1983) Gamma-glutamyl transpeptidase activity in isolated cells and in various regions of the mouse brain during early development and aging. *Physiologia Bohemoslovaca* **32**, 1–10.

[33] K. Rambabu, T. N. Pattabiraman, and A. P. Rao (1980) Gamma glutamyl transpeptidase in amniotic fluid and blood during pregnancy. *Indian J. Med. Res.* **71**, 738–741.

[34] O. Yalcin, E. Sürmen, and F. Eryürek (1989) Activity of gamma-glutamyl transpeptidase in human fetal membranes. *Biol. Neonate* **56**, 1–5.

[35] J. D. Schulman, S. I. Goodman, J. W. Mace, A. D. Patrick, F. Tietze, and E. J. Butler (1975) Glutathionuria: Inborn error of metabolism due to tissue deficiency of gamma-glutamyl transpeptidase. *B. B. R. C.* **65**, 68–74.

[36] P. N. Konrad, F. Richards, W. N. Valentine, and D. E. Paglia (1972) γ-Glutamyl-cysteine synthetase deficiency: A case of hereditary hemolytic anemia. *N. Engl. J. Med.* **286**, 557–561.

[37] D. Acheampong-Mensah (1976) Activity of γ-glutamyl transpeptidase in serum of patients receiving anticonvulsant or anticoagulant therapy. *Clin. Biochem.* **9**, 67–70.

[38] Y. Mochizuki and K. Furukawa (1983) Histochemical investigation of hepatic gamma-glutamyl transpeptidase of rats treated with high dose of phenobarbital. *Acta Histochem. Cytochem.* **16**, 155–162.

[39] D. Ratanasavanh, A. Tazi, M. M. Galteau, and G. Siest (1979) Localization of gamma-glutamyltransferase in subcellular fractions of rat and rabbit liver: Effect of phenobarbital. *Biochem. Pharmacol.* **28,** 1363–1365.

[40] I. Cepelak and B. Straus (1983) Effect of phenobarbital on gamma-glutamyltransferase activity in serum and liver of rats. *Acta Pharm. Jugosl.* **33,** 273–277.

[41] E. Ivanov, L. Krustev, D. Adjarov, K. Chernev, I. Apostolov, P. Dimtrov, E. Drenska, M. Stefanova, and V. Pramatarova (1976) Studies on the mechanism of the changes in serum and liver γ-glutamyl transpeptidase activity II. Experimental hexachlorobenzene prophyria in rabbits. *Enzyme* **21,** 8–20.

[42] D. Ratanasavanh, J. Magdalou, B. Antoine, M.-M. Galteau, and G. Siest (1981) Gamma-glutamyltransferase activity of liver plasma membranes in phenobarbital treated rabbits. *Pharmacol. Res. Comm.* **13,** 909–919.

[43] J. Sano, H. Kawada, N. Yamaguchi, M. Kawakita, and K. Kobayashi (1981) Effects of phenytoin on serum γ-glutamyl transpeptidase activity. *Epilepsia* **22,** 331–338.

[44] S. J. Sulakhe and W. W. Lautt (1987) A characterization of γ-glutamyl-transpeptidase in normal perinatal, premalignant and malignant rat liver. *Int. J. Biochem.* **19,** 23–32.

[45] N. Sawabu, M. Nakagen, M. Yoneda, H. Makino, S. Kameda, K. Kobayashi, N. Hattori, and M. Ishi (1978) Novel γ-glutamyl transpeptidase isoenzyme specifically found in sera of patients with hepatocellular carcinoma. *Gann* **69,** 601–605.

[46] P. J. Dierickx (1981) Urinary gamma-glutamyl transferase as an indicator of acute nephrotoxicity in rats. *Arch. Toxicol.* **47,** 209–215.

[47] D. Adjarov, E. Ivanov, and D. Keremidchiev (1982) Gamma-glutamyl transferase: A sensitive marker in experimental hexachlorobenzene intoxication. *Toxicology* **23,** 73–77.

[48] E. Reyes (1980) The effects of alcohol on γ-glutamyl transpeptidase: A membrane bound enzyme. *Proc. West. Pharmacol. Soc.* **23,** 433–436.

[49] E. Reyes and W. D. Cooke (1980) Effects of alcohol on brain γ-glutamyl transpeptidase, in *Alcoholism: A Perspective.* F. S. Messiha and G. S. Tyner, eds. PJD, Westbury, NY, pp. 433–440.

[50] D. E. Freer and B. E. Statland (1977) Effects of ethanol (0.75 g/kg body weight) on the activities of selected enzymes in sera of healthy young adults: 2 interindividual variations in response of γ-glutamyltransferase to repeated ethanol challenges. *Clin. Chem.* **23,** 2099–2101.

[51] M. Nishimura and R. Teschke (1983) Alcohol and gamma-glutamyltransferase. *Klin Wochenschr.* **61,** 265–275.

[52] E. Reyes (1985) Role of γ-glutamyl transpeptidase in alcoholism. *Neurobehav. Toxicol. Teratol.* **7,** 171–175.

[53] E. Reyes and W. R. Miller (1980) Serum gamma-glutamyl transpeptidase as a diagnostic aid in problem drinkers. *Addict. Behav.* **5,** 59–65.

[54] E. Reyes, W. R. Miller, C. A. Taylor, and C. T. Spalding (1978) The activity of γ-glutamyl transpeptidase in the serum of problem drinkers. *Proc. West. Pharmacol. Soc.* **21,** 289–297.

[55] R. Teschke, J. Rauen, and G. Strohmeyer (1980) Alcoholic liver disease: Assessment of various stages by determination of the adult and fetal form of gamma-glutamyltransferase (GGT) activity in serum. *Inser* **95,** 215–220.

[56] J. Morland, N. E. Huseby, M. Sjoblom, and J. H. Stromme (1977) Does chronic alcohol consumption really induce hepatic microsomal gamma-glutamyltransferase activity? *Biochem. Biophys. Res. Commun.* **77,** 1060–1066.

[57] P. J. M. J. Kok, B. Seidel, H. C. Holtkamp, and J. Huisman (1981) A new procedure for the visualization of multiple forms of gamma-glutamyl transferase (GGT): Results in normals, patients receiving enzyme inducing drugs and patients having liver parenchymal lesions. *Clin. Chim. Acta* **214,** 642–645.

[58] H. Ishii, Y. Ebihara, F. Okuno, Y. Munakata, T. Takagi, M. Arai, S. Shigeta, and M. Tsuchiya (1986) γ-Glutamyl transpeptidase activity in liver of alcoholics and its histochemical localization. *Alcohol. Clin. Exp. Res.* **10,** 81–85.

[59] R. Teschke, A. Brand, and G. Strohmeyer (1977) Induction of hepatic microsomal gamma-glutamyltransferase activity following chronic alcohol consumption. *Biochem. Biophys. Res. Commun.* **75,** 718–723.

[60] G. Larsson, C. Ottenblad, L. Hagenfeldt, A. Larsson, and M. Forsgren (1983) Evaluation of serum γ-glutamyl transferase as a screening method for excessive alcohol consumption during pregnancy. *Am. J. Obstet. Gynecol.* **147,** 654–657.

[61] H. Ishii (1988) Alcohol-induced enhancement of intestinal γ-glutamyl transpeptidase activity in rats and humans: A possible role in increased serum γ-glutamyl transpeptidase activity in alcoholics. *Alcohol. Clin. Exp. Res.* **12,** 111–115.

[62] K. Rambabu, Y. Matsuda, and N. Katunuma (1986) Studies on turnover rates of rat γ-glutamyltranspeptidase after chronic ethanol administration in vivo. *Biochem. Med. Metabol. Biol.* **35,** 335–344.

[63] E. Reyes, J. M. Rivera, and L. J. Lewis (1980) The effect of oral alcohol administration on brain γ-glutamyl transpeptidase. *Soc. Neurosci.* **6,** 47 (Abstract).

[64] S. Yamada, J. S. Wilson, and C. S. Lieber (1985) The effects of ethanol and diet on hepatic and serum γ-glutamyltranspeptidase activities in rats. *J. Nutr.* **115,** 1285–1289.

[65] G. Gadeholt, J. Aarbakke, E. Dybing, M. Sjoblom, and J. Morland (1980) Hepatic microsomal drug metabolism, glutamyl transferase activity and in vivo antipyrine half-life in rats chronically fed and ethanol diet, a control diet and a chow diet. *JPET* **213,** 196–203.

[66] H. Speisky and Y. Israel (1990) Gamma-glutamyl transferase ectoactivity in the intact rat liver: Effect of chronic alcohol consumption. *Alcohol* **7,** 339–347.

[67] R. Barouki, N. Perrot, J. Bouguet, M. N. Chobert, V. Toffis, M. Pav-Preux, C. S. Yang, P. Beaune, and J. Hanoune (1989) Glucocorticoid hormones prevent the induction of gamma-glutamyl transpeptidase by ethanol in a rat hepatoma cell line. *Biochem. Pharmacol.* **38,** 677–684.

[68] B. Leluyer, P. Leroux, J. P. Goulle, and J. P. Chabrolle (1987) Gamma glutamyl transferase et syndrome d' alcoolesme foetal. *Bulletin de la Cociete Francaise d'Alcoologie* **9,** 48–52.

[69] K. D. Garcia, J. Wolfe, and E. Reyes (1987) Effect of the *in utero* administration of alcohol on the ontogenic development of gamma glutamyl transpeptidase in brain and liver. *Alcohol. Clin. Exp. Res.* **11,** 209.

[70] K. Garcia, E. Reyes, J. Wolfe, and D. Sandoval (1986) Effects in utero administration of phenobarbitol on gamma glutamyl transferase transpeptidase. *Alcohol* **3,** 153-155.

[71] E. Reyes and R. W. Murray (1985) Gamma glutamyl transpeptidase as a sensitive marker of fetal alcohol exposure. *Neurobehav. Toxicol. Teratol.* **7,** 177–180.

[72] E. Reyes, J. M. Rivera, L. C. Saland, and H. M. Murray (1983) Effects of maternal administration of alcohol on fetal brain development. *Neurobehav. Toxicol. Teratol.* **5,** 263–267.

[73] E. Reyes, J. Wolfe, and M. Marquez (1989) Effects of prenatal alcohol on γ-glutamyl transpeptidase in various brain regions. *Physiol. Behav.* **46,** 49–53.

[74] E. Reyes, J. Wolfe, and D. D. Savage (1988) The effects of prenatal alcohol exposure on radial arm maze performance in adult rats. *Res. Comm. Sub. Abuse* **8,** 165.

[75] R. Glockner and M. Kretzschmar (1989) Perinatal activity of hepatic gamma-glutamyltranspeptidase in rats from large and small litters. *Biol. Neonate* **56,** 237–240.

[76] J. Y. Bertholet (1981) Mating method to produce accurate timed pregnancies. *Lab Animal Sci.* **31,** 180.

[77] S. B. Rosalki and D. Tarlow (1974) Optimized determination of γ-glutamyl-transferase by reaction rate analysis. *Clin. Chem.* **20,** 1121–1124.

[78] O. H. Lowry, N. J. Rosenbrough, A. L. Farr, and R. J. Randall (1951) Protein measurement with folin phenol reagent. *J. Biol. Chem.* **193,** 265–275.

Free Radicals
and Alcohol Liver Injury

Lester A. Reinke
and Paul B. McCay

Introduction

A role for free radicals in the development of alcoholic liver damage has been suspected since the early 1960s, when DiLuzio and associates reported that antioxidants protected rats from fatty liver induced by a large acute dose of ethanol.[1–3] Subsequent investigations from the same group indicated that ethanol administration led to the formation of lipid peroxides in the liver[4] and liver homogenates.[5] Because free radicals have long been known to initiate lipid peroxidation, these early findings indicated that ethanol administration could lead to free radical generation through some undetermined mechanism.

Occasional negative results[6–8] have caused the role of lipid peroxidation in the development of alcoholic liver disease to be controversial. Nevertheless, the results of recent experiments have demonstrated that free radical intermediates are indeed produced after acute and chronic administration of alcohol to experimental animals. In this chapter, evidence supporting ethanol-induced free radical formation in vivo, and possible mechanisms for the generation of these radicals, will be discussed.

From: *Drug and Alcohol Abuse Reviews, Vol. 2: Liver Pathology and Alcohol*
Ed: R. R. Watson ©1991 The Humana Press Inc.

Definition of a Free Radical

A free radical is generally defined as a molecule that contains one or more unpaired electrons. There are many known examples of stable free radicals, such as diphenylpicrylhydrazyl and potassium nitrosodisulfonate (Fremy's salt). However, the presence of unpaired electrons usually confers a large degree of chemical reactivity to the molecule. As a result, most free radicals are highly reactive with a short half-life.

Radicals can be formed through a variety of physical or chemical reactions. In biological systems, many drugs or other xenobiotics can be metabolized to free radical intermediates, which may initiate cellular injury. Although the literature usually focuses on undesirable effects of free radicals, potentially beneficial reactions include antineoplastic[9,10] and antiparasitic[11] actions.

The unpaired electrons are usually visualized as being located in specific regions of a molecule. For this reason, radicals are often spoken of as being "carbon-centered," "oxygen-centered," and so forth, to indicate the localization of the electron.

Detection of Free Radicals

Because of their usually high degree of reactivity, free radicals are difficult to detect directly. This is particularly true in biological systems, where radicals may react with any number of molecules in the cellular milieu to produce a variety of secondary reaction products. However, the most widely used methods to study free radical reactions in biology are based on measurement of products of biological origin, such as intermediates of lipid peroxidation, which may have been formed through such types of reactions. Other evidence may involve altered activity of enzyme systems capable of generating, or catabolizing, free radical intermediates. Specific examples from the alcohol literature will be given in the following section.

In addition, spin trapping techniques and electron paramagnetic resonance have been utilized to directly demonstrate that alcohol administration initiates free radical formation in vivo. This data will be reviewed later in this chapter.

Possible Roles of Oxygen Radicals
in Alcoholic Liver Disease

A role for oxygen radicals in the pathogenesis of alcoholic tissue injury has been indicated in a number of studies. In order to gain an appreciation of this research, it is first necessary to discuss some of the more prominent types of oxygen radicals and means by which they may be formed.

Radicals Derived from Oxygen

Oxygen itself is a diradical, and its reactivity is highly regulated in the body. The normal fate for oxygen is reduction to water by cytochrome oxidase, a process that does not involve any free radical intermediates. However, oxygen can also be metabolized in a series of one-electron reductions, yielding superoxide anion and hydrogen peroxide as intermediates of toxicological concern. Superoxide anion $[O_2(^\cdot)^-]$ is a radical that dismutates to hydrogen peroxide either spontaneously, or as a result of the catalytic action of superoxide dismutase.[12] The superoxide radical has relatively low reactivity, but is nevertheless thought to be an important toxicological intermediate.[13] Hydrogen peroxide $[H_2O_2]$ is a strong oxidant, but its concentration in cells is normally kept low by the actions of catalase and glutathione peroxidase.[14] Many theories of "oxidative stress" propose that more highly reactive free radical metabolites of oxygen, such as the hydroxyl radical [$^\cdot$OH], are formed, and may actually be the cause of tissue damage.

Although the hydroxyl radical could be formed in a variety of chemical reactions, the Haber-Weiss and Fenton reactions have received considerable attention. In the Haber-Weiss reaction, superoxide anion reacts with hydrogen peroxide to form the hydroxyl radical:

$$O_2(^\cdot)^- + H_2O_2 + H^+ \longrightarrow H_2O + O_2 + {}^\cdot OH \tag{1}$$

This reaction is not thought to have great biological significance because its rate is extremely slow in the absence of contaminating trace minerals.

In the Fenton reaction, ferrous ions catalyze the breakdown of hydrogen peroxide to form hydroxyl radicals as one of the products:

$$H_2O_2 + Fe^{2+} + H^+ \longrightarrow H_2O + Fe^{3+} + {}^\cdot OH \tag{2}$$

Ions of certain other transition elements, such as copper, can replace iron in this reaction.

A related reaction sequence that is thought to have great biological relevance is often referred to as the iron-catalyzed Haber-Weiss reaction. In this scheme, ferric iron is reduced by superoxide anion, and the resulting ferrous iron then reacts with hydrogen peroxide to form the hydroxyl radi-

Table 1

Possible Sources of Hepatic Oxygen Radical Formation
Following Acute or Chronic Ethanol Exposure[a]

Enhanced activity of cellular systems capable of generating oxygen radicals:

    Isozymes of cytochrome P-450[20–23]
    NADPH-cytochrome P-450 reductase[19,104]
    Conversion of xanthine dehydrogenase to xanthine oxidase[35,36]
    "Leakage" during mitochondrial electron transport[39,40]
    Increased "redox cycling"[31]
    Phagocytic migration[45,46]

Increased iron-dependent radical generation, as a result of:

    Increased hepatic iron stores[47,48]
    Release of iron from storage sites[51,52]

Decreased capacity of cellular "antioxidants":

    Glutathione[56–58,60,77]
    Superoxide dismutase[67,68,75]
    Catalase[66,68,69]
    α-Tocopherol[62,63]
    Vitamin A[64,65]

[a]References to representative studies are set in superscript.

cal and regenerate ferric iron. Because hydrogen peroxide is formed by dismutation of superoxide, this mechanism has the potential of producing large amounts of hydroxyl radicals when superoxide is generated continually. The relationships that exist among oxidative tissue injury and iron or related transition metals have been recently reviewed by Halliwell and Gutteridge.[15,16]

Evidence Associating Alcohol Exposure with Oxygen Radical Generation

Oxygen radicals associated with alcohol administration have never been directly detected in vivo using spin trapping and electron paramagnetic resonance techniques. Nevertheless, there are numerous reports in the literature that strongly suggest an association between alcohol use and oxygen radical formation. The major proposed sources for such oxygen radicals are outlined in Table 1, and related concepts are discussed in the following sections. The table is not intended to be exhaustive, and reviews are cited where it is feasible.

Activity of Enzymes that Lead
to Oxygen Radical Generation

Monooxygenase Enzymes. The monooxygenase enzymes of the endoplasmic reticulum are thought to be among the major intracellular sources of oxygen radicals. These enzymes have important roles in the oxidation and reduction of many endogenous and exogenous compounds, and utilize the cytochrome P-450 enzymes as terminal oxidases. Hydrogen peroxide formation by the microsomal enzymes has been known for many years.[17] The cytochrome P-450 enzymes are now thought to be the major sources of this hydrogen peroxide, which most likely arises after dismutation of superoxide anion released from an oxygenated, ferrous heme iron intermediate.[18] In addition, the flavoprotein NADPH-cytochrome P-450 reductase, which transfers electrons from NADPH to the cytochrome P-450 enzymes, has also been shown to be a source of superoxide anions.[19]

Chronic ethanol administration was first reported to induce the activity of the hepatic drug-metabolizing enzymes by Rubin and Lieber in 1968,[20] and this finding has been confirmed in many laboratories. More recently, a unique ethanol-inducible isozyme of cytochrome P-450 has been characterized from livers of various species, including humans.[21–23] Because microsomes from ethanol-treated rats have been shown to generate superoxide anion and hydrogen peroxide at higher rates than microsomes from pair-fed controls,[24,25] it is conceivable that similar reactions could occur in the intact liver. Extensive studies from the laboratories of Cederbaum[19,26–28] and Ingelman-Sundberg[25,29,30] have produced convincing evidence that hydroxyl radicals produced by liver microsomes have a role in the oxidation of ethanol and other xenobiotics, and that ethanol feeding stimulates this process. In addition, rates of hydroxyl radical generation during redox cycling of paraquat and related compounds may also be increased by ethanol feeding.[31]

The induction of the monooxygenase enzymes by ethanol can also increase the hepatotoxicity of drugs or other chemicals that are metabolized to reactive intermediates.[32,33] Some of these reactive metabolites could be free radicals, but very few studies have been performed to test whether ethanol exposure increases free radical formation that is detectable by electron paramagnetic resonance methods. In one such report, ethanol feeding was found to increase rates of trichloromethyl radical formation from carbon tetrachloride in isolated microsomes and in vivo.[34] Ethanol also markedly potentiated the hepatotoxicity of carbon tetrachloride, but this effect was not well correlated with the rates of trichloromethyl radical formation,[34] suggesting that other biological effects of ethanol were also involved.

Xanthine Oxidase. Xanthine oxidase is another enzyme that is capable of forming both superoxide anion and hydrogen peroxide under appropriate conditions. Oei[35] and Sultatos[36] have demonstrated that some of this enzyme is converted from its normal dehydrogenase form to its oxidase form following ethanol administration. During ethanol intoxication, acetaldehyde or xanthine and hypoxanthine could serve as substrates for the intracellular generation of superoxide anion and/or hydrogen peroxide by xanthine oxidase.[35–37] This topic is reviewed in greater detail in another chapter of this volume.

Mitochondrial Electron Transport Chain. The mitochondrial electron transport chain normally exhibits tight coupling between electron flow and energy production, but small amounts of superoxide anion and hydrogen peroxide can be formed at various steps.[38] In the case of mitochondrial injury, this "leakage" of electrons may be enhanced. In this respect, it is interesting to note that chronic ethanol exposure has been shown to cause damage to mitochondria[39] and stimulate mitochondrial superoxide formation.[40] Mitochondrial lipid peroxidation has also been reported after acute ethanol intoxication.[41,42]

Phagocytic White Blood Cells. Phagocytic white blood cells infiltrate the liver in alcoholic liver disease,[43] and these cells are well known for their ability to produce superoxide anion during a "respiratory burst."[44] It has also been shown that ethanol metabolism by hepatocytes seems to result in the formation of a chemoattractant substance for the white blood cells, which may also involve the participation of oxygen radicals.[45,46] This topic is also reviewed in another section of this volume.

Roles of Iron

Because of the well-known role of iron to catalyze the generation of hydroxyl radicals,[15,16,28] observations that alcohol feeding increases hepatic iron stores,[47,48] or that iron loading increases the toxicity of alcohol,[49,50] are often interpreted as evidence that oxygen radicals, such as the hydroxyl radical, could be generated at unusually high rates.

Iron is normally found in storage forms such as ferritin, in which it is chemically nonreactive. For this reason, the mobilization of iron from its storage sites during ethanol intoxication becomes an important consideration, and this topic has been recently reviewed by Shaw.[51,52]

Iron may also participate in free radical reactions in mechanisms that are not related to hydroxyl radical production. For example, iron-dependent lipid peroxidation has been postulated to occur through complexes of iron and oxygen called perferryl $[Fe^{2+}O_2]$ or ferryl $[Fe^{2+}O]$ ions, which could participate in the direct generation of alkoxy radicals.[53]

Sinaceur et al. have demonstrated that the iron-chelating agent deferoxamine (desferrioxamine) decreased the rate of ethanol clearance in alcohol-treated rats.[54] This effect was interpreted as evidence that ethanol oxidation dependent on the formation of hydroxyl radicals had been interrupted.[54] Deferoxamine also diminished the degree of lipid peroxidation in the cerebellum following an acute ethanol dose,[55] but a protective effect of iron chelation was not observed in the liver.

Changes in Cellular Antioxidants

Changes in certain cellular systems, which can be broadly grouped as "antioxidants," have been cited as evidence that alcohol initiates free radical events in the liver. The first evidence is that free radicals are expected to react readily with thiols and other natural antioxidants, and should then cause decreases in their concentration. Acute alcohol administration has long been known to lower hepatic levels of glutathione,[56–58,60] although increases may occur after chronic alcohol administration.[59] Increased biliary concentrations of glutathione dissulfide following ethanol feeding have been interpreted as evidence for "oxidative stress."[61] These and other interactions between ethanol and glutathione are reviewed elsewhere in this volume. Alcohol administration has also been reported to decrease the hepatic concentrations of α-tocopherol[62,63] and vitamin A,[64,65] vitamins that are thought to have roles in protection of cells from radical-induced injury. In addition to possible radical-induced depletion, alcohol may interfere with the normal biosynthesis or metabolism of these natural antioxidants, thereby rendering cells more susceptible to oxidative damage.

Alcohol administration to experimental animals has also been reported to affect the hepatic activities of some forms of superoxide dismutase,[66–68,75] catalase,[66–69] and glutathione peroxidase.[68,70,71] Although increases in the activity of some of these enzymes have been observed in some studies, decreased activities have been more commonly reported. Because alcohol appears to increase the hepatic generation of toxic metabolites of oxygen, as discussed in an earlier section, unchanged or decreased activity of the enzyme systems that degrade superoxide anion and hydrogen peroxide could further predispose the liver to oxidative damage.

Lipid Peroxidation

Lipid peroxidation is thought to occur subsequent to the interaction of free radicals with polyunsaturated fatty acids in biological membranes. In this process, a radical abstracts a hydrogen atom from a methylene carbon between two unconjugated double bonds, forming a secondary carbon-centered radical [R-C(·)H-R'] from the fatty acid. Subsequent reactions include rearrangement of the fatty acid chain to form a conjugated diene, and addition of oxygen to form a hydroperoxy radical [R-COO·]. This series of reactions is propagated by continued hydrogen atom abstraction by both the primary and secondary radicals, and results in the formation of a variety of carbon-centered and oxygen-centered radicals. Fragments of the fatty acid chains may be further metabolized to low mol wt alkanes and aldehydes. When lipid peroxidation is extensive, widespread damage to cellular membranes, proteins, and organelles can occur.[72,73]

Many of the studies which have implicated free radicals in deleterious effects of alcohol have utilized "lipid peroxidation" to indicate free radical generation. There are many reports that alcohol increases levels of malondialdehyde,[2,37,41,74,75] conjugated dienes,[76–78] volatile hydrocarbons such as ethane and pentane,[79–82] loss of polyunsaturated fatty acids,[77,83] or chemiluminescence[24] in various experimental designs. Evidence of this type has been the topic of several recent reviews,[56,84,85] and is discussed in greater detail elsewhere in this volume.

Exerimental Protection
or Potentiation of Alcohol Toxicity

As discussed in preceding sections, alcohol has been shown to affect cellular enzymes and antioxidants in ways that are consistent with free radical-induced mechanisms. This relationship has also been studied by experimentally altering these cellular systems and then assessing the effects on alcohol toxicity.

For example, when hepatic glutathione concentrations were experimentally depleted by the administration of phorone,[86] enhanced toxicity of ethanol, indicated by increased release of liver enzymes from perfused livers, was observed. Conversely, when rats were pretreated with cysteine, mercaptopropionylglycine, or methionine, alcohol-induced toxicity was antagonized.[77,87,88] These data give additional support to a protective role of glutathione and related thiols against alcohol toxicity, which could involve free radical intermediates.

As indicated in an earlier section, the first evidence that ethanol might cause free radical formation in the liver was that antioxidants prevented the development of fatty liver from an acute dose of ethanol.[1-3] This experimental result has been confirmed and extended through the use of a number of different types of antioxidants, including coenzyme Q,[89,90] and various synthetic products.[65,91,92]

Relationship to Hypoxic Liver Damage

Several laboratories have reported increased rates of hepatic oxygen uptake following acute[93] or chronic[94,95] ethanol administration. When oxygen concentrations and the pyridine nucleotide oxidation-reduction state were measured from the surface of perfused rat livers, alcohol was found to increase the oxygen gradient across the liver lobule.[96] Tissue damage, evidenced by "blebbing," was observed in the perivenous region of livers from ethanol-treated rats when oxygen delivery was further decreased by lowering the perfusion flowrate.[96] Yamada et al. have also found that ethanol feeding enhanced lipid peroxidation following hepatic ischemia.[74]

The relationship between hypoxia and ethanol has been studied further by Younes and Strubelt. These investigators have found that hypoxia increased ethanol-induced lipid peroxidation in perfused livers, and that the infusion of superoxide dismutase, catalase, deferoxamine, and allopurinol all had protective effects.[97-99] These data support a protective effect of allopurinol against alcohol toxicity in laboratory rats,[37,55] and provide additional evidence that oxygen radicals, perhaps related to xanthine oxidase activity, could have a role in initiating tissue damage. The relationship between hypoxia and ethanol-induced liver injury bears many similarities to the model of ischemia-reperfusion injury developed by McCord and associates,[100] in which oxygen radicals appear to have important pathological roles.

Limitations of Indirect Evidence
for Alcohol-Induced Radical Generation

Experimental results outlined earlier, which suggest the participation of free radicals in cellular toxicity, are widely employed because they are usually relatively simple, or can be conducted with instruments normally found in the scientific laboratory. Although these approaches provide valuable data, caution must be observed in interpreting the results. For example, lipid peroxidation is a natural consequence of cell death, so the detection of malondialdehyde does not necessarily indicate that free radicals are being actively generated by a metabolic process in living cells. Although deferoxamine is an efficient iron chelating agent, its protective effects could conceivably be explained by interactions with superoxide anion[101] or hydroxyl radicals.[102] In addition, deferoxamine can be oxidized to a nitroxide radical that has been shown to inactivate alcohol dehydrogenase.[103]

It should be noted that there are many studies that have failed to show associations between alcohol use and lipid peroxidation, glutathione, and so on, or that acute and chronic ethanol administration may produce opposite effects. These contradictory reports are presumed to be related to differences in methodology or experimental design, and have not been discussed in the preceding sections. Complex relationships that exist among alcohol exposure and other experimental variables, such as the strain of animal or the diet,[104] require that great care is used in interpretation of data.

Even if radicals are formed, these indirect methods do not necessarily indicate what type of radicals are present, or their relative rates of formation. Because of these limitations, many investigators have begun to utilize methods in which free radicals can be directly detected. Electron paramagnetic resonance and spin trapping methods have provided a means of directly demonstrating that ethanol administration initiates free radical reactions in vivo.

Electron Paramagnetic Resonance Spectroscopy

General Considerations

Electron paramagnetic resonance (EPR) spectroscopy, which is often referred to as electron spin resonance (ESR) spectroscopy, is a magnetic resonance technique that allows the direct study of certain paramagnetic species. The method depends on the interaction of the magnetic moment of an unpaired electron spinning on its axis with a large, external, homogeneous magnetic field. The electron will align either with, or against, the external field, and these two orientations are not of equal energy. If electromagnetic radiation is applied at a frequency that corresponds to the energy separation of the two levels, energy is absorbed or emitted by the electron, allowing transitions from one energy level to another. The absorption or emission of energy is detected by the EPR spectrometer as the magnetic field is varied.

The electron also interacts with the nucleus of the atom. When the nucleus also possesses magnetic spin, the interaction of the magnetic spins of the electron and nucleus gives rise to multiple spectral lines, which may serve to identify the free radical species that is present. Thus, EPR spectroscopy is a valuable method for the study of certain types of chemical systems in which reasonably stable free radicals are produced. In addition, the height (intensity) of the spectral lines is proportional to the number of unpaired electrons in the sample, which allows comparison of free radical formation in different experimental designs.

The high reactivity of most radical species in solution does not permit their direct detection by EPR. This problem has been overcome, in part, by the development of the spin trapping technique in the late 1960s.

Spin Trapping

Spin trapping is a technique whereby a short-lived reactive free radical is trapped through an addition reaction to form a more persistent radical, referred to as a spin adduct:

$$R^{\bullet} + \text{Spin Trap} \longrightarrow \text{Spin Adduct}$$

The usefulness of spin trapping requires that the spin trap be stable under conditions of the reaction in which the radical is generated; that there is a favorable rate of reaction between the radical and the spin trap under the test conditions; and that the spin adduct is sufficiently stable to allow for its detection by EPR analysis. Interactions between the magnetic spins of the unpaired electron and nuclei in the spin trap result in unique spectral lines that may help to identify the initial, nonpersistent radical that has been trapped.

The most common spin traps presently in use have nitrone or nitroso functionalities. In general, the nitrones have proven to be more useful for biological applications, because the nitroso compounds tend to be photochemically and thermally unstable.[105] The structures of spin trapping agents that have proven to be useful in studies with alcohol are shown in Fig. 1.

The free electron of the spin adduct is resonance stabilized by the nitrogen and oxygen atoms of the nitroxide function. The EPR spectrum of

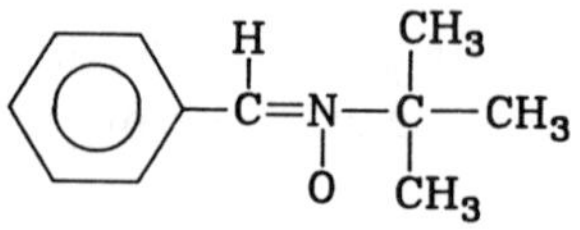

I

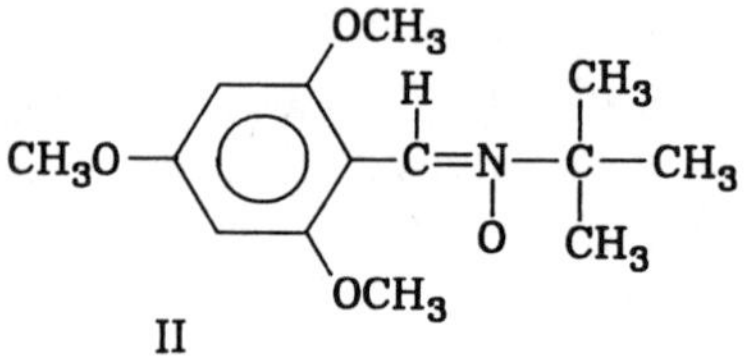

II

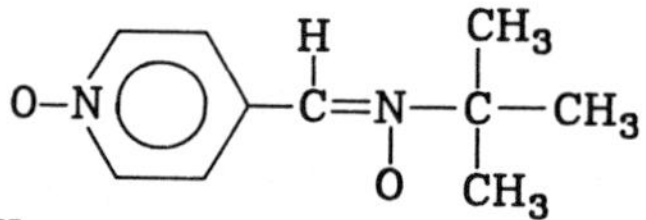

III

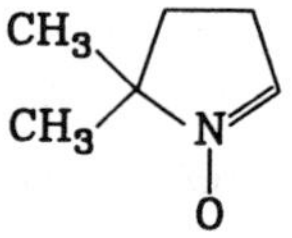

IV

Fig. 1. Spin traps used in alcohol studies. The chemical names of the spin traps, their abbreviations, and representative references for their use in alcohol studies, are as follows: I. α-Phenyl-*N*-*t*-butylnitrone, PBN.[116,127] II. α-2,4,6-Trimethoxyphenyl-*N*-*t*-butylnitrone, MO$_3$PBN.[116] III. α-(4-Pyridyl 1-oxide)-*N*-*t*-butylnitrone, POBN.[115,129] IV. 5,5-Dimethylpyrolline-*N*-oxide, DMPO.[118,127]

a nitrone spin adduct would be expected to consist of at least six spectral lines, because of interactions between the unpaired electron and nuclei present in the spin trap. These concepts are illustrated in Fig. 2, which indicates the structure of the 1-hydroxyethyl spin adduct of the spin trap PBN. The nitrogen atom of the nitroxide function possesses a nuclear spin equal to 1, and would split the signal of the free electron into a triplet. This splitting, measured in Gauss, is termed the nitrogen hyperfine splitting constant, a_N (Fig. 2). In addition, the β-hydrogen, with a spin of 1/2, will split each of the spectral lines, and the distance between the peaks is termed the β-hydrogen hyperfine splitting constant, a_H. The values for a_N and a_H are in many cases unique for a type of spin adduct, and may help to assign the identity of the radical that has been trapped. The hyperfine splitting constants are also affected by the polarity of the solvent. An extensive listing of hyperfine splitting constants for commonly studied spin adducts in different solvents has been published.[106]

Application to Biological Problems

As stated earlier, free radicals are often not sufficiently stable in solution to permit their direct measurement by EPR methods. This problem is accentuated in biological systems, where radical intermediates

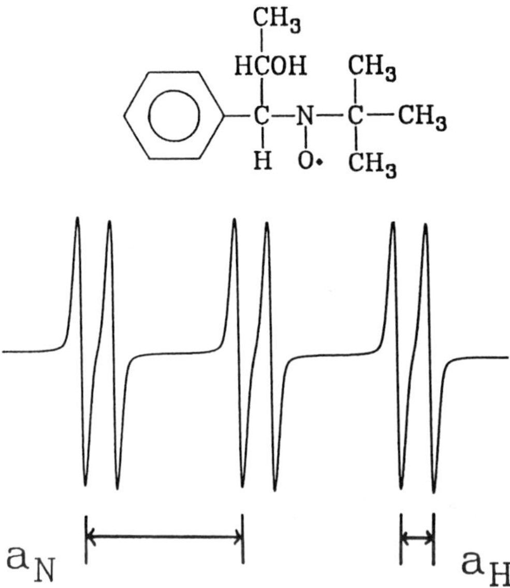

Fig. 2. Structure of the 1-hydroxyethyl radical adduct of PBN and a representative EPR spectrum. The chemical structure is the 1-hydroxyethyl radical adduct of PBN, with the unpaired electron indicated on the nitrone function. Measurements of the hyperfine splitting constants for nitrogen (a_N) and the β-hydrogen (a_H) are indicated on the EPR spectrum shown. Note that four measurements for a_N and three measurements for a_H can be obtained from each spectrum. The spectrum shown is a computer simulation of the 1-hydroxyethyl radical adduct of PBN in water, using hyperfine splitting constants of 16.1 Gauss and 3.3 Gauss for a_N and a_H, respectively.

may be formed in a rich milieu of organic molecules with which they can react quickly. In addition, cells contain a variety of natural antioxidants, such as vitamin E or glutathione, which serve to react with, and detoxify, free radicals.

For these reasons, spin trapping has been a particularly useful method to study free radicals in subcellular fractions, whole cells, and even in living animals. The best example is probably that of halogenated hydrocarbons such as carbon tetrachloride. The trichloromethyl radical and carbon dioxide anion radical have both been proven to be metabolites of carbon tetrachloride in vitro and in vivo through the use of spin trapping experiments.[107–110] Various biological applications of the spin trapping technique have been recently reviewed.[105,111–113]

Radicals Derived from Ethanol

1-Hydroxyethyl Radical Formation by Liver Microsomes

When hepatic microsomes are incubated with ethanol, NADPH, and appropriate spin trapping agents, carbon-centered spin adducts can be detected by EPR analysis of the incubation systems.[114–119] An example of these results is shown in Fig. 3. In this experiment, microsomes were incubated with ethanol and the spin trapping agent phenyl-*N-t*-butylnitrone (PBN), and the reaction mixture was then extracted with toluene. In order to prove the identity of this radical, 1-^{13}C-ethanol was used in the incubation system. The resulting EPR spectrum contained twelve spectral lines instead of six (Fig. 3). The explanation for the altered spectrum is that ^{13}C has a nuclear spin of 1/2, and will cause additional splitting if and only if the initial radical was centered on the atom bearing the carbon isotope, so that it is covalently bound to the spin trap, and is thus close enough to the free electron to influence its spectral pattern. Isotopic labeling is a commonly employed method to prove the identity of radicals that have formed spin adducts.

Reaction Mechanism

The mechanism for 1-hydroxyethyl radical formation in hepatic microsomes is presently uncertain. Spin trapping experiments have demonstrated that the reaction is sensitive to cytochrome P-450 inhibitors such as SKF 525-A and metyrapone (Fig. 4). Catalase caused 50% inhibition of the rate of 1-hydroxyethyl radical formation (Fig. 4), indicating a role of hydrogen peroxide. In the presence of deferoxamine (1 m*M*), only weak EPR signals were observed, which most likely indicates an important role of iron in the reaction mechanism, but could be explained in part by other biological effects of deferoxamine.[120] Furthermore, rates of ethanol radical formation can be stimulated by addition of iron chelates such as ADP-Fe^{3+}, or inhibition of catalase activity by azide (Fig. 4). Taken together, these data clearly indicate that iron and hydrogen peroxide have an important role in the microsomal formation of 1-hydroxyethyl radicals. One interpretation of these data is that hydroxyl radicals could be formed through a Fenton type of reaction (Eq. 2), and then abstract a hydrogen atom from ethanol (Eq. 3):

$$CH_3CH_2OH + {}^{\bullet}OH \longrightarrow H_2O + CH_3C(^{\bullet})HOH \qquad (3)$$

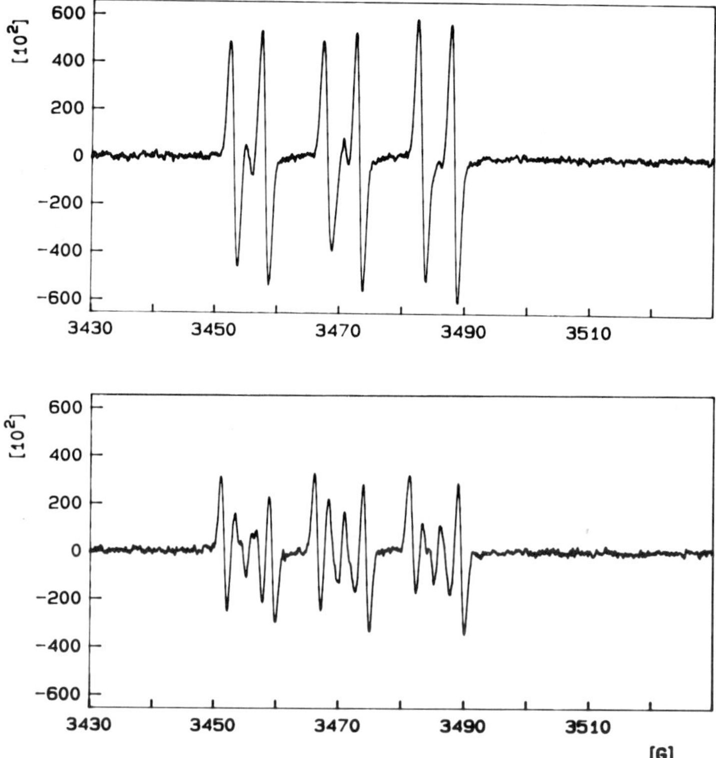

Fig. 3. Formation of the 1-hydroxyethyl radical adduct of PBN by hepatic microsomes. Hepatic microsomes were incubated with ethanol, 50 m*M*; PBN, 30 m*M*; and an NADPH-generating system.[116] After 30 min of incubation, toluene extracts were prepared and analyzed by EPR spectroscopy. In the lower panel, 1-^{13}C-ethanol was used, and the additional spectral lines are caused by the ^{13}C covalently bound to PBN (*see* Fig. 2). The numbers on the horizontal axis represent the magnetic field (in Gauss) and relative signal intensity is shown on the vertical axis. In this experiment, the measured hyperfine splitting constants were 15.0 G and 5.0 G for nitrogen and hydrogen, respectively.

However, the incomplete inhibition by catalase, sensitivity to cytochrome P-450 inhibitors, and related observations[115,117] suggest that some of the radical could be formed directly by the cytochrome P-450 enzymes.

In summary, spin trapping studies have proven that ethanol is metabolized in hepatic microsomes to the 1-hydroxyethyl radical. This reaction is dependent on NADPH and cytochrome P-450, but the mechanism may

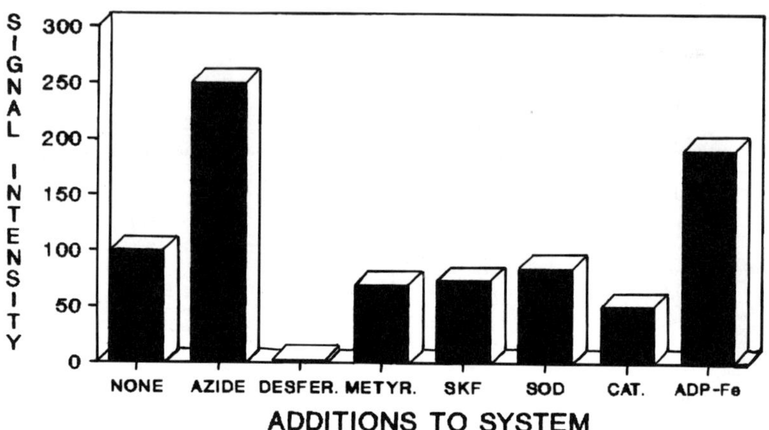

Fig. 4. Effect of various additions on rates of 1-hydroxyethyl radical formation in liver microsomes. Experiments were performed as indicated in Fig. 3, and the signal intensity in the control incubation (no additions) was assigned a value of 100. The final concentrations of the various additions were as follows: Sodium azide, 1 mM; Desferyl (DESFER., deferoxamine), 1 mM; metyrapone (METYR), 1 mM; SKF-525A (SKF), 1 mM; superoxide dismutase (SOD), 100 U/mL; catalase (CAT), 100 U/mL; ADP, 0.4 mM, plus FeCl$_3$, 0.012 mM (ADP-Fe). Values are means of two measurements, using the same microsomal preparation.

involve both direct catalytic formation and an oxygen radical intermediate, which is presumed to be the hydroxyl radical. Once formed, the 1-hydroxyethyl radical probably adds molecular oxygen and rearranges to produce acetaldehyde. The proportion of microsomal ethanol metabolism that may arise through an ethanol radical intermediate is currently unknown, but acetaldehyde appears to be produced directly by cytochrome P-450, as well as through mechanisms involving hydroxyl radicals.[19,27–30]

Possible Consequences
of Ethanol Radical Formation

Because ethanol is a well-known "scavenger" of the hydroxyl radical (Eq. 3), it has been suggested that ethanol should be considered as an antioxidant. For example, antioxidant properties have been cited to explain the protective effects of ethanol against methamphetamine-induced neuronal damage[121] or radiation-induced hemolysis.[122] These data seem to argue against a role of "oxidative stress" in alcohol toxicity. However, it is possible that highly reactive hydroxyl radicals, if they are formed in liver cells, could react indiscriminately at sites that are easily repaired, or have no long-term adverse effects in the cell. But if another less reactive radical, such as the 1-hydroxyethyl radical were formed, it could diffuse to more distant sites before reacting with critical target molecules.

Some support for this hypothesis has been provided by Ahmad and Sun,[118,119] who demonstrated that the addition of ascorbate to microsomal incubations increased both the production of the 1-hydroxyethyl radical and lipid peroxidation. The proposed mechanism was that ascorbyl radicals could generate ethanol radicals by hydrogen atom abstraction, and that the 1-hydroxyethyl radicals were the reactive intermediates that stimulated lipid peroxidation.[118,119]

Rates of microsomal 1-hydroxyethyl radical formation are inducible by ethanol feeding,[115,116] indicating that this metabolite of ethanol could be formed in relatively high concentrations in individuals who ingest large amounts of ethanol. More recently, this radical species has been detected in spin trapping studies in vivo (*see* section on "Spin Trapping of Alcohol-Induced Free Radicals in Liver").

Other Free Radical Metabolites of Ethanol

The ethoxy radical [$CH_3CH_2O^\bullet$] was the first free radical that was proposed to explain the occurrence of alcohol-induced lipid peroxidation, but hydrogen atom abstraction from oxygen is less likely than from carbon because of greater bond dissociation energy.[123] Other radicals could also be formed,[123] but none of these other free radical metabolites of ethanol have been observed in spin trapping studies with liver microsomes or in vivo.

Spin Trapping of Alcohol-Induced Free Radicals in Liver

Experiments with Rats Fed Ethanol in Liquid Diets

The first direct evidence that ethanol initiates free radical events in the liver was reported in 1987, when Reinke et al. demonstrated that the EPR spectra of liver extracts from rats that had been fed ethanol for 2 wk contained evidence of nitroxide radical adducts.[116] In these experiments, rats had been offered liquid diets containing ethanol and fat as 36 and 35% of total calories, respectively. The rats were then given the spin trapping agent

2,4,6-trimethoxyphenyl-*N*-*t*-butyl nitrone (MO$_3$PBN, Fig. 1) by ip injection. Thirty minutes after the administration of the spin trap, livers were removed and organic extracts were prepared. The predominant spin adducts detected had characteristics typical of carbon-centered lipid radicals of MO$_3$PBN (Fig. 5). Minor components of these spectra were interpreted as evidence of oxygen-centered adducts, with some possible contribution of adducts of demethylated metabolites of the spin adduct.[116] Liver extracts from rats that had been pair-fed liquid diets free of ethanol did not contain spin adducts under these conditions. It is interesting to note that similar lipid radical adducts have been observed in liver extracts of rats given an acute dose of carbon tetrachloride.[124]

If the fat content of the liquid diet was decreased to only 12% of total calories, the intensity of the EPR spectrum was also diminished (Fig. 5). Because the intensity of the EPR signal is proportional to the number of unpaired electrons in the sample, these data indicate that high levels of dietary fat increase the generation of free radicals in the liver. These observations are in good agreement with previous reports that high levels of dietary fat potentiate alcoholic liver injury,[125,126] and give additional evidence for a role of free radicals in the hepatotoxicity of ethanol. Because high levels of dietary fat also have a "permissive effect" on the induction of cytochrome P-450,[104] and rates of 1-hydroxyethyl radical formation were greatest in microsomes from rats fed ethanol in a high fat diet,[116] these data also suggest a role of the ethanol radical in the formation of the lipid radicals trapped in vivo.

In summary, data obtained with ethanol-fed rats have indicated that ethanol initiates free radical reactions in the liver, and that these processes are enhanced when the diet is also rich in fat. The spin adducts detected are presumed to be from lipid radicals. Unfortunately, they cannot be identified further by currently available methods. It is also important to note that the adducts detected are of radicals that were formed secondary to the attack of some other more highly reactive radical on endogenous compounds, which are probably membrane lipids.

Radicals Observed
During Acute Ethanol Intoxication

Types of Spin Adducts Detected

A number of studies have been conducted in order to detect free radical intermediates that may be formed in vivo after the administration of

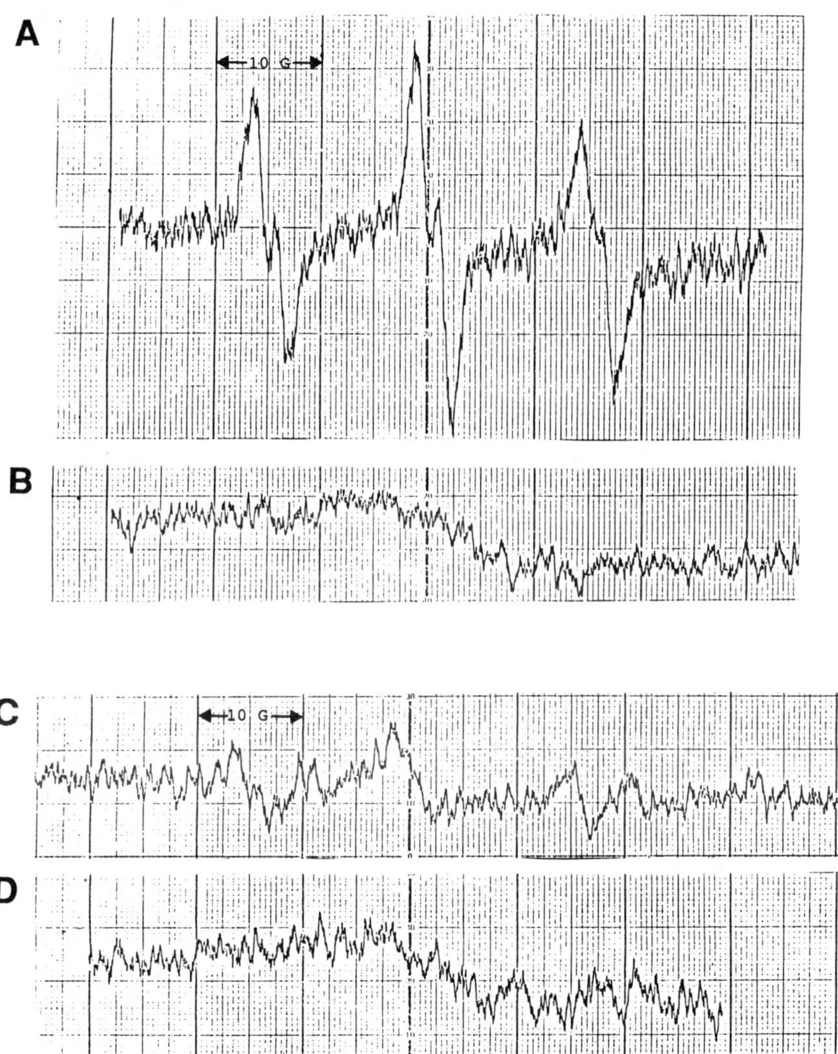

Fig. 5. EPR spectra of lipid extracts of livers of rats fed liquid ethanol-containing diets or control diets for two weeks. Rats were given the spin trapping agent 2,4,6-trimethoxyphenyl-*N-t*-butylnitrone 30 min before livers were removed and extracts were prepared for EPR analyses.[116] The treatments of the individual rats were as follows: **A** = ethanol-fed, high fat diet; **B** = control, high fat diet; **C** = ethanol-fed, low fat diet; **D** = control, low fat diet. For the spectra in **A** and **C**, a_N = 15.0 G; a_H = 2.0 G.

ethanol. In the first of these experiments, rats that had been fed ethanol in combination with a diet that was also rich in fat were given an intraperitoneal dose of 1-^{13}C-ethanol, along with the spin trapping agent PBN.[116] After 30 min, liver extracts were prepared and subjected to EPR analyses. Extracts of livers and hearts from rats that had received both ethanol and PBN contained spin adducts that appeared to be from mixtures of carbon-centered and oxygen-centered radicals, whereas no spin adducts were detected in extracts from rats that had received PBN only.[116] Because the EPR signals of the carbon-centered adducts were not affected by the presence of ^{13}C in the ethanol molecule, it was concluded that the adducts detected could not be 1-hydroxyethyl radicals and were probably from lipid radicals.

These experiments were extended through the use of 5,5-dimethyl-pyrolline-*N*-oxide (DMPO, Fig. 1), a spin trapping agent that forms relatively stable adducts with the hydroxyl radical and superoxide anion, and also combines readily with the 1-hydroxyethyl radical. Hepatic microsomes were found to form the 1-hydroxyethyl radical adduct of DMPO, and the identity of this adduct was proven through the use of 1-^{13}C-ethanol.[117] When ^{13}C-labeled ethanol and DMPO were injected into rats, liver extracts again contained spectra of carbon-centered lipid adducts, but did not contain evidence of the 1-hydroxyethyl radical.[127] In these experiments, similar ethanol-dependent spectra were also detected in the heart, lungs, and spleen of ethanol-treated rats, but not in organs of rats that had received DMPO only.[127]

The question of free radicals that are generated during ethanol intoxication has been more recently reexamined through the use of computer analysis of the EPR spectra. When PBN was administered along with an oral dose of ethanol, and EPR spectra of liver extracts were accumulated through multiple scans to improve the signal-to-noise ratio, at least three adducts could be observed in liver extracts (Fig. 6). Computer simulations indicated that the predominant adduct is apparently from a carbon-centered lipid radical (Fig. 6E), and its hyperfine splitting constants (*see legend*) are similar to adducts that have been reported to form during the microsomal metabolism of carbon tetrachloride.[128] Another component (Fig. 6D) is most likely an oxygen-centered lipid radical adduct.[128] In addition, some spectra contain evidence of a third component (Fig. 6C), with wider hyperfine splitting constants that give the appearance of "shoulders" at the extremes of the spectrum. This adduct has been tentatively identified as the 1-hydroxyethyl adduct, based on its hyperfine splitting constants (*see legend*). Com-

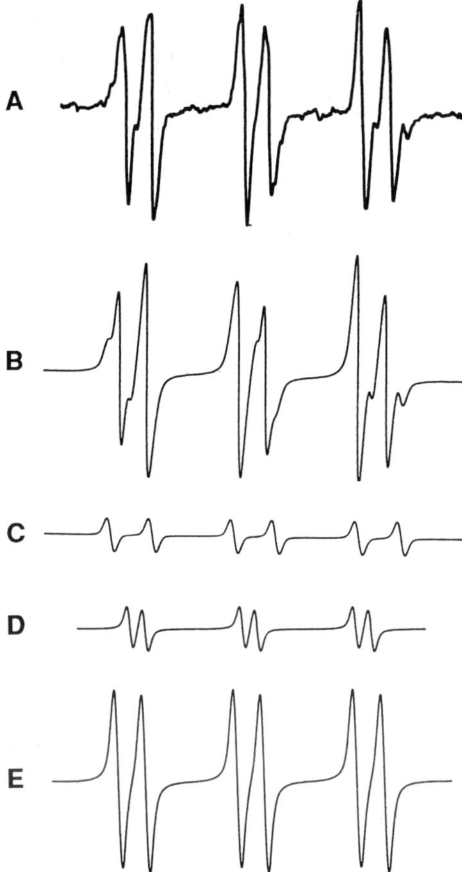

Fig. 6: Computer analysis of an EPR spectrum of a liver extract from an ethanol-treated rat. A fasted rat was given diethylmaleate (1 mL/kg, ip, diluted in corn oil) to deplete hepatic glutathione levels. After 30 min, the rat was given PBN (125 mg/kg, ip) and ethanol (2.5 g/kg, p.o.). After an additional 30 min, the rat was anesthetized, and a chloroform extract of the liver was prepared, evaporated to dryness, and dissolved in toluene. The EPR spectrum of the extract is shown in **A**, and **B** shows a computer simulation of the spectrum of the extract. The individual components of the spectrum in **B** are as follows: **C** a_N = 15.04 G; a_H = 5.05 G, similar to the 1-hydroxyethyl adduct of PBN in toluene (*see legend to Fig. 3*). **D** a_N = 13.70 G; a_H = 1.83 G. **E** a_N = 14.49 G; a_H = 3.30 G.

puter simulations have indicated that this third component, which we believe to be the 1-hydroxyethyl radical adduct of PBN, constitutes less than 10% of the total spin adducts of PBN represented in Fig. 6. In most experiments, the spectral contribution of this component is much smaller. When the weak signal of the ethanol adduct is further split through the use of 1-^{13}C-ethanol, it becomes even more difficult to detect. The weakness of the signal, along with spectral overlap with the carbon-centered lipid radical, probably explain the failure to detect the ethanol adduct of PBN in earlier studies.[116]

Knecht et al. have recently reported the detection of the 1-hydroxyethyl radical adduct of the spin trapping agent α-(4-pyridyl 1-oxide)-*N*-*t*-butyl-nitrone (POBN, Fig. 1) in the bile of deermice that are deficient in alcohol dehydrogenase.[129] This observation provides additional evidence that ethanol is metabolized to the 1-hydroxyethyl radical in vivo, and it must be considered as a possible intermediate that initiates free radical reactions that result ultimately in the trapping of lipid radicals.

Additional information has been obtained on the nature of the carbon-centered lipid adducts formed during ethanol intoxication through the use of PBN that contains deuterium on the phenyl ring and *t*-butyl groups (*see* Fig. 1). The hydrogen atoms in nondeuterated PBN do not contribute to the EPR spectrum, but their nuclear spin causes broadening of the spectral lines and loss of resolution.[130] When ethanol was administered along with deuterated PBN, a complex spectrum was observed in extracts of liver, but no signal was observed if PBN was given with an oral dose of saline (Fig. 7). When the spectrum in Fig. 7 was further analyzed through a computer simulation, two components were observed (Fig. 8). The major component (Fig. 8B) is a carbon-centered adduct, with a 1:2:1 splitting pattern from hydrogen atoms on a methylene carbon covalently bound to PBN. This splitting pattern indicates that the radical trapped must be of a primary alkyl [R-C(·)H$_2$] type.[130] Deuterated PBN did not reveal additional information about the nature of the oxygen-centered adduct (Fig. 8C). It is possible that this radical is formed after the addition of oxygen to the carbon-centered adduct; or it could arise through an independent sequence of events. The 1-hydroxyethyl radical adduct is present in concentrations that are too low to be observed under the spectrometer conditions necessary to resolve the splitting pattern of the primary alkyl radical adduct (Figs. 7 and 8).

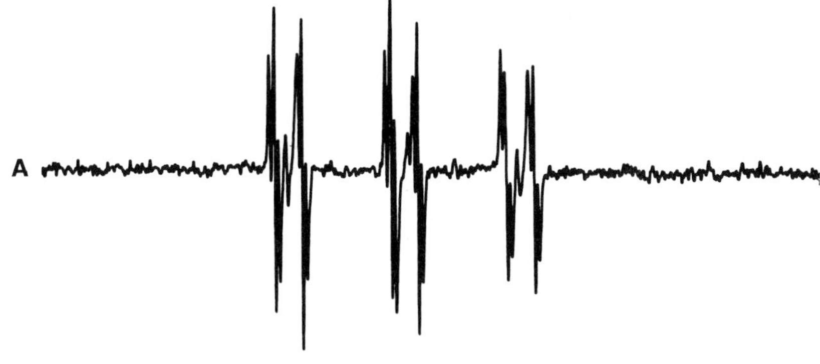

Fig. 7. EPR spectra of liver extracts from ethanol-treated or control rats using deuterated PBN as a spin trap. Representative spectra obtained when rats were given PBN (135 mg/kg, ip) containing deuterium on the phenyl and *t*-butyl groups (PBN-d$_{14}$, *see ref. 130*), and either **A** ethanol (5 g/kg, p.o.), or **B** saline (10 mL/kg, p.o.). Other procedures were as indicated in the legend to Fig. 6. Both spectra were obtained under identical spectrometer conditions, with a scan width of 100 G.

Acetaldehyde

Acetaldehyde is the primary product of ethanol metabolism, and it is substantially more toxic than ethanol. However, concentrations of acetaldehyde during ethanol intoxication are normally quite low, primarily because of the action of mitochondrial and cytosolic aldehyde dehydrogenases. Nevertheless, acetaldehyde has been implicated in the development of ethanol-induced liver disease because it is known to form adducts with liver proteins,[131] deplete glutathione,[132] stimulate chemiluminescence in perfused livers,[133] and serve as a substrate for xanthine oxidase.[35,36] For these reasons, we have also evaluated possible roles of acetaldehyde in the initiation of free radical reactions in vivo.

When acetaldehyde was administered to rats along with PBN, carbon-centered lipid radicals could be detected in extracts of the liver and the heart.[127] Hepatic microsomes also metabolize acetaldehyde to a free radical,

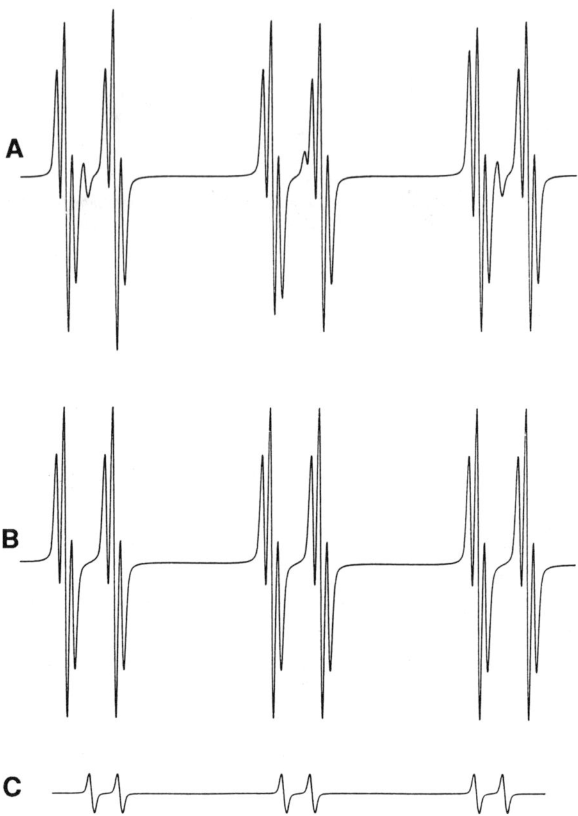

Fig. 8. Computer simulations of spectra observed in liver extracts of rats treated with ethanol and deuterated PBN. Figure 8A shows a computer simulation of a spectrum similar to that shown in Fig. 7A, except that a 50-G scan width was used to increase the detail of the spectral components. The major component **B** has splitting constants of $a_N = 14.45$ G, $a_H = 3.30$ G. The additional spectral lines in **B**, which produce a 1:2:1 pattern, are caused by two hydrogen atoms on the initial radical, and have γ-hydrogen splitting constants of 0.53 G. This pattern identifies component **B** as a primary alkyl (R-C($\cdot$)H$_2$ adduct.[130] Component **C** has characteristics of an oxygen-centered lipid adduct ($a_N = 13.50$ G; $a_H = 1.80$ G).

which is thought to be the acetyl radical.[134] However, experiments with ^{13}C-labelled acetaldehyde have demonstrated that the adducts detected in vivo do not contain acetaldehyde carbon, and have different hyperfine splitting constants than adducts induced by ethanol administration.[127]

Although acetaldehyde also initiates free radical reactions when administered to rats, supraphysiological concentrations are required before these radicals can be detected. Thus, although a role for acetaldehyde in free radical reactions during alcohol intoxication cannot be excluded altogether, the high concentrations required to initiate these events makes an important role for acetaldehyde unlikely.

Alcohol-Induced Free Radicals in Extrahepatic Tissues

Free radical formation and lipid peroxidation following ethanol administration have been proposed as a mechanism for damage to a number of extrahepatic tissues, such as the heart,[135] gastric mucosa,[136] testes,[137] and brain.[138] Because lipid peroxidation is usually, if not always, associated with the formation of free radicals, these data suggest that ethanol may also initiate free radical reactions in these extrahepatic tissues.

Very few studies have been designed to directly test for free radical formation following ethanol exposure in extrahepatic tissues. When an acute dose of ethanol was administered along with PBN to rats that had also been fed ethanol in liquid diets for a period of 2 wk, PBN spin adducts of lipid radicals were detected in extracts of heart.[116] Similarly, if ethanol was administered along with the spin trapping agent DMPO, spin adducts of carbon-centered radicals were detected in extracts of heart, lung, and spleen of ethanol-fed rats.[127] Tissues extracts prepared from rats that received DMPO or PBN, but no ethanol, were consistently negatively. When ethanol-fed rats were given the spin trapping agent trimethoxy-PBN without an acute ethanol dose, no radical adducts were detected in extracts of lung, spleen, or kidney.[116]

Little is known of the mechanisms of ethanol-induced free radical reactions in the extrahepatic tissues. As discussed in earlier sections, data obtained in experiments with the liver has often implicated ethanol metabolism in the generation of free radicals. Evidence that free radical reactions may occur in tissues that are low in alcohol dehydrogenase activity or cytochrome P-450 content suggests that other mechanisms may be involved in the initiation of these events.

Summary

Studies with spin trapping and EPR spectroscopy have demonstrated that the acute and chronic administration of ethanol to laboratory rats and mice results in the formation of free radical intermediates in the liver and other body organs. The major radical adducts that have been detected are of biological origin, and are presumed to be lipid radicals, but methods for their identification are not currently available.

The mechanism for the initiation of ethanol-induced free radical production in the liver is also not known. A substantial number of literature reports have implicated oxygen radical formation as an early event in the process of lipid peroxidation following alcohol exposure. Potential sources of these oxygen radicals include the monooxygenase enzyme system of the endoplasmic reticulum, xanthine oxidase, "leakage" of electrons from the mitochondrial electron transport chain, or phagocytic white blood cells. In addition, ethanol is metabolized by hepatic microsomes to the 1-hydroxy-ethyl radical, and this free radical species has also been detected in vivo. Either oxygen radicals or the ethanol radical may attack membranes or other cellular components to form the lipid radicals that have been detected by the spin trapping methods.

Finally, the significance of free radical formation following ethanol exposure is uncertain. Because free radicals are highly reactive, any set of circumstances that results in their formation is assumed to pose a toxic insult to cells. On the other hand, because occasional drinking seems to pose no great health hazard, it is clear that the body is capable of detoxifying the radicals, or repairing damage that they may produce, quite readily.

The relationships that exist between free radical formation and mechanisms of cell death are poorly understood and are being intensely studied in many areas of toxicological research. As the mechanisms of free radical toxicity become better elucidated, our understanding of the role of free radicals in alcoholic tissue damage will also become more clear.

References

[1] N. R. DiLuzio (1964) Prevention of the acute ethanol-induced fatty liver by the simultaneous administration of anti-oxidants. *Life Sci.* **3,** 113–119.

[2] N. R. DiLuzio and F. Costales (1965) Inhibition of the ethanol and carbon tetrachloride induced fatty liver by antioxidants. *Exp. Mol. Pathol.* **4,** 141–154.

[3] N. R. DiLuzio and G. H. Kalish (1966) Enhanced peroxidation of lipid in the pathogenesis of acute ethanol-induced liver injury. *Gastroenterology* **50,** 392–396.

[4] N. R. DiLuzio (1968) The effect of acute ethanol intoxication on liver and plasma lipid fractions in the rat. *Am. J. Physiol.* **194,** 453–460.

[5] M. Comporti, A. Hartman, and N. R. DiLuzio (1967) Effect of in vivo and in vitro ethanol administration on liver lipid peroxidation. *Lab. Invest.* **16,** 616–624.

[6] S. Hashimoto and R. O. Recknagel (1968) No chemical evidence of hepatic peroxidation in acute ethanol toxicity. *Exp. Mol. Pathol.* **8**, 225–242.

[7] M. Pesh-Imam and R. O. Recknagel (1977) Lipid peroxidation and the concept of antioxygenic potential: Vitamin E changes in acute experimental CCl_4-, $BrCCl_3$-, and ethanol-induced liver injury. *Toxicol. Appl. Pharmacol.* **42**, 463–475.

[8] T. Inomata, G. A. Rao, and H. Tsukamoto (1987) Lack of evidence for increased lipid peroxidation in ethanol-induced centrilobular necrosis of rat liver. *Liver* **7**, 233–239.

[9] I. H. Goldberg, L. Kappen, and D. F. Chin (1988) Roles of oxygen and oxygen substitutes in DNA sugar damage by antitumor antibiotics, in *Oxygen Radicals in Biology and Medicine*. M. G. Simic, K. A. Taylor, J. F. Ward, and C. von Sonntag, eds. Plenum, New York, pp. 745–757.

[10] B. K. Sinha (1989) Free radicals in anticancer drug pharmacology. *Chem. Biol. Interact.* **69**, 293–317.

[11] R. Docampo (1990) Sensitivity of parasites to free radical damage by antiparasitic drugs. *Chem. Biol. Interact.* **73**, 1–27.

[12] J. M. McCord and I. Fridovitch (1969) Superoxide dismutase: An enzymic function for erythrocuprein (hemocuprein). *J. Biol. Chem.* **244**, 6049–6055.

[13] I. Fridovitch (1983) Superoxide radical: An endogenous toxicant. *Ann. Rev. Pharmacol. Toxicol.* **23**, 239–257.

[14] D. P. Jones, L. Eklow, H. Thor, and S. Orrenius (1981) Metabolism of hydrogen peroxide in isolated hepatocytes: Relative contributions of catalase and glutathione peroxidase in decomposition of endogenously generated H_2O_2. *Arch. Biochem. Biophys.* **210**, 505–516.

[15] B. Halliwell and J. M. C. Gutteridge (1984) Oxygen toxicity, oxygen radicals, transition metals and disease. *Biochem. J.* **219**, 1–14.

[16] B. Halliwell and J. M. C. Gutteridge (1988) Iron as a biological prooxidant. *ISI Atlas Sci. Biochem.* **1**, 48–52.

[17] A. G. Hildebrandt and I. Roots (1975) Reduced nicotinamide adenine dinucleotide phosphate (NADPH)-dependent formation and breakdown of hydrogen peroxide during mixed function oxidation reactions in liver microsomes. *Arch. Biochem. Biophys.* **171**, 385–397.

[18] D. Dolphin (1988) The generation of radicals during the normal and abnormal functioning of cytochromes P-450, in *Oxygen Radicals in Biology and Medicine*. M. G. Simic, K. A. Taylor, J. F. Ward, and C. von Sonntag, eds. Plenum, New York, pp. 491–500.

[19] G. W. Winston and A. I. Cederbaum (1983) NADPH-dependent production of oxy radicals by purified components of the rat liver mixed function oxidase system. I. Oxidation of hydroxyl radical scavenging agents. *J. Biol. Chem.* **258**, 1508–1513.

[20] E. Rubin and C. S. Lieber (1968) Hepatic microsomal enzymes in man and rat: Induction and inhibition by ethanol. *Science* **162,** 690–691.

[21] D. R. Koop, E. T. Morgan, G. E. Tarr, and M. J. Coon (1982) Purification and characterization of a unique isozyme of cytochrome P-450 from liver microsomes of ethanol-treated rabbits. *J. Biol. Chem.* **257,** 8472–8480.

[22] I. Johansson, G. Ekstrom, B. Scholte, D. Puzyck, H. Jornvall, and M. Ingelman-Sundberg (1988) Ethanol-, fasting-, and acetone-inducible cytochromes P-450 in rat liver: Regulation and characteristics of enzymes belonging to the IIB and IIE gene subfamilies. *Biochemistry* **27,** 1925–1934.

[23] J. M. Lasker, J. Raucy, S. Kubota, B. P. Bloswick, M. Black, and C. S. Lieber (1987) Purification and characterization of human liver cytochrome P-450-ALC. *Biochem. Biophys. Res. Commun.* **148,** 232–238.

[24] A. Boveris, C. G. Fraga, A. I. Varsavsky, and O. R. Koch (1983) Increased chemiluminescence and superoxide production in the liver of chronically ethanol-treated rats. *Arch. Biochem. Biophys.* **227,** 534–541.

[25] G. Ekstrom and M. Ingelman-Sundberg (1989) Rat liver microsomal NADPH-supported oxidase activity and lipid peroxidation dependent on ethanol-inducible cytochrome P-450 (P-450IIEl). *Biochem. Pharmacol.* **38,** 1313–1319.

[26] S. M. Klein, G. Cohen, C. S. Lieber, and A. I. Cederbaum (1983) Increased microsomal oxidation of hydroxyl radical scavenging agents and ethanol after chronic consumption of ethanol. *Arch. Biochem. Biophys.* **223,** 425–432.

[27] G. W. Winston and A. I. Cederbaum (1983) NADPH-dependent production of oxy radicals by purified components of the rat liver mixed function oxidase system. II. Role in the microsomal oxidation of ethanol. *J. Biol. Chem.* **258,** 1514–1519.

[28] A. I. Cederbaum (1989) Oxygen radical generation by microsomes: Role of iron and implications for alcohol metabolism and toxicity. *Free Rad. Biol. Med.* **7,** 559–567.

[29] M. Ingelman-Sundberg and I. Johansson (1981) The mechanism of cytochrome P-450-dependent oxidation of ethanol in reconstituted membrane vesicles. *J. Biol. Chem.* **256,** 6321–6326.

[30] G. Ekstrom, T. Cronholm, and M. Ingelman-Sundberg (1986) Hydroxyl-radical production and ethanol oxidation by liver microsomes isolated from ethanol-treated rats. *Biochem. J.* **233,** 755–761.

[31] O. Beloqui and A. I. Cederbaum (1985) Microsomal interactions between iron, paraquat, and menadione: Effect on hydroxyl radical production and alcohol oxidation. *Arch. Biochem. Biophys.* **242,** 187–196.

[32] O. Strubelt (1984) Alcohol potentiation of liver injury. *Fund. Appl. Toxicol.* **4,** 144–151.

[33] C. S. Lieber (1988) Metabolic effects of ethanol and its interaction with other

drugs, hepatotoxic agents, vitamins, and carcinogens: A 1988 update. *Sem. Liver Dis.* **8,** 47–68.

[34] L. A. Reinke, E. K. Lai, and P. B. McCay (1988) Ethanol feeding stimulates trichloromethyl radical formation from carbon tetrachloride in liver. *Xenobiotica* **18,** 1311–1318.

[35] H. H. H. Oei, H. C. Zoganas, J. M. McCord, and S. W. Schaffer (1986) Role of acetaldehyde and xanthine oxidase in ethanol-induced oxidative stress. *Res. Commun. Chem. Pathol. Pharmacol.* **51,** 195–203.

[36] L. G. Sultatos (1988) Effects of acute ethanol administration on the hepatic xanthine dehydrogenase/oxidase system in the rat. *J. Pharmacol. Exp. Ther.* **246,** 946–949.

[37] S. Kato, T. Kawase, J. Alderman, N. Inatomi, and C. S. Lieber (1990) Role of xanthine oxidase in ethanol-induced lipid peroxidation in rats. *Gastroenterology* **98,** 203–210.

[38] H. J. Forman and A. Boveris (1982) Superoxide radical and hydrogen peroxide in mitochondria, in *Free Radicals in Biology,* vol. V. W. A. Pryor, ed. Academic, New York, pp. 65–90.

[39] A. I. Cederbaum and E. Rubin (1975) Molecular injury to mitochondria produced by ethanol and acetaldehyde. *Fed. Proc.* **34,** 2045–2051.

[40] J. Sinaceur, C. Ribiere, D. Sabourault, and R. Nordman (1985) Superoxide formation in liver mitochondria during ethanol intoxication: Possible role in alcohol hepatotoxicity, in *Free Radicals in Liver Injury.* G. Poli, K. H. Cheeseman, M. U. Dianzani, and T. F. Slater, eds. IRL Press, Oxford, UK, pp. 175–177.

[41] H. Rouach, M. Clement, M. T. Orfanelli, B. Janvier, J. Nordman, and R. Nordman (1983) Hepatic lipid peroxidation and mitochondrial susceptibility to peroxidative attacks during ethanol inhalation and withdrawal. *Biochim. Biophys. Acta* **753,** 439–444.

[42] M. Uysal, G. Ozdemirler, G. Kutalp, and H. Oz (1989) Mitochondrial and microsomal lipid peroxidation in rat liver after actue acetaldehyde and ethanol intoxication. *J. Appl. Toxicol.* **9,** 155–158.

[43] J. K. Boitnett and W. C. Maddrey (1981) Alcoholic liver disease: Interrelationships among histologic features and the histologic effects of prednisolone therapy. *Hepatology* **1,** 599–612.

[44] R. L. Baehner, L. A. Boxer, and L. M. Ingraham (1982) Reduced oxygen byproducts and white blood cells, in *Free Radicals in Biology,* vol. V. W. A. Pryor, ed. Academic, New York, pp. 91–113.

[45] H. D. Perez, F. J. Roll, D. M. Bissell, S. Shak, and I. M. Goldstein (1984) Chemotactic activity for polymorphonuclear leukocytes by cultured rat hepatocytes exposed to ethanol. *J. Clin. Invest.* **74,** 1350–1357.

[46] F. J. Roll, M. Alexander, and H. D. Perez (1989) Generation of chemotactic

activity for neutrophils by liver cells metabolizing ethanol. *Free Rad. Biol. Med.* **7,** 549–555.

[47] J. Sanchez, M. Casas, and R. Rama (1988) Effect of chronic ethanol administration on iron metabolism in the rat. *Eur. J. Haematol.* **41,** 321–325.

[48] R. Mazzanti, K. S. Srai, E. S. Debnam, A. M. Boss, and P. Gentilini (1987) The effect of chronic ethanol consumption on iron absorption in rats. *Alcohol Alcohol.* **22,** 47–52.

[49] A. Valenzuela, V. Fernandez, and L. A. Videla (1983) Hepatic and biliary levels of glutathione and lipid peroxides following iron overload in the rat: Effect of simultaneous ethanol administration. *Toxicol. Appl. Pharmacol.* **70,** 87–95.

[50] H. Rouach, M. K. Park, M. T. Orfanelli, B. Janvier, P. Brissot, M. Bourel, and R. Nordman (1988) Effects of ethanol on hepatic and cerebellar lipid peroxidation and endogenous antioxidants in naive and chronic iron overloaded rats. *Adv. Biosci.* **71,** 49–54.

[51] S. Shaw, E. Jayatilleke, and C. S. Lieber (1988) Lipid peroxidation as a mechanism of alcoholic liver injury; Role of iron mobilization and microsomal induction. *Alcohol* **5,** 135–140.

[52] S. Shaw (1989) Lipid peroxidation, iron mobilization and radical generation induced by alcohol. *Free Rad. Biol. Med.* **7,** 541–547.

[53] G. Minotti and S. D. Aust (1989) The role of iron in oxygen radical mediated lipid peroxidation. *Chem. Biol. Interact.* **71,** 1–19.

[54] J. Sinaceur, C. Ribiere, C. Abu-Murad, J. Nordman, and R. Nordman (1983) Reduction in the rate of ethanol elimination in vivo by desferrioxamine and diethylenetriamine pentaacetic acid: Suggestion for involvement of hydroxyl radicals in ethanol oxidation. *Biochem. Pharmacol.* **32,** 2371–2373.

[55] M. K. Park, H. Rouach, M. T. Orfanelli, B. Janvier, and R. Nordman (1988) Influence of allopurinol and desferrioxamine on the ethanol-induced oxidative stress in rat liver and cerebellum. *Adv. Biosci.* **71,** 135–139.

[56] L. A. Videla and A. Valenzuela (1982) Alcohol ingestion, liver glutathione and lipoperoxidation: Metabolic interrelations and pathological implications. *Life Sci.* **31,** 2395–2407.

[57] C. M. MacDonald, J. Dow, and M. R. Moore (1977) A possible protective role for sulphydryl compounds in acute alcoholic liver injury. *Biochem. Pharmacol.* **26,** 1529–1531.

[58] B. H. Lauterburg, S. Davies, and J. R. Mitchell (1984) Ethanol suppresses hepatic glutathione synthesis in rats in vivo. *J. Pharmacol. Exp. Ther.* **230,** 7–11.

[59] S. Morton and M. C. Mitchell (1985) Effects of chronic ethanol feeding on glutathione turnover in the rat. *Biochem. Pharmacol.* **34,** 1559–1563.

[60] H. Speisky, A. MacDonald, G. Giles, H. Orrego, and Y. Israel (1985) Increased loss and decreased synthesis of hepatic glutathione after acute ethanol administration: Turnover studies. *Biochem. J.* **225,** 565–572.

[61] H. Sies, O. R. Koch, E. Martino, and A. Boveris (1979) Increased biliary glutathione disulfide release in chronically ethanol-treated rats. *FEBS Lett.* **103**, 287–290.

[62] G. E. A. Bjorneboe, A. Bjorneboe, B. F. Hagen, J. Morland, and C. A. Drevon (1987) Reduced hepatic α-tocopherol content after long-term administration of ethanol to rats. *Biochim. Biophys. Acta* **918**, 236–241.

[63] T. Kawase, S. Kato, and C. S. Lieber (1989) Lipid peroxidation and antioxidant defense systems in rat liver after chronic ethanol feeding. *Hepatology* **10**, 815–821.

[64] M. A. Leo and C. S. Lieber (1982) Hepatic vitamin A depletion in alcoholic liver injury in man. *N. Engl. J. Med.* **307**, 597–601.

[65] P. R. Ryle, A. Hodges, and A. D. Thomson (1986) Inhibition of ethanol induced hepatic vitamin A depletion by administration of N-N'-diphenyl-p-phenylene-diamine (DPPD). *Life Sci.* **38**, 695–702.

[66] C. Ribiere, J. Sinaceur, J. Nordman, and R. Nordman (1983) Liver superoxide dismutases and catalase during ethanol inhalation and withdrawal. *Pharm. Biochem. Behav.* **18 (Suppl. 1)**, 263–266.

[67] C. L. Keen, T. Tamura, B. Lonnerdal, L. S. Hurley, and C. H. Halsted (1985) Changes in hepatic superoxide dismutase activity in alcoholic monkeys. *Am. J. Clin. Nutr.* **41**, 929–932.

[68] N. J. Schisler and S. M. Singh (1989) Effect of ethanol in vivo on enzymes which detoxify oxygen free radicals. *Free Rad. Biol. Med.* **7**, 117–123.

[69] E. G. DeMaster, E. Kaplan, and E. Chesler (1981) The differential response of tissue catalase activity to chronic ethanol administration in the rat. *Alcohol. Clin. Exp. Res.* **5**, 45–48.

[70] C. M. MacDonald (1973) The effects of ethanol on hepatic lipid peroxidation and on the activities of glutathione reductase and peroxidase. *FEBS Lett.* **35**, 227–230.

[71] G. Aykac, M. Uysal, A. S. Yalcin, N. Kocak-Toker, A. Sivas, and H. Oz (1985) The effect of chronic ethanol ingestion on hepatic lipid peroxide, glutathione, glutathione peroxidase and glutathione transferase in rats. *Toxicology* **36**, 71–76.

[72] C. Richter (1987) Biophysical consequences of lipid peroxidation in membranes. *Chem. Phys. Lipids* **44**, 175–189.

[73] F. R. Ungemach (1987) Pathobiochemical mechanisms of hepatocellular damage following lipid peroxidation. *Chem. Phys. Lipids* **45**, 171–205.

[74] S. Yamada, K. Fujiwara, N. Masaki, Y. Ohta, Y. Sato, and H. Oka (1988) Evidence for potentiation of lipid peroxidation in the rat liver after chronic ethanol feeding. *Scand. J. Clin. Lab. Invest.* **48**, 627–632.

[75] J. Harata, M. Nagata, E. Sasaki, I. Ishiguro, Y. Ohta, and Y. Murakami (1983) Effect of prolonged alcohol administration on activities of various enzymes scavenging activated oxygen radicals and lipid peroxide level in the liver of rats. *Biochem. Pharmacol.* **32**, 1795–1798.

[76] R. Fink, M. R. Clemens, D. H. Marjot, P. Patsalos, C. Cawood, A. G. Norden, S. A. Iversen, and T. L. Dormandy (1985) Increased free-radical activity in alcoholics. *Lancet* **ii,** 291–294.

[77] S. Shaw, E. Jayatilleke, W.A. Ross, E. R. Gordon, and C. S. Lieber (1981) Ethanol-induced lipid peroxidation: Potentiation by long-term alcohol feeding and attenuation by methionine. *J. Lab. Clin. Med.* **98,** 417–424.

[78] A. Valenzuela, N. Fernandez, V. Fernandez, G. Ugarte, and L. A. Videla (1980) Effect of acute ethanol ingestion on lipoperoxidation and on the activity of the enzymes related to peroxide metabolism in rat liver. *FEBS Lett.* **111,** 11–13.

[79] U. Koster, D. Albrecht, and H. Kappus (1977) Evidence for carbon tetrachloride- and ethanol-induced lipid peroxidation *in vivo* demonstrated by ethane production in mice and rats. *Toxicol. Appl. Pharmacol.* **41,** 639–648.

[80] R. E. Litov, D. L. Gee, J. E. Downey, and A. L. Tappel (1981) The role of lipid peroxidation during chronic and acute exposure to ethanol as determined by pentane expiration in the rat. *Lipids* **16,** 52–57.

[81] H. Remmer, W. Kessler, H. Einsele, T. Hintze, G. Diaz de Toranzo, A. M. Gharaibeh, and H. Frank (1989) Ethanol promotes oxygen-radical attack on proteins but not on lipids. *Drug Metab. Rev.* **20,** 219–232.

[82] A. Muller and H. Sies (1982) Role of alcohol dehydrogenase activity and of acetaldehyde in ethanol-induced ethane and pentane production by isolated perfused rat liver. *Biochem. J.* **206,** 153–156,

[83] H. Rouach, M. Clement, M. T. Orfanelli, B. Janvier, and R. Nordman (1984) Fatty acid composition of rat liver mitochondrial phospholipids during ethanol inhalation. *Biochim. Biophys. Acta* **795,** 125–129.

[84] M. U. Dianzani (1985) Lipid peroxidation in ethanol poisoning: A critical reconsideration. *Alcohol Alcohol.* **20,** 161–173.

[85] M. Comporti (1985) Lipid peroxidation and cellular damage in toxic liver injury. *Lab. Invest.* **53,** 599–623.

[86] O. Strubelt, M. Younes, and R. Pentz (1987) Enhancement by glutathione depletion of ethanol-induced acute hepatotoxicity in vitro and in vivo. *Toxicology* **45,** 213–233.

[87] M. V. Torrielli, L. Gabriel, and M. U. Dianzani (1978) Ethanol-induced hepato-toxicity; experimental observations on the role of lipid peroxidation. *J. Pathol.* **126,** 11–25.

[88] C. Hirayama, Y. Kishimoto, T. Wakushima, and Y. Murawaki (1983) Mechanism of the protective action of thiol compounds in ethanol-induced liver injury. *Biochem. Pharmacol.* **32,** 321–325.

[89] T. Yuki, K. Yoshitoku, Y. Nakagawa, H. H. Park, H. Senmaru, K. Kagawa, T. Okanoue, and T. Takino (1987) Effect of coenzyme Q_{10} (Co-Q_{10}) on hepatic lipid peroxidation and glutathione metabolism in alcohol-treated rats. *Sulfur Amino Acids* **10,** 221–227.

[90] R. E. Beyer (1988) Inhibition by coenzyme Q of ethanol- and carbon tetra-chloride-stimulated lipid peroxidation in vivo and catalyzed by microsomal and mitochondrial systems. *Free Rad. Biol. Med.* **5,** 297–303.

[91] L. A. Videla, V. Fernandez, A. Valenzuela, and G. Ugarte (1981) Effect of (+)-cyanidanol-3 on the changes in liver glutathione content and lipoperoxidation induced by acute ethanol administration in the rat. *Pharmacology* **22,** 343–348.

[92] P. R. Ryle, J. Chakraborty, and A. D. Thomson (1987) Effects of cysteine and antioxidants on the hepatic redox-state, acetaldehyde, and triglyceride levels after acute ethanol dosing. *Alcohol Alcohol.* **(Suppl. 1),** 289–293.

[93] T. Yuki and R. G. Thurman (1980) The swift increase in alcohol metabolism. Time course for the increase in hepatic oxygen uptake and the involvement of glycolysis. *Biochem. J.* **186,** 119–126.

[94] L. Videla, J. Bernstein, and Y. Israel (1973) Metabolic alterations produced in the liver by chronic ethanol administration: Increased oxidative capacity. *Biochem. J.* **134,** 507–514.

[95] R. G. Thurman, W. R. McKenna, and T. B. McCaffrey (1976) Pathways responsible for the adaptive increase in ethanol uilization following chronic treatment with ethanol: Inhibitor studies with the hemoglobin-free perfused rat liver. *Mol. Pharmacol.* **12,** 156–166.

[96] R. G. Thurman, S. Ji, T. Matsumura, and J. J. Lemasters (1984) Is hypoxia involved in the mechanism of alcohol-induced liver injury? *Fund. Appl. Toxicol.* **4,** 125–133.

[97] M. Younes and O. Strubelt (1987) Enhancement of hypoxic liver damage by ethanol. Involvement of xanthine oxidase and the role of glycolysis. *Biochem. Pharmacol.* **36,** 2973–2977.

[98] M. Younes and O. Strubelt (1987) Alcohol-induced hepatotoxicity; a role for oxygen free radicals. *Free Rad. Res. Commun.* **3,** 19–26.

[99] M. Younes, H. Wagner, and O. Strubelt (1989) Enhancement of acute ethanol hepatotoxicity under conditions of low oxygen supply and ischemia/reperfusion: The role of oxygen radicals. *Biochem. Pharmacol.* **38,** 3573–3581.

[100] J. M. McCord (1985) Oxygen-derived free radicals in post-ischemic tissue injury. *N. Engl. J. Med.* **312,** 159–163.

[101] J. Sinaceur, C. Ribiere, J. Nordman, and R. Nordman (1984) Desferrioxa-mine: A scavenger of superoxide radicals? *Biochem. Pharmacol.* **33,** 1693–1694.

[102] S. Hoe, D. A. Rowley, and B. Halliwell (1982) Reactions of ferrioxamine and desferrioxamine with the hydroxyl radical. *Chem. Biol. Interact.* **41,** 75–81.

[103] M. J. Davies, R. Donkor, C. A. Dunster, C. A. Gee, S. Jonas, and R. L. Willson (1987) Desferrioxamine (Desferal) and superoxide free radicals. Formation of an enzyme-damaging nitroxide. *Biochem. J.* **246,** 725–729.

[104] J. G. Joly and C. Hetu (1975) Effects of chronic ethanol administration in the

rat: Relative dependency on dietary lipids. I. Induction of hepatic drug-metabolizing enzymes in vitro. *Biochem. Pharmacol.* **24,** 1475–1480.

[105] M. J. Perkins (1980) Spin trapping. *Adv. Phys. Org. Chem.* **17,** 1–64.

[106] G. R. Buettner (1987) Spin trapping: ESR parameters of spin adducts. *Free Rad. Biol. Med.* **3,** 259–303.

[107] J. L. Poyer, R. A. Floyd, P. B. McCay, E. G. Janzen, and E. R. Davis (1978) Spin-trapping of the trichloromethyl radical produced during enzymic NADPH oxidation in the presence of carbon tetrachloride or bromotrichloromethane. *Biochim. Biophys. Acta* **539,** 402–409.

[108] E. K. Lai, P. B. McCay, T. Noguchi, and K. L. Fong (1979) *In vivo* spin-trapping of trichloromethyl radicals formed from CCl_4. *Biochem. Pharmacol.* **28,** 2231–2235.

[109] H. D. Connor, R. G. Thurman, M. D. Galizi, and R. P. Mason (1986) The formation of a novel free radical metabolite from CCl_4 in the perfused rat liver and in vivo. *J. Biol. Chem.* **261,** 4542–4548.

[110] J. M. Rau, L. A. Reinke, and P. B. McCay (1990) Direct observation of spintrapped carbon dioxide radicals in hepatocytes exposed to carbon tetrachloride. *Free Rad. Res. Comm.* **9,** 197–204.

[111] E. G. Janzen (1984) Spin trapping. *Methods Enzymol.* **105,** 188–198.

[112] M. J. Davies and T. F. Slater (1988) The use of electron-spin-resonance techniques to detect free-radical formation and tissue damage. *Proc. Nutr. Soc.* **47,** 397–405.

[113] C. Mottley and R. P. Mason (1989) Nitroxide radical adducts in biology: Chemistry, applications, and pitfalls, in *Biological Magnetic Resonance,* vol. 8. L. J. Berliner and J. Reuben, eds. Plenum, New York, pp. 489–546.

[114] E. Albano, A. Tomasi, L. Goria-Gatti, G. Poli, V. Vannini, and M. U. Dianzani (1987) Free radical metabolism of alcohols by rat liver microsomes. *Free Rad. Res. Comm.* **3,** 243–249.

[115] E. Albano, A. Tomasi, L. Goria-Gatti, and M. U. Dianzani (1988) Spin trapping of free radical species produced during the microsomal metabolism of ethanol. *Chem. Biol. Interact.* **65,** 223–234.

[116] L. A. Reinke, E. K. Lai, C. M. DuBose, and P. B. McCay (1987) Reactive free radical generation in vivo in heart and liver of ethanol-fed rats; correlation with radical formation in vitro. *Proc. Natl. Acad. Sci. USA* **84,** 9223–9227.

[117] L. A. Reinke, J. M. Rau, and P. B. McCay (1990) Possible roles of free radicals in alcoholic tissue damage. *Free Rad. Res. Comm.* **9,** 205–211.

[118] F. F. Ahmad, D. L. Cowan, and A. Y. Sun (1988) Potentiation of ethanol-induced lipid peroxidation of biological membranes by vitamin C. *Life Sci.* **43,** 1169–1176.

[119] F. F. Ahmad, D. L. Cowan, and A. Y. Sun (1989) Spin trapping studies of the influence of alcohol on lipid peroxidation, in *Molecular Mechanisms of Alcohol.*

G. Y. Sun, P. K. Rudeen, W. G. Wood, Y. H. Wei, A. Y. Sun, eds. Humana, Clifton, NJ, pp. 257–277.

[120] B. Halliwell (1989) Protection against tissue damage in vivo by desferrioxamine: What is its mechanism of action? *Free Rad. Biol. Med.* **7,** 645–651.

[121] M. J. DeVito and G. C. Wagner (1989) Methamphetamine-induced neuronal damage: A possible role for free radicals. *Neuropharmacology* **28,** 1145–1150.

[122] G. G. Miller and J. A. Raleigh (1983) Action of some hydroxyl radical scavengers on radiation-induced haemolysis. *Int. J. Rad. Biol. Stud. Phys. Chem. Med.* **43,** 411–419.

[123] T. F. Slater (1988) Free radical mechanisms in tissue injury with special reference to the cytotoxic effects of ethanol and related alcohols. *Adv. Biosci.* **71,** 1–9.

[124] P. B. McCay, E. K. Lai, J. L. Poyer, C. M. DuBose, and E. G. Janzen (1984) Oxygen- and carbon-centered free radical formation during carbon tetrachloride metabolism. Observation of lipid radicals in vivo and in vitro. *J. Biol. Chem.* **259,** 2135–2143.

[125] E. Baraona and C. S. Lieber (1979) Effects of ethanol on lipid metabolism. *J. Lipid Res.* **20,** 289–315.

[126] S. W. French, K. Miyamoto, and H. Tsukamoto (1986) Ethanol-induced hepatic fibrosis in the rat; role of the amount of dietary fat. *Alcohol. Clin. Exp. Res.* **10 (Suppl.),** 13S-19S.

[127] L. A. Reinke, E. K. Lai, and P. B. McCay (1988) Administration of ethanol or acetaldehyde to rats results in the generation of free radicals in liver, heart, and other organs, in *Biomedical and Social Aspects of Alcohol and Alcoholism.* K. Kuriyama, A. Takada, H. Ishii, eds. Elsevier, Amsterdam, pp. 663–666.

[128] E. G. Janzen, R. A. Towner, and D. L. Haire (1987) Detection of free radicals generated from the in vitro metabolism of carbon tetrachloride using improved ESR spin trapping techniques. *Free Rad. Res. Comm.* **3,** 357–364.

[129] K. T. Knecht, B. U. Bradford, R. P. Mason, and R. G. Thurman (1990) In vivo formation of a free radical metabolite of ethanol. *Mol. Pharmacol.* **38,** 26–30.

[130] E. G. Janzen, U. M. Oehler, D. L. Haire, and Y. Kotake (1986) ENDOR spectra of aminoxyls. Conformational study of alkyl and aryl spin adducts of deuterated *alpha*-phenyl-N-*tert*-butylnitrone (PBN) based on proton and *beta*-^{13}C hyperfine splittings. *J. Am. Chem. Soc.* **108,** 6858–6863.

[131] T. J. Mauch, T. M. Donohue, R. K. Zetterman, M. F. Sorrel, and D. J. Tuma (1986) Covalent binding of acetaldehyde selectively inhibits the catalytic activity of lysine-dependent enzymes. *Hepatology* **6,** 263–269.

[132] L. A. Videla, V. Fernandez, and A. deMarinis (1982) Liver lipoperoxidative pressure and glutathione status following acetaldehyde and aliphatic alcohols pretreatments in the rat. *Biochem. Biophys. Res. Comm.* **104,** 965–970.

[133] E. Cadenas and H. Sies (1985) Oxidative stress: Excited oxygen species and enzyme activity. *Adv. Enz. Regul.* **23,** 217–237.

[134] L. A. Reinke, E. K. Lai, C. M. DuBose, and P. B. McCay (1988) In vivo generation of free radicals in the heart and other organs of rats treated with ethanol or acetaldehyde. *FASEB J.* **2,** A1388 (abstract).

[135] I. Edes, A. Toszegi, M. Csanady, and B. Bozoky (1986) Myocardial lipid peroxidation in rats after chronic alcohol ingestion and the effects of different antioxidants. *Cardiovasc. Res.* **20,** 542–548.

[136] A. Terano, H. Hiraishi, S. Ota, J. Shiga, and T. Sugimoto (1989) Role of superoxide and hydroxyl radicals in rat gastric mucosal injury induced by ethanol. *Gastroenterol. Jpn.* **24,** 488–493.

[137] E. Rosenblum, J. S. Gavaler, and D. H. Van Thiel (1985) Lipid peroxidation: A mechanism for ethanol-associated testicular injury in rats. *Endocrinology* **116,** 311–318.

[138] R. Nordman (1987) Oxidative stress from alcohol in the brain. *Alcohol Alcohol.* **(Suppl. 1),** 75–82.

Effects of Ethanol
on Glutathione Metabolism

Mack C. Mitchell, David S. Raiford, and Ariane Mallat

Introduction

Glutathione (GSH), the most abundant nonprotein thiol in cells, plays a pivotal role in protecting cells against damage from reactive drug metabolites, free radicals, peroxides, and other toxic oxygen species. Within the last decade, there has been substantial progress in understanding the metabolism of glutathione, its functions in cellular detoxification processes, and how these processes are altered by both acute and chronic alcohol consumption. Some evidence suggests that alcohol-related changes in glutathione homeostasis and detoxification may contribute directly or indirectly to the pathogenesis of tissue damage from alcohol. This chapter will summarize briefly the salient features of glutathione metabolism and current understanding of how these are altered by alcohol consumption in experimental animals and in humans.

Biosynthesis of Glutathione

Glutathione is a tripeptide, γ-glutamylcysteinylglycine, which is synthesized from its constituent amino acids in a two-step process.[1–3] The first and rate-limiting enzymatic reaction is catalyzed by γ-glutamylcysteine

From: *Drug and Alcohol Abuse Reviews, Vol. 2: Liver Pathology and Alcohol*
Ed: R. R. Watson ©1991 The Humana Press Inc.

synthetase.[4] The reaction utilizes ATP,[5] which is hydrolyzed to ADP and inorganic phosphate as indicated by reaction (1):

$$\text{L-cysteine} + \text{L-glutamate} + \text{ATP} \longleftrightarrow \text{L-}\gamma\text{-glutamylcysteine} + \text{ADP} + P_i \quad (1)$$

The second step in synthesis, catalyzed by glutathione synthetase, also utilizes ATP as indicated by reaction (2):

$$\text{L-}\gamma\text{-glutamylcysteine} + \text{glycine} + \text{ATP} \longleftrightarrow \text{glutathione} + \text{ADP} + P_i \quad (2)$$

The enzyme γ-glutamylcysteine synthetase is inhibited by nonallosteric interaction of glutathione at the γ-glutamyl binding site.[6] Concentrations of GSH normally present in cells exceed the approximate K_i of 2.3 mM for this inhibition. Decreasing intracellular levels of glutathione has been shown to increase its rate of synthesis in vivo,[7] whereas a lack of cysteine can limit synthesis of γ-glutamylcysteine.[1,2,8] Cystine must first be reduced to cysteine since only the reduced moiety can be used in this reaction. Interestingly, intracellular concentrations of cysteine (<200 μM) are generally much lower than those not only of glutathione (~5 mM) but also of many other amino acids including glutamate and glycine.[3,8] The reasons for the low concentrations of cysteine are not entirely clear but may be related to its tendency to undergo redox cycling, generating reactive oxygen species in the process.[9]

Many cells express a sodium-independent uptake mechanism that has high affinity for glutamate and cystine (the disulfide).[10] This carrier-mediated process has greater affinity for cystine than the A, ASC, or L systems, which have been described, and probably accounts for the majority of cystine entry into cells. Adult hepatocytes do not express this transport system to the extent seen in many other tissues. By contrast, cysteine is taken up rapidly by hepatocytes by a sodium-dependent process with characteristics of the ASC system.[11] The uptake of cysteine is, in general, much more rapid than that of cystine.[3] The adult liver expresses the enzymes of the transsulfuration (cystathionine) pathway, which transfers the sulfur moiety of methionine to serine forming cysteine as shown in Fig. 1. Unpublished studies from our laboratory using high specific activity [^{35}S]-methionine indicate that cysteine formed through this pathway does not accumulate within hepatocytes but is rapidly used for synthesis of glutathione. Almost no radioactivity could be detected within the intracellular cysteine pool under these conditions. Other published studies have indi-

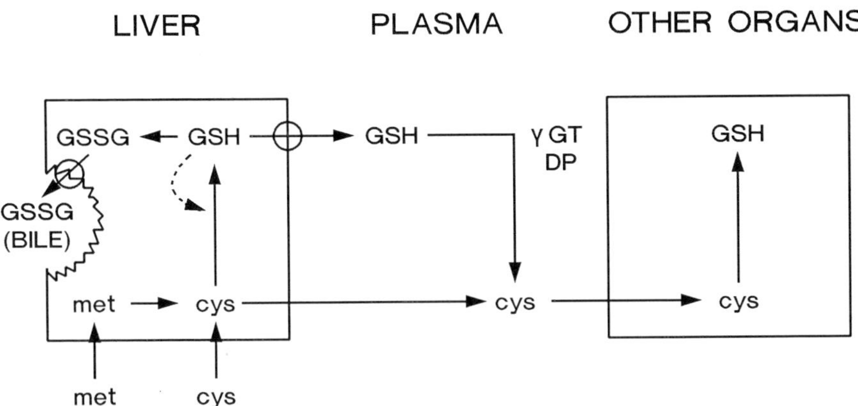

Fig. 1. Transsulfuration of methionine to cysteine. The carbon skeleton of cysteine is derived from serine and the sulfur atom originates from methionine. Once formed, cysteine is converted rapidly to glutathione.

cated the importance of methionine as a sulfur donor for glutathione synthesis in the liver.[12,13]

Turnover and Hepatic Efflux of Glutathione

The turnover of glutathione varies in different tissues.[1,2] Catabolism of glutathione begins with cleavage of the γ-glutamyl moiety in a reaction catalyzed by γ-glutamyltranspeptidase (GGT).[1] This membrane-bound enzyme is located primarily on the apical surface of epithelial cells and may play a role in the recovery and uptake of the amino acid components of glutathione.[1,14] Some investigators have postulated a role for GGT in the formation and subsequent transport and utilization of γ-glutamylcyst(e)ine in glutathione synthesis in the kidney and possibly other organs.[15] There is little evidence that GGT influences the intracellular concentration of GSH since GGT is confined to the plasma membrane and GSH exists predominantly within the cytosol and mitochondria.[2]

The hepatic turnover of glutathione in the rat depends mostly on the efflux of GSH into the bile and circulation.[2,16,17] Efflux of GSH across the plasma membrane of hepatocytes occurs by a carrier-mediated process.[18,19] This process, which has been characterized extensively by Kaplowitz and his colleagues, is saturable,[18,19] exhibits transstimulation in hepatic membrane vesicles,[20,21] and is inhibited by a variety of organic anions including unconjugated bilirubin.[22] Efflux of GSH has been demonstrated in the perfused liver, in isolated hepatocytes, and in membrane vesicles, as well as in intact animals. Sinusoidal (basolateral) efflux (10–15 nmol/min/g liver) of GSH is greater than biliary (apical) (3–5 nmol/min/g liver) under conditions that maintain polarity of the hepatocytes. Since GGT is localized primarily on the apical membrane, it may function in recovery of the amino acid components of glutathione following its efflux into bile.[23] Thus, the extent of biliary efflux of GSH may be greater than that reflected by the recovery of GSH from bile. This hypothesis is supported by the demonstration of large amounts of glutamate and cysteinylglycine in bile.[23] The concentration gradient for glutathione across the sinusoidal membrane is much higher than that across the canalicular membrane. Concentrations in the cytosol are approx 5 mM compared with 3 mM in bile[23] and 10–50 µM in plasma.[24]

Considerable interest has been focused on the role of circulating GSH and on the regulation of hepatic efflux of glutathione. Hepatic efflux accounts for most of the GSH ln the plasma.[24] The half-life of GSH in the plasma is surprisingly short, approx 2–3 min in the rat and in humans.[25,26] This finding suggests that the entry into and clearance of GSH from the circulation is a very dynamic process (Fig. 2). Those tissues with the highest activity of GGT remove the greatest amount of the sulfur moiety of GSH.[26] They include the kidney, small intestinal mucosa, and pancreas. The function(s) of GSH within the plasma has not yet been completely elucidated. One postulated function is the transport of the sulfur moiety of GSH from the liver to other organs.[27] This role for GSH was proposed since the liver is the primary tissue with the capacity for transsulfuration of methionine to cysteine.[13] Other proposed functions include maintenance of the thiol redox state of enzymes or other proteins and protection against oxidant stress.

Sinusoidal efflux of GSH is enhanced by infusion of physiological concentrations of hormones that initiate phosphoinositide hydrolysis, such as the α_1-adrenergic agonist phenylephrine, vasopressin, and angiotensin II.[28] The increase in sinusoidal efflux of GSH is accompanied by a decrease in biliary efflux of GSH (D. S. Raiford et al., unpublished observations). Infusion of phorbol dibutyrate, an agent that activates protein kinase C, also increased sinusoidal and decreased biliary efflux of GSH, suggesting a role

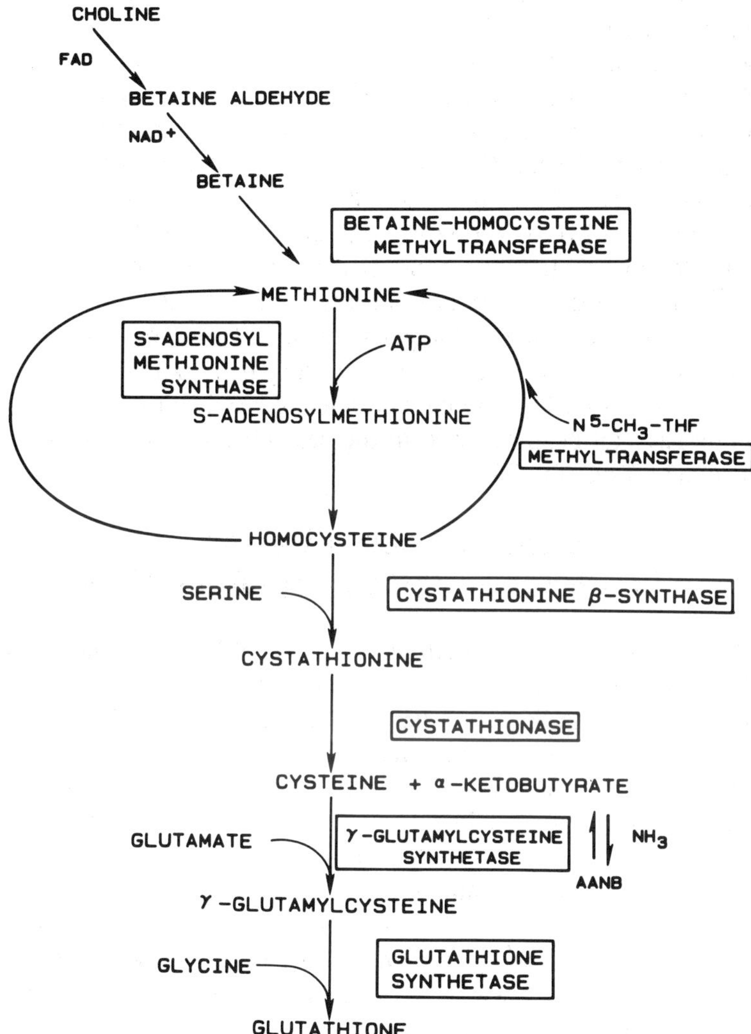

Fig. 2. Interorgan metabolism of glutathione. GSH is transported into plasma by carrier-mediated process. Clearance from plasma is rapid with a half-life of 2–3 min. The uptake of the sulfur moiety of GSH is greatest by those organs with γ-glutamyltranspeptidase (γ-GT) on the membrane. Final cleavage of the cysteinylglycine is catalyzed by dipeptidase (DP), prior to uptake of constituent amino acids.

for protein kinase C in the regulation of GSH efflux in response to vasopressor and stress hormones (D. S. Raiford et al., unpublished observations). One mechanism postulated to explain these effects is increased permeability of tight junctions, which occurs in response to vasopressor hormones.[29] However, no change in permeability of tight junctions occurred in response to infusion of phorbol ester (D. S. Raiford et al., unpublished observations). The reported effects of glucagon and other hormones that elevate cAMP and of dibutyryl cAMP on efflux of GSH are conflicting. Several reports have indicated that glutathione turnover and efflux are increased by these agents[30,31] whereas others have not confirmed these findings.[28,32] The physiological significance of these changes is unclear. However, during pathological states, the effects of these hormones may be important. Circulatory and septic shock as well as selenium deficiency[26] and chronic ethanol consumption[33] have all been reported to increase plasma GSH levels and/or the sinusoidal efflux of GSH.

Compartmentalization and Cellular Functions of Glutathione

The concentration of glutathione varies in different tissues ranging from 2–10 μmol/g wet wt. Hepatic concentrations are usually 4–6 μmol/g.[2,3] Overnight fasting decreases hepatic GSH by approx 25–30%.[2,3,18,30] Decreased availability of cysteine and increased hepatic efflux both contribute to lowering GSH levels.[2,18,30] More than 95% of glutathione is in the reduced form, whereas only a small percentage is present as the disulfide.[1–3] Approximately 10% of total glutathione is compartmentalized in mitochondria.[34] The hepatic mitochondrial pool of GSH has a longer half-life (30 h compared to 2–3 h) than the cytosolic pool.[34,35] Mitochondrial GSH is synthesized in the cytosol and transported into the mitochondria against a concentration gradient, with final concentrations of 10 mM in mitochondria, compared with 5 mM in cytosol.[34] The high concentrations of GSH in mitochondria are postulated to prevent oxidation of protein thiols during mitochondrial electron transport.[36]

Depletion of glutathione enhances the toxicity of many drugs and susceptibility to injury from oxidant stress.[8] In part, this increased susceptibility is owing to the participation of GSH in a number of detoxification processes, which are discussed in the following section. Glutathione may also be important in protecting critical protein thiol groups from oxidation and in the regulation of some enzymes[37] and other cellular processes including condensation of microtubules.[38]

Glutathione-Dependent Detoxification Processes

Glutathione is directly involved in several detoxification processes, either as a cofactor in enzyme-catalyzed reactions or through direct interaction with reactive electrophiles. These reactions are diagrammed in Fig. 2. The thiol group in glutathione is nucleophilic and reacts readily with many electrophiles. Although these reactions may proceed spontaneously, usually they are catalyzed by the glutathione *S*-transferases. At least seven distinct proteins with GSH *S*-transferase activity have been purified from rat liver.[39] Some are localized to the nucleus, mitochondria, or the smooth endoplasmic reticulum, although the majority are found in the cytosol, where they account for 5–10% of cytosolic proteins. A full discussion of these enzymes and their properties has been published recently.[39] The products of these reactions are covalent adducts of GSH and the substrate, which is most often an electrophile, in a thioether linkage. These conjugates are transported out of the cell, primarily into bile in the case of the liver.[2] They are subject to further metabolism by γ-glutamyltranspeptidase, which produces a mercapturic acid conjugate after cleavage of the γ-glutamyl moiety.[40]

Reduction of organic peroxides and H_2O_2 catalyzed by glutathione peroxidase represents the major source of GSSG within cells. GSSG is rapidly reduced to GSH by glutathione reductase with concomitant oxidation of the pyridine nucleotide, NADPH (Fig. 3). This two-step enzymatic reduction is the major pathway for the enzymatic reduction of both hydrogen and organic hydroperoxides.[41] The maximum activity of glutathione peroxidase is four- to fivefold higher (~40 μmol/min/g liver) than that of glutathione reductase (8–10 μmol/min/g liver).[8] This difference occasionally results in the accumulation of GSSG within cells. For this reason the intracellular ratio of GSSG/GSH is frequently used to provide an indication of oxidant stress.[42] Alterations in the thiol redox state may interfere with several enzymatic reactions and with calcium homeostasis in the cell and in mitochondria.[36,42] GSSG is subsequently transported out of cells, preferentially across the canalicular (apical) membrane of hepatocytes.[16] This transporter appears to be identical with the one that transports GSH conju-

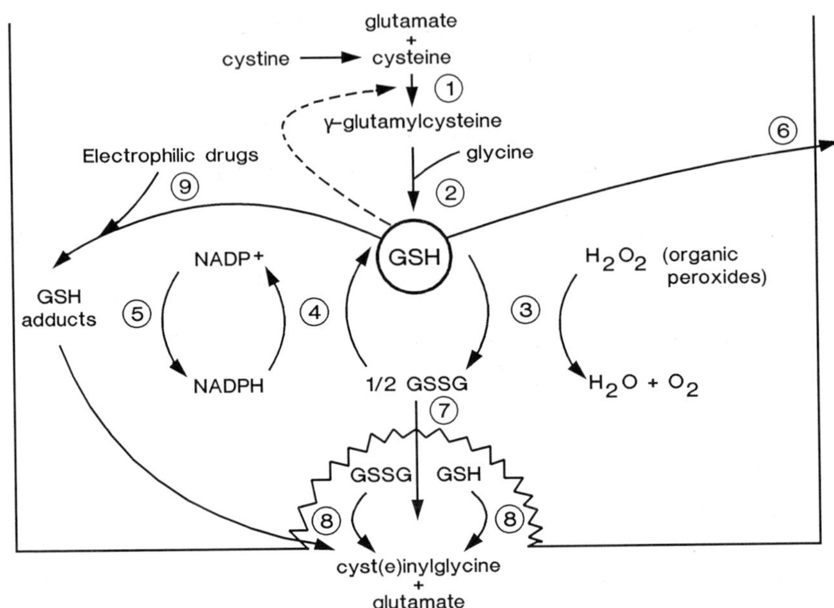

Fig. 3. Intrahepatic metabolism of glutathione. GSH is synthesized from constituent amino acids in a two-step process catalyzed by (1) γ-glutamylcysteine synthetase and (2) glutathione synthetase. It serves as a cofactor for the reduction of H_2O_2 and organic peroxides catalyzed by (3) glutathione peroxidase. Oxidized GSSG is reduced to GSH by (4) glutathione reductase with concomitant oxidation of NADPH to NADP+, which is subsequently reduced by (5) various dehydrogenases. GSH is transported across the (6) sinusoidal membrane and GSSG across the (7) canalicular membrane by carrier-mediated transport. GSH and GSSG in bile may be hydrolyzed to cyst(e)inylglycine and glutamate by (8) γ-glutamyltranspeptidase. GSH also serves as a cosubstrate for (9) glutathione *S*-transferases to form conjugates with electrophilic drugs or their metabolites and with other compounds, such as leukotrienes.

gates.[43–45] Whether this transporter also transports reduced GSH as well is the subject of controversy.[44,45]

Induction
of Cellular Detoxification Processes

The enzymes that utilize GSH as a cofactor are included among the Phase II drug metabolizing enzymes. Other Phase II enzymes include NADPH quinone reductase, glucuronyl transferases, and epoxide hydrolases. Most of these enzymes have substrates that are electrophilic, some of which are metabolites formed by cytochrome P-450. Like many of the Phase I enzymes, such as cytochrome P-450, the activities of these enzymes may be induced by their substrates and by other compounds.[46] The mechanism of induction is not completely understood, but does not appear to involve a receptor-mediated process. Some compounds will induce both Phase I and Phase II enzymes, whereas others selectively induce only Phase II enzymes.[47] It is of interest that chronic ethanol feeding induces not only cytochrome P-450, but also induces many of these Phase II drug metabolizing enzymes, as discussed later in this chapter.

Although the structures of agents that induce Phase II enzymes are quite diverse, a common characteristic of these inducers is that the compounds themselves or their oxidative metabolites are electrophilic.[46,47] The spectrum of inducing agents is broad and includes compounds with α, β-unsaturated ketone structures, such as quinones, phenolic antioxidants, and other electrophiles that are substrates for glutathione *S*-transferases. These inducing agents appear not only to induce the glutathione *S*-transferases and quinone reductase,[46] but also to increase glutathione levels in cells.[48,49] The induction of each of these enzymes may involve a common mechanism, rather than independent induction of each separately. Whether the genes encoding these enzymes share common regulatory sequences remains to be determined. Conceivably, the induction process may be initiated through a common signal transduction pathway.

Acute Effects of Ethanol
on Glutathione Levels and Metabolism

The effects of acute or chronic ethanol exposure on biological processes often differ and in many instances are opposite. In this regard, many of the effects of chronic exposure to ethanol may be viewed as adaptive responses or as tolerance to the acute effects. The effects of ethanol on glutathione metabolism follow this general pattern, and thus will be discussed separately.

Effects of Ethanol
on Hepatic GSH Levels

The acute administration of large doses (3–5 g/kg) of alcohol to rodents lowers hepatic levels of GSH by 25–50% over 3–5 hrs.[50–62] Decreases in GSH content of kidneys, heart, and brain have also been reported following an ethanol challenge.[52–54] The decrease in glutathione levels is reminiscent of that seen after administration of a variety of electrophiles or drugs that are metabolized to electrophiles, such as acetaminophen. Depletion of GSH following these agents results from the formation of GSH conjugates with these drugs. Based on this finding, some investigators have speculated that oxidation of ethanol to acetaldehyde would produce a more electrophilic compound that could react with GSH.[53,55,64] However, the decrease observed after ethanol differs from that following administration of electrophiles in two ways. First, the degree of depletion of GSH after administration of ethanol is never as extensive as that which occurs after electrophiles. Second, the time course of depletion as a result of ethanol is not as rapid as that which is a result of an electrophile. These differences suggest that the effects of alcohol are not completely explained by the formation of a conjugate of acetaldehyde or ethanol with GSH.

Interaction of Acetaldehyde with GSH

There is some evidence that acetaldehyde can react with GSH in vitro, forming first a semimercaptal with the sulfhydryl group of the cysteine residue and later cyclizing to form a thiazolidine.[65–67] Whether the reaction is quantitatively important is not clear. Based on rates of nonenzymatic conjugation at concentrations of acetaldehyde and GSH typically present in alcoholics (70 μM and 4 mM, respectively), Speisky and his colleagues calculated that this reaction could account for only 6% of the rate at which glutathione is depleted from the livers of rats given ethanol.[59] The conjugation of acetaldehyde with thiols proceeds much more rapidly with cysteine[67] or cysteinylglycine[68] than with GSH.

Further evidence for involvement of acetaldehyde in depletion of GSH was obtained in isolated hepatocytes. In this experimental model, ethanol lowered GSH levels within 3 h, an effect that was enhanced by the presence of disulfiram to inhibit oxidation of acetaldehyde.[69] Direct administration of acetaldehyde (0.3 g/kg) decreased hepatic GSH by 25%.[70] In human volunteers, administration of 0.2 g/kg of ethanol transiently lowered plasma levels of GSH, but not cysteine.[71] In subjects taking disulfiram, a similar dose of ethanol lowered both cysteine and GSH levels, with the decreases in cysteine preceding the decrease in plasma GSH, suggesting possible reaction of acetaldehyde with cysteine. Together, the results of these studies indicate that acetaldehyde can react with nonprotein thiols although direct proof of the in vivo formation of a stable conjugate of acetaldehyde and GSH is lacking. In part, this lack of evidence may be attributed to the instability of the adducts that are formed. Improvements in current analytical techniques will be required before this issue can be clarified.

Effects of Ethanol on Synthesis of GSH

The rate of depletion of hepatic GSH following ethanol administration is consistent with inhibition of glutathione synthesis by ethanol. Two published studies indicate that the hepatic synthesis of GSH in rats is inhibited in vivo by a single large dose of ethanol.[58,59] Both studies monitored the incorporation of radiolabeled cysteine into GSH as an index of glutathione synthesis. Ethanol could interfere with synthesis of GSH by a direct effect on the enzymes involved in synthesis, by inhibition of uptake of the amino acid precursors, or by depletion of one of the precursors, such as cysteine. However, no effect of ethanol on hepatic levels of cysteine was observed.[58,59] In isolated hepatocytes, the rate of recovery of GSH levels following depletion by the electrophile diethyl maleate was similar in the presence and absence of 80 mM of ethanol,[61] although in vivo administration of ethanol decreased the rate of recovery of GSH in vitro[61] and decreased activity of γ-glutamylcysteine synthetase.[62] Recent unpublished studies from our laboratory have not found evidence of inhibition of glutathione synthesis by ethanol in cultured primary hepatocytes or hepatoma cells using either [^{35}S]-cysteine or [^{35}S]-methionine as precursors for GSH. The inconsistencies between the results of in vivo and in vitro studies suggest that the effects of ethanol on synthesis of glutathione may be mediated indirectly through the effects of hormones or other more complex processes that are not reproduced in isolated or cultured hepatocytes.

Effects of Acute Administration of Ethanol on Hepatic Efflux of GSH

Administration of single doses of ethanol to rats increased the concentration of GSH in the hepatic veins.[55,59,63] However, infusion of high concentrations (50–200 mM) of ethanol into the perfused rat liver or exposure of isolated rat hepatocytes to ethanol did not increase efflux of GSH in vitro.[72] These observations are best explained by an indirect effect of ethanol on GSH efflux, which may be mediated by the release of hormones, such as catecholamines with α_1-agonist properties, which have been shown to increase efflux of GSH.[28] Furthermore, previous reports have indicated that ethanol can potentiate release of catecholamines from the adrenal glands.[73] Several studies have suggested that ethanol decreases the biliary efflux of GSH both in vivo and from the perfused rat liver[58,74,75] (M. C. Mitchell et al., unpublished observations). The mechanism and significance of this observation are both unclear, but suggest that ethanol may modulate hepatic transport processes either directly or indirectly.

Effects of Ethanol on Lipid Peroxidation and Thiol Redox State

Some studies have suggested that administration of single large doses of ethanol increases formation of lipid peroxides,[50,54,56,57] which could result in oxidation of GSH to GSSG during reduction by glutathione peroxidase. Once formed, GSSG is either reduced rapidly or exported from the cell.[16] Under some circumstances the rate of reduction of peroxides may exceed that of the reduction of GSSG.[36] However, it seems highly unlikely that the rate of lipid peroxidation following administration of ethanol in vivo would be sufficient to exceed the capacity of glutathione reductase to the extent necessary to deplete GSH.

Chronic Effects of Ethanol on Glutathione Levels and Metabolism

Effects of Chronic Administration of Ethanol on Heptatic GSH Levels

Although all studies have reported decreases in GSH levels following acute administration of ethanol, the effects of long-term ethanol feeding on hepatic GSH levels have been conflicting. Most studies have found similar or slightly increased levels of glutathione in the livers of rats fed liquid diets containing ethanol.[33,75–87] GSH levels in other tissues are generally unchanged. A smaller number have observed lower levels of GSH in ethanol-fed rats compared to pair-fed controls.[52,53,72,88] In some of these studies, levels of GSH were measured in hepatocytes freshly isolated from rats that were fasted overnight.[88] The differences in methodology may explain, in part, the discordant findings in reported studies. Although the steady-state levels of the GSH remain relatively unchanged by chronic ethanol feeding, there is some evidence that such treatment may decrease the mitochondrial pool to 40–50% of the levels in pair-fed control rats.[88] Acute ethanol administration can also lower mitochondrial GSH (M. C. Mitchell et al., unpublished observations). The implications of the decreases in mitochondrial GSH remain to be eluciated. It is tempting to speculate that changes in this pool of glutathione may permit oxidant damage to the enzymes of the electron transport chain. The adverse effects of chronic ethanol feeding on mitochondrial function are well recognized. Interestingly, cysteine may prevent some of the ethanol-related damage to mitochondria.[89]

Effects of Ethanol on Hepatic Turnover and Efflux of GSH

Although steady-state levels of GSH are important in determining susceptibility to drug-induced or oxidant injury to cells, they do not provide information about glutathione homeostasis. The hepatic turnover of glutathione was approximately twofold higher in rats fed ethanol for 6 wk compared with pair-fed controls, whereas steady-state levels were similar in both groups.[79] In addition, the rate of synthesis of glutathione in vitro was significantly higher in the liver homogenates from ethanol-fed rats compared to controls.[79] Further studies indicated that the sinusoidal efflux of GSH was increased to a similar extent in the perfused livers of ethanol-fed rats, suggesting that the increase in turnover was related to the increased rate of hepatic efflux[80] (Fig. 4). These findings were confirmed by other investigators not only for the perfused liver, but also for freshly isolated hepatocytes.[72]

Indirect evidence for increased synthesis of GSH after ethanol feeding is provided by reported increases in the activities of S-adenosylmethionine synthetase and cystathionine synthetase.[90] The activities of these enzymes are pivotal in regulating the flux of methionine through the transsulfuration pathway. Chronic ethanol feeding also increased hepatic production and plasma levels of α-amino-n-butyric acid (AANB), an amino acid that is in equilibrium with α-ketobutyrate, a byproduct of the transsulfuration pathway[91] (Fig. 1). Together, these observations suggest increased requirements for and/or synthesis of glutathione in rats fed ethanol.

The stimulus for increased hepatic synthesis and efflux of glutathione remains uncertain. Plasma levels of GSH and cysteine were higher whereas plasma clearance of GSH was similar in ethanol-fed rats compared with

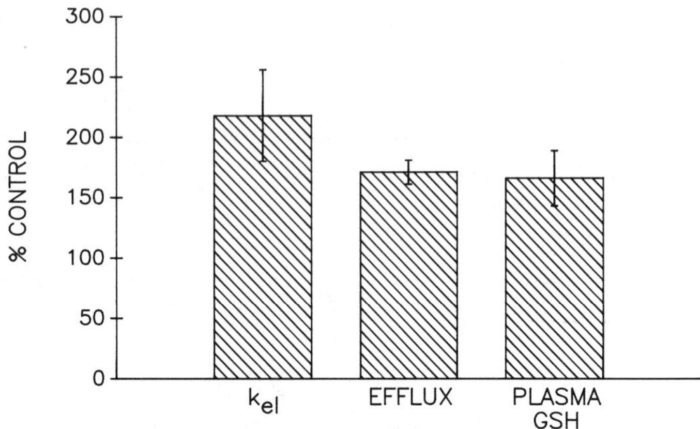

Fig. 4. Effects of ethanol on glutathione turnover and efflux. The bars represent the turnover (k_{el}) (ref. *79*), sinusoidal efflux (ref. *80*), and plasma GSH levels (ref. *33*) in rats fed ethanol for 6 wk expressed as a percent of the values for pair-fed controls.

pair-fed controls[33] (Fig. 4). Furthermore, the uptake of ^{35}S by extrahepatic tissues was similar in both groups.[33] Since the extrahepatic utilization of glutathione is not altered by chronic ethanol feeding, these observations suggest that the increased sinusoidal efflux of GSH is a result of an ethanol-mediated effect on the liver. That this may be a direct effect is supported by unpublished studies from our laboratory that have confirmed that increased efflux of glutathione occurs in primary hepatocyte cultures following 7–10 d of exposure to 100 m*M* ethanol.

Effects of Ethanol on GSH-Dependent Detoxification Enzymes

There are several reports that have shown that chronic ethanol feeding increases the activities of glutathione *S*-transferases[33,78,82,86,92] and glutathione reductase.[33] The increases in the activities of these enzymes and in the levels of GSH resemble the induction of Phase II drug metabolism in response to an electrophilic challenge. As noted earlier, the majority of inducing agents are substrates for the glutathione *S*-transferases. Recently published studies by Lange and his colleagues indicate that ethanol may be a substrate for an acidic glutathione *S*-transferase,[93] which is identical to the previously described fatty acid ethyl ester synthetase.[94] It is interesting to speculate that the interaction of ethanol with the glutathione *S*-transferases is involved in the induction of these enzymes during chronic ethanol feeding. Although the activities of the GSH *S*-transferases are increased by chronic ethanol feeding, reported changes in the activity of glutathione peroxidase are conflicting. Most studies have found similar values,[85,86] whereas others have observed decreased[79] or increased activity.[82]

Hepatic γ-glutamyltranspeptidase (GGT) is increased both in alcoholics[95,96] and in rats chronically fed ethanol.[97–100] Despite the importance of GGT in catabolism of glutathione,[1] the significance of the increases in GGT after chronic ethanol feeding is unclear. Although hepatic efflux of GSH is believed to account for the turnover of GSH in the rat, there was a good correlation between the rate of hepatic turnover of GSH and the GGT activity after 6 wk of ethanol feeding.[79] Additional evidence has been presented for a role for hepatic basolateral GGT in degradation of circulating GSH particularly in the guinea pig.[101] After chronic ethanol feeding, the degradation of GSH infused into the perfused rat liver was enhanced along with basolateral and total homogenate activity of GGT.[102] Although it is conceivable that the enzyme may participate in the clearance of GSH from the circulation, there was no direct evidence of increased uptake of $[^{35}S]$-GSH by the livers of ethanol-fed rats compared to controls.[33] Additional work will be needed to clarify the role of this enzyme in glutathione homeostasis.

Effects of Alcohol on Glutathione Levels and Metabolism in Humans

Relatively few studies have examined the effects of a single dose of alcohol on glutathione levels in human volunteers. In one study, 0.2 g/kg of ethanol lowered plasma GSH levels in alcoholics and in healthy volunteers.[70] Other studies have measured the levels of GSH and/or GSSG in liver biopsies from alcoholics with clinical signs of liver disease and compared them to levels in otherwise healthy individuals undergoing cholecystectomy. Most alcoholics with liver disease have hepatic levels of GSH that are 30–50% lower than those in healthy individuals.[103–107] In those instances in which the severity of liver damage was quantitated, there was no correlation between the severity of liver injury caused by alcohol and the levels of GSH.[105,106] Following 2 wk of abstinence from ethanol, GSH levels increased to a greater degree in those patients without hepatic necrosis.[105]

This observation suggests a degree of reversibility, although the mechanism underlying this effect is unclear.

Interpreting the lower levels of hepatic GSH in alcoholics is difficult. There are many potentially confounding factors that are not easily assessed. Since alcoholism and alcoholic liver disease are often associated with generalized malnutrition or selective nutritional deficiencies,[108] it is necessary to consider this variable. Duration of abstinence may also affect hepatic GSH levels. The effects of ethanol on GSH metabolism in animals do not persist indefinitely.[78] Thus, some of the observed differences in alcoholics may reflect the effects of prior alcohol consumption followed by abstinence.[105] Furthermore, it is difficult to separate the effects of ethanol from those of liver disease. Patients with nonalcoholic liver disease also have lower hepatic levels of glutathione.[107] In rodents, which do not develop damage beyond the stage of fatty liver, it is easier to identify those effects that are caused by ethanol feeding itself. One explanation for the decrease in GSH levels in patients with cirrhosis is decreased transsulfuration of methionine to cysteine (and glutathione).[109] The defect in transsulfuration appears to be a consequence of cirrhosis, since in alcoholics without liver disease increases in plasma α-aminobutyric acid provide evidence of increased flux through this pathway.[110,111] There is additional evidence that the defect is at the level of *S*-adenosylmethionine (SAM) synthetase.[112] Supplying SAM in the diet increased hepatic GSH levels in patients with both alcoholic and nonalcoholic cirrhosis and in baboons fed ethanol.[113,114] Thus, although it is relatively easy to measure GSH levels in alcoholics with and without liver disease, interpretation of these finding requires caution.

Consequences of Altered Glutathione Metabolism Caused by Alcohol

In general, lower levels of hepatic GSH increase susceptibility to damage caused by free radicals, reactive oxygen species, electrophiles, and lipid peroxides.[8] Although there is evidence that alcoholics are at increased risk of liver injury from acetaminophen[115–117] and presumably other drugs that have similar toxicologic properties,[118] the mechanism underlying this enhanced risk is not completely clear.[117] The increased risk can be reproduced in rodents[119] and in primates fed ethanol for several weeks.[120] Under these conditions, there is an increased rate of oxidation of acetaminophen to an electrophilic metabolite that can deplete GSH, bind to cellular proteins, initiate oxidant stress, and damage hepatocytes.[119] Because this enhanced susceptibility does not require prior lowering of GSH levels in response to ethanol feeding, many have assumed that increased activity of certain isozymes of cytochrome P-450 was the predominant effect of ethanol accounting for the enhanced toxicity. Under conditions resulting in increased oxidation of drugs, there is an increase in the requirements for GSH to provide detoxification of the electrophilic drug metabolites. For example, following administration of bromobenzene, a drug with a mechanism of toxicity similar to acetaminophen, the amount of oxidized metabolites excreted as derivatives of GSH may exceed the amount of GSH present at the time of administration indicating the importance of newly synthesized GSH in drug detoxification.[121] As mentioned, chronic ethanol feeding increases the loss of GSH through nondetoxification pathways (sinusoidal efflux).[72,80] Under those circumstances in which there is an increased requirement for GSH in detoxification reactions, this loss and/or inability to increase further the rate of synthesis may prevent adequate replenishment of glutathione stores. In addition to increasing susceptibility to drug-induced injury, chronic ethanol feeding may also render the liver more susceptible to oxidant stress from other sources, including ischemia and reperfusion or even those normal metabolic processes that produce reactive oxygen species.[122]

Whether changes in glutathione levels or metabolism increase ethanol-related damage is a matter of speculation. Ethanol-induced injury to the liver and other organs occurs in fewer than half of all alcoholics. In this regard, the toxicity of ethanol resembles an idiosyncratic reaction more than a direct toxic reaction. Although it is conceivable that some of the toxicity of ethanol may involve a free radical-mediated mechanism or other source of oxidant stress, there is insufficient evidence to conclude that the adaptive changes in glutathione metabolism are central to this process. Although there is some evidence that GSH may have a role in the detoxification of ethanol or acetaldehyde, much remains to be learned about its significance in preventing organ damage caused by ethanol. The effects of chronic ethanol consumption on glutathione metabolism may provide a necessary, but not sufficient condition for the ultimate toxicity of ethanol within an otherwise predisposed individual.

References

[1] A. Meister and M. E. Anderson (1983) Glutathione. *Ann. Rev. Biochem.* **52,** 711–760.

[2] N. Kaplowitz, T. Y. Aw, and M. Ookhtens (1985) The regulation of hepatic glutathione. *Ann. Rev. Pharm. Toxicol.* **25,** 715–744.

[3] S. Deneke and B. L. Fanburg (1989) Regulation of cellular glutathione. *Am. J. Physiol.* **257,** L163–173.

[4] R. Sekura and A. Meister (1977) γ-glutamylcysteine synthetase. Further purification, "half of the sites" reactivity subunits and specificity. *J. Biol. Chem.* **252,** 2599–2605.

[5] S. Yanari, J. E. Snoke, and K. Bloch (1953) Energy sources in glutathione synthesis. *J. Biol. Chem.* **201,** 561–571.

[6] P. G. Richman and A. Meister (1975) Regulation of γ-glutamylcysteine synthetase by nonallosteric feedback inhibition by glutathione. *J. Biol. Chem.* **250,** 1422–1426.

[7] B. H. Lauterburg, Y. Vaishnav, W. G. Stillwell, and J. R. Mitchell (1980) The effects of age and glutathione depletion on hepatic glutathione turnover in vivo determined by acetaminophen probe analysis. *Pharmacol. Exp. Ther.* **213,** 54–58.

[8] D. J. Reed and M. W. Fariss (1984) Glutathione depletion and susceptibility. Pharmacol. Rev. **36,** 25S–35S.

[9] B. A. Arrick, W. Griffo, Z. Cohn, and C. Nathan (1985) Hydrogen peroxide from cellular metabolism of cystine. *J. Clin. Invest.* **76,** 567–574.

[10] S. Bannai (1984) Transport of cystine and cysteine in mammalian cells. *Biochim. Biophys. Acta* **779,** 289–306.

[11] M. S. Kilberg, H. N. Christensen, and M. E. Handlogten (1979) *Biochem. Biophys. Res. Commun.* **88,** 747–751.

[12] N. Tateishi, T. Higashi, A. Naruse, K. Hikita, and Y. Sakamoto (1981) Relative contributions of sulfur atoms of dietary cysteine and methionine to rat liver glutathione and proteins. *J. Biochem.* **90,** 1603–1610.

[13] D. J. Reed and S. Orrenius (1977) The role of methionine in glutathione biosynthesis by isolated hepatocytes. *Biochem. Biophys. Res. Commun.* **77,** 1257–1264.

[14] S. S. Tate and A. Meister (1974) Interaction of γ-glutamyl transpeptidase with amino acids, dipeptides, and derivatives and analogs of glutathione. *J. Biol. Chem.* **249,** 7593–7602.

[15] M. E. Anderson and A. Meister (1983) Transport and direct utilization of γ-glutamylcyst(e)ine for glutathione synthesis. *Proc. Natl. Acad. Sci.* **80,** 707–711.

[16] G. A. Bartoli and H. Sies (1978) Reduced and oxidized glutathione efflux from the liver. *FEBS Lett.* **86,** 89–91.

[17] B. H. Lauterburg, J. D. Adams, and J. R. Mitchell (1984) Hepatic glutathione

homeostasis in the rat: Efflux accounts for glutathione turnover. *Hepatology* **4,** 586–590.

[18] M. Ookhtens, K. Hobdy, M. C. Corvasce, T. Y. Aw, and N. Kaplowitz (1985) Sinusoidal efflux of glutathione in the perfused rat liver. Evidence for a carrier-mediated process. *J. Clin. Invest.* **75,** 258–265.

[19] T. Y. Aw, M. Ookhtens, C. Ren, and N. Kaplowitz (1986) Kinetics of glutathione efflux from isolated rat hepatocytes. *Am. J. Physiol.* **250,** G236–243.

[20] M. Inoue, R. Kinne, T. Tran, and I. M. Arias (1984) Glutathione transport across hepatocyte plasma membranes: Analysis using isolated rat liver sinusoidal-membrane vesicles. *Eur. J. Biochem.* **138,** 491–495.

[21] T. Y. Aw, M. Ookhtens, J. F. Kuhlenkamp, and N. Kaplowitz (1987) Trans-stimulation and driving forces for GSH transport in sinusoidal membrane vesicles from rat liver. *Biochem. Biophys. Res. Commun.* **143,** 377–382.

[22] M. Ookhtens, I. Lyon, J. Fernandez-Checa, and N. Kaplowitz (1988) Inhibition of glutathione efflux in the perfused rat liver and isolated hepatocytes by organic anions and bilirubin. *J. Clin. Invest.* **82,** 608–616.

[23] N. Ballatori, R. Jacob, C. Barrett, and J. L. Boyer (1988) Biliary catabolism of glutathione and differential reabsorption of its amino acid constituents. *Am. J. Physiol.* **254,** G1–G7.

[24] J. D. Adams, B. H. Lauterburg, and J. R. Mitchell (1983) Plasma glutathione and glutathione disulfide in the rat: Regulation and response to oxidative stress. *J. Pharmacol. Exp. Ther.* **227,** 749–754.

[25] A. Wendel and P. Cikryt (1980) The level and half-life of glutathione in human plasma. *FEBS Lett.* **120,** 209–211.

[26] K. E. Hill and R. F. Burk (1985) Effect of selenium deficiency on the disposition of plasma glutathione. *Arch. Biochem. Biophys.* **240,** 166–171.

[27] T. Higashi, N. Tateishi, A. Naruse, and Y. Sakamoto (1977) A novel physiological role of liver glutathione as a reservoir of cysteine. *J. Biochem.* **82,** 117–124.

[28] H. Sies and P. Graf (1985) Hepatic thiol and glutathione efflux under the influence of vasopressin, phenylephrine and adrenaline. *Biochem. J.* **226,** 545–549.

[29] P. J. Lowe, K. Miyal, H. Steinbach, and W. G. M. Hardison (1988) Hormonal regulation of hepatocyte tight junctional permeability. *Am. J. Physiol.* **255,** G454–G461.

[30] B. H. Lauterburg and J. R. Mitchell (1981) Regulation of hepatic glutathione turnover in rats *in vivo* and evidence for kinetic homogeneity of the hepatic glutathione pool. *J. Clin. Invest.* **67,** 1415–1424.

[31] S. Lu, C. Garcia-Ruiz, J. Kuhlenkamp, M. Ookhtens, and N. Kaplowitz (1990) Hormonal regulation of GSH efflux. *Clin. Res.* **38,** 424A.

[32] T. L. Wright, G. Fitz, and T. D. Boyer (1988) Hepatic efflux of glutathione by

the perfused rat liver: Role of membrane potential difference. *Am. J. Physiol.* **255,** G547–G555.

[33] D. J. Callans, L. S. Wacker, and M. C. Mitchell (1987) Effects of ethanol feeding and withdrawal on plasma glutathione elimination in the rat. *Hepatology* **7,** 496–501.

[34] O. W. Griffith and A. Meister (1985) Origin and turnover of mitochondrial glutathione. *Proc. Natl. Acad. Sci. USA* **82,** 4668–4672.

[35] M. J. Meredith and D. J. Reed (1982) Status of the mitochodrial pool of glutathione in the isolated hepatocyte. *J. Biol. Chem.* **257,** 3747–3753.

[36] D. J. Reed (1990) Glutathione: Toxicological implications. *Ann. Rev. Pharmacol. Toxicol.* **30,** 603–631.

[37] D. M. Ziegler (1985) Role of reversible oxidation reduction of enzyme thiols-disulfides in metabolic regulation. *Ann. Rev. Biochem.* **54,** 305–329.

[38] J. M. Oliver, D. F. Albertini, and R. D. Berlin (1976) Effects of glutathione oxidizing agents on microtubule assembly and microtubule-dependent surface properties of human neutrophils. *J. Cell. Biol.* **71,** 921–932.

[39] T. D. Boyer (1989) The glutathione *S*-transferases: An update. *Hepatology* **9,** 486–496.

[40] E. Boyland and L. F. Chasseud (1969) The role of glutathione and glutathione *S*-transferases in mercapturic acid biosynthesis. Advan. Enzymol. **32,** 172–219.

[41] H. Sies and K. H. Summer (1975) Hydroperoxide-metabolising systems in rat liver. *Eur. J. Biochem.* **57,** 503–512.

[42] G. Bellomo and S. Orrenius (1985) Altered thiol and calcium homeostasis in oxidative hepatocellular injury. *Hepatology* **5,** 876–882.

[43] M. Inoue, R. Kinne, T. Tran, and I. Arias (1983) The mechanism of biliary secretion of reduced glutathione. Analysis of transport process in isolated rat-liver canalicular membrane vesicles. *Eur. J. Biochem.* **134,** 467–471.

[44] G. Lindwall and T. D. Boyer (1987) Excretion of glutathione conjugates by primary cultured rat hepatocytes. *J. Biol. Chem.* **262,** 5151–5158.

[45] R. P. Elferink, R. Ottenhoff, W. Liefting, J. deHaan, and P. L. Jansen (1989) Hepatobiliary transport of glutathione and glutathione conjugate in rats with hereditary hyperbilirubinemia. *J. Clin. Invest.* **84,** 476-483.

[46] P. Talalay, M. J. De Long, and H. J. Prochaska (1987) Molecular mechanisms in protection against carcinogenesis, in *Cancer Biology and Therapeutics*. J. G. Cory and A. Szentivanyi, eds. Plenum, New York, pp. 197–216.

[47] H. J. Prochaska, M. J. De Long, and P. Talalay (1985) On the mechanisms of induction of cancer-protective enzymes: A unifying proposal. *Proc. Natl. Acad. Sci.* **82,** 8232–8236.

[48] S. Bannai (1989) Induction of cystine and glutamate transport activity in human fibroblasts by diethylmaleate and other electrophilic agents. *J. Biol. Chem.* **259,** 2435–2440.

[49] S. M. Deneke, D. F. Baxter, S. T. Phelps, and B. L. Fanburg (1989) Increase in endothelial cell glutathione and precursor amino acid uptake by diethyl maleate and hyperoxia. *Am. J. Physiol.* **257**, L265–L271.

[50] A. Takada, F. Ikegami, Y. Okumura, Y. Hasumura, R. Kanayama, and J. Takeuchi (1970) Effect of alcohol on the liver of rats. *Lab. Invest.* **23**, 421–428.

[51] C. M. MacDonald, J. Dow, and M. R. Moore (1977) A possible protective role for sulphydryl compounds in acute alcoholic liver injury. *Biochem. Pharmacol.* **26**, 1529–1531.

[52] V. Fernández and L. A. Videla (1981) Effect of acute and chronic ethanol ingestion on the content of reduced glutathione of various tissues of the rat. *Experientia* **37**, 392–394.

[53] C. Guerri and S. Grisolía (1980) Changes in glutathione in acute and chronic alcohol intoxication. *Pharmacol. Biochem. Behav.* **13**, 53–61.

[54] Y. Kera, S. Komura, Y. Ohbora, T. Kiriyama, and K. Inoue (1985) Ethanol induced changes in lipid peroxidation and nonprotein sulfhydryl content. *Res. Comm. Chem. Pathol. Pharmacol.* **47**, 203–209.

[55] L. A. Videla, V. Fernández, N. Fernández, and A. Valenzuela (1981) On the mechanism of the glutathione depletion induced in the liver by acute ethanol ingestion. *Subst. Alcohol Actions/Misuse* **2**, 153–160.

[56] N. Koçak-Toker, M. Uysal, G. Aykaç, S. Yalçin, A. Sivas, and H. Oz (1983) Effect of acute ethanol intoxication on the liver lipid peroxide and glutathione levels in the rat. *IRCS Med. Sci.* **11**, 915,916.

[57] L. A. Videla, V. Fernández, A. Valenzuela, and G. Ugarte (1981) Effect of (+)-cyanidanol-3 on the changes in liver glutathione content and lipoperoxidation induced by acute ethanol administration in the rat. *Pharmacology* **22**, 343–348.

[58] B. H. Lauterburg, S. Davies, and J. R. Mitchell (1984) Ethanol suppresses hepatic glutathione synthesis in rats *in vivo. J. Pharmacol. Exp. Ther.* **230**, 7–11.

[59] H. Speisky, A. MacDonald, G. Giles, H. Orrego, and Y. Israel (1985) Increased loss and decreased synthesis of hepatic glutathione after acute ethanol administration. *Biochem. J.* **225**, 565–572.

[60] H. Speisky, D. Bunout, H. Orrego, H. G. Giles, A. Gunasekara, and Y. Israel (1985) Lack of changes in diene conjugate levels following ethanol induced glutathione depletion or hepatic necrosis. *Res. Comm. Chem. Pathol. Pharmacol.* **48**, 77–90.

[61] H. Speisky, Y. Kera, K. E. Penttilä, Y. Israel, and K. O. Lindros (1988) Depletion of hepatic glutathione by ethanol occurs independently of ethanol metabolism. *Alcohol. Clin. Exp. Res.* **12**, 224–228.

[62] J. Gonzalez, M. E. Muñoz, M. I. Martin, P. S. Collado, J. Fermoso, and A. Esteller (1988) Influence of acute ethanol administration on hepatic glutathione metabolism in the rat. *Alcohol* **5**, 103–106.

[63] S. R. Paredes, P. A. Kozicki, H. Fukuda, M. V. Rossetti, and A. M. Del C.

Batlle (1987) *S*-adenosyl-L-methionine: Its effect on aminolevulinate dehydratase and glutathione in acute ethanol intoxication. *Alcohol* **4,** 81–85

[64] L. A. Videla and A. Valenzuela (1982) Alcohol ingestion, liver glutathione and lipoperoxidation: Metabolic interrelations and pathological implications. *Life Sci.* **31,** 2395–2407.

[65] M. P. Schubert (1936) Compounds of thiol acids with aldehydes. *J. Biol. Chem.* **114,** 341–350.

[66] M. P. Schubert (1937) Reactions of semimercaptals with amino compounds. *J. Biol. Chem.* **121,** 539–548.

[67] L. Wlodek (1988) The reaction of sulfhydryl groups with carbonyl compounds. *Acta Biochimica Polonica* **35,** 307–316.

[68] Y. Kera, T. Kiriyama, and S. Komura (1985) Conjugation of acetaldehyde with cysteinylglycine, the first metabolite in glutathione breakdown by γ-glutamyltranspeptidase. *Agents and Actions* **17,** 48–52.

[69] J. Viña, J. M. Estrela, C. Guerri, and F. J. Romero (1980) Effect of ethanol on glutathione concentration in isolated hepatocytes. *Biochem. J.* **188,** 549–552.

[70] L. A. Videla, V. Fernández, and A. de Marinis (1982) Liver lipoperoxidative pressure and glutathione status following acetaldehyde and aliphatic alcohols pretreatments in the rat. *Biochem. Biophys. Res. Commun.* **104,** 965–970.

[71] J.-M. Burgunder, J. Nelles, M. Bilzer, and B. H. Lauterburg (1988) Ethanol decreases plasma sulphydryls in man: Effect of disulfiram. *Eur. J. Clin. Invest.* **18,** 420–424.

[72] J. C. Fernández-Checa, M. Ookhtens, and N. Kaplowitz (1987) Effect of chronic ethanol feeding on rat hepatocytic glutathione. Compartmentation, efflux, and response to incubation with ethanol. *J. Clin. Invest.* **80,** 57–62.

[73] R. H. Johnson, G. Eisenhofer, and D. G. Lambie (1986) The effects of acute and chronic ingestion of ethanol on the autonomic nervous system. *Drug Alcohol Depend.* **18,** 319–328.

[74] C.-P. Siegers, U. Jeb, and M. Younes (1983) Effects of phenobarbital, GSH-depletors, CCl_4 and ethanol on the biliary efflux of glutathione in rats. *Arch. Int. Pharmacodyn.* **266,** 315–325.

[75] G. Vendemiale, E. Jayatilleke, S. Shaw, and C. S. Lieber (1984) Depression of biliary glutathione excretion by chronic ethanol feeding in the rat. *Life Sci.* **34,** 1065–1073.

[76] J. M. Hassing, A. L. Hupka, S. J. Stohs, and P. C. Yoon (1979) Hepatic glutathione levels in D-penicillamine-fed ethanol-dependent rats. *Res. Comm. Chem. Pathol. Pharmacol.* **25,** 389–394.

[77] E. Kaplan, E. G. DeMaster, and H. T. Nagasawa (1980) Effect of pargyline on hepatic glutathione levels in rats treated acutely and chronically with ethanol. *Res. Comm. Chem. Pathol. Pharmacol.* **30,** 577–580.

[78] C. Hétu, L. Yelle, and J.-G. Joly (1982) Influence of ethanol on hepatic

glutathione content and on the activity of glutathione *S*-transferases and epoxide hydrase in the rat. *Drug Metab. Dis.* **10,** 246–250.

[79] S. Morton and M. C. Mitchell (1985) Effects of chronic ethanol feeding on glutathione turnover in the rat. *Biochem. Pharmacol.* **34,** 1559–1563.

[80] J. L. Pierson and M. C. Mitchell (1986) Increased hepatic efflux of glutathione after chronic ethanol feeding. *Biochem. Pharmacol.* **35,** 1533–1537.

[81] S. Shaw, E. Jayatilleke, W. A. Ross, E. R. Gordon, and C. S. Lieber (1981) Ethanol-induced lipid peroxidation: Potentiation by long-term alcohol feeding and attenuation by methionine. *J. Lab. Clin. Med.* **98,** 417–424.

[82] G. Aykaç, M. Uysal, A. S. Yalçin, N. Koçak-Toker, A. Sivas, and H. Öz (1985) The effect of chronic ethanol ingestion on hepatic lipid peroxide, glutathione, glutathione peroxidase and glutathione transferase in rats. *Toxicology* **36,** 71–76.

[83] J. T. Työppönen and K. O. Lindros (1986) Combined vitamin E deficiency and ethanol pretreatment: Liver glutathione and enzyme changes. *Int. J. Vit. Nutr. Res.* **56,** 241–245.

[84] M. Uysal, M. Keyer-Uysal, N. Koçak-Toker, and G. Aykaç (1986) The effect of chronic ethanol ingestion on brain lipid peroxide and glutathione levels in rats. *Drug Alcohol Depend.* **18,** 73–75.

[85] J. Harata, M. Nagata, E. Sasaki, I. Ishiguro, Y. Ohta, and Y. Murakami (1983) Effect of prolonged alcohol administration on activities of various enzymes scavenging activated oxygen radicals and lipid peroxide level in the liver of rats. *Biochem. Pharmacol.* **32,** 1795–1798.

[86] M. E. Muñoz, M. I. Martin, J. Fermoso, J. Gonzalez, and A. Esteller (1987) Effect of chronic ethanol feeding on glutathione and glutathione-related enzyme activities in rat liver. *Drug Alcohol Depend.* **20,** 221–226.

[87] T. Kawase, S. Kat, and C. S. Lieber (1989) Lipid peroxidation and antioxidant defense systems in rat liver after chronic ethanol feeding. *Hepatology* **10,** 815–821.

[88] J. C. Fernandez-Checa, M. Ookhtens, and N. Kaplowitz (1989) Effects of chronic ethanol feeding on rat hepatocytic glutathione. Relationship of cytosolic glutathione to efflux and mitochondrial sequestration. *J. Clin. Invest.* **83,** 1247–1252.

[89] A. I. Cederbaum and E. Rubin (1976) Protective effect of cysteine on the inhibition of mitochondrial functions by acetaldehyde. *Biochem. Pharmacol.* **25,** 963–973.

[90] J. D. Finkelstein, J. P. Cello, and W. E. Kyle (1974) Ethanol-induced changes in methionine metabolism in rat liver. *Biochem. Biophys. Res. Commun.* **61,** 525–531.

[91] S. Shaw and C. S. Lieber (1980) Increased hepatic production of alpha-amino-*n*-butyric acid after chronic alcohol consumption in rats and baboons. *Gastroenterology* **78,** 108–113.

[92] R. M. David and D. E. Nerland (1983) Induction of mouse liver glutathione *S*-transferase by ethanol. *Biochem. Pharmacol.* **32,** 2809–2811.

[93] P. S. Bora, C. A. Spilburg, and L. G. Lange (1989) Metabolism of ethanol and carcinogens by glutathione transferases. *Proc. Natl. Acad. Sci. USA* **86,** 4470–4473.

[94] P. S. Bora, C. A. Spilburg, and L. G. Lange (1989) Identification of a satellite fatty acid ethyl ester synthase from human myocardium as a glutathione *S*-transferase. *J. Clin. Invest.* **84,** 1942–1946.

[95] R. Teschke, M. Neuefeind, M. Nishimura, and G. Strohmeyer (1983) Hepatic gamma-glutamyltransferase activity in alcoholic fatty liver: comparison with other liver enzymes in man and rats. *Gut* **24,** 625–630.

[96] E. Ivanov, D. Adjarov, M. Etarska, T. Stankushev, K. Brumbarov, and M. Kerimova (1980) Elevated liver gamma-glutamyl transferase in chronic alcoholics. *Enzyme* **25,** 304–308.

[97] G. Gadeholt, J. Aarbakke, E. Dybing, M. Sjöblom, and J. Mørland (1980) Hepatic microsomal drug metabolism, glutamyl transferase activity and *in vivo* antipyrine half-life in rats chronically fed an ethanol diet, a control diet and a chow diet. *J. Pharmacol. Exp. Ther.* **213,** 196–203.

[98] H. Ishii, S. Yasuraoka, Y. Shigeta, S. Takagi, T. Kamiya, F. Okuno, K. Miyamoto, and M. Tsuchiya (1978) Hepatic and intestinal gamma-glutamyltranspeptidase activity: Its activation by chronic ethanol administration. *Life Sci.* **23,** 1393–1398.

[99] R. Teschke and A. S. Petrides (1982) Hepatic gamma-glutamyltransferase activity: Its increase following chronic alcohol consumption and the role of carbohydrates. *Biochem. Pharmacol.* **31,** 3751–3756.

[100] S. Yamada, J. S. Wilson, and C. S. Lieber (1985) The effects of ethanol and diet on hepatic and serum γ-glutamyltranspeptidase activities in rats. *J. Nutr.* **115,** 1285–1290.

[101] H. Spiesky, N. Shackel, G. Varghese D. Wade, and Y. Israel (1990) Role of hepatic γ-glutamyltransferase in the degradation of circulating glutathione: Studies in the intact guinea pig perfused liver. *Hepatology* **11,** 843–849.

[102] H. Speisky, A. Gunasekara, G. Varghese, and Y. Israel (1987) Basolateral gamma-glutamyltransferase ectoactivity in rat liver: Effects of chronic alcohol consumption. *Alcohol Alcohol.* **1 (Suppl),** 245–249.

[103] S. Shaw, K. P. Rubin, and C. S. Lieber (1983) Depressed hepatic glutathione and increased diene conjugates in alcoholic liver disease. Evidence of lipid peroxidation. *Dig. Dis. Sci.* **28,** 585–589.

[104] K. W. Woodhouse, F. M. Williams, E. Mutch, P. Wright, O. F. W. James, and M. D. Rawlins (1983) The effect of alcoholic cirrhosis on the activities of microsomal aldrin epoxidase, 7–ethoxycoumarin-*O*–DE-ethylase and epoxide hydrolase, and on the concentrations of reduced glutathione in human liver. *Br. J. Clin. Pharmacol.* **15,** 667–672.

[105] L. A. Videla, H. Iturriaga, M. E. Pino, D. Bunout, A. Valenzuela, and G.

Ugarte (1984) Content of hepatic reduced glutathione in chronic alcoholic patients: Influence of the length of abstinence and liver necrosis. *Clin. Sci.* **66**, 283–290.

[106] S. A. Jewell, D. Di Monte, A. Gentile, A. Guglielmi, E. Altomare, and O. Albano (1986) Decreased hepatic glutathione in chronic alcoholic patients. *J. Hepatol.* **3**, 1–6.

[107] E. Altomare, G. Vendemiale, and O. Albano (1988) Hepatic glutathione content in patients with alcoholic and non alcoholic liver diseases. *Life Sci.* **43**, 991–998.

[108] M. C. Mitchell and H. F. Herlong (1986) Alcohol and nutrition: Caloric value, bioenergetics, and relationship to liver damage. *Ann. Rev. Nutr.* **6**, 457–474.

[109] R. K. Chawla, F. W. Lewis, M. H. Kutner, D. M. Bate, R. G. B. Roy, and D. Rudman (1984) Plasma cysteine, cystine, and glutathione in cirrhosis. *Gastroenterology* **87**, 770–776.

[110] A. M. Diehl, M. C. Mitchell, H. F. Herlong, J. J. Potter, L. Wacker, and E. Mezey (1986) Changes in plasma amino acids during sobriety in alcoholic patients with and without liver disease. *Am. J. Clin. Nutr.* **44**, 453–460.

[111] S. Shaw, and C. S. Lieber (1978) Plasma amino acid abnormalities in the alcoholic. Respective role of alcohol, nutrition, and liver injury. *Gastroenterology* **74**, 677–682.

[112] A. M. Duce, P. Ortiz, C. Cabrero, and J. M. Mato (1988) S-adenosyl-L-methionine synthetase and phospholipid methyltransferase are inhibited in human cirrhosis. *Hepatology* **8**, 65–68.

[113] G. Vendemiale, E. Altomare, T. Trizio, C. LeGrazie, C. DiPadova, M. T. Salerno, V. Carrieri, and O. Albano (1989) Effects of oral S-adenosyl-L-methionine on hepatic glutathione in patients with liver disease. *Scand. J. Gastroenterol.* **24**, 407–415.

[114] C. S. Lieber, A. Casini, L. M. DeCarli, C. I. Kim, N. Lowe, R. Sasaki, and M. A. Leo (1990) S-adenosyl-L-methionine attenuates alcohol-induced liver injury in the baboon. *Hepatology* **11**, 165–172.

[115] C. J. McClain, J. P. Kromhout, F. J. Peterson, and J. L. Holtzman (1980) Potentiation of acetaminophen hepatotoxicity by alcohol. *JAMA* **244**, 251–253.

[116] L. B. Seeff, B. A. Cuccherini, H. J. Zimmerman, E. Adler, and S. B. Benjamin (1986) Acetaminophen hepatotoxicity in alcoholics. *Ann. Int. Med.* **104**, 399–404.

[117] B. H. Lauterburg and M. E. Velez (1988) Glutathione deficiency in alcoholics: Risk factor for paracetamol hepatotoxicity. *Gut* **29**, 1153–1157.

[118] A. C. Smith, F. W. Freeman, and R. D. Harbison (1981) Ethanol enhancement of cocaine-induced hepatotoxicity. *Biochem. Pharmacol.* **30**, 453–458.

[119] C. Sato, Y. Matsuda, and C. S. Lieber (1981) Increased hepatotoxicity of acetaminophen after chronic ethanol consumption in the rat. *Gastroenterology* **80**, 140–148.

[120] E. Altomare, M. A. Leo, C. Sato, G. Vendemiale, and C. S. Lieber (1984) Interaction of ethanol with acetaminophen metabolism in the baboon. *Biochem. Pharmacol.* **33,** 2207–2212.

[121] N. Zampaglione, D. J. Jollow, J. R. Mitchell, B. Stripp, M. Hamrick, and J. R. Gillette (1973) Role of detoxifying enzymes in bromobenzene-induced liver necrosis. *J. Pharmacol. Exp. Ther.* **187,** 218–227.

[122] M. Younes and O. Strubelt (1977) Enhancement of hypoxic liver damage by ethanol. *Biochem. Pharmacol.* **36,** 2973–2977.

Liver Cancer

Role of Alcohol
and Other Factors

Siraj I. Mufti

Introduction

An association between long-term chronic alcohol consumption and increased risk of cancers in humans has long been suspected. Numerous epidemiological studies have related national or regional per capita alcohol consumption to age-adjusted cancer mortality.[1–5] Prospective cohort studies of groups of people who consume great quantities of alcoholic beverages, for example brewery workers who get drinks free of charge, have shown an increased cancer risk.[6–9] These conclusions are supported by case-control studies where patients with malignant disease are examined for the relative risk of cancer.[10–16] Additional evidence for association is provided by studies among traditional abstainers, such as Seventh Day Adventists and Mormons.[17,18] These studies indicate that the sites frequently associated with increased cancer risk are the mouth, pharynx, larynx esophagus, and liver. Other sites associated with alcohol abuse are the pancreas,[19] breast,[20] stomach,[21–24] and colon.[15,25–30]

This chapter will first discuss the main etiological factors for liver cancer, i.e., hepatitis virus infection and alcohol consumption and their possible interactions, and then focus on the mechanisms underlying alcohol-related cancers. In addition to these, several other etiological factors

From: *Drug and Alcohol Abuse Reviews, Vol. 2: Liver Pathology and Alcohol*
Ed: R. R. Watson ©1991 The Humana Press Inc.

have been identified, for example, aflotoxin, α-1-antitrypsin deficiency, thorothrast administration, and the use of androgenic or anabolic steroids,[31,32] but their relative contributions are not clear. Infection by hepatitis B is generally regarded to be the major causative factor.[33] In the US and other low-risk areas of Western countries, alcohol appears to contribute significantly, although it may act in combination with other factors.

Incidence of Liver Cancer

There is a great deal of variation in incidence of primary liver cancer in different parts of the world. In the US and most Western countries it is relatively uncommon and has an incidence rate of about 4/100,000,[34] accounting for about 1% of total cancer deaths. However, in sub-Saharan Africa and Southeast Asia the incidence of liver cancer is high. Hepatocellular carcinoma (HCC) incidence is about 50 or more per 100,000 in Africa and the Far East; in Hong Kong and Taiwan it is the second most common malignant tumor.[35–37]

Hepatocellular carcinoma (HCC) accounts for 70–90% of primary liver cancers (PLC) and is one of the ten most prevalent cancers in the world.[38] HCC arises in parenchymal liver cells whereas cholangiocarcinoma (CC) arises in bile duct cells and accounts for only 10–15% of primary liver cancers. HCC is uncommon before the age of 40 and a peak incidence normally occurs in the fifth decade.[39–46] The WHO reports a median male:female ratio of autopsy diagnosed cases of HCC to be generally about 5:1,[38] whereas CC occurs almost equally in the two sexes. In a cohort study of 1100 patients in Birmingham, Great Britain between 1948 and 1971, Prior[9] found that there was an eightfold increase of liver cancers in men with alcohol consumption. The differential incidence in sexes has stimulated interest for determining the underlying mechanism involved. The differences may simply be a result of low normal consumption of alcohol by women compared to men. Alternatively, the differences may reflect differences in metabolism between the two sexes. For example, Nagasue et al.[47] suggested that HCC is testosterone-dependent and therefore, more frequent in males. Male alcoholics have also been shown to have lower levels of cytosolic acetaldehyde dehydrogenase[48] or their pathways of ethanol metabolism may differ.[49] However, it is not clear whether these differences precede or result from liver damage. Also, no differences in blood concentrations of acetaldehyde have been found between siblings of alcoholics and their matched controls.[50]

Etiology of Liver Cancer

Association with Viral Infection

Cirrhosis of almost any kind appears to favor the development of primary liver cancer and cirrhotic lesions resulting from infection of hepatitis B virus appear to play a prominent role in such developments. For example, Geer et al.[51] found that 90% of their PLC patients in a referral hospital in Hawaii tested positive for hepatitis antigen reaction. Gibson et al.[52] in a postmortem study in Hong Kong found that 55% of 196 hepatitis B surface antigen-positive (HBsAg$^+$) cirrhotics had HCC, but only 27% of 121 HBsAg$^-$ had a liver tumor. Furthermore, it appears that there are racial and genetic differences in incidence of HBV infections, which could explain the differences in incidence of HCC. For example, Peters et al.,[53] in an autopsy study in Los Angeles, found that 46% of the Oriental patients with HBsAg$^+$ cirrhosis had liver cancers, whereas only 10–25% of patients from other races that were exposed to HBsAg had such cancers. In areas of South Africa, nonCaucasians developing some form of cirrhosis have a 40–50% risk of developing liver cancer,[54] whereas for comparable incidence of cirrhosis in Chicago the risk of liver cancer is only 5%.[55] Lam et al.[56] in Hong Kong observed that 18% of Chinese patients without liver cancer and 82% of patients with liver cancer had HBsAg$^+$ reactions. Additional support for association of HBV and HCC is provided by the observation that liver cancer patients with hepatitis positive reactions in these studies were younger than those without positive reactions for hepatitis.

There is a large amount of evidence indicating involvement of HBV in HCC. The areas in Asia and Africa with a high incidence of PLC also have a high incidence of HBV infection. Several case control and cohort studies from various parts of the world have indicated an association between HCC and chronic HBV infection[57–75] as shown by the presence of HBsAg. The most notable of these studies is a prospective study of 22,707 Chinese men in Taiwan showing that the relative risk of HCC in carriers of HBsAg was 223.[57] However, the best estimates of relative risks in most studies are in the range of 20 or so. In general, it has been estimated that as much as 80% of HCC patients have HBsAg in their serum; others have antibodies to HBV antigens.[76] There is evidence that HCC could occur in the absence of HBV or hepatitis A virus (HAV) infections and strong evidence for this comes from Japan. In Japan, the incidence of liver cancer and mortality associated with it has been increasing since 1975. Indeed, in

1985 liver cancer was the third most common cause of cancer deaths among males in Japan following gastric and lung cancers,[76,77] and this despite the fact that prevalence of chronic HBV infection has been on a rapid decline.[78–80] Tanaka et al.[81] noted that whereas about 40% of HCC patients in 1968–1977 were HBsAg[+], only 21% were so in their current study, suggesting that factors other than chronic HBV infection are playing an increasingly important role in causation. Patients with a history of blood transfusion showed a significantly elevated relative risk of 3 to 4.9, and most of these were noncarriers of HBV as determined by HBsAg and antibody to hepatitis B core antigen (anti-HBc) titers. Actually, the patients had received blood transfusions nearly 30 yr prior to interview. It is likely that infections with unknown viruses may have produced chronic carrier non-A non-B hepatitis state in these patients. Although several follow-up studies have shown development of chronic hepatitis and liver cirrhosis[82–84] but not of HCC,[85–88] this is probably a result of the limited period of study. Tanaka et al.[81] estimate that 15% of male HCC in Japan could be attributed to such non-A non-B hepatitis infections in blood transfusions.

HBV genome has been detected both in the hepatic DNA of carriers and of patients with HCC[88,89] further supporting the role of virus in the etiology of neoplasm. The child of a mother who is a chronic carrier carries an especially high risk of developing HCC and the risk is even higher if the father is negative for surface antibodies to the virus indicating that he is immunologically defective.[90]

Association with Alcohol

In most Western countries, the incidence of hepatitis infection is low and alcohol consumption is considered the major cause of cirrhosis (for example, *see* ref. *91*), which may lead to the development of HCC. A few noteworthy examples of association of alcohol with cirrhosis are as follows. During prohibition in the US the number of deaths as a result of cirrhosis was substantially reduced. Similarly, in Paris with wine rationing during 1942–1948, the number of deaths from cirrhosis decreased from 35 to 6 per 100,000. Furthermore, deaths as a result of cirrhosis at these and other places have increased with rising alcohol consumption.[92] However, not all alcoholics develop cirrhosis. Most of the available studies suggest that only about 20% of alcoholics develop cirrhosis and the incidence appears to depend on the duration and dose of drinking. For example, more than 50% of the patients drinking 200 g of ethanol daily for 20 yr were found cirrhotic in a study by Christofferson and Nielson.[93]

It is not clear whether alcohol causes cirrhosis and/or liver cancer by itself or by an indirect effect, such as through a nutritional deficiency that is caused by alcohol consumption. Nutritional deficiencies are common in alcoholics. In experimental dogs and rats, the development of cirrhosis has been found to depend not only on the dose and duration of alcohol administration, but also on the nutritional composition of the diet.[94] For example, diets low in choline, methionine, vitamin B_{12}, folate, and protein favor cirrhosis and it can be prevented by dietary supplementation. The proposition for a direct effect of ethanol is favored by the observation that ethanol is hepatotoxic. Since humans consume far larger quantities of alcohol and for very long durations of time, hepatotoxicity may be a major factor. However, liver lesions are apparent in humans only after consuming large quantities, e.g., 160 g ethanol corresponding to 40% of total caloric intake for a period of 15 yrs. Effects of ethanol are not readily apparent in experimental animals because their life-span is short and because they are averse to drinking alcohol and can only be induced to consume relatively small quantities, but precirrhotic changes, e.g., increased collagen synthesis, have been observed.[95] Furthermore, Lieber and DeCarli[96] have shown that baboons, which can consume quantities of ethanol that are comparable to human drinking, develop cirrhosis. However, these studies have been criticized on the grounds that the diet was not nutritionally adequate and the results have not been reproduced by others.[97,98] Therefore, the controversy regarding direct and indirect role of ethanol in cirrhosis still remains to be resolved. The difficulty of reproducing cirrhosis in rodents may be the reason for the failure to induce experimental liver cancers with alcohol administration, as discussed later.

Several earlier case control studies in the US[99,100] and Japan[101,102] have suggested a positive association of drinking with HCC. Most cohort studies have also shown a weak or moderately positive correlation with drinking.[6,8,103,104] A study in Japan has shown a considerably high risk with Shochu or strong Japanese spirits.[105] Yu and Henderson[99,100,106] and Austin et al.[100] in case control studies in Los Angeles and Hong Kong found that drinkers of more than 65 cumulative drinks per year exhibited twofold increased risk of primary hepatocellular carcinoma compared to nondrinkers. Drinkers of 80+ g ethanol per day had a relative risk of 3.3 after adjusting for cigaret smoking. Kono and his colleagues[104] studying mortalities among

5130 male Japanese physicians, starting in 1965 and followed for 19 yr, found that liver cancer was significantly related to alcohol consumption. Yu et al.[104] have reviewed case control and prospective studies on the relationship of chronic alcohol abuse and alcoholic cirrhosis as factors in pathogenesis of PLC observing that the relative risk estimates varied from 2.0 to 8.0 for various studies in the US and Japan. In one study, Tanaka et al.[81] found a relatively low risk of 2.0 with heavy drinking, but argued that although the relative risk does not appear to be great yet, it may present a substantial proportion of HCC, because drinking is very common among Japanese males. The positive correlation between alcohol consumption and HCC is particularly significant among HBsAg-negative subjects with no history of blood transfusion, but who had been drinking heavily in their younger years. The current upward trend of HCC among Japanese males, despite a reduction in HBV infection, could be explained as a result of increasing alcohol consumption. Additional support for association with alcohol is provided in studies by Ohnishi and coworkers[108,109] indicating that the average age of HCC patients who drank moderately or heavily was significantly younger than those who did not drink regardless of the state of HBV seromarkers. The observation is justified since most of the patients died within 2 yr with only a small fraction surviving more than 5 yr.

Yu et al.,[107] in a case control study of 165 PLC cases and 465 matched controls from several US hospitals, found a significant dose response in elderly females and a similar, but somewhat weaker pattern was evident in males. Specifically, females over 50 who ingested more than one drink per day had approximately twofold increase in risk compared to those who consumed lesser quantities.

In Scandinavian countries, including Finland and Sweden, the incidence of HBV infection is low[110] and alcohol consumption is considered the most important predisposing factor for HCC.[111] Similarly, in Italy, the incidence of HBV infection varies, but there is in general high daily alcohol intake.[112] Karhunen and Penttila[115] studied consecutive autopsy series of 95 males age 35–69 yr in Helsinki, Finland and found that parenchymal hyperplastic nodules of clear cells occurred in 11.6% and liver dysplasia in 7.4% of the subjects.[113] Hyperplastic nodules of clear cells were found significantly associated with liver cirrhosis, liver enlargement, and heavy alcohol consumption.

Although primary liver cancer is associated with cirrhotic liver, there are a few reports of occurrence of HCC in noncirrhotic liver. For example,

Lieber and his coworkers[114] examined 48 autopsy cases of HCC in Bronx, New York from 1947 to 1978 and found that in 15 cases (or 31%) there was no evidence of cirrhosis. Furthermore, most estimates of cirrhotic liver developing into cancer are low. The reports of the proportion of alcoholic cirrhotics developing cancer vary from 5 to 30%.[115,116] The estimates may be low because many cirrhotic patients die before cancer could be clinically diagnosable. It may also be caused by misdiagnosis at necropsy since a few cancerous nodules, in a grossly distorted and nodular cirrhotic liver, could be easily missed.

Interaction of Virus Infection and Alcohol (and of Other Factors)

There is considerable variation in HCC occurrence, HBV infection, and alcohol consumption between countries and incidence data have been analyzed to provide clues to the etiology of HCC. For example, Qiao et al.[117] studied the relationship between prevalence of HBsAg, mean annual per capita alcohol consumption, and primary liver cancer (PLC) death rates in 30 countries. They observed that HBsAg prevalence was associated significantly with the logarithm of PLC death rate (simple correlation coefficient = 0.44, $p < 0.05$). The correlation increased further following adjustment for a country's mean annual per capita alcohol consumption (partial correlation coefficient = 0.53, $p < 0.01$). A logarithmic linear relationship was also found between per capita alcohol consumption and the PLC death rate after adjusting for prevalence of HBsAg (partial correlation coefficient = 0.38, $p < 0.05$). Both correlation and regression analyses showed a more significant association of prevalence of HBsAg than of alcohol consumption with PLC death rates. However, the two variables were independently correlated in a stepwise multiple regression model and an interaction between the two could not be demonstrated. Thus, these findings support the view that chronic hepatitis B infection is the major factor for the most common form of PLC and that alcohol contributes significantly and independently, although probably to a lesser extent than hepatitis B.

In studies carried out by Ohnishi and his colleagues[108,109] it was observed that the average age of HCC patients who drank moderately or heavily was significantly lower, regardless of HBV reactivity. Since it is generally thought that in Japan the HBV negative patients carry the chronic non-A

non-B hepatitis, a conclusion could be drawn that habitual alcohol ingestion may promote development of HCC in people who contract infections
by these agents. Ubakata et al.[118] compared cancer incidence among mi-
grant Koreans in Japan, native Koreans, and native Japanese and found that
liver cancer was most prominent among Koreans in Japan, whereas the liver
cancer risk among native Koreans and Japanese was similar. The prevalence of HBsAg positives was higher among Koreans compared to Japanese, but alcohol consumption was higher among Korean migrants than
among Japanese, which was higher than native Koreans. Therefore, the liver
cancer risk among these populations paralleled the combination of alcohol
consumption and prevalence of HBV carriers. Similarly, Villa et al.[112] studied
646 consecutive patients in Italy; 58 of these had chronic active hepatitis,
428 had cirrhosis, and 160 had HCC. They found that although there was
HBsAg, HBV DNA positivity in 23 to 41% of patients, alcohol consumption was equal in all categories and HCC was apparent in more than 90%
of cirrhotics, suggesting that these factors may cooperate in the development of HCC probably through their potential for causing cirrhosis.

Other examples of interaction of alcohol with infection by hepatitis B
are as follows. Ohnishi et al.[108] observed that cirrhosis developed 8–10 yr
earlier in both HBsAg positive and negative patients if they were habitual
drinkers and there was a similar stimulation of HCC with continued drinking, especially in those individuals who carried HBs antigens. These and
similar other studies suggest that alcohol may act as a tumor promoter in
chronic hepatitis B carriers.[119,120] Support for the aforementioned is provided by the observations of Brechot et al.,[121] who found that there were
integrated HBV sequences in the HCC DNA of alcoholics even though the
HBV serum markers were not detected.

A number of other studies indicate that the liver cancer incidence may
be increased by a combination of other factors. For example, Geer et al.[51]
observed that 60–65% of their patients were heavy users of alcohol and
cigarets. Yu et al.[99] found that, whereas for nonsmoking subjects consuming 80 g of ethanol per day the relative risk of developing hepatocellular
carcinoma was 4.2, it increased to 14.0 for smokers drinking the same
amount of ethanol. Hirayama[122] analyzed results of a large cohort study
carried out in Japan during 1966–1982 and found a close association of
liver cancer with smoking and drinking. For liver cirrhosis, daily smoking
was of a lesser importance compared to daily drinking with a relative risk
of 1.17 and 1.82, respectively. However, for liver cancer, the risk from daily

smoking in this study was higher than from daily drinking with relative risks of 3.14 and 1.89. Results such as these are important in explaining the increase in liver cancer mortality that is limited to Japanese men despite a decrease in hepatitis B carriers. Other studies have attempted to relate other dietary factors, e.g., a study correlated consumption of pork and wine with increased incidence of hepatocellular carcinoma.[123]

However, it may be noted that cirrhosis associated with alcohol or nutrition is of hobnail or finely nodular type, whereas cirrhosis most associated with liver cancer risk is of postnecrotic or macronodular type. There is a good deal of evidence indicating that chronic carriers of HBV tend to develop macronodular cirrhosis, which may progress to HCC. Therefore, it appears that the risk of developing liver cancer with alcoholic or nutritional cirrhosis is not very high unless it occurs in association with other factors, particularly hepatitis B infection. Occurrence of cirrhosis and primary liver cancer in different social classes in England and Wales agrees with this conclusion.[124] However, Arrigoni et al.[125] observed that in Italy HCC occurred as commonly in patients with alcoholic cirrhosis who were not infected with HBV as in those who were.

Alcohol-Related Experimental Hepatocarcinogenesis: The Underlying Mechanisms

A large number of studies have been carried out to determine the direct and indirect effects of ethanol on carcinogenesis. However, ethanol, the major component of alcoholic beverages, has not been shown to be carcinogenic in any of the experimental animal models and there is little evidence of liver cancer induced by high or intermittent daily dose of ethanol. For example, Ketcham et al.[126] administered 20% ethanol to CDBA/2F$_1$ female mice for up to 15 mo and found no effect on longevity, primary tumor incidence at any site, or the growth or spread of tumor implants. Moderate, fatty infiltration of liver parenchymal cells was seen after 1 yr, but the change regressed in a subsequent alcohol-free period. Kurastune et al.[127] observed no tumor in 108 male and 42 female CF$_1$ mice given intermittently 43% solution of ethanol and observed for up to 34 mo. Similar results were observed in 100 male ddN mice given intermittently a 19.5% ethanol solution for up to 22 mo. Gibel[128] exposed 40 Sprague-Dawley rats to 0.5 mL of 50% ethanol once daily for up to 20 mo and found that apart from slight changes in 10% of animals after 6 mo of treatment, no adverse effects on the liver were apparent. Similarly, Schmahl[129] maintained Sprague-Dawley rats on 30 mL/kg of 25% ethanol in drinking water for 5 d per wk for up to 780 d and found no evidence of hepatotoxicity or liver tumors. Recently, Tanaka and coworkers[130] found that treating ACI/N rats with ethanol alone for 56 wk did not induce any tumors. Herrold[131] administered 0.5 mL 50% ethanol twice a week to five each male and female hamsters for a period of 10–11 mo and then followed the animals for life without observing any adverse effect on the liver. Hollander and Higginson[132] gave 10% ethanol to 19 male and 33 female mastomys for 2 mo and then increased the ethanol to 20% for the remainder of their life-spans (up to 30 mo) and found that incidence of malignant carcinoid stomach tumors, which this species is prone to, was not adversely affected by ethanol nor did the animals develop primary liver tumors.

Since, as discussed earlier, ethanol by itself is not carcinogenic, ethanol effects have been studied in association with known carcinogens. A large number of studies have been done using nitrosamines to induce tumors. *N*-nitrosamines are organ specific carcinogens and, therefore, are often used to induce tumors at sites that are associated with alcohol consumption in humans. The relevance of these studies is based on the evidence that considerable human exposure occurs to preformed nitrosamines or their precursors from a variety of environmental sources, e.g., tobacco chewing and tobacco smoking. Also, nitrosamines could be synthesized endogenously from interaction of breakdown products of proteins with nitrate/nitrite contaminants in foods. Since different coenzymes of the cytochrome P-450 system metabolize different nitrosamines differently, the distribution of these coenzymes in different organs could be the major determinant of the differences in organ specificity by nitrosamines.[133–135] That ethanol could affect organ specificity of nitrosamines is evidenced by the observations of Swann and his colleagues.[136–138] These investigators observed that ethanol interferes with first pass clearance and thus influences the pharmacokinetics of nitrosamines by affecting their distribution in extrahepatic tissues. Other organs that do not possess as adequate a DNA repair capability as liver and are more susceptible to carcinogens are thus exposed to the damaging effects of carcinogens. However, the aforementioned conclusions were drawn using dimethylnitrosamine (NDMA) and first pass clearance of other nitrosamines, e.g., dimethylnitrosamine (NDEA), is not as efficient as that of NDMA.[138,139] The results are further complicated by the observation that ethanol competes with nitrosamines for the active site on the demethylase enzyme[140,141] and that the extent of inhibition depends on the relative liphophilicity of the specific nitrosamine.

A number of investigators, including ourselves, have reviewed the effect of ethanol on carcinogenesis.[114,142,143] In general, the results obtained depend on the carcinogen used, its dose and time of exposure, and on the amount of ethanol fed and its schedule of administration. Most studies of the concurrent feeding of ethanol did not indicate an increase. For example, Schmahl and his colleagues[144,145] did not observe an increase in hepatic tumors when rats were fed commercial brandy with administration of nitrosodiethylamine (NDEA) or with methylphenylnitrosamine. Further, Habs and Schmahl[146] found that simultaneous administration of ethanol with a low dose of NDEA significantly reduced the incidence of liver tumors, but not of esophageal tumors. Teschke et al.[147] did not observe an increase in the number of tumors or a change in target organ when rats were fed an ethanol diet in 4 cycles of 3 wk followed by 2 wk of chow with doses of dimethylnitrosamine given in the latter period. In contrast to the aforementioned, Schwarz et al.[148] found an increase in preneoplastic lesions indicated by γ-glutamyltransferase-altered foci when NDEA was administered at the same time as 10% ethanol in drinking water.

The carcinogenicity of substances other than nitrosamines may be affected variously by ethanol. For example, Radlike et al.[149] found that hepatocarcinogenicity of vinyl chloride is increased by concurrent ethanol administration. Yamamoto et al.[150] did not find any increase in tumors induced by 2-fluorenyl-acetamide. Similarly, Yanagi et al.[151] did not find any significant difference in rat hepatic lesions initiated with 3-methyl-4-dimethylaminoazobenzene that could be ascribed to 5, 10, or 15% of ethanol in drinking water. Misslbeck et al.[152] investigating tumor promoting effect of ethanol after initiation by aflatoxin (AF) B1 found that ethanol had no effect on the development of γ-glutamyl transpeptidase (GGT)-positive foci. However, recently, Tanaka et al.[130] reported that AFB_1 induced altered foci and liver cell tumors were significantly increased by giving ACI/N male inbred rats 10% ethanol in drinking water as a tumor promoter.

Similar are the results on effect of ethanol on tumor promotion, ethanol being administered following treatment by a carcinogen. Takada et al.[153] observed that 20% ethanol in drinking water used as a promoter increased the number of GGT-altered foci induced by NDEA. However, Schwarz et al.[147] found no effect of 10% ethanol in drinking water on the promotion of GGT-altered foci. On the other hand in studies by Driver and McLean,[154] even 5% ethanol in drinking water starting 1 wk after a single dose of 30 mg/ kg NDEA significantly increased hepatocellular carcinoma, equal in effect to 1000 µg/mL sodium phenobarbitone given for 15 mo.

In recently completed studies where ethanol constituting 36% of total caloric intake as part of Lieber-DeCarli[155] isocaloric liquid diet was administered posttreatment with NDEA, we observed neither an increase in liver tumors nor in GGT-altered foci that could be attributed to tumor promoting effects of ethanol.[156] These studies were prompted by our earlier studies that indicated an increase in esophageal tumors occurring only when ethanol was administered postinitiation by methylbenzylnitrosamine (NMB_zA).[157] Following these studies, we observed that whereas an increase in generation of lipid peroxidation products as measured by ethane exhalation, diene conjugates, and fluorescent lipid products that was observed with administration of ethanol was unaffected by NMB_zA treatment, such an increase was obliterated with NDEA treatment. Also, with NDEA treatment there was a corresponding increase in hepatic glutathione, the peroxidation scavengers. Similarly, there was a drastic reduction in cytochrome P-450 levels and a significant decrease in concentration of cytochrome c reductase in NDEA-treated ethanol-fed rats indicating an absence of reactive oxygen intermediates that are normally generated by ethanol in microsomal ethanol oxidizing system.[156,157–160] These studies implicate free radicals generated by ethanol in its tumor promoting effects, a finding that is in line with tumor promoting effects of a variety of tumor promoters.[161]

At this point, some comments on experimentally induced vs naturally occurring liver cancer are relevant. First, it must be understood that compared to humans, liver cancer is a relatively common disease in rodents. Popper[162] has expounded upon these differences. The differences may be a result of longer lives of humans and their hepatocytes present an increase by a factor of approx 30 compared to rodents.[163] Since the number of mitotic cycles in the life of different species is almost the same, it means that far less mitoses occur in human than in rodent liver, decreased by the same factor of 30. Thus dividing DNA is exposed to carcinogens less often in humans than in rodents. Another possible reason for the difference in occurrence of liver cancer in rats and humans is that the larger size of human liver allows less hepatic oxygen production. The rate of metabolism of carcinogens, depending on the specific variant of cytochrome P-450, is higher in rodents than in humans.[164] Also, the larger liver size allows less amount of oxidizable material in humans than in rodents.[165] For these reasons, care must be taken when extrapolating from rodents to humans.

Also, it is important to note differences in human vs chemically induced experimental liver tumors. Whereas human hepatic tumors are predominantly HCC, chemically induced tumors are angiosarcomas, which are relatively uncommon in humans. The chemical induction is also characterized by an absence of fibrosis or cirrhosis in the surrounding tissue. However, whereas rats and mice have no parallel viral hepatopathogenesis, woodchuck may present a suitable model since it can be infected with a closely resembling hepadna virus leading to the development of chronic viral hepatitis, which progresses to macronodular cirrhosis and eventually to hepatocellular carcinoma.[168–174]

Conclusions

There is plenty of evidence indicating an association of hepatitis virus infection with HCC yet the causal relationship with liver cancer has still to be clearly demonstrated. For example, available evidence indicates that integration of HBV genome into host DNA occurs, but the transforming potential of HBV has yet to be shown. Similarly, the nature of non-A non-B hepatitis (or hepatitis C virus, HCV) infection and its mode of transmission must be clearly understood. A number of studies have implicated alcohol in causing HCC in countries where consumption of alcohol is high, but the role of alcohol without the confounding effects of other factors, nutrition in particular, remains to be clearly defined. Similarly, the role of nutrition and smoking must also be determined. Apparently liver cancer, like most other cancers, is the result of the interaction of a number of factors, and the relative contribution of each factor and the interaction of these factors need be established. An experimental animal species like woodchuck that could be infected with a closely related hepatitis virus causing HCC provides a useful model for the study of underlying molecular mechanisms involved. It is anticipated that with the availability of modern genetic, biochemical, and immunological techniques answers to some of these questions will become apparent in the near future.

Acknowledgment

Part of the research described in this chapter was carried out by grant No. CA51088 from the National Institutes of Health.

References

[1] D. Schwartz, J. Lellouch, R. Flamant, and P. F. Denoix (1962) Alcohol et cancer-resultats d'une enquete retrospective. *Revue Fr. Etud. Clin. Biol.* **7**, 590–604.

[2] Finnish Foundation for Alcohol Studies and World Health Organization (Europe) (1977) *International Statistics on Alcoholic Beverages, Production, Trade and Consumption,* vol. 27. Finnish Foundation for Alcohol Studies, Helsinki.

[3] A. J. Tuyns (1982) Incidence trends of laryngeal cancer in relation to national alcohol and tobacco consumption, in *Trends in Cancer Incidence, Causes and Practical Implications.* K. Magnus, ed. Hemisphere, Washington, DC., pp. 199–214.

[4] N. E. Breslow and J. E. Enstrom (1974) Geographic correlations between cancer mortality rates and alcohol-tobacco consumption in the United States. *J. Natl. Cancer Inst.* **53,** 631–639.

[5] A. J. Tuyns (1970) Cancer of the oesophagus: Further evidence of the relation to drinking habits in France. *Int. J. Cancer* **5,** 152–156.

[6] T. Hakulinen, L. Lehtimaki, M. Lehtonen, and L. Teppo (1974) Cancer morbidity among two male cohorts with increased alcohol consumption in Finland. *J. Natl. Cancer Inst.* **52,** 1711–1714.

[7] R. R. Monson and J. L. Lyons (1975) Proportional mortality among alcoholics. *Cancer* **36,** 1077–1079.

[8] O. M. Jensen (1979) Cancer morbidity and causes of death among Danish brewery workers. *Int. J. Cancer* **23,** 454–463.

[9] P. Prior (1988) Long term cancer risk in alcoholics. *Alcohol Alcohol.* **23,** 163–171.

[10] R. G. Vincent and F. Marchetta (1963) The relationship of the use of tobacco and alcohol to cancer of the oral cavity, pharynx, and larynx. *Am. J. Surg.* **106,** 501–505.

[11] I. Martinez (1969) Factors associated with cancer of the esophagus, mouth and pharynx in Puerto Rico. *J. Natl. Cancer Inst.* **42,** 1069–1094.

[12] K. J. Rothman and A. Z. Keller (1972) The effect of joint exposure to alcohol and tobacco on risk of cancer of the mouth and pharynx. *J. Chron. Dis.* **25,** 711–716.

[13] A. J. Tuyns, G. Pequignot, O. M. Jensen, and Y. Pomeau (1975) La consommation individuelle de bossons alcoolisees et de tabac dans un echantilon de la population en We-et-Vitaine. *Rev. Alcohol.* **21,** 105–110.

[14] J. G. Feldman, M. Hazan, M. Nagarajen, and B. Kissin (1975) A case-control investigation of alcohol, tobacco and diet in head and neck cancer. *Prev. Med.* **4,** 444–463.

[15] R. R. Williams and J. W. Horm (1977) Association of cancer sites with tobacco and alcohol consumption and socio-economic status of patients: Interview study for the Third National Cancer Survey. *J. Natl. Cancer Inst.* **58,** 525–547.

[16] E. L. Wynder (1977) The dietary environment and cancer. *J. Am. Diet. Assoc.* **71,** 385–392.

[17] F. R. Lemon, R. T. Walden, and R. W. Woods (1964) Cancer of the lung and mouth in Seventh-Day Adventists. Preliminary report on a population study. *Cancer* **17,** 486–497.

[18] J. L. Lyon, J. W. Gardner, M. R. Klauber, and C. R. Smart (1977) Low cancer incidence and mortality in Utah. *Cancer* **39,** 2608–2618.

[19] C. E. Burch and A. Ansari (1968) Chronic alcoholism and carcinoma of the pancreas: A correlative hypothesis. *Arch. Intern. Med.* **122,** 273–275.

[20] L. Rosenberg, S. Shapiro, D. Slone, D. W. Kaufman, S. P. Helmrich, D. S. Miettinen, P. D. Stolley, M. Levy, N. B. Rosenshein, D. Schottenfeld, and R. L. Engle (1982) Breast cancer and alcoholic beverage consumption. *Lancet* **1,** 267–271.

[21] W. C. MacDonald (1972) Clinical and pathological features of adenocarcinoma of the gastric cardia. *Cancer* **29,** 724–732.

[22] W. Haenszel, M. Kurihara, M. Segi, and R. K. C. Lee (1972) Stomach cancer among Japanese in Hawaii. *J. Natl. Cancer Inst.* **49,** 969–988.

[23] J. Hoey, C. Montvernay, and R. Lambert (1981) Wine and tobacco: Risk factors for gastric cancer in France. *Am. J. Epidemiol.* **113,** 668–674.

[24] D. Trichopoulos, G. Ouranos, N. E. Day, A. Tzonou, O. Manousos, C. H. Papadimitriou, and A. Trichopoulos (1985) Diet and cancer of the stomach: A case-control study in Greece. *Int. J. Cancer* **36,** 291–297.

[25] J. D. Potter, A. J. McMichael, and J. M. Hartshorne (1982) Alcohol and beer consumption in relation to cancers of bowel and lung: An extended correlation analysis. *J. Chron. Dis.* **35,** 833–842.

[26] E. Bgelke (1974) Frequency of use of alcoholic beverages and incidence of cancer of the large bowl and other sites. Prospective study of 12,000 Norwegian men. Meeting on Alcohol and Cancer. IARC, Lyon, France.

[27] M. W. Hinds, L. N. Kolonel, J. Lee, and T. Hirohata (1980) Associations between cancer incidence and alcohol/cigarette consumption among five ethnic groups in Hawaii. *Br. J. Cancer* **41,** 929–940.

[28] D. Kozarevic, N. Vojvodic, T. Gordon, C. T. Kaelber, D. McGee, and W. Zukel (1983) Drinking habits and death: The Yugoslavia cardiovascular disease study. *Int. J. Epidemiol.* **12,** 145–155.

[29] J. D. Potter and A. J. McMichael (1986) Diet and cancer of the colon and rectum: A case control study. *J. Natl. Cancer Inst.* **76,** 557–569.

[30] J. E. Engstrom (1977) Colorectal cancer and beer drinking. *Br. J. Cancer* **35,** 674–683.

[31] P. P. Anthony, C. L. Vagel, and L. F. Barker (1973) Liver cell dysplasia: A premalignant condition. *J. Clin. Pathol.* **26,** 217–223.

[32] P. P. Anthony (1976) Precursor lesions for liver cell cancer in humans. *Cancer Res.* **36,** 2579–2583.

[33] W. Szmuness (1978) Hepatocellular carcinoma and the hepatitis B virus. *Prog. Med. Virol.* **24,** 40–69.

[34] D. Sandler, R. Sandler, and L. Horney (1983) Primary liver cancer mortality in the United States. *J. Chron. Dis.* **36,** 227–236.

[35] M. Kew and E. Geddes (1982) Hepatocellular carcinoma in rural Southern Africa Blacks. *Medicine* **61,** 98–108.

[36] C. Lai, K. Lam, K. Wong, P. Wu, and D. Todd (1981) Clinical features in Hong Kong. *Cancer* **47,** 2746–2755.

[37] Hong Kong Government. Hong Kong annual department report. Hong Kong Government Printer, Hong Kong, 1985.

[38] World Health Organization. Prevention of liver cancer: Report of WHO meeting. World Health Organization Technical Report Series. World Health Organization, Geneva. 1983, pp. 7,8.

[39] L. Pagliaro, R. Simonetti, A. Craxi, C. Spano, M. Filippazzo, U. Palazzo, S. Patti, G. Giannuoli, A. Marraffa, M. Colombo, M. Tommasini, S. Bellentani, E. Villa, F. Manenti, N. Caporaso, M. Coltorti, C. Del Vecchio-Blanco, P. Farsi, A. Smedile, and G. Verme (1981) Alcohol and HBV infection as risk factor for hepatocellular carcinoma in Italy: A multicentric, controlled study. *Hepatogastroenterology* **30,** 48–50.

[40] P. Attali, S. Prod'homme, G. Pellettier, L. Papoz, C. Buffet, and J. Etienne (1985) Carcinomes hepato-cellulaires en France. Aspects cliniques, biologiques at virologoques chez 197 malades. *Gastroent. Clin. Biol.* **9,** 396–402.

[41] R. Chlebowski, M. Tong, J. Weissman, J. Block, K. Ramming, J. Weiner, J. Bateman, and J. Chlebowski (1984) Hepatocellular carcinoma: Diagnostic and prognostic features in North American patients. *Cancer* **53,** 2701–2706.

[42] G. Luna, L. Florence, and R. Johansen (1985) Hepatocellular carcinoma: A 5-year institutional experience. *Am. J. Surg.* **149,** 591–594.

[43] S. Zaman, W. Melia, R. Johnson, B. Portman, P. Johnson, and R. Williams (1985) Risk factors in development of hepatocellular carcinoma in cirrhosis: Prospective study of 613 patients. *Lancet* **i,** 1357–1360.

[44] H. Hsu, J. Sheu, Y. Lin, D. Chen, C. Lee, L. Hwang, and R. Beasley (1985) Prognostic histologic features of resected small hepatocellular carcinoma (HCC) in Taiwan. A comparison with resected large HCC. *Cancer* **56,** 672–680.

[45] J. Sheu, J. Sung, D. Chen, P. Yang, M. Lai, C. Lee, H. Hsu, C. Chuang, P. Yang, T. Wang, J. Lin, and C. Lee (1985) Growth rate of asymptomatic hepatocellular carcinoma and its clinical implications. *Gastroenterology* **89,** 259–266.

[46] N. Nagasue, H. Yukaya, T. Hamada, S. Hirose, R. Kanashima, and R. Inokuchi (1984) The natural history of hepatocellular carcinoma. A study of 100 untreated cases. *Cancer* **54,** 1461–1465.

[47] N. Nagasue, H. Kukaya, Y. C. Chang, Y. Ogawa, H. Kohno, and A. Ito (1986)

Active uptake of testosterone by androgen receptors of hepatocellular carcinoma in humans. *Cancer* **57,** 2162–2167.

[48] M. Thomas, S. Halsall, and T. J. Peters (1982) Role of acetaldehyde dehydrogenase in alcoholism, demonstration of persistent reduction of cytosolic activity in abstaining patients. *Lancet* **2,** 1057–1059.

[49] D. D. Rutstein, R. L. Veech, R. J. Nickerson, M. E. Felver, A. A. Vernon, L.L. Needham, P. Kishore, and S. B. Thacker (1983) 2,3-Butanediol, an unusual metabolite in the serum of severely alcoholic men during acute intoxication. *Lancet* **2,** 534–537.

[50] K. Ward, D. Weir, J. M. McCrodden, and K. F. Tipton (1983) Blood acetaldehyde levels in relatives of alcoholics following ethanol ingestion. *IRCS Medical Science* **10,** 950.

[51] D. A. Geer, Y. M. Lee, V. P. Brooks, and J. L. Berenberg (1987) Primary liver cancer in a referral hospital in Hawaii. *J. Surg. Oncol.* **35,** 235–240.

[52] J. P. Gibson, P. C. Wu, J. C. Ho, and I. J. Lauder (1980) HB_sAg, hepatocellular carcinoma and cirrhosis in Hong Kong: A necropsy study 1963–1976. *Br. J. Cancer* **42,** 370–377.

[53] R. L. Peters, A. P. Afroudakis, and D. Tatter (1977) The changing incidence of association of hepatitis B with hepatocellular carcinoma in California. *Am. J. Clin. Pathol.* **68,** 1–7.

[54] J. G. Thompson (1961) Primary carcinoma of the liver in the three ethnic groups in Capetown. *Acta U.I.C.C.* **17,** 632–638.

[55] Stuart, H. L. (1965) Geographic distribution of hepatic cancer in primary hepatoma, in *Primary Hepatoma.* W. J. Burdette, ed. University of Utah Press, Salt Lake City.

[56] K. C. Lam, M. C. Yu, J. W. C. Leung, and B. E. Henderson, (1982) Hepatitis B virus and cigarette smoking: Risk factors for hepatocellular carcinoma in Hong Kong. *Cancer Res.* **42,** 5246–5247.

[57] R. P. Beasley, L. Y. Hwang, C. C. Lin, and C. S. Chien (1981) Hepatocellular carcinoma and hepatitis B virus: A prospective study of 22,707 men in Taiwan. *Lancet* **2,** 1129–1131

[58] A. L. Lingao, E. O. Domingo, and K. Nishioka (1981) Hepatitis B virus profile of hepatocellular carcinoma in the Phillipines. *Cancer* **48,** 1590–1595.

[59] G. M. MacNab, J. M. Urbanowicz, E. W. Geddes, and M. C. Kew (1976) Hepatitis-B surface antigen and antibody in Bantu patients with primary hepatocellular cancer. *Br. J. Cancer* **33,** 544–548.

[60] M. J. Simons, E. H. Yap, M. Yu, and K. Shanmugaratnam (1972) Australia antigen in Singapore Chinese patients with hepatocellular carcinoma and comparison groups: Influence of technique sensitivity on differential frequencies. *Int. J. Cancer* 10, 320–325.

61 M. J. Tong, S. C. Sun, B. T. Shaeffer, N. K. Chang, K. J. Lo, and R. T. Peters (1971) Hepatitis-associated antigen and hepatocellular carcinoma in Taiwan. *Ann. Intern. Med.* **75,** 687–691.

62 H. C. Hsu, W. S. Lin, and M. J. Tsai (1983) Hepatitis-B surface antigen and hepatocellular carcinoma in Taiwan: With special reference to types and localization of HB_sAg in tumor cells. *Cancer* **52,** 1825–1832.

63 D. Trichopoulos, E. Tabor, R. J. Gerety, E. Xirouchaki, L. Sparros, and N. Munoz (1978) Hepatitis B and primary hepatocellular carcinoma in a European population. *Lancet* **2,** 1217–1219.

64 A. Nomura, G. N. Stemmermann, and R. D. Wasnich (1982) Presence of hepatitis B surface antigen before primary hepatocellular carcinoma. *JAMA* **247,** 2247–2249.

65 L. J. Sandlow and M. A. Spellberg (1980) Primary hepatic carcinoma: Its incidence and relationship to HB_sAg. *Am. J. Gastroenterol.* **74,** 512–515.

66 C. Brechot, M. Hadchouel, and J. Scotto (1981) State of hepatitis B virus DNA in hepatocytes of patients with hepatitis B surface antigen-positive and -negative liver diseases. *Proc. Natl. Acad. Sci. USA* **78,** 3906–3910.

67 T. C. Wu, M. J. Tong, B. Hwang, S. D. Lee, and M. M. Hu (1987) Primary hepatocellular carcinoma and hepatitis B infection during childhood. *Hepatology* **7,** 46–48.

68 C. Brechot, B. Nalpas, A. M. Courouce, G. Duhamel, P. Callard, F. Carnot, P. Tiollais, and P. Berthelot (1982) Evidence that hepatitis B virus has a role in liver-cell carcinoma in alcoholic liver disease. *N. Engl. J. Med.* **306,** 1384–1387.

69 D. Trichopoulos, J. Kremastinou, and A. Tzonou. Does hepatitis B virus cause hepatocellular carcinoma? in *Factors in Human Carcinogenesis.* B. Armstrong and H. Bartsch, eds. IARC Scientific Publication No. 39, International Agency for Research on Cancer, Lyon, France, 1982, pp. 317–332.

70 A. M. Prince and P. Alcabes (1982) The risk of development of hepatocellular carcinoma in hepatitis B virus carriers in New York. A preliminary estimate using death-records matching. *Hepatology* **2,** 15S–20S.

71 M. J. P. Arthur, A. J. Hall, and R. Wright (1984) Hepatitis B, hepatocellular carcinoma, and strategies for prevention. *Lancet* **1,** 607–610.

72 T. Iuma, N. Saitoh, K. Nobutomo, M. Nambu, and K. Sakuma (1984) A prospective cohort study of hepatitis B surface antigen carriers in a working population. *Gann* **75,** 571–573.

73 F. S. Yeh, C. C. Mo, S. Luo, B. E. Henderson, M. J. Tong, and M. C. Yu (1985) A serological case-control study of primary hepatocellular carcinoma in Guangxi, China. *Cancer Res.* **45,** 872,873.

74 A. J. Hall, P. O. Winter, and R. Wright (1985) Mortality of hepatitis B positive blood donors in England and Wales. *Lancet* **1,** 91–93.

75 D. Trichopoulos, N. E. Day, E. Kaklamani, A. Tzonou, N. Munoz, X.

Zavitsanos, Y. Koumantaki, and D. Trichopoulou (1987) Hepatitis B virus, tobacco smoking and ethanol consumption in the etiology of hepatocellular carcinoma. *Int. J. Cancer* **39,** 45–49.

[76] P. Cook-Mozaffari and S. J. Van Rensburg (1984) Cancer of the liver. *Br. Med. Bull.* **40,** 342–345.

[77] Statistics and Information Department, Minister's Secretariat. Mortality statistics from malignant neoplasms 1972–1984, Special report of vital statistics in Japan. Ministry of Health and Welfare, Tokyo, 1986.

[78] Osaka Perfecture Department of Health. Osaka Medical Association and Center for Adult Diseases. Cancer registry in Osaka, 44th Report. Osaka Cancer Registry, Osaka, 1987.

[79] Liver Cancer Study Group of Japan (1979) Survey and follow-up study of primary liver cancer in Japan, Report 4. *Acta Hepatol. Jpn.* **20,** 433–441.

[80] Liver Cancer Study Group of Japan (1986) Survey and follow-up study of primary liver cancer in Japan, Report 7. *Acta Hepatol. Jpn.* **27,** 1161–1169.

[81] K. Tanaka, T. Hirohata, and S. Takeshita (1988) Blood transfusion, alcohol consumption, and cigarette smoking in causation of hepatocellular carcinoma: A case-control study in Fukuoka, Japan. *Gann* **79,** 1075–1082.

[82] K. Kiyosawa, Y. Akahane, A. Nagata, Y. Koike, and S. Furuta (1982) The significance of blood transfusion in non-A, non-B chronic liver disease in Japan. *Vox. Sang.* **43,** 45–52.

[83] G. Realdi, A. Alberti, M. Rugge, A. M. Rigoli, F. Tremolada, L. Schivazappa, and A. Ruol (1982) Long-term follow-up of acute and chronic non-A, non-B post-transfusion hepatitis: Evidence of progression to liver cirrhosis. *Gut* **23,** 270–275.

[84] R. L. Koretz, O. Stone, M. Mousa, and G. L. Gitnick (1985) Non-A, non-B posttransfusion hepatitis — a decade later. *Gastroenterology* **88,** 1251–1254.

[85] R. H. Resnick, K. Stone, and D. Antonioli (1983) Primary hepatocellular carcinoma following non-A, non-B posttransfusion hepatitis. *Dig. Dis. Sci.* **28,** 908–911.

[86] J. H. Gilliam, K. R. Geisinger, and J. E. Richter (1984) Primary hepatocellular carcinoma after chronic non-A, non-B posttransfusion hepatitis. *Ann. Intern. Med.* **101,** 794,795.

[87] K. Kiyosawa, Y. Akahane, A. Nagata, and S. Furuta (1984) Hepatocellular carcinoma after non-A, non-B posttransfusion hepatitis. *Am. J. Gastroenterol.* **79,** 777–781.

[88] D. A. Shafritz and M. C. Kew (1981) Identification of integrated hepatitis B virus DNA sequences in human hepatocellular carcinomas. *Hepatology* **1,** 1–8.

[89] A. M. Prince (1981) Hepatitis B virus and hepatocellular carcinoma: Molecular biology provides further evidence for an etiologic association. *Hepatology* **1,** 73–75.

[90] B. Larouze, W. T. London, G. Saimot, H. G. Werner, E. D. Lustbader, M.

Payet, and B. S. Blumberg (1976) Host responses to hepatitis B infection in patients with primary hepatic carcinoma and their families. A case control study in Senegal, West Africa. *Lancet* **2**, 534–538.

[91] W. K. Lelbach (1975) Quantitative aspects of drinking in alcoholic liver cirrhosis, in *Alcoholic Liver Pathology*. J. M. Khanna, Y. Israel, and T. H. Kalan, eds. Addiction Research Foundation, Toronto, Canada, pp. 1–18.

[92] G. Klatskin (1961) Alcohol and its relation to liver damage. *Gastroenterology* **41**, 443–451.

[93] P. Christofferson and K. Nielsen (1972) Histological changes in human liver biopsies from chronic alcoholics. *Acta Pathologica et Microbiologica Scand.* (Section A) **80**, 557–565.

[94] W. S. Hartroft (1975) On the etiology of alcoholic liver cirrhosis, in *Alcoholic Liver Pathology*. J. M. Khanna, Y. Israel, and H. Kalant, eds. Addiction Research Foundation, Toronto, Canada, pp. 189–197.

[95] H. M. Middleton, G. D. Dunn, and S. Schenker (1975) Alcohol-induced liver injury: Pathogenic considerations, in *The Liver: Normal and Abnormal Functions*. F. F. Becker, ed. Marcel Decker, New York, pp. 647–677.

[96] C. S. Lieber and L. M. DeCarli (1976) Animal models of ethanol dependence and liver injury in rats and baboons. *Fed. Proc.* **35**, 1232–1236.

[97] A. E. Rogers, J. G. Fox, and J. C. Murphy (1981) Ethanol and diet interactions in male rhesus monkeys. *Drug-Nutrient Interact.* **1**, 3–14.

[98] S. W. French, B. Reuber, T. J. Ihrig, N. C. Benson, E. Mezey, and C. H. Halsted (1982) Effect of chronic ethanol feeding on hepatic mitochondria in the monkey. *Fed. Proc.* **41**, 709.

[99] C. M. Yu, T. Mack, R. Hanisch, R. L. Peters, B. E. Henderson, and M. C. Pike (1983) Hepatitis, alcohol consumption, cigarette smoking and hepatocellular carcinoma in Los Angeles. *Cancer Res.* **43**, 6077–6079.

[100] H. Austin, E. Delzell, S. Grufferman, R. Levine, A. S. Morrison, P. D. Stolley, and P. A. Cole (1986) Case-control study of hepatocellular carcinoma and the hepatitis B virus, cigarette smoking, and alcohol consumption. *Cancer Res.* **46**, 962–966.

[101] A. Oshima, H. Tsukuma, T. Hiyama, I. Fujimoto, H. Yamano, and M. Tanaka (1984) Follow-up study of HB_sAg-positive blood donors with special reference to effect of drinking and smoking on development of liver cancer. *Int. J. Cancer* **34**, 775–779.

[102] Y. Inaba, N. Maruchi, M. Matsuda, N. Yoshihara, and S. Yamamoto (1981) A case-control study in liver cancer and liver cirrhosis in Yamanashi perfecture. *Jpn. J. Public Health* **28**, 362–369.

[103] T. Hirayama (1981) A large-scale cohort study on the relationship between diet and selected cancers of digestive organs. *Banbury Rep.* **7**, 409–426.

[104] S. Kono, M. Ikeda, S. Tokudome, M. Nishizumi, and M. Kurastune (1987) Cigarette smoking, alcohol and cancer mortality: A cohort study of male Japanese physicians. *Gann* **78,** 1323–1328.

[105] A. Shibata, T. Hirohata, H. Toshima, and H. Tashiro (1986) The role of drinking and cigarette smoking in the excess deaths from liver cancer. *Gann* **77,** 287–295.

[106] M. C. Yu and B. E. Henderson (1986,1987) Correspondence re. Harland Austin et al. A case-control study of hepatocellular carcinoma and the hepatitis B virus, cigarette smoking, and alcohol consumption. *Cancer Res.* **46,** 962–966, *Cancer Res.* **47,** 654,655.

[107] H. Yu, R. E. Harris, G. C. Kabat, and E. L. Wynder (1988) Cigarette smoking, alcohol consumption and primary liver cancer: A case-control study in the U.S.A. *Int. J. Cancer* **42,** 325–328.

[108] K. Ohnishi, S. Iida, S. Iwama, N. Goto, F. Nomura, M. Takashi, A. Mishima, K. Kono, K. Kimura, H. Musha, K. Kotota, and K. Okuda (1982) The effect of habitual alcohol intake in the development of liver cirrhosis and hepato-cellular carcinoma: Relation to hepatitis B surface antigen carriage. *Cancer* **49,** 672–677.

[109] K. Ohnishi, H. Terabayashi, T. Unuma, A. Takahashi, and K. Okuda (1987) Effects of habitual alcohol intake and cigarette smoking on the development of hepatocellular carcinoma. *Alcohol. Clin. Exp. Res.* **11,** 45–48.

[110] T. Helske (1974) Carriers of hepatitis B antigen and transfusion hepatitis in Finland. *Scand. J. Haematol.* Suppl. **22,** 1–65.

[111] L. Hardell, N. O. Bengtsson, U. Jonsson, S. Eriksson, and L. G. Larsson (1984) Aetiological aspects of primary liver cancer with special regard to alcohol, organic solvents and acute intermittent porphyria—an epidemiologic investigation. *Br. J. Cancer* **50,** 389–397.

[112] E. Villa, G. M. Baldini, C. Pasquinelli, M. Malegari, E. Cariani, G. Chirico, and F. Manenti (1988) Risk factors for hepatocellular carcinoma in Italy. Male sex, hepatitis B virus, non-A, non-B infection, and alcohol. *Cancer* **62,** 611–615.

[113] P. J. Karhunen and A. Penttila (1987) Preneoplastic lesions of human liver. *Hepato-gastroenterol.* **34,** 10–15.

[114] C. S. Lieber, H. K. Seitz, A. J. Garro, and T. M. Worner (1979) Alcohol related diseases and carcinogenesis. *Cancer Res.* **39,** 2863–2886.

[115] C. M. Leevy, R. Gellene, and M. Ning (1964) Primary liver cancer in cirrhosis of the alcoholic. *Ann. NY Acad. Sci.* **114,** 1026–1040.

[116] A. J. Tuyns. Alcohol et cancer. Monographie hors serie. IARC Monographs, Lyon, France, 1978.

[117] Z. Qiao, M. L. Halliday, J. G. Rankin, and R. A. Coates (1988) Relationship between hepatitis B surface antigen prevalence, per capita alcohol consump-

tion and primary liver cancer death rate in 30 countries. *J. Clin. Epidemiol.* **41,** 787–792.

[118] T. Ubakata, A. Oshima, K. Morinaga, T. Hiyama, S. Kamiyama, A. Shimada, and J. Kim (1987) Cancer patterns among Koreans in Japan, Koreans in Korea and Japanese in Japan in relation to life style factors. *Gann* **78,** 437–446.

[119] J. Nei (1981) Primary hepatic cancers in alcoholics. *J. Kanazawa Med. Univ.* **6,** 1–6.

[120] A. Takada, J. Nei, S. Takase, and Y. Matsuda (1986) Effects of ethanol in experimental hepatocarcinogenesis. *Hepatology* **6,** 65–72.

[121] C. Brechot, S. Pasquinelli, P. Saadi, M. Deugnier, P. Simon, P. Brissot, and M. Bourel (1985) Liver hepatitis B virus DNA sequences in the liver of patients with hepatocellular carcinoma and primary haemochromatosis. *Hepatology* **5,** 970.

[122] T. Hirayama (1989) A large scale cohort study on risk factors for primary liver cancer, with special reference to the role of cigarette smoking. *Cancer Chemother. Pharmacol.* **23 (Suppl.),** S114–S117.

[123] A. Nanji and S. W. French (1985) Hepatocellular carcinoma: Relationship to wine and pork consumption. *Cancer* **56,** 2711,2712.

[124] F. J. Roe (1987) Liver tumors in rodents: Extrapolation to man. *Adv. Vet. Sci. Comp. Med.* **31,** 45–68.

[125] A. Arrigoni, P. Zago, D. Mazzucco, A. Andriulli, and M. Rizzetto (1985) Cirrhosis and liver cancer. *Lancet* **2,** 277.

[126] A. S. Ketcham, H. Wexler, and N. Mantel (1963) Effects of alcohol in mouse neoplasia. *Cancer Res.* **23,** 667–670.

[127] M. Kuratsune, S. Kohchi, A. Horie, and M. Nishizumi (1971) Test of alcoholic beverages and ethanol solutions for carcinogenicity and tumor promoting activity. *Gann* **62,** 395–405.

[128] W. Gibel (1961) Experimentelle untersuchungen zur synkarzinogenese beim osophaguskarzinom. *Arch. Geschwulstforsch.* **30,** 181–185.

[129] D. Schmahl (1976) Investigations on esophageal carcinogenicity by methyl-phenyl-nitrosamine and ethyl alcohol in rats. *Cancer Lett.* **1,** 215–218.

[130] T. Tanaka, A. Nishikawa, H. Iwata, Y. Mori, A. Hara, I. Hirono, and H. Mori (1989) Enhancing effect of ethanol on aflatoxin B_1-induced hepatocarcinogenesis in male ACI/N rats. *Jpn. J. Cancer Res.* **80,** 526–530.

[131] K. Herrold (1969) Aflatoxin induced lesions in Syrian hamsters. *Br. J. Cancer* **23,** 655–660.

[132] C. F. Hollander and J. Higginson (1971) Spontaneous cancers in Praomys (Mastomys) natalenis. *J. Natl. Cancer Inst.* **46,** 1343–1355.

[133] F. P. Guengerich (1982) Isolation and purification of cytochrome P-450 and the existence of multiple forms, in *Hepatic Cytochrome P-450 Monooxygenase System.* J. B. Schenkman and D. Kupfer, eds. International Encyclopedia of Pharmacology and Therapeutics (Section 108), Pergamon, Oxford, pp. 497–521.

[134] G. E. Labuc and M. Arther (1982) Esophageal and hepatic microsomal metabolism of *N*-nitrosomethylbenzylamine in the rat. *Cancer Res.* **42**, 3181–3186.

[135] Y. Y. Tu and C. S. Yang (1985) Demethylation and denitrosation of nitrosamines by cytochrome P-450 isozymes. *Arch. Biochem. Biophys.* **242**, 32–40.

[136] M. I. Diaz Gomez, P. F. Swann, and P. N. Magee (1977) The absorption and metabolism in rats of small oral doses of dimethylnitrosamine. *Biochem. J.* **164**, 497–500.

[137] P. F. Swann (1982) Metabolism of nitrosamines: Observations on the effect of alcohol on nitrosamine metabolism and on human cancer (Banbury Report 12), Cold Spring Harbor Laboratory, Cold Spring Harbor, NY, 53–68.

[138] P. F. Swann, A. M. Coe, and R. Mace (1984) Ethanol and dimethylnitrosamine and dimethylnitrosamine metabolism in the rat. Possible relevance to the influence of ethanol on human cancer incidence. *Carcinogenesis* **5**, 1337–1343.

[139] P. N. Magee, R. Montesano, and R. Preussmann (1976) N nitroso compounds and related carcinogens, in *Chemical Carcinogens.* C. E. Searle, ed. ACS Monograph 173, American Chemical Society, Washington, DC, pp. 491–625.

[140] J. C. Phillips, B. G. Lake, S. D. Gangolli, P. Grasso, and A. G. Lloyd (1977) Effects of pyrazole and 3-amino-1,2,4-triagote on the metabolism and toxicity of dimethylnitrosamine in the rat. *J. Health Cancer Inst.* **58**, 629–633.

[141] M. Schwarz, K. E. Appel, D. Schrenk, and W. Kunz (1980) Effect of ethanol on microsomal metabolism of dimethylnitrosamine. *J. Cancer Res. Clin. Oncol.* **97**, 233–240.

[142] N. G. Misslbeck and T. C. Campbell (1985) The role of ethanol in the etiology of primary liver cancer. *Adv. Nutr. Res.* **7**, 129–135.

[143] S. I. Mufti, H. R. Darban, and R. R. Watson (1989) Alcohol, cancer and immunomodulation. *CRC Critical Rev. Oncol/Hematol.* **9**, 243–261.

[144] D. Schmahl, C. Thomas, W. Sattler, and G. F. Scheld (1965) Experimental studies of syncarcinogenesis. III. Attempts to induce cancer in rats by administering dimethylnitrosamine and CCl_4 (or ethyl alcohol) simultaneously. In addition, an experimental contribution regarding "alcoholic cirrhosis." *Z. Krebsforsch* **66**, 526–532.

[145] D. Schmahl (1976) Investigations on esophageal carcinogenicity by methylphenyl-nitrosamine and ethyl alcohol in rats. *Cancer Lett.* **1**, 215–229.

[146] M. Habs and D. Schmahl (1981) Inhibition of the hepatocarcinogenic activity of dimethylnitrosamine (DENA) by ethanol in rats. *Hepato-Gastroenterol.* **28**, 242–244.

[147] R. Teschke, M. Minzlaff, H. Oldiges, and H. Frenzel (1983) Effect of chronic alcohol consumption on human incidence due to dimethylnitrosamine administration. *J. Cancer Res. Clin. Oncol.* **106**, 58–64.

[148] M. Schwarz, A. Buchmann, G. Wiesbeck, and W. Kinz (1983) Effect

of ethanol on early nitrosamine carcinogenesis in rat liver. *Cancer Lett.* **20,** 305–312.

[149] M. J. Radlike, K. L. Stemmen, P. G. Brown, E. Larson, and E. Bingham (1977) Effect of ethanol and vinyl chloride on the induction of liver tumours: Preliminary report. *Environ. Health Perspect.* **21,** 153–155.

[150] R. S. Yamamoto, J. Korzis, and J. H. Weisburger (1967) Chronic ethanol ingestion and the hepatocarcinogenicity of N-hydroxy-N-2–fluorenylacetamide. *Int. J. Cancer* **2,** 337–343.

[151] S. Yanagi, M. Yamashita, Y. Hiasa, and T. Kamiya (1989) Effect of ethanol on hepatocarcinogenesis initiated in rats with 3'-methyl-4-dimethylaminoazobenzene in the absence of liver injuries. *Int. J. Cancer* **44,** 681–684.

[152] N. G. Misslbeck, T. C. Campbell, and D. A. Roe (1984) Effect of ethanol consumed in combination with high or low fat diets on the postinitiation phase of hepatocarcinogenesis in the rat. *J. Nutr.* **114,** 2311–2323.

[153] A. Takada, J. Nei, S. Takase, and Y. Matsuda (1986) Effects of ethanol on experimental hepatocarcinogenesis. *Hepatology* **6,** 65–72.

[154] H. E. Driver and A. E. M. McLean (1986) Dose-response relationships for initiation of rat liver tumours by dimethylnitrosamine and promotion by phenobarbitone or alcohol. *Fd. Chem. Toxic.* **24,** 242–245.

[155] C. S. Lieber and L. M. DeCarli (1982) The feeding of alcohol in liquid diets: Two decades of applications and 1982 update. *Alcohol. Clin. Exp. Res.* **6,** 523–531.

[156] S. I. Mufti and I. G. Sipes (1991) A reduction in mixed function oxidases and in tumor promoting effects of ethanol in a NDEA-initiated hepatocarcinogenesis model. *Adv. Exp. Med. Biol.* **283,** 347–352.

[157] S. I. Mufti, G. Becker, and I. G. Sipes (1989) Effect of chronic dietary ethanol consumption on the initiation and promotion of chemically-induced esophageal carcinogenesis in experimental rats. *Carcinogenesis* **10,** 313–319.

[158] J. Szebeni, C. D. Eskelson, S. Mufti, R. R. Watson and I. G. Sipes (1986) Inhibition of ethanol induced ethane exhalation by carcinogenic pretreatment of rats 12 months earlier. *Life Sci.* **39,** 2589–2591.

[159] S. I. Mufti (1991) Free radicals generated in ethanol metabolism may be responsible for tumor promoting effects of ethanol. *Adv. Exp. Med. Biol.* **283,** 777–783.

[160] S. I. Mufti and C. D. Eskelson (1991) Lack of tumor promoting effects of ethanol in a hepatocarcinogenesis model and association of free radicals generation by ethanol with its tumor promoting effects (in preparation).

[161] E. S. Copeland (1983) A National Institutes of Health Workshops report, Free radicals in promotion—a chemical pathology study section workshop. *Cancer Res.* **43,** 5631–5637.

[162] H. Popper (1988) Viral versus chemical hepatocarcinogenesis. *J. Hepatol.* **6,** 229–238.

[163] G. M. Martin (1977) Cellular aging. 1. A review — clonal senscence. *Am. J. Pathol.* **89,** 484–511.

[164] D. V. Parke and C. Ioannides (1984) Reactive intermediates and oxygen toxicity in liver inury, in *Mechanisms of Hepatocyte Injury and Death.* D. Kappler, H. Popper, L. Bianchi and W. Reutter, eds. MTP Press, Lancaster, pp. 37–48.

[165] R. G. Cutler (1985) Peroxide-producing potential of tissues: Inverse correlation with longevity of mammalian species. *Proc. Natl. Acad. Sci. USA* **82,** 4798–4802.

[166] B. N. Ames, R. Magaw, and L. S. Gold (1987) Ranking possible carcinogenic hazards. *Science* **236,** 271–280.

[167] P. H. Abelson (1987) Cancer phobia. *Science* **237,** 473.

[168] J. Summers (1981) Three recently described animal virus models for human hepatitis B virus. *Hepatology* **1,** 179–183.

[169] H. Popper, M. A. Gerber, and S. N. Thung (1982) The relation of hepatocellular carcinoma to infections with hepatitis B and related viruses in man and animals. *Hepatology* **2,** 1S–9S.

[170] R. L. Snyder, G. V. Tyler, and J. Summers (1982) Chronic hepatitis and hepatocellular carcinoma associated with woodchuck hepatitis virus. *Am. J. Pathol.* **107,** 422–425.

[171] H. Popper, J. W. Shi, J. L. Gerin, D. C. Wong, B. H. Hoyer, U. T. London, D. L. Sly, and R. H. Purcell (1981) Woodchuck hepatitis and hepatocellular carcinoma: Correlation of histologic with virologic observations. *Hepatology* **1,** 91–98.

[172] W. S. Robinson, P. L. Marion, and R. H. Miller (1984) The hepadna viruses of animals. *Semin. Liver Dis.* **4,** 347–360.

[173] G. V. Tyler, R. L. Snyder, and J. Summers (1986) Experimental infection of the woodchuck (Marmota monax) with woodchuck hepatitis virus. *Lab. Invest.* **55,** 51–55.

[174] H. Popper, L. Roth, R. H. Purcell, B. C. Tennant, and J. L. Gerin (1987) Hepatocarcinogenicity of the woodchuck hepatitis virus. *Proc. Natl. Acad. Sci. USA* **84,** 866–870.

Alcohol and Hepatic Protein Modification

Renee C. Lin and Lawrence Lumeng

Alcohol Metabolism

Although a small percentage of alcohol, after ingestion, can be excreted unchanged in breath and urine, most of its elimination is carried out by enzymatic oxidation. Studies with experimental animals have shown that the liver is the principal organ responsible for alcohol elimination.[1] Enzyme systems known to catalyze the oxidation of ethanol in vivo include: alcohol dehydrogenase (ADH), microsomal ethanol-oxidizing system (MEOS), and catalase. In individuals who do not abuse alcohol, ADH is quantitatively the most important enzyme responsible for the conversion of ethanol to acetaldehyde.[2] But because MEOS is inducible by chronic alcohol consumption,[3] it can contribute significantly to the elimination of alcohol in chronic alcoholics. The role of catalase in ethanol oxidation in vivo remains controversial.

Acetaldehyde is the product of ADH-, MEOS-, and catalase-mediated reactions. Once formed during ethanol oxidation, acetaldehyde is very effectively removed by aldehyde dehydrogenase. Thus the acetaldehyde concentration in tissues and in circulation is low during ethanol oxidation. Blood acetaldehyde concentrations are about 1–30 μM in humans consuming alcohol[4] and may be higher in persons chronically abusing alcohol and patients with liver disease.[4,5] Since the liver is the major site of ethanol

From: *Drug and Alcohol Abuse Reviews, Vol. 2: Liver Pathology and Alcohol*
Ed: R. R. Watson ©1991 The Humana Press Inc.

oxidation, acetaldehyde concentration in hepatic tissue is likely to be higher than that in circulation.[6] However, acetaldehyde is highly reactive; thus its accumulation in the body after alcohol drinking may produce many pathophysiological abnormalities.[7] Biochemical studies in both humans and experimental animals have provided evidences indicating that acetaldehyde might be directly or indirectly hepatotoxic.

Binding of Acetaldehyde to Proteins In Vitro

Stable vs Unstable Protein-Acetaldehyde Adducts

When incubated in vitro at 37°C with [^{14}C]acetaldehyde, many proteins have been found to form radioactive protein-acetaldehyde adducts (-AA). These proteins include: plasma proteins,[8] albumin,[8,9] erythrocyte membrane proteins,[10] tubulin,[11] hepatic proteins,[12] a number of enzymes with critical lysine residues,[13] and hemoglobin.[8,14,15] Both stable and unstable (Schiff's bases) protein-AAs are formed during in vitro incubation. Stable adducts are not reversible by treatment with trichloroacetic acid or gel filtration. Unstable protein-AAs can be stabilized by adding reducing agents, e.g., sodium borohydride or sodium cyanoborohydride, to the incubation mixture. A physiological reducing agent, L-ascorbic acid, has also been shown to be effective in inducing a slow but continuous formation of stable protein-acetaldehyde adducts in experiments in vitro.[16] Using bovine serum albumin (BSA) as the model protein, Tuma et al.[16] have reported that, even in the absence of ascorbate, the proportion of stable BSA-AA increased in the incubation mixture as a function of time but the rate of stable adduct formation was slower than with the presence of ascorbic acid. Thus, it appears that unstable BSA-AA can be stabilized even in the absence of added reducing agents either through chemical rearrangements or by spontaneous reduction. Interestingly, Tuma et al.[17] have also presented evidence showing that the chemical reactions that result in stable adduct formation in the presence of NaCNBH$_3$ or ascorbic acid are not identical (*see* the following section).

Another approach to study the in vitro formation of protein-AAs has been used by Medina et al.[18] These investigators obtained radiolabeled proteins by incubating [^{14}C]ethanol with rat liver slices in the presence of protein synthesis inhibitors. Radiolabeling of proteins decreased when pyrazole, an inhibitor of ADH,[19–21] was added to the incubation mixture. On the other hand, adding cyanamide, an inhibitor of aldehyde dehydrogenase,[22,23] increased the radiolabeling of proteins by [14C]ethanol. Their experiments thus demonstrate that the amount of acetaldehyde generated by hepatic ethanol oxidizing enzymes is sufficient to produce hepatic protein-AAs.

Chemical Forms of Protein-Acetaldehyde Adducts

Unstable protein-AAs formed in vitro have been identified to be Schiff's bases from the reaction between acetaldehyde and the ε-amino group of lysine residues.[9,15,16] Stevens et al.[15] incubated human globin with [14C]acetaldehyde in the presence of $NaCNBH_3$. The radioactive globin-AA derived from this treatment was subjected to amino acid analysis. The chromatographic pattern was compared with synthesized standards of borohydride-reduced [14C]acetaldehyde conjugated amino acids. In addition to acetaldehyde-modified lysine, Stevens et al.[15] found two other major peaks with radioactivities corresponding to acetaldehyde modified valine and tyrosine. Tuma et al.[17] also showed that lysine participates in the formation of stable protein-AA. The latter investigators further demonstrated that different lysine residues in protein were variably modified when high or low concentrations of acetaldehyde were used to modify BSA. Moreover, they found that although both $NaCNBH_3$ and ascorbic acid increased stable acetaldehyde adduct formation by way of reacting with lysine residues, [14C]acetaldehyde modified polylysine or [14C]acetaldehyde modified BSA mediated by ascorbic acid reduction produce an extra radioactive modified lysine residue that is chemically different from the *N*-ethylysine formed by $NaCNBH_3$ reduction. These results indicate that several chemical modifications can occur for the same amino acid residue in peptides under different in vitro reaction conditions.

San George and Hoberman[24] reported that when acetaldehyde was allowed to react with hemoglobin at neutral pH and 37°C, these components formed stable adducts that could not be reduced by sodium borohydride. These investigators[24] delineated the sites of acetaldehyde attachment and found them to involve the free amino groups of the *N*-terminal valine residues of the α and β chains of hemoglobins. Reaction with β chains was preferred over α chains. These investigators performed ^{13}C-NMR analysis of the adducts formed between hemoglobin and [1,2-^{13}C] acetaldehyde. They

Table 1
Protein-Acetaldehyde Adducts Detected In Vivo

Target protein	Detection method	Reference
The 37-kDa rat liver protein	Immunoblot	Lin et al.[31]
Rat liver cytP450IIE1	Immunoblot	Behrens et al.[32]
Human serum proteins	ELISA, immunoblot	Lin et al.[34]
Hemoglobin	HPLC	Lumeng et al.[14]
	ELISA	Niemela et al.[30]
Rat liver plasma proteins	HPLC	Barry et al.[35]

observed that acetaldehyde reacted with the amino termini of hemoglobin to form stable cyclic imidazolidinone derivatives. On the other hand, Stevens et al.[15] showed that, in addition to valine and lysine, tyrosine residues of hemoglobin were also sites that reacted with acetaldehyde to form stable adducts in vitro. The nature of interaction between acetaldehyde and tyrosine residues of peptides remains unknown.

Using equilibrium dialysis, Hernandez-Munoz et al.[25] more recently showed that the binding of acetaldehyde to red blood cells was inhibited by pyridoxal phosphate and *N*-ethylmaleimide. These researchers suggested that both amino and thiol groups are involved in reaction with acetaldehyde, probably by condensing acetaldehyde with cysteine residues to form thiazolidine.[26,27] Earlier, Li and Lumeng[28] presented a body of evidences implicating competition between acetaldehyde and pyridoxal phosphate for protein binding and they postulated that this mechanism is important in mediating increased degradation of pyridoxal phosphate in alcohol-induced vitamin B-6 deficiency.

Formation of Protein-Acetaldehyde Adducts In Vivo

Formation of several protein-AAs in vivo has been detected recently by several laboratories using different approaches (Table 1). Using a HPLC system with a high resolution power, Lumeng and Minter[14] were able to separate human hemoglobin into as many as 13 peaks. After incubation with acetaldehyde, hemoglobin exhibited 2 distinct fast-moving peaks when eluted with HPLC. The peak areas increased in a dose-dependent manner according to acetaldehyde concentrations in the incubation mixture. When blood samples collected from mice fed alcohol chronically were fractionated by the HPLC system, the fast moving peaks corresponding to those of hemoglobin-AA prepared in vitro were significantly elevated in the alcohol-fed mice when compared with their pair-fed controls. These findings indicated for the first time the formation of hemoglobin-AA in vivo. However, the HPLC method was not sensitive enough to detect the presence of hemoglobin-AA in human alcoholics.

In 1986, Israel and his coworkers[29] succeeded in raising antibodies that specifically recognized acetaldehyde-containing epitopes in protein-AAs. These investigators prepared their antigen by incubating keyhole limpet hemocyanin with acetaldehyde for 1 h and then incubating the mixture with the addition of $NaCNBH_3$ for an additional 3 h. When the antigen was repeatedly injected into rabbits, the animals produced antibodies against hemocyanin-AA. These antihemocyanin-AA antibodies cross-reacted with both plasma protein-AAs and erythrocyte protein-AAs but did not cross-react with the respective unmodified carrier proteins. Thus, they are the first to demonstrate that a small hapten such as acetaldehyde can bind to proteins to form immunogenic epitopes. Using antibodies raised in this manner, Niemela and Israel[30] reported higher activity in red blood cell lysate of human alcoholic patients than that of control subjects when tested with enzyme-linked immunosorbent assay (ELISA). Their findings suggest the presence of hemoglobin-AA in alcoholic patients.

Our group raised antiprotein-AA antibodies in rabbits using hemocyanin-AA and myoglobin-AA prepared according to the protocol of Israel et al.[29] as antigens. Liver extracts were prepared from rats pair-fed the alcohol-containing and the alcohol-free liquid diets chronically. The liver extracts were then subjected to sodium dodecyl polyacrylamide gel electrophoresis (SDS-PAGE). Protein bands in the gel were electrotransferred to a piece of nitrocellulose paper, which was subsequently immunoblotted with antiprotein-AA antibodies. Both antihemocyanin-AA IgG and antimyoglobin-AA IgG detected a protein-AA in the liver of rats that were fed alcohol but not in those fed the control diet. The protein-AA has an apparent mol wt of 37,000 (37 kDa).[31] The adduct is stable and does not require borohydride reduction to stabilize it. Repeated acute administrations of ethanol by ip injections over 24 h did not produce the 37-kDa protein-AA. Chronic administration of alcohol by forced feeding of ethanol in a liquid diet required approx 1 wk to produce this protein-AA in vivo.

Later, Behrens et al.[32] presented evidence that cytP450IIIEl (or microsomal ethanol oxidizing system, MEOS) can also form acetaldehyde adducts in vivo. Although the detection methods (i.e., immuoblotting) employed by our laboratory and by Behrens et al.[32] were similar, antigens used to raise the antibodies for immunoblotting were prepared differently. Behrens et al.[32] used a higher acetaldehyde concentration, a longer incubation time and a lower concentration of $NaCNBH_3$ than those used by Israel et al.[29] or Lin et al.[31] The different incubation conditions probably produce adducts of different chemical modifications. Antibodies raised with these antigens, in turn, may recognize different -AA epitopes. It is therefore not entirely too surprising to note that Behrens et al. could not detect any cytosolic protein-AA, e.g., the 37-kDa liver protein-AA, and that we failed to detect any protein-AAs in microsomes.[33] This also leaves open the possibility that more hepatic protein-AAs with other different epitopes derived from reaction with acetaldehyde may exist. It is also likely that more protein-AAs may form in the liver with prolonged alcohol consumption and with advanced liver disease.

When measured with ELISA method, we were able to show that the serum samples of some alcoholic patients reacted more strongly with antiprotein-AA IgG than the samples of nondrinking control subjects.[34] Immunoblotting of serum samples from alcoholics revealed at least two serum protein-AAs with apparent mol wt of 50,000 and 103,000, respectively. Mol wt of these proteins do not correspond to that of serum albumin. Interestingly, although antihemocyanin-AA IgG reacts more strongly with the 37-kDa liver protein-AA when compared with antimyoglobin-AA IgG,[31] the reverse is true for serum protein-AAs.[34] This, again, supports the notion that different carrier proteins can produce -AAs of different chemical forms with acetaldehyde under the identical reaction conditions.

In another report,[35] a seemingly unstable liver plasma membrane protein-AA from the alcohol-fed rat was detected when the liver cell membranes were prepared by a rapid (Percoll) method and assessed by reversed phase liquid chromatography. However, the membrane proteins involved were not characterized, and their mol wt were not reported. The implication of this finding remains unclear and will need further confirmation.

Further Studies of the 37-kDa Protein-Acetaldehyde Adduct

Formation in the Liver of the Alcohol-Fed Rat

To study the formation of hepatic protein-AAs in vivo, male Wistar rats were pair-fed alcohol-containing and alcohol-free AIN'76 or the Lieber-DeCarli liquid diets for up to 7 wk. Both AIN'76 and the Lieber-DeCarli diets contain 1000 KCal/L. The major difference between these two diets is in the fat content. The Lieber-DeCarli diet contains 35% fat whereas the AIN'76 diet contains only 12% fat. The former also contains slightly lower protein (18%) compared to the AIN'76 diet (22%). Ethanol constitutes 35% of total calories in the alcohol-containing diets. The control diet is isocalorically substituted with maltose dextrins. At the end of the feeding periods, rats were sacrificed and liver extracts were prepared. Liver proteins were subjected to SDS-PAGE and electrotransferred to nitrocellulose paper. Protein-AA bands were revealed by enzyme-linked immunoblotting with antihemocyanin-AA IgG.[33] As shown in Fig. 1, no protein-AA band was detected in the liver extract of a rat fed the control diet (lane C). On the other hand, liver extracts from rats fed either the alcohol-containing Lieber-DeCarli diet (lane A) or the alcohol-containing AIN'76 diet (lanes 9 and 10) exhibited the same 37-kDa protein-AA band of approximately the same intensity. No other protein-AA band was found in either diet. The 37-kDa protein-AA band could be detected as early as 1 wk after feeding the alcohol-containing diet. Therefore, the 37-kDa protein is highly susceptible to chemical modification during alcohol-feeding, and the formation of this protein-AA is not affected by higher fat and lower protein contents in the Lieber-DeCarli diet. The 37-kDa protein-AA degraded in vivo when alcohol was removed from the liquid diet. Only 50% of the initial band intensities remained 4 d after rats were switched to the alcohol-free diet.[33] The 37-kDa protein is a liver cytosolic protein. When liver subcellular fractions from an alcohol-fed rat were prepared and blotted for protein-AA, the 37-kDa protein-AA was found only in the crude homogenate (Fig. 2, lane 1) and the cytosol fraction (Fig. 2, lane 4). The mitochondrial fraction and the microsomal fraction (Fig. 2, lane 3 and lane 4, respectively) showed only nonspecific binding with the antihemocyanin-AA IgG (Fig. 2A) as well as the unimmunized rabbit IgG (Fig. 2B).

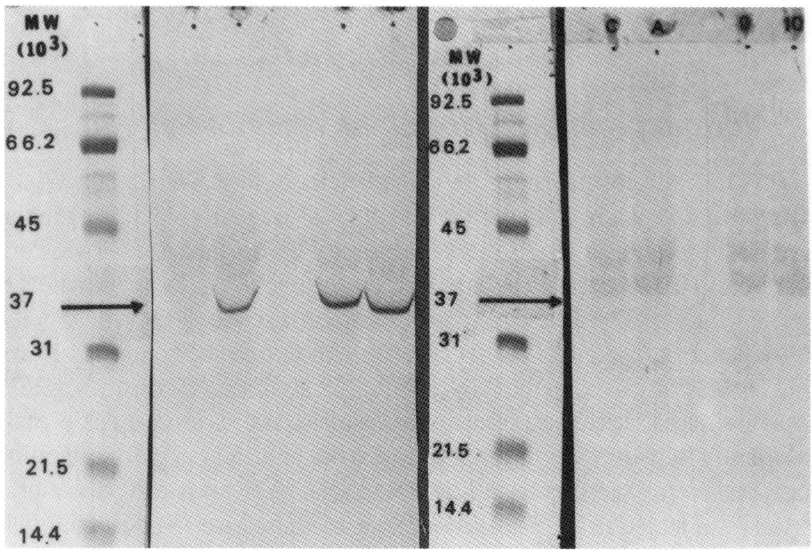

Fig. 1. Formation of the 37-kDa liver protein-AA in rats fed alcohol-containing liquid diet. Mle Wistar rats were pair-fed the alcohol-containing and the isocaloric alcohol-free (control) AIN'76 or Lieber-DeCarli liquid diets for 7 wk. Soluble liver proteins were subjected to SDS-PAGE, electrotransferred to nitrocellulose paper, then detected for protein-AA by immunoblotting with antihemocyanin-AA IgG. Lane C was soluble liver proteins of a rat fed the control Lieber-DeCarli diet, lane A was from a rat fed the alcohol-containing Lieber-DeCarli diet, lanes 9 and 10 were from rats fed the alcohol-containing AIN'76 diet. The left panel was immunoblotted with antihemocyanin-AA IgG whereas the right panel was immunoblotted with unimmunized control rabbit IgG (from Lin and Lumeng,[33] reprinted with permission).

In order to further understand the mechanism of the formation of the liver 37-kDa protein-AA, cyanamide (inhibitor of aldehyde dehydrogenase) and pyrazole (inhibitor of alcohol dehydrogenase and a known inducer of the MEOS) were added to the liquid diet. After 3 wk on the alcohol-containing and the control AIN'76 liquid diets supplemented with cyanamide (100 mg/L) or pyrazole (2 mM), blood samples were obtained from rats and measured for ethanol and acetaldehyde levels. Microsomal fraction was isolated from the fresh liver and immunoblotted for cytP450IIE1. The 37-kDa protein-AA band and the cytP450IIE1 band obtained by immunoblot were quantitated by using a densitometer and expressed as arbitrary unit.

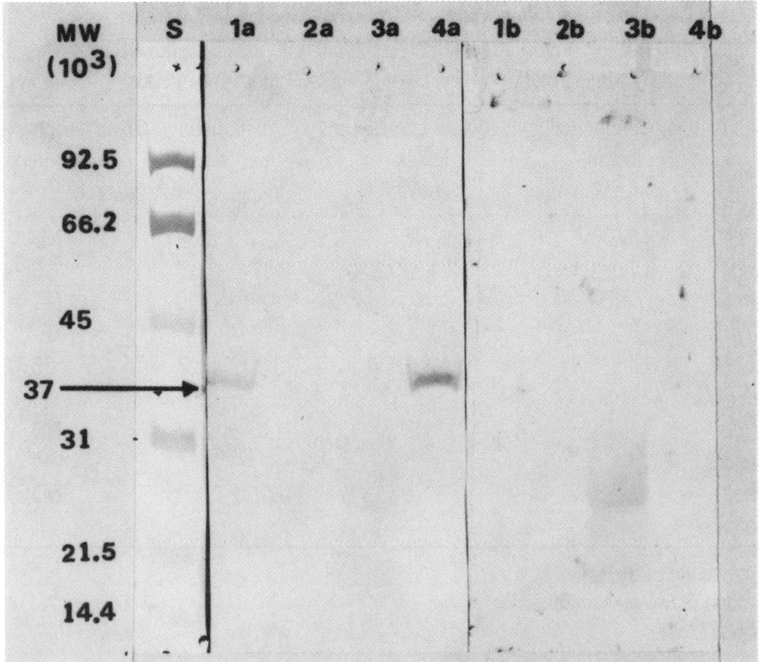

Fig. 2. Subcellular localization of the 37-kDa liver protein-AA. Subcellular fractions were prepared from the liver of a rat fed the alcohol-containing AIN'76 diet for 7 wk. Protein-AA was detected by immunoblotting as described in Fig. 1. Lanes denoted by **a** were immunoblotted with antihemocyanin-AA IgG, whereas lanes denoted by **b** were immunoblotted with control rabbit IgG. S: mol wt standards, 1: crude homogenate, 2: mitochondria, 3: microsomes, 4: cytosol (from Lin and Lumeng,[33] reprinted with permission).

Results are summarized in Table 2. Cyanamide inhibits aldehyde dehydrogenase activity.[22,23] Rats fed the cyanamide supplemented alcohol-containing AIN'76 liquid diet showed no change in blood alcohol levels but their blood acetaldehyde level were about 5 times higher than those fed alcohol only. When the diet was supplemented with pyrazole, an inhibitor of ADH,[19–21] the blood alcohol levels in rats were elevated but the blood acetaldehyde levels fell below the detectable limit. The intensities of the 37-kDa protein-AA band obtained from livers of rats fed these alcohol-containing diets with different supplements closely correlated with the blood

Table 2
Effects of Cyanamide and Pyrazole on Blood Ethanol
and Acetaldehyde Levels, the Hepatic Content of CytP450IIE1
and the Formation of the Liver 37-kDa Protein-AA in Rats

Diets	Blood ethanol[a] levels (mM)	Blood acetaldehyde[a] levels (mM)	CytP450IIE1[a] contents	37-kDa Protein-AA[b] contents
			(arbitrary unit)	
A. Control	ND[c]	ND	1.73 ± 0.08	ND
B. Alcohol	6.7 ± 1.1	2.1 ± 0.8	3.17 ± 0.33[d]	5.94
C. Control +cyanamide	ND	ND	1.70 ± 0.20	ND
D. Alcohol +cyanamide	6.1 ± 0.8	11.1 ± 5.4	3.20 ± 0.07	26.52
E. Control +pyrazole	ND	ND	1.67 ± 0.17	ND
F. Alcohol +pyrazole	11.2 ± 0.9[e]	ND	4.05 ± 0.17[e]	ND

a: Mean values $\pm$ SEM, $n = 4$.
b: Average of two measurements.
c: Not detectable.
d: $p < 0.05$; CytP450IIE1 contents, B vs A.
e: $p < 0.05$; Blood alcohol concentrations and CytP450IIE1 contents, F vs B.

acetaldehyde levels observed. Whereas supplementing with cyanamide increased the band intensity four- to fivefold, supplementing with pyrazole completely abolished the formation of the 37-kDa protein-AA. Our data therefore provide evidence that the formation of the liver 37-kDa protein-AA is dependent on ADH activities and on acetaldehyde concentrations in plasma (most likely in liver also). Feeding alcohol to rats increased liver cytP450IIE1 content nearly twofold. Feeding pyrazole or cyanamide to the rat had little effects on this microsomal protein. However, supplementing pyrazole to the alcohol-containing diet enhanced cytP460IIE1 content more than with feeding alcohol alone, yet the formation of the 37-kDa protein-AA was blocked. On the other hand, supplementing cyanamide to the alcohol-containing diet did not change cytP450IIE1 content when the intensity of the 37-kDa protein-AA band was greatly increased. Thus, the extent of formation of the 37-kDa protein-AA was dissociated from MEOS activities. We found undetectable blood acetaldehyde concentrations in pyrazole supplemented alcohol-fed rat. We therefore concluded that acetaldehyde produced by MEOS is not used for the formation of the cytosolic 37-kDa protein-AA.

The identity of the 37-kDa protein remains to be determined. We have, nevertheless, obtained evidences that rule out ADH and aldehyde dehydrogenase as the 37-kDa liver protein.[33] Thus, the 37-kDa protein is not directly involved in the production and degradation of acetaldehyde in the liver.

Formation in Cultured Rat Hepatocytes Treated with Ethanol

To study the formation of protein-AA in cultured hepatocytes, liver cells were isolated from rats that had been fed regular laboratory rat chow and cultured as monolayers in hormone-defined[36] and trace mineral enriched[37] serum-free Waymouth's medium. Hepatocytes cultured under the aforementioned condition maintained at least 70 and 40%, respectively, of the initial ADH and MEOS activities after 4 d.[38] For treatment, ethanol was added to the culture medium, which was changed daily and incubated in an incubator humidified with a pan containing ethanol solution of the same concentration. Soluble proteins were extracted from cultured hepatocytes and immunotransblotted with antihemocyanin-AA IgG as described earlier. When cells were treated with 40 mM ethanol, the 37-kDa protein-AA could be detected after 3 d of incubation. The intensity of the 37-kDa protein-AA increased to near maximum on the fourth day and remained stable for at least two more days (Fig. 3). It is not understood why there was a time lapse (3 d) before the 37-kDa protein-AA could be detected in hepatocytes treated with ethanol.[38] We have found that the acetaldehyde concentrations that accumulated in the culture media were the same for 1-d-old and 4-d-old cells. Therefore, the delay in the protein-AA formation must not be due to insufficient acetaldehyde in cells. Several possible explanations are under investigation.

It was apparent that the intensities of the 37-kDa protein-AA bands formed in cells paralleled the medium acetaldehyde concentrations that resulted from ethanol treatment (Fig. 4). Ethanol concentration as low as 5 mM was effective and the maximal effect was at approximately 10 mM. These blood ethanol concentrations are pharmacologically relevant during alcohol consumption. Adding cyanamide (50 μM) further increased the in-

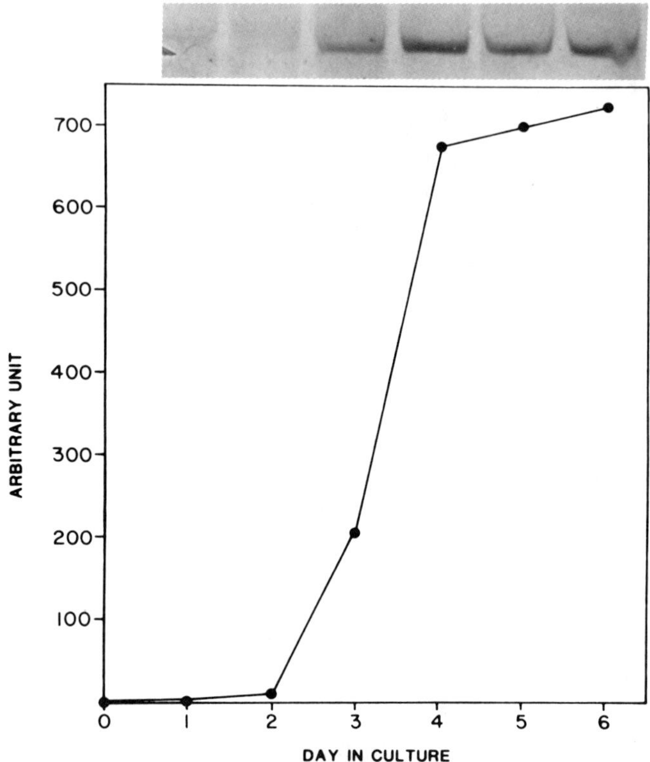

Fig. 3. Time-course for the formation of the 37-kDa protein-AA in cultured rat hepatocytes. Hepatocytes were cultured in serum-free Waymoutlh's medium containing 40 m*M* ethanol. Cells were harvested daily for up to 6 d to detect for the 37-kDa protein-AA. Half-tone photograph is the immunoblot using antihemocyanin-AA IgG. The intensities of the bands were determined by using a densitometer and were expressed as arbitrary units (from Lin et al.,[38] reprinted with permission).

tensity of the protein-AA band by more than twofold. Adding 4-methyl-pyrazole (10 µ*M*) completely blocked the formation of the protein-AA in cultured liver cells, although cytP450IIEl increased by twofold when cells were treated by ethanol and 4-methylpyrazole simultaneously. Therefore, our results with cultured hepatocytes are in agreement with those obtained in vivo, i.e., formation of the 37-kDa protein-AA in hepatocytes is dependent on acetaldehyde concentrations and ADH activities but not MEOS.

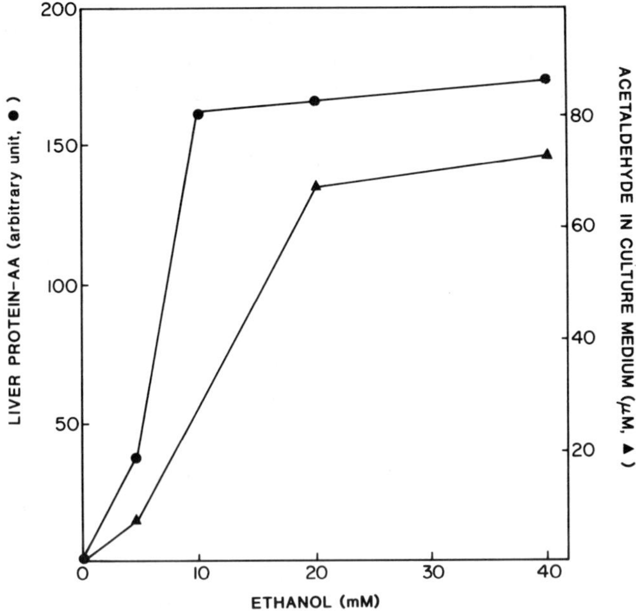

Fig. 4. Correlation of the 37-kDa protein-A and acetaldehyde concentrations in the culture medium. Hepatocytes were cultured in serum-free Waymouth's medium containing various concentrations of ethanol as indicated. Intensities of the 37-kDa protein-A bands were determined by densitometry as in Fig. 3. Acetaldehyde concentrations in the culture medium were determined by gas chromatography (from Lin et al.,[38] reprinted with permission).

Clinical Implications of the In Vivo Formation of Liver Protein-Acetaldehyde Adducts

About 20% of alcoholic patients develop advanced liver disease. The pathogenesis of alcoholic liver injury remains mostly unknown. Chronic alcohol consumption often leads to liver enlargement, due to accumulation of lipids, proteins, and water in hepatocytes.[39] The increase in liver proteins is mainly explained by induction of protein synthesis and by inhibiting export of secretory proteins.[40] It has been reported that when rat liver slices were incubated with 10 mM ethanol, the secretion of albumin and serum glycoproteins prelabeled with either [^{14}C]leucine or [^{14}C]fucose decreased.[41]

The inhibition of hepatic secretion of albumin and glycoproteins by acute and chronic alcohol administration has also been demonstrated in vivo.[42–44] Furthermore, the ethanol-induced impairment of hepatic protein secretion was prevented by ip injection of pyrazole prior to ethanol administration,[43] and was enhanced by pretreating animals with cyanamide.[44] These results indicate that the effect of ethanol on the protein secretion is mediated by acetaldehyde, the metabolite of ethanol in the liver. One possible site of the protein export system in liver that is rendered defective by ethanol ingestion is the microtubular system. Hepatic microtubules have been found to be decreased and morphologically altered after chronic alcohol feeding.[45–47] Tuma et al.[48] and Jennett et al.[49] reported that tubulin, covalently modified by acetaldehyde in vitro, exhibited decreased ability to form microtubules. These investigators hypothesized that a similar interaction in vivo can lead to functional deficiency of the tubulin/microtubule system. However, the formation of tubulin-acetaldehyde adducts in vivo has yet to be demonstrated. A possible but yet unexplored cause for the impairment of hepatic protein secretion is the covalent modification of secretory proteins per se, e.g., chemical modification by acetaldehyde. If a protein destined for export forms an adduct with acetaldehyde prior to secretion, it may acquire an altered conformation that will prevent its normal processing through the cellular secretory mechanism. This disturbance may result in the retention of export proteins in hepatocytes. Another detrimental effects of protein-acetaldehyde adducts may result from the binding of acetaldehyde to proteins in amino acid residues essential for their biological functions.[13] In sum, the interference of either hepatic protein secretion and/or hepatic enzyme function mediated by protein-AA formation can potentially lead to liver damage in the long run.

There is an almost universal increase in immunoglobulins in alcoholics[50–56] even without evidence of liver disease.[57] The hypothesis that immune response plays a pathogenic role in the development of alcoholic liver disease has recently been proposed.[58,59] Immune responses in alcoholic liver disease are now better characterized.[59] Israel et al.[29] have demonstrated that proteins modified with haptens as small as acetaldehyde are immunogenic. They have further reported that mice fed alcohol chronically developed antibodies that recognized acetaldehyde-modified epitopes.[29] Using ELISA method and hemagglutination assay, respectively, Niemela et al.[60] and Hoerner et al.[61] have reported that the serum of alcoholic patients showed significantly higher antibody titers against protein-AAs prepared in vitro than the serum of control subjects. The elevation of circulating antiprotein-AA antibodies seems to correlate with severity of liver disease with the highest titers being in patients with alcoholic hepatitis. It is uncertain, however, whether the appearance of these antibodies is the consequence or the cause of liver injury. It will be of great interest to identify which of the protein-AAs formed in vivo (hepatic as well as extrahepatic) can serve as neoantigens that trigger auto-antibody production.

Acknowledgment

Work performed in the authors' laboratories was supported by Grants from the National Institute on Alcohol Abuse and Alcoholism (AA06991 and AA07647) and by VA Merit Review Funds. The authors thank Michael Fillenwarth, Ron Minter, and Rebecca Smith for their excellent technical assistance, and Brenda Edwards for the preparation of the manuscript.

References

[1] R. D. Hawkins and H. Kalant (1972) The metabolism of ethanol and its metabolic effects. *Pharmacol. Rev.* **24,** 67–157.

[2] T. K. Li (1977) Enzymology of human alcohol metabolism, in *Advances in Enzymology,* vol. 45. A. Meister, ed. Wiley, New York, pp. 427–483.

[3] C. S. Lieber and L. M. DeCarli (1972) The role of the hepatic microsomal ethanol oxidizing system (MEOS) for ethanol metabolism in vivo. *J. Pharmacol. Exp. Ther.* **181,** 279–287.

[4] M. A. Korsten, S. Matsuzaki, L. Feinman, and C. S. Lieber (1975) High blood acetaldehyde levels after ethanol administration: Difference between alcoholic and nonalcoholic subjects. *N. Engl. J. Med.* **292,** 386–389.

[5] C. J. P. Eriksson (1980) Elevated blood acetaldehyde levels in alcoholics and their relatives: A reevaluation. *Science* **207,** 1383–1384.

[6] K. O. Lindros and C. J. P. Eriksson (1975) The role of acetaldehyde in the actions of ethanol. *Finn. Found. Alcohol Stud.* **23,** 67–81.

[7] M. Salaspuro and K. Lindros (1985) Metabolism and toxicity of acetaldehyde, in *Alcohol Related Diseases in Gastroenterology.* H. K. Seitz and B. Kommerell, eds. Springer–Verlag, Berlin, pp. 105–123.

[8] L. Lumeng, R. G. Minter, and T. K. Li (1982) Distribution of stable acetaldehyde adducts in blood under physiological conditions. *Fed. Proc.* **41,** 765.

[9] T. M. Donohue, D. J. Tuma, and M. F. Sorrell (1983) Acetaldehyde adducts with proteins: Binding of ^{14}C–acetaldehyde to serum albumin. *Arch. Biochem. Biophys.* **220,** 239–246.

[10] K. C.Gaines, J. M. Salhany, W. Tuma, and M. F. Sorrell (1977) Reactions of acetaldehyde with human erythrocyte membrane proteins. *FEBS Lett.* **75,** 115–119.

[11] R. B. Jennett, D. J. Tuma, and M. F. Sorrell (1980) Effect of ethanol and its metabolites. *Pharmacology* **21,** 363–368.

[12] F. Nomura and C. S. Lieber (1981) Binding of acetaldehyde to rat liver microsomes: Enhancement after chronic alcohol consumption. *Biochem. Biophys. Res. Commun.* **100,** 131–137.

[13] T. J. Mauch, T. M. Donohue, R. K. Zetterman, and M. F. Sorrell (1985) Covalent binding of acetaldehyde to lysine-dependent enzymes can inhibit catalytic activity. *Hepatology* **5,** 1056.

[14] L. Lumeng and R. G. Minter (1985) Formation of acetaldehyde-hemoglobin adducts in vitro and in vivo demonstrated by high performance liquid chromatography. *Alcohol. Clin. Exp. Res.* **9,** 209.

[15] V. J. Stevens, W. J. Fantl, C. B. Newman, R. V. Sims, A. Cerami, and C. Peterson (1981) Acetaldehyde adducts with hemoglobin. *J. Clin. Invest.* **67,** 361–369.

[16] D. J. Tuma, T. M. Donohue, V. A. Medina, and M. F. Sorrell (1984) Enhancement of acetaldehyde-protein adduct formation of L-ascorbate. *Arch. Biochem. Biophys.* **234,** 377–381.

[17] D. J. Tuma, M. R. Newman, T. M. Donohue, and M. F. Sorrell (1987) Covalent binding of acetaldehyde to proteins: Participation of lysine residues. *Alcohol. Clin. Exp. Res.* **11,** 578–584.

[18] V. A. Medina, T. M. Donohue, M. F. Sorrell, and D. J. Tuma (1985) Covalent binding of acetaldehyde to hepatic proteins during ethanol oxidation. *J. Lab. Clin. Med.* **105,** 5–10.

[19] T. K. Li and H. Theorell (1969) Human liver alcohol dehydrogenase: Inhibition by pyrazole and pyrazole analogs. *Acta Chem. Scand.* **23,** 892–902.

[20] M. Reynier (1969) Pyrazole inhibition and kinetic studies of ethanol and oxidation catalyzed by rat liver alcohol dehydrogenase. *Acta Chem. Scand.* **23,** 1119–1129.

[21] L. Goldberg and U. Ryberg (1969) Inhibition of ethanol metabolism in vivo by administration of pyrazole. *Biochem. Pharmacol.* **18,** 1749–1762.

[22] J. E. Peachey and E. M. Seller (1981) The disulfiram and calcium carbimide acetaldehyde-mediated ethanol reactions. *Pharmacol. Ther.* **15,** 89–97.

[23] J. M. Ritchie (1985) The aliphatic alcohols, in *The Pharmacological Basis of Therapeutics,* 7th Ed. A. G. Gilman, L. S. Goodman, and A. Gilman, eds. Macmillan, New York, pp. 372–386.

[24] R. C. San George and H. D. Hoberman (1986) Reaction of acetaldehyde with hemoglobin. *J. Biol. Chem.* **261,** 6811–6821.

[25] R. Hernandez-Munoz, E. Baroana, I. Blacksberg, and C. S. Lieber (1989) Characterization of the increased binding of acetaldehyde to red blood cells in alcoholics. *Alcohol. Clin. Exp. Res.* **13,** 654–659.

[26] H. Speisky, A. MacDonald, G. Giles, H. Orrego, and Y. Israel (1985) Increased loss and decreased synthesis of hepatic glutathione after acute ethanol administration. *Biochem. J.* **225,** 565–572.

[27] A. I. Cederbaum and E. Rubin (1976) Protective effect of cysteine on the inhibition of mitochondrial function by acetaldehyde. *Biochem. Pharmacol.* **25,** 963–973.

[28] T. K. Li and L. Lumeng (1985) Vitamin B-6 metabolism in alcoholism and alcoholic liver disease, in *Vitamin B-6: It's Role in Health and Disease.* R. D. Reynolds and J. E. LeKlem, eds. Alan Liss, New York, pp. 257–269.

[29] Y. Israel. E. Hurwitz, O. Niemela, and R. Arnon (1986) Monoclonal and polyclonal antibodies against acetaldehyde–containing epitopes in acetaldehyde-protein adducts. *Proc. Natl. Acad. Sci. USA* **83,** 7923–7927.

[30] O. Niemela and Y. Israel (1987) Immunological detection of acetaldehyde containing epitopes (ACES) in human hemoglobin: A new test in alcoholism. *Alcohol. Clin. Exp. Res.* **11,** 23.

[31] R. C. Lin, R. S. Smith, and L. Lumeng (1988) Detection of a protein-acetalde-hyde adducts in the liver of rats fed alcohol chronically. *J. Clin. Invest.* **81,** 615–619.

[32] U. J. Behrins, M. Hoerner, J. M. Lasker, and C. S. Lieber (1988) Formation of acetaldehyde adducts with ethanol-inducible P450IIEl in vivo. *Biochem. Biophys. Res. Commun.* **154,** 584–590.

[33] R. C. Lin and L. Lumeng (1989) Further studies on the 37-KD liver protein-acetaldehyde adduct that forms in vivo during chronic alcohol ingestion. *Hepatology* **10,** 807–814.

[34] R. C. Lin, L. Lumeng, S. Shahidi, T. Kelly, and D. Pound (1990) Protein-acetaldehyde adducts in serum of alcoholic patients. *Alcohol. Clin. Exp. Res.* **14,** 438–443.

[35] R. E. Barry, A. J. K. Williams, and J. D. McGivan (1987) The detection of acetaldehyde/liver plasma membrane protein adduct formed in vivo by alcohol feeding. *Liver* **7,** 364–368.

[36] R. Enat, D. M. Jefferson, N. Ruiz-Opazo, Z. Gatmaitan, L. A. Leinwand, and L. M. Reid (1984) Hepatocyte proliferation in vitro: Its dependence on the use of serum-free hormonally defined medium and substrata of extracellular matrix. *Proc. Natl. Acad. Sci. USA* **81,** 1411–1415.

[37] D. W. Crabb and T. K. Li (1985) Expression of alcohol dehydrogenase in primary monolayer cultures of rat hepatocytes. *Biochem. Biophys. Res. Commun.* **128,** 12–17.

[38] R. C. Lin, M. J. Fillenwarth, R. G. Minter, and L. Lumeng (1990) Formation of the 37KD protein-acetaldehyde adduct in primary cultured rat hepatocytes exposed to alcohol in vitro. *Hepatology* **11,** 401–407.

[39] E. Baroana, M. A. Leo, S. A. Borowsky, and C. S. Lieber (1975) Alcoholic hepatomegaly: Accumulation of protein in liver. *Science* **190,** 794,795.

[40] E. Baroana, M. A. Leo, S. A. Borowsky, and C. S. Lieber (1977) Pathogenesis of alcohol-induced accumulation of protein in the liver. *J. Clin. Invest.* **60,** 546–554.

[41] D. J. Tuma, R. B. Jennett, and M. F. Sorrell (1981) Effect of ethanol on the synthesis and secretion of hepatic secretory glycoproteins and albumin. *Hepatology* **1,** 590–598.

[42] M. F. Sorrell, J. M. Nauss, T. M. Donohue, and D. J. Tuma (1983) Effects of chronic ethanol administration on hepatic glycoprotein secretion in the rat. *Gastroenterology* **84,** 580–586.

[43] G. D. Volentine, D. J. Tuma, and M. F. Sorrell (1984) Acute effects of ethanol on hepatic glycoprotein secretion in the rat in vivo. *Gastroenterology* **84,** 225–229.

[44] G. D. Volentine, K. A. Ogden, D. K. Kortje, D. J. Tuma, and M. F. Sorrell (1987) Role of acetaldehyde in the ethanol-induced impairment of hepatic glycoprotein secretion in the rat in vivo. *Hepatology* **7,** 490–495.

[45] Y. Matsuda, E. Baroana, M. Salaspuro, and C. S. Lieber (1979) Effect of ethanol on liver microtubules and Golgi apparatus. *Lab. Invest.* **41,** 455–463.

[46] T. Okanoue, O. Ou, and M. Ohta (1984) Effect of chronic alcohol administration on the cytoskeleton of rat hepatocytes — including morphometric analysis. *Acta Hepatol. Japonica* **25,** 210–213.

[47] E. Baroana, F. Finkelman, and C. S. Lieber (1984) Reevaluation of the effects of alcohol consumption on rat liver microtubules. *Res. Commun. Clin. Pathol. Pharmacol.* **44,** 265–278.

[48] D. J. Tuma, R. B. Jennett, and M. F. Sorrell (1987) The interaction of acetaldehyde with tubulin. *Ann. NY Acad. Sci.* **492,** 277–286.

[49] R. B. Jennett, M. F. Sorrell, A. Saffari-Abbas, J. L. Ockner, and D. J. Tuma (1989) Preferential covalent binding of acetaldehyde to the α-chain of purified rat liver tubulin. *Hepatology* **9,** 57–62.

[50] T. Feizi (1968) Immunoglobulins in chronic liver disease. *Gut* **9,** 193–198.

[51] I. D. Wilson, G. Onstad, and R. C. Williams (1969) Serum immunoglobulin concentrations in patients with alcoholic liver disease. *Gastroenterology* **57,** 59–68.

[52] K. Akdamar, A. C. Epps, L. T. Mauma, and R. D. Sparks (1972) Immunoglobulin changes in liver disease. *Ann. NY Acad. Sci.* **197,** 101–107.

[53] R. A. Thompson, R. Carter, R. P. Stokes, A. M. Geddes, and J. A. D. Goodall (1973) Serum immunoglobulins, complement component levels and auto-antibodies in liver disease. *Clin. Exp. Immunol.* **14,** 335–346.

[54] R. J. Baily, N. Krasner, A. L. W. F. Eddleston, R. Williams, D. E. H. Tee, D. Doniach, L. A. Kennedy, and J. R. Batchelor (1976) Histocompatibility antigens, autoantibodies and immunoglobulins in alcoholic liver disease. *Br. Med. J.* **2,** 727–731.

[55] E. Van Epps, G. Husby, R. C. Williams, and R. G. Strickland (1976) Liver disease a prominent cause of serum IgE elevation. *Clin. Exp. Immunol.* **23**, 444–450.

[56] H. Iturriaga, T. Pereda, A. Estevez, and G. Ugarte (1977) Serum Immunoglobulin A changes in alcoholic patients. *Ann. Clin. Res.* **9**, 3943.

[57] P. A. Drew, P. M. Clifton, J. T. LaBrooy, and D. J. C. Shearman (1984) Polyclonal B cell activation in alcoholic patients with no evidence of liver dysfunction. *Clin. Exp. Immunol.* **57**, 479–486.

[58] H. Orrego, Y. Israel, and I. M. Blendis (1981) Alcoholic liver disease: Information in search of knowledge? *Hepatology* **1**, 267–283.

[59] R. D. Johnson and R. Williams (1986) Immune responses in alcoholic liver disease. *Alcohol. Clin. Exp. Res.* **10**, 471–486.

[60] O. Niemela, F. Klajner, H. Orrego, E. Vidins, L. Blendis, and Y. Israel (1987) Antibodies against acetaldehyde-modified protein epitopes in human alcoholics. *Hepatology* **7**, 1210–1214.

[61] M. Hoerner, U. J. Behrins, T. M. Worner, I. Blackberg, L. F. Braly, F. Schaffner, and C. S. Lieber (1988) The role of alcoholism and liver disease in the appearance of serum antibodies against acetaldehyde adducts. *Hepatology* **8**, 569–574.

Fatty Acid Ethyl Esters, Alcohol, and Liver Changes

Puran S. Bora and Louis G. Lange

Introduction

More than 25 years ago the World Health Organization concluded that an important association existed between excessive drinking of alcohol and development of tumors of the pharynx, esophagus, stomach, and liver.[1] There are at least 10 million alcoholics in the US, costing the economy over $100 billion annually,[2] but no generally accepted mechanism has been proposed that accounts for the propensity of certain individuals to drink to excess or to develop alcohol-related damage to organs.

Organs other than the liver develop alcohol-induced damage, especially the heart, pancreas, and brain. Since these organs lack or show minimal oxidative metabolism to ethanol and therefore are free of substantial acetaldehyde production,[3–5] the mechanism of this alcohol-related injury is unknown. Selectivity of organ damage, such as the occurrence of alcohol-induced cardiomyopathy in the absence of liver or pancreatic disease,[6] to these extrahepatic organs occurs despite a common exposure to blood containing similar concentrations of acetaldehyde derived from the liver.[7] Selective damage to organs that lack oxidative alcohol metabolism, therefore, suggests the existence of mechanisms of alcohol-induced organ injury that

From: *Drug and Alcohol Abuse Reviews, Vol. 2: Liver Pathology and Alcohol*
Ed: R. R. Watson ©1991 The Humana Press Inc.

are intrinsic to extrahepatic organs themselves. We have now documented over the past five years that ethanol is metabolized to fatty acid ethyl esters (FAEE) in many human organs.[8–11] These esters, which are produced *in situ*, may be one candidate for mediating some of the noted alcohol-induced end organ disease. Recent observations on the relationship of fatty acid ethyl ester Synthase III (major) to hepatic glutathione *S*-transferase demonstrate that nonoxidative ethanol metabolism may also be important in the liver, where its interaction with oxidative alcohol metabolism drug detoxification and carcinogen inactivation may occur.

Fatty Acid Ethyl Esters and End Organ Damage

The observation that FAEEs are synthesized at high rates in the pancreas, brain, heart, and other organs that lack oxidative ethanol metabolism[10,11] provided a plausible link between the observed tissue damage and the ingestion of alcohol.[12] FAEEs are formed in myocardium principally from nonesterified fatty acid.[13] Since ethyl esters are bound less readily to protein than is nonesterified fatty acid[14] and because FAEEs synthesized in myocardium tissue slices bind substantially to mitochondria, FAEEs may act in a toxic fatty acid shuttle to induce mitochondrial dysfunction in vivo after prolonged alcohol abuse.[14]

Several factors may modulate FAEEs induced mitochondrial damage. First, factors that regulate the equilibrium concentration of soluble fatty acid could be important. Second, the activity of intracellular enzyme(s) that catalyze the synthesis of FAEEs may be influenced both by small molecular effectors or potentially by isoenzymes with inherent differences in catalytic properties. Third, the amount of ethanol ingested and its rate of clearance, i.e., factors related to the type of hepatic alcohol dehydrogenase present, would modify the concentration of ethanol in myocardium available for esterification.

Recently, Mair et al.[15] have shown that chronic FAEEs exposure can decrease hepatic protein secretion in vitro. They have suggested that the effects of ethanol on protein metabolism may be owing to disaggregation of membrane-bound ribosomes. Thus, the FAEEs may possibly mediate, at least in part, the decrease in hepatic protein secretion noted after chronic ethanol exposure, possibly by interfering with the function of membrane-bound ribosomes. Furthermore, since alcohol abuse is chronic, synergystic metabolic insults to hepatic mitochondria may occur,[14] resulting in impaired energy production as well as reductions in protein synthesis. Whether such potential cellular injury may occur in other organs, such as the brain, remains open to experimental scrutiny.

Fatty Acid Ethyl Ester Synthase Assay

Formation of FAEE from ethanol is enzymatically mediated and can be determined as described by Mogelson and Lange[16] by incubating samples containing enzyme with 0.4 mM [^{14}C]oleate (20,000 dpm/nmol) and 200 mM ethanol in 60 mM sodium phosphate buffer, pH 7.2, in a total volume of 0.17 mL in capped vials at 37°C. At the end of the incubation interval, the reaction is terminated by the addition of 2 mL of cold acetone containing a known amount of ethyl [^{3}H]oleate and 0.6 μmol of carrier ethyl oleate. Volumes are reduced by evaporation under a stream of nitrogen at 37°C, and residual lipids in acetone chromatographed on silica plates (Analabs, North Haven, CT) developed with petroleum ether/diethyl ether/acetic acid (75/5/1). After visualization of lipids with iodine vapor, fatty acid ethyl ester spots were scraped, and the lipid eluted with acetone and assayed for radioactivity. ^{14}C Counts are adjusted for yield as determined by recovery of ^{3}H, and after subtraction of blanks, results are expressed as nmol of fatty acid ethyl ester formed per mL per h. Assays for enzymatic synthesis of fatty acid ethyl esters were linear with respect to expended time (up to 45 min) and added enzyme (up to 0.02 mg/mL).[16–18] Rates of synthase activity in various organ homogenates may vary from 468 nmol/g/h for pancreas to 7 nmol/g/h for aorta.[8]

Mogelson et al.[19] have shown that the rate of synthesis of FAEEs facilitated by FAEE synthase is caused by an augmentation of reaction rate that reflects a reduction in ΔG, attributable to a positive entropy change. Accumulation of product, FAEE, is a consequence of the thermodynamically favorable self-association of monomeric molecules into a hydrocarbon phase to provide an overall favorable equilibrium constant for the formation of aggregated product from soluble reactants. Thus, the unusual reaction in which the lipid precursor is free fatty acid—not fatty acid CoA—is driven by positive entropic changes and lipid product self-association.

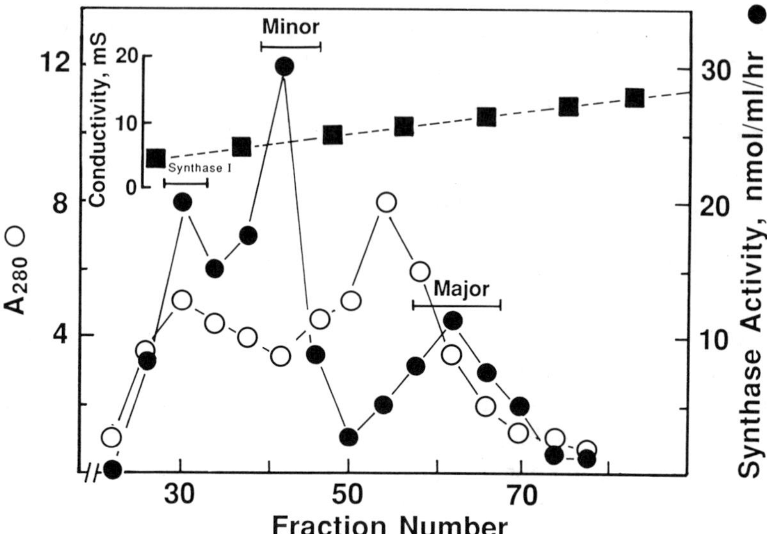

Fig. 1. DEAE-Cellulose Chromatography. Enzyme activity from human myo-cardium was fractionated at 40 mL/h in 1 m*M* BME, 10 m*M* Tris, pH 8.0. The column was developed with a linear salt gradient running from buffer to 400 m*M* NaCl (■). Fractions (6 mL) were collected and monitored for protein (O) and syn-thase activity (●). (Reproduced from the *Journal of Clinical Investigation*, 1989, **84,** 1943 by copyright permission of the American Society for Clinical Investigation.)

Purification and Characterization of Fatty Acid Ethyl Ester Synthases

All organs thus far examined in rabbit or humans have a typical set of synthases in the soluble fraction from homogenates. When fractionated on DEAE-cellulose (2 × 18 cm) in 1 m*M* of BME, 10 m*M* Tris, pH 8.0, these chromatograph as a minor and major synthase.[14] In some organs, e.g., human myocardium, a third peak of FAEE synthase activity is consistently and reproducibly observed, migrating ahead of the minor synthase (Fig. 1). The nomenclature of these species has now been designated as follows: when chromatography is carried out as just described, Synthase I, eluting at 5 mS; minor synthase (II) eluting at 7 mS; and the major synthase (III) eluting at 11 mS.

Fatty Acid Ethyl Ester Synthase I

A typical purification scheme for the human myocardial Synthase I would be as follows. In order to concentrate the fatty acid ethyl ester Synthase I pool (45 mL) from the DEAE-cellulose column, solid ammonium sulfate was added to 70% of saturation. The precipitate was collected by centrifugation, dialyzed against 1 mM BME, 10 mM Tris, 50 mM phosphate, pH 7.0, and applied to a Sephadex G-100 column (2.5 × 72 cm). The enzyme was recovered in 75% yield as a single, broad peak.

An octyl Sepharose column (1 × 7 cm) was equilibrated with 1 mM BME, 10 mM Tris, 50 mM phosphate, pH 7.0, and those Sephadex G-100 fractions with activity greater than 2 nmol/mL/h were applied at 20 mL/h. After washing the resin with 0.10% sodium cholate in the same buffer, the column was developed further with a linear cholate gradient running from 0.10 to 0.20% and the enzyme emerged at 0.13% cholate in 70% yield.

Fractions containing enzyme activity greater than 2 nmol/mL/h were pooled and applied to FPLC Superose-12, equilibrated with 1 mM BME, 10 mM Tris, 50 mM sodium phosphate, pH 7.0. Enzymatic activity emerged at an elution volume corresponding to a mol mass of 52 kDa. SDS-PAGE of this material (35 μg) showed a single band of mol mass 26 kDa when stained either with silver or Coomassie Blue. The enzyme therefore is a dimer, consisting of two 26 kDa subunits. Synthase I showed significant crossreactivity to antibody raised against homogeneous human heart fatty acid ethyl ester Synthase III, both by solid phase radioimmunoassay and immunoblot.

An overall yield of 9% was obtained for the 1118-fold purified enzyme when assayed in the presence of 0.2M ethanol and 0.91 mM oleic acid. Myocardium contains approx 20 μg of the fatty acid ethyl ester Synthase I per g of tissue.[18]

Several chromatography experiments were performed to confirm that Synthase I is a GST. First, the DEAE-cellulose fractions (active as Synthase I, total activity 700 nmol/mL/h) were assayed for GST activity with 1 mM 1-chloro-2, 4-dinitrobenzene as substrate, and this activity cochromatographed with the Synthase I activity. Using this chromophoric substrate, the pooled fractions had a total activity of 40 mL/min/mol enzyme. These fractions were concentrated by ammonium sulfate (70% saturation) and dialyzed against 1 mM BME, 10 mM Tris, and 50 mM sodium phosphate, pH 7.0. The enzyme was applied to a Sephadex G-100 and eluted with 1 mM

BME, 10 mM Tris, and 50 mM sodium phosphate, pH 7.0. A single peak of synthase activity (total pool activity, 434 nmol/mL/h) was observed in 62% yield and a single peak of GST activity cochromatographed (total pool activity, 24 mol/min/mol enzyme) in 60% yield. Finally, the pool from the Sephadex G-100 column was dialyzed against phosphate-buffered saline, pH 7.4, and was applied to S-hexylglutathione agarose, previously equilibrated with phosphate-buffered saline, pH 7.4. After applying the sample, the column was washed with this buffer until the effluent was free of protein. The enzyme was eluted by raising the pH to 9.6 (4°C) with 0.05M Tris buffer containing 5 mM GSH. These fractions were active for both Synthase I (total activity 118 nmol/mL/h, yield 17%) and GST (8 mol/min/h enzyme) with 20% yield. SDS-PAGE of this material showed a single band at 26 kDa, further indicating that Synthase I may be one of the members of GSTs. Therefore, it is important to note that GST may play a role in the liver as an ethanol-detoxification enzyme.

The substrate specificity of the fatty acid ethyl ester Synthase I was examined by measuring the rate of ethyl ester synthesis in the presence of fatty acids of different chain length and degree of saturation. The following ^{14}C-labeled fatty acids were used: palmitate, stearate, oleate, linoleate, and arachidonate. In all cases, linear Lineweaver-Burke plots were found and the maximum rates of synthesis (V_{max}) were observed with linoleate and oleate, 222 nmol/mg/h and 200 nmol/mg/h, respectively. Saturated fatty acids had the lowest rates of ethyl ester synthesis, with rates of 36 and 32 nmol/mg/h for stearate and palmitate, respectively. In contrast, binding affinities (K_m) for these fatty acid substrates were all nearly the same, 0.40 mM to 0.59 mM at a fixed oleate concentration of 0.91 mM; the V_{max} and K_m for ethanol were 59 nmol/mg/h and 0.30M, respectively. Importantly, the homogeneous Synthase I was also active as a GST with the standard substrate 1-chloro-2, 4-dinitrobenzene (1 mM) as substrate (8 mol/min/mol enzyme) and 1,2-dichloro-4-nitrobenzene (5.93 mol/min/mol enzyme).

Fatty Acid Ethyl Ester Synthase II

The second peak eluted at a conductivity of 7 mS and accounted for 60% of recovered total activity. After DEAE-cellulose chromatography, the Synthase II pool (550 mL) was dialyzed against 5 mM sodium phosphate, pH 7.2 and applied to hydroxylapatite (5 × 16 cm). All the synthase activity was bound. Elution with a linear phosphate gradient (5–250 mM) produced two

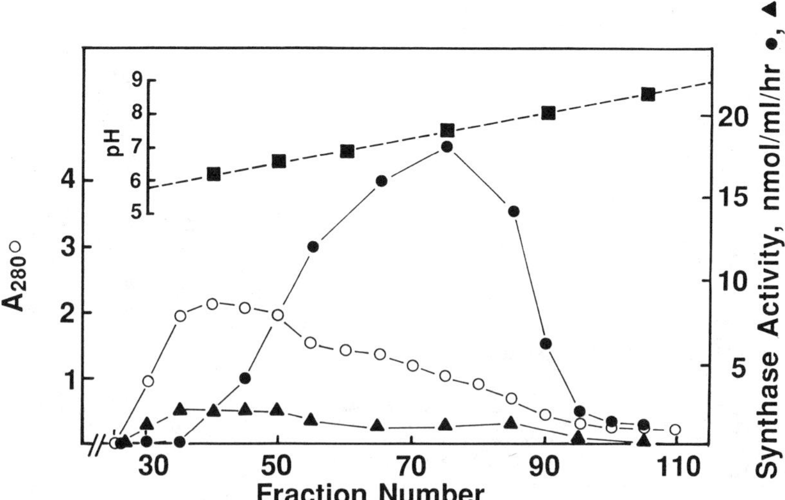

Fig. 2. CM-Cellulose Chromatography. Protein was applied at 36 mL/h on CM-cellulose (5 ¥ 60 cm) equilibrated with 5 mM citrate buffer, pH 5.8. When the A$_{280}$ was less than 0.1, a pH gradient from pH 5.8 to pH 8.8 (■) was applied. Fractions (4 mL) were monitored for A$_{280}$ (○) and fatty acid ethyl ester synthase activity, +CaCl$_2$ (5 mM) (●), and –CaCl$_2$ (▲).

peaks of enzyme activity, but since the first peak contained less than 10% of the applied activity, further studies were performed only on the second peak.

The pooled activity (600 mL) was dialyzed against 5 mM citrate buffer, pH 5.8 and then applied to CM-cellulose (5 × 16 cm) equilibrated with the same buffer. All the activity was bound and the column was developed with a pH gradient running from 5 mM citrate, pH 5.8 to 10 mM Tris, pH 8.8. When the fractions were assayed, little or no activity was found; however, after addition of 5 mM CaCl$_2$ to each fraction, synthase activity was restored, with an overall recovery of 60% (Fig. 2).

Fractions from CM-cellulose chromatography with activity greater than 1 nmol/mL/h were pooled, dialyzed against 1 mM BME, 10 mM Tris, pH 8.0, and applied in 5-mL aliquots to FPLC Mono Q column. The resin was washed with a linear sodium chloride gradient (0–220 mM) and then with a steep gradient to 2M sodium chloride. Active enzyme was eluted at 1M NaCl.

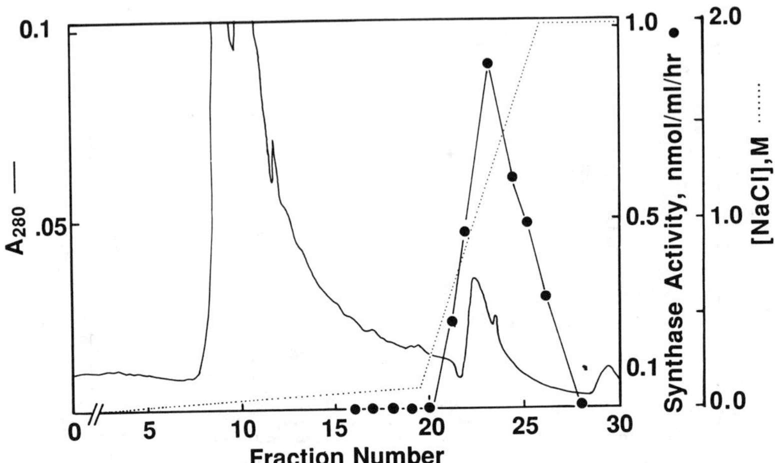

Fig. 3. FPLC Mono Q Chromatography. Protein was applied at 1 mL/min to a Mono Q column equilibrated with 1 mM BME, 10 mM Tris, pH 8.0. Protein was first eluted with a shallow NaCl gradient, 0–220 mM (- - -) followed by a steep gradient running to 2.0M (- - -) NaCl. Fractions (1 mL) were monitored for A_{280} (—) and fatty acid ethyl ester synthase activity in the presence of 5 mM CaCl$_2$ (●).

When assays were performed in the presence of 5 mM calcium chloride (Fig. 3), more than 63% of the activity initially applied to Mono Q was recovered, and again, little activity was detected if calcium was omitted from the assay.

The purification of the fatty acid ethyl ester Synthase II from human myocardium is summarized in Table 1. The enzyme was purified 596-fold with an overall yield of 6%, and SDS-PAGE showed that the product from the Mono Q column contained two closely migrating polypeptides (Fig. 4), one with a mol mass of 67 kDa and the other of 65 kDa. These polypeptides copurified during further attempts to separate them. Their relationship to cholesterol esterase, mol mass 67 kDa,[13] is under investigation.

Fatty Acid Ethyl Ester
Synthase II Calcium Requirement

To investigate the effect of metals on synthase activity, the enzyme was incubated with EDTA and EGTA. One millimolar EGTA reduced the enzyme activity by 90%, and 5 mM EGTA totally inhibited the enzyme. Importantly, calcium ions (7 mM) are able to restore enzymatic activity fully.

Table 1
Purification of Human Myocardial Fatty Acid Ethyl Ester Synthase II

Step	Total protein, mg	Total activ., nmol/h	SA, nmol/mg/h	Purif., X-fold	Yield, %
Cytosol[a]	53,694	25,200	.5	1	100
DEAE-cellulose	5162	13,718	2.7	5	54
Hydroxylapatite	2522	18,925	7.5	15	75
Carboxylmethyl cellulose	602	8904	14.8	30	35
Mono Q	4.95	1476	298.2	596	6

[a]Synthase II activity in the cytosol was calculated from the proportions of Synthase III and Synthase II activities as determined after DEAE-cellulose chromatography.

To determine the K_A for calcium binding, synthase activity was measured in the presence of increasing concentrations of Ca^{2+}. As the added calcium concentration increased from 0 to 5 mM, the activity increased eightfold with an apparent binding constant of 3 mM. Above 5 mM Ca^{2+}, less activation was observed so that at 20 mM Ca^{2+} the activity was only four times greater than the no-calcium control. Other divalent metal ions, such as Mg^{2+} and Zn^{2+}, had no effect on enzyme activity. These results suggest that Synthase II contains a weak binding site for calcium that enhances enzymatic activity. In view of the documented alterations of intracellular calcium homeostasis that occur during alcohol abuse,[20] pathophysiological significance of this finding cannot be ignored.

Fatty Acid Ethyl Ester Synthase III

Human myocardium FAEE Synthase III was purified to homogeneity by sequential DEAE-cellulose, gel permeation, hydrophobic interaction, and immunoaffinity chromatographies. In brief, human heart soluble fraction was applied to DEAE-cellulose (5 × 16 cm) in 1 mM BME, 10 mM Tris, pH 8.0. All the activity was bound, and after extensive washing, the column was developed further with a linear salt gradient running from starting buffer to 400 mM NaCl, 1 mM BME, 10 mM Tris, pH 8.0. The activity eluted at a conductivity of 11 mS, and this pool was precipitated with ammonium sulfate (70% of saturation), dialyzed against 1 mM BME, 10 mM Tris, 50 mM

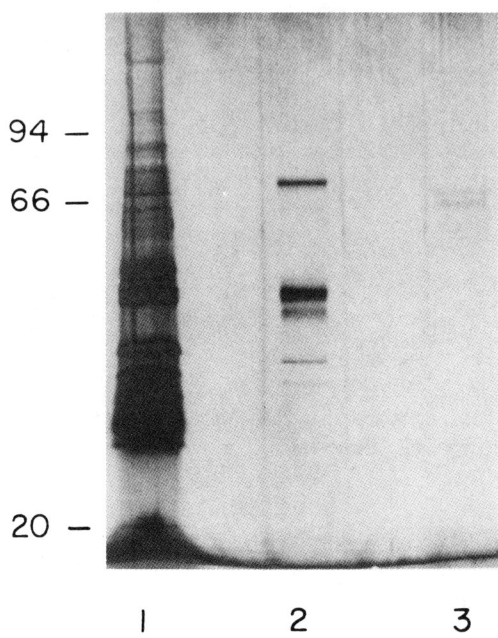

Fig. 4. SDS-PAGE of FAEE Synthase II Purification. Lane 1, hydroxylapatite chromatography; Lane 2, CM-cellulose chromatography; and Lane 3, Mono Q chromatography. This gel was stained with silver; similar results were noted after Coomassie brilliant blue staining.

sodium phosphate, pH 7.0 and applied to a Sephadex G-100 column (2.5 × 72 cm). Active enzyme from G-100 was applied at 20 mL/h to octyl-Sepharose CL-4B (1.0 × 6.0 cm) equilibrated with 1 mM BME, 10 mM Tris, 50 mM sodium phosphate, pH 7.0. The resin was washed with 0.1% cholate and was developed further with a linear sodium cholate gradient (0.1–0.25%). The enzyme emerged as a single peak (85% yield) at approx 0.15% (w/v) sodium cholate. SDS-PAGE of this peak showed a single band of mol mass 26 kDa, containing only a trace amount of albumin. The fractions eluting from octyl Sepharose having synthase activity greater than 2 nmol/mL/h were then pooled and applied to an antihuman albumin affinity column (0.9 × 7 cm) equilibrated with 1 mM BME, 10 mM Tris, 50 mM sodium phosphate, pH 7.0. Synthase activity washed through the column with full retention of enzyme activity, and SDS-PAGE of the preparation demonstrated the presence of a single polypeptide with a mol mass of 26 kDa.[21–25]

Table 2
Comparison of the *N*-Terminal
Amino Acid Sequences of FAEE Synthase and GSTs

Human heart FAEE synthase	Rat hepatocellular carcinoma GST-P[a]	Human heart acidic GST[b]
A	P	P
P	P	P
Y	Y	Y
T	T	T
V	I	V
V	V	V
Y	Y	Y
F	F	F
P	P	P
V	V	V
R	R	R
G	G	G
R	R	R
X	C	X
K	E	A
A	A	A
L	T	L
R	R	R
M	M	M
L	L	L
X	L	L
A	A	A
D	D	D

[a] Ref. 26; [b] Ref. 27.

Homology with Hepatic
Glutathione *S*-Transferases

Homogeneous FAEE Synthase III from human myocardium was subjected to sequence analysis, and 23 amino acids from its *N*-terminus were determined without ambiguity, except for the 14th and 21st amino acids (Table 2). This sequence revealed greater than 80% identity with that of the *N*-terminal sequence for rat glutathione *S*-transferase (GST-P),[26] with variations at residues 1, 5, 15, and 17, some of which may reflect species differences (Table 2). It is also virtually identical to that of an acidic GST recently purified to homogeneity from human heart.[27]

The amino acid compositions of FAEE Synthase III and two GSTs are quite similar. These structural studies thus show that the FAEE Synthase III from human myocardium is very similar to the GSTs, which constitute an important defense mechanism against numerous ingested xenobiotics and carcinogens (22).

Common Catalytic Properties
of FAEE Synthase III
and Glutathione S-Transferase

Using the standard FAEE synthase assay,[16,18] GST was found to catalyze the formation of ethyl ^{14}C-oleate with saturation kinetics when incubated with $0.2M$ ethanol and oleic acid, ranging in concentration from 0.1 to 2 mM. The corresponding Lineweaver-Burke plot was linear, and V_{max} and K_m were 98 nmol ethyl oleate formed/mg/h and 0.48 mM, respectively. These values are close to those previously found for human heart FAEE synthase: 105 nmol/mg/h and 0.23 mM. Similarly, the reaction was studied in the presence of a fixed concentration of oleic acid 0.91 mM, and increasing concentrations of ethanol from 25 mM to $2M$. In this case, the enzyme is active at physiological concentrations of ethanol. K_m for ethanol was $0.65M$, and the V_{max} was 56 nmol/mg/h. These values are nearly the same as those found when this reaction was catalyzed by human heart FAEE synthase.[22]

FAEE synthase is also able to catalyze the formation of glutathione conjugates. Human myocardial FAEE synthase (26 kDa, single protein on SDS-PAGE) was incubated with 1 mM glutathione and increasing concentrations of 1-chloro-2, 4-dinitrobenzene from 0.2 to 2 mM. Following the same assay conditions as those used for GST,[28] the synthase demonstrated high transferase activity with saturation kinetics. The corresponding Lineweaver-Burke plot was linear, and V_{max} and K_m were found to be 67 mol/min/mol enzyme and 5 mM, respectively. These results are similar to those reported for rat hepatic GST, given the different organs of origin and the known variation of GST activity reported during isolation.[29,30] Inhibition of human myocardial FAEE Synthase III catalyzed formation of FAEE was also observed in the presence of 1-chloro-2, 4-dinitrobenzene. This substrate for the standard GST assay inhibited the rate of synthesis of ethyl oleate, with 50% and 90% inhibition occurring at 25 and 300 µM, respectively. Thus, the myocardial synthase recognizes a typical GST substrate as both an inhibitor and substrate, evidence confirming the hypothesis that the Synthase III is a GST.

Induction of Fatty Acid Ethyl Ester Synthase

Two male rabbits were placed on a liquid diet containing 36% of the calories as ethanol, and two other male rabbits were fed control diet without ethanol. At the end of a 10-d feeding period, the rabbits were sacrificed and the liver homogenates were assayed for FAEE synthase activity. Cystolic synthase activity of rabbits fed ethanol diet was sevenfold higher than synthase activity noted in the the control rabbit.

When this cytosol was passed through DEAE-cellulose, the unbound activity was washed through by 10 mM Tris, pH 8.0, containing 1 mM BME, and the bound activity was eluted by a linear gradient of sodium chloride from 0 to 0.4M. There was a threefold increase in the activity of Synthase III compared to the control group. Since we have shown that Synthase III is a member of the GSTs[22] and it is also known that GSTs are induced by ethanol and phenobarbital,[31] the induction of FAEE synthase by ethanol is in keeping with past knowledge of the glutathione S-transferases and its newly identified biological substrate, ethanol.[22,31,32] Pickett et al.[32] have demonstrated that a transcriptional activation of GST subunit genes (3 and 4) occurred after administration of phenobarbital to rat and was sufficient to account for the elevation of the mRNAs. Thus, ethanol is capable of modifying its own hepatic metabolism by activating specific GST genes through a presently unknown mechanism.

Conclusion

Previous investigations suggest that alcohol metabolism may be under genetic control, and related to the presence of different amounts or types of ethanol metabolizing enzymes.[33,34] Since no other pathway for alcohol metabolism exists in the heart, fatty acid ethyl ester synthase may be one of the gene products underlying a genetic vulnerability to the effects of alcohol in this and other organs, such as the brain.[8,9,18] Recent genetic studies using peripheral human leukocytes have shown that this synthase activity is heritable in an autosomal recessive pattern for high activity,[35,36] a pattern expected for a gene controlling the production of a toxic agent.

It will now be possible to examine this hypothesis in segregation studies using the cloned Synthase III to enable restriction fragment-length polymorphism studies of families containing an alcoholic proband. Thus, the present results provide a foundation for subsequent protein sequence studies, cloning, and genetic studies of the fatty acid ethyl ester synthase system in humans. Because it is present in those organs commonly injured by alcohol, we may now evaluate a genetic link between alcohol consumption and specific end organ damage, which may have a monogenic etiology in some cases.

Inclusion of an alcohol metabolizing enzyme within the group comprising the GSTs also bears importantly on the long appreciated relationship between alcohol abuse and the propensity to develop tumors of the pharynx, esophagus, stomach, and liver.[37,38] These organs are exposed to high concentrations of ethanol (100–500 mM), where excessive fatty acid ethyl ester generation may occur. Because GSTs are the major route for elimination of endogenous and ingested carcinogens, cometabolism of ethanol and carcinogens by these enzymes may affect end product concentrations and biological half-lives of either or both. Thus, environmental and genetic influences on the rates of ethanol metabolism and xenobiotic transformation may be interrelated since numerous agents, such as ethanol, phenobarbital, and thyroid hormone, may induce the glutathione S-transferases.

Abbreviations

BME, 2-mercaptoethanol; EDTA, ethylenediamine tetraacetic acid; EGTA, ethyleneglycol-bis-(beta-amino ethyl ether)-N,N,N^1,N^1 tetraacetic acid; FAEE, fatty acid ethyl ester; GSH, glutathione; GST, glutathione S-transferases; SDS-PAGE, sodium dodecylsulfate-polyacrylamide gel electrophoresis; Tris, tris(hydroxymethyl) aminomethane.

References

[1] World Health Organization (1964) Association between drinking and carcinogenesis. *World Health Bulletin* **9,** 16,17.

[2] L. J. West (1984) Alcoholism. *Ann. Intern. Med.* **100,** 405–416.

[3] C. S. Lieber and L. M. DeCarli (1968) Ethanol oxidation by hepatic microsomes: Adaptive increase after ethanol feeding. *Science* **162,** 917,918.

[4] A. Lochner, R. Cowley, and A. Brink (1969) Effect of ethanol on metabolism and junction of perfused rat heart. *Am. Heart J.* **78,** 770–780.

[5] H. H. Raskin and L. Sokoloff (1972) Enzyme catalysing ethanol metabolism in neutral and somatic tissue of the rat. *J. Neurochem.* **19,** 273–282.

[6] L. M. Lefkowitch and J. Fenoglio (1983) Liver disease in alcoholic cardiomyopathy: Evidence against cirrhosis. *Hum. Pathol.* **14,** 457–463.

[7] C. J. Ericksson and H. W. Sippel (1977) The distribution and metabolism of acetaldehyde in rats during ethanol oxidation-I. The distribution of acetaldehyde in liver, brain, blood and breath. *Biochem. Pharmacol.* **26,** 241–247.

[8] E. A. Laposata and L. G. Lange (1986) Presence of non-oxidative ethanol metabolism in human organs commonly damaged by ethanol abuse. *Science* **231,** 497–499.

[9] E. A. Laposata, D. E. Scherrer, C. Mazow, and L. G. Lange (1987) Metabolism of ethanol by human brain to fatty acid ethyl esters. *J. Biol. Chem.* **262,** 4653–4657.

[10] E. A. Laposata, D. E. Scherrer, and L. G. Lange (1989) Fatty acid ethyl esters in adipose tissue. *Arch. Pathol. Lab. Med.* **113,** 762–766.

[11] D. J. S. Riley, E. M. Kyger, C. A. Spilburg, and L. G. Lange (1990) Pancreatic cholesterol esterases. Purification and characterization of human pancreatic fatty acid ethyl ester synthase. *Biochemistry* **29,** 3848–3852.

[12] L. G. Lange, S. R. Bergman, and B. E. Sobel (1981) Identification of fatty acid ethyl esters as products of rabbit myocardial ethanol metabolism. *J. Biol. Chem.* **256,** 12,968–12,973.

[13] L. G. Lange (1982) Nonoxidative ethanol metabolism. Formation of fatty acid ethyl esters by cholesterol esterase. *Proc. Natl. Acad. Sci. USA* **79,** 3954–3957.

[14] L. G. Lange and B. E. Sobel (1983) Mitochondrial dysfunction induced by fatty acid ethyl esters, myocardial metabolites of ethanol. *J. Clin. Invest.* **72,** 724–731.

[15] D. C. Mair, M. E. Donnell, and E. A. Laposata (1990) Fatty acid ethyl esters, a family of ethanol metabolites, mediate changes in protein secretion in HEP G2 cells. *Clin. Res.* **38,** 264A (abstract).

[16] S. Mogelson and L. G. Lange (1984) Nonoxidative ethanol metabolism in rabbit myocardium purification to homogeneity of fatty acid ethyl ester synthase. *Biochemistry* **23,** 4075–4081.

[17] P. M. Kinnunen and L. G. Lange (1984) Identification and quantification of fatty acid ethyl esters in biological specimens. *Anal. Biochem.* **140,** 567–576.

[18] P. S. Bora, C. A. Spilburg, and L. G. Lange (1989) Identification of a satellite fatty acid ethyl ester synthase from human myocardium as a glutathione *S*-transferase. *J. Clin. Invest.* **84,** 1942–1946.

[19] S. Mogelson, S. J. Pieper, and L. G. Lange (1984) Thermodynamic bases for fatty acid ethyl ester synthase catalyzed esterification of free fatty acid with ethanol and accumulation of fatty acid ethyl esters. *Biochemistry* **23,** 4082–4087.

[20] J. B. Hoek, A. P. Thomas, R. Rubin, and E. Rubin (1987) Ethanol-induced mobilization of calcium by activation of phosphoinositide-specific phospholipase C in intact hepatocytes. *J. Biol. Chem.* **262,** 682–691.

[21] P. S. Bora, C. A. Spilburg, and L. G. Lange (1989) Purificaton to homogeneity and characterization of major fatty acid ethyl ester synthase from human myocardium. *FEBS Lett.* **258,** 236–239.

[22] P. S. Bora, C. A. Spilburg, and L. G. Lange (1989) Metabolism of ethanol and carcinogens by glutathione transferases. *Proc. Natl. Acad. Sci. USA* **86,** 4470–4473.

[23] P. S. Bora, C. A. Spilburg, and L. G. Lange (1989) Co-metabolism of ethanol and carcinogens by GSH transferases. *Clin. Res.* **37,** 247A (abstract).

[24] P. S. Bora, C. A. Spilburg, and L. G. Lange (1989) Ethanol and carcinogen metabolism by glutathione *S*-transferases. *Clin. Res.* **37,** 897A (abstract).

[25] P. S. Bora and L. G. Lange (1991) Homogeneous Synthase I from human myocardium is a glutathione *S*-transferase. *Ann. NY Acad. Sci.* (in press).

[26] Y. Suguoka, T. Kano, A. Okuda, M. Sakai, T. Kitagawa, and M. Muramatsu (1985) Cloning and the nucleotide sequence of rat glutathione *S*-transferase P cDNA. *Nucleic Acids Res.* **13,** 6049–6057.

[27] A. M. Caccuri, C. Dillio, D. Campagnone, D. Barra, and G. Frederici (1989) Acidic glutathione transferase from human heart characterization and *N*-terminal sequence determination. *Biochem. Med. Metab. Biol.* **40,** 123–132.

[28] W. R. Habig, M. J. Rabst, and W. B. Jakoby (1974) Glutathione *S*-transferase: The first enzymatic step in metcapturic acid formation. *J. Biol. Chem.* **249,** 7130–7139.

[29] G. Wistow and J. Piatigoslay (1987) Recruitment of enzymes as lens structural proteins. *Science* **236,** 1554–1556.

[30] S. Tomarev and R. D. Zinovieva (1988) Squid major lens polypeptides are homologous to glutathione *S*-transferases subunits. *Nature (Lond.)* **336,** 86–88.

[31] R. M. David and D. E. Nerland (1983) Induction of mouse liver glutathione *S*-transferase by ethanol. *Biochem. Pharmacol.* **32,** 2809–2811.

[32] C. B. Pickett, C. A. Tetakowsky-Hopkins, C. F. G. Ding, and V. D. M. Ding (1987) Sequence analysis and regulation of rat liver glutathione *S*-transferase mRNAs. *Xenobiotica* **17,** 317–323.

[33] C. R. Cloninger, M. Bohman, and S. Sigvardsson (1981) Inheritance of alcohol abuse. *Arch. Gen. Psychiatry* **38,** 861–868.

[34] D. W. Goodwin (1987) Genetic influence in alcoholism. *Adv. Intern. Med.* **32,** 283–297.

[35] M. Wright, K. J. Bieser, P. M. Kinnunen, and L. G. Lange (1987) Nonoxidative ethanol metabolism in human leukocytes: Detection of fatty acid ethyl ester synthase activity. *Biochem. Biophys. Res. Commun.* **142,** 979–985.

[36] S. B. Gilligan, L. G. Lange, T. Reich, and C. R. Cloninger (1987) Nonoxidative ethanol metabolism in alcoholic pedigrees. *Am. J. Hum. Genet.* **41,** A255 (abstr).

[37] C. S. Lieber, H. K. Seitz, and H. J. Gaoro (1987) Alcohol-related diseases and carcinogenesis. *Cancer Res.* **39,** 2863–2867.

[38] J. E. Engstrom (1977) Colorectal cancer and beer drinking. *Br. J. Cancer Res.* **35,** 679–684.

Ethanol, Lipoprotein Metabolism, and Fatty Liver

M. R. Lakshman, Stuart J. Chirtel, and Pradeep Ghosh

Introduction

Persistent excessive intake of ethanol can lead to liver cell injury and eventually to cirrhosis of the liver after prolonged abuse over many years. There are individual variations in susceptibility to alcohol toxicities. Hepatocellular necrosis results in a wide variety of clinical symptoms ranging from a relatively asymptomatic enlargement of the liver to massive fatty infiltration that ultimately leads to hepatic failure.[1,2] As the process of alcohol-mediated injury progresses, liver fibrosis and eventually cirrhosis ensue, resulting in total failure of the liver functions. The pathogenesis of alcohol-induced toxicity generally begins with specific episodes of hepatocellular injury accompanied by varying degrees of fatty liver.[3] As the alcohol abuse continues, this degenerative process manifests itself into liver cell dysfunction, chronic inflammation, and structural distortion leading to the proliferation of fibrous tissue, which ultimately culminates into the cirrhosis of the liver and death.

Accumulation of fat in the liver is predominant in alcoholic hepatitis and alcoholic cirrhosis. Biochemically, the onset of steatosis and hyperlipidemia represent the initial effects of ethanol on lipid metabolism. Profound changes in the concentration and composition of plasma lipids and

From: *Drug and Alcohol Abuse Reviews, Vol. 2: Liver Pathology and Alcohol*
Ed: R. R. Watson ©1991 The Humana Press Inc.

lipoproteins occur at each phase of alcohol-induced liver injury. Metabolic derangements in the liver and peripheral tissues resulting in the excessive accumulation of triglycerides are among the leading pathological manifestations of chronic alcohol abuse. Some of the abnormalities in lipid and lipoprotein metabolism both in the liver and peripheral tissues associated with various stages of chronic alcohol abuse are (a) moderate to excessive increases in plasma triglycerides, (b) defective metabolism of triglyceride-rich (TGR) lipoproteins, and (c) defective regulation of hepatic *de novo* lipid synthesis. The exact mechanism(s) underlying the ethanol-induced fatty liver are not completely understood in spite of intensive work in this area (for review, *see* refs. 4,5).

Plasma Lipoproteins

The plasma lipoproteins are water soluble macromolecules formed by complexing various lipids, such as cholesterol, triglycerides, and phospholipids with specific apoproteins. They facilitate the transport of the hydrophobic lipid molecules to various parts of the body in the aqueous environment of the blood. They are classified based on their particle size, hydrated density, and electrophoretic mobility. They are generally divided into five major classes, namely, chylomicrons, very low-density lipoproteins (VLDL), intermediate-density lipoproteins (IDL), low-density lipoproteins (LDL), and high-density lipoproteins (HDL).

Chylomicrons are the largest of these lipoproteins (mol wt, 100×10^6; density, 0.95 g/mL; electrophoretic mobility, origin). They are synthesized by the intestine to transport dietary triglycerides and cholesterol via the lymphatic route into systemic circulation. VLDL are the second largest (mol wt, 6×10^6; density, <1.006 g/mL; electrophoretic mobility, pre-Beta). They transport triglycerides and cholesterol of hepatic origin for redistribution to various tissues. IDL are generated from VLDL as a result of partial hydrolysis of their triglycerides by the action of lipoprotein lipase (mol wt, 3–4 $\times$ 10^6; density, 1.006–1.019 g/mL). Since triglycerides are the major component of chylomicrons, VLDL, and IDL, these lipoproteins are referred to as triglyceride-rich (TGR) lipoproteins. LDL are smaller than VLDL or IDL and are essentially the end products of VLDL catabolism at least in humans (mol wt, 2×10^6; density, 1.019–1.063 g/mL; electrophoretic mobility, Beta). High-density lipoproteins (HDL) are the smallest of the lipoproteins and are produced both by the liver and the intestine (mol wt,

Table 1
Major Plasma Apoproteins[a]

Apoproteins	Density class	Mol mass kDa	Origin	Carbohydrate residues
A-I	HDL	28	Liver, intestine	No?
A-II	HDL	18	Liver	No?
B-100	CM,VLDL,IDL,LDL	500	Liver, intestine	Yes
B-48	CM,VLDL,IDL	250	Intestine	Yes
C	CM,VLDL,HDL	10	Liver	Yes
E_{2-4}	CM,VLDL,HDL	34	Liver	Yes

[a]CM: Chylomicrons; VLDL: Very low-density lipoproteins; LDL: Low-density lipoproteins; IDL: Intermediate-density lipoproteins; HDL: High-density lipoproteins.

$0.2–0.4 \times 10^6$; density, 1.063–1.21; electrophoretic mobility, Alpha). HDL are involved in the reverse cholesterol transport from the peripheral tissues to the liver for excretion. They also serve as a reservoir for the exchange of apoproteins E and C with chylomicrons and VLDL. The various lipoproteins are in a dynamic state of synthesis and degradation, and their plasma and tissue levels are regulated by the relative contributions of these two metabolic processes. Details of the characteristics, metabolism, and metabolic roles of various lipoproteins in health and disease are beyond the scope of this chapter. Furthermore, excellent review articles already exist in this area.[6–8] Nonetheless, the present chapter will give an overview of the chemistry and metabolism of apolipoproteins, and then focus on the synthesis and metabolism of lipoproteins in relation to alcohol abuse.

Apolipoproteins

The major apolipoproteins of the various classes of lipoproteins and their origin and properties are listed in Table 1. Briefly, although intestinal chylomicrons, VLDL, and IDL contain both apo B-100 and apo B-48, the hepatic VLDL exclusively consists of apo B-100. The major apoproteins of HDL are apo A-I and apo A-II. In addition, all of these lipoproteins contain apo-C and apo-E. In contrast, LDL has exclusively apo B-100.

Apo B-100 has 4536 amino acids, whereas apo B-48 has 2152, which are closely related in their structures. Apo B-100 is synthesized from 14.1-kb mRNA, whereas apo B-48 is also synthesized from the same mRNA with an in-frame stop codon UAA at the nucleotide residue #6666 instead of the normal codon CAA.[9–12] This stop codon is not present in the genomic DNA, but is introduced by a novel RNA editing mechanism at the translational level so that both proteins are synthesized from the same gene. Both are required structural constituents for the secretion of triglyceride-rich lipoproteins from both liver and intestine. Apo B-100 has been proven to be atherogenic, whereas the evidence for the atherogenic property of apo B-48 is only indirect.[13]

Apo A-I is an activator of lecithin-cholesterol acyltransferase (LCAT) and apo A-II may be an activator of hepatic lipoprotein lipase.[14] Apo C-II is an activator of extrahepatic lipoprotein lipase.[15,16] Apo-E exists as three isoproteins, apo E_2, apo E_3, and apo E_4. Apo E_3 is considered as the normal isoprotein, apo E_2 is formed by substitution of cysteine for arginine at position #158, and apo E_4 is derived from apo E_3 by substitution of arginine for cysteine at position #112.[17] Human Type III hyperlipoproteinemia is characterized by increased plasma apo E_2, whereas apo E_4 is increased in patients with high LDL levels.[13,18,19]

Both apo B and apo E are glycoproteins.[6] Apo B-100 is composed of multiple subunits of mol wt 10,000 and has 8–10% of its mass as carbohydrate.[20] It contains mannose chains as well as other complex oligosaccharides consisting of *N*-acetylglucosamine, galactose, fucose, and sialic acid residues. Apo E is a basic protein of mol wt 34,000 and is primarily synthesized by the liver, although a number of other tissues also synthesize it, albeit in smaller amounts.[21–25] It is synthesized with an 18 amino acid signal peptide, which is cotranslationally cleaved[26] and then glycosylated.[27] The protein is secreted in highly sialylated form,[26,28] but 80% of it exists in asialo form in the plasma, presumably because of postsecretory desialylation. This implies that glycosylation may play a significant role in cellular processing of apo E. Among the known functions of carbohydrate moieties of glycoproteins are: (a) maintenance of physicochemical properties of the molecule; (b) proteolytic processing and stabilization against proteolysis; and (c) mediation of biological activity.[5] As a ligand for the LDL receptor, apo E directs the delivery of triglycerides and cholesterol from lipoproteins to cells. As a component of HDL, apo E may also play a role in the efflux of cholesterol from cells (reverse cholesterol transport). Apoprotein A-I, the major protein of HDL, is synthesized by the liver and the intestine. It is a single polypeptide with a mol wt of 28,000 and does not have any carbohydrate residues. Besides being the structural backbone of HDL to carry the lipids and possibly function in reverse cholesterol transport, the other major function of apo A-I is to serve as a cofactor in the activation of LCAT activity. Increased plasma apo A-I concentration correlates negatively with the incidence of heart disease. Apoprotein A-II is the second major apoprotein of HDL. It exists as a dimer with a mol wt of 17,400 and also lacks any carbohydrate residues. Apo A-II may play a role as a cofactor in the action of hepatic lipoprotein lipase.

Current Trends in the Metabolism of TGR-Lipoproteins

In view of the fact that TGR lipoproteins are significantly altered as a result of alcohol abuse, a summary of current trends in TGR lipoprotein metabolism is depicted in Fig. 1. Dietary triglycerides and cholesterol emerge as lymph chylomicrons after intestinal absorption. At this stage, they contain predominantly apoprotein (apo) B with some apo E and apo A. Once they enter the systemic circulation, lymph chylomicrons acquire a net transfer of apo E and apo C from the circulating HDL_2 resulting in the formation of native chylomicrons and HDL_3. The catabolism of circulating chylomicrons takes place in two phases.[29-32] In the first phase, extrahepatic lipoprotein lipases (LPL) are activated by the apo C-II component of chylomicrons. The active LPL partially hydrolyze the triglyceride moiety of chylomicrons to yield chylomicron remnants. The remnants are depleted of triglyceride, phospholipids, and apo C, and enriched with cholesterol and apo E.[32,33] At the same time, phospholipids and apo C are transferred back to HDL_3 to regenerate HDL_2.[34] In the second phase, the remnants are rapidly taken up by the liver via a high affinity receptor mediated process.[29,30,35-40] Apoproteins E are involved in the recognition and uptake of the remnants by the liver, whereas apo C proteins are inhibitory to this process.[41-46] Subsequent metabolism of the remnants inside the liver leads to the feedback inhibition of hepatic lipid synthesis. The metabolism of VLDL follows an identical pathway to that of chylomicrons.

Receptor-Mediated Uptake of TGR-Lipoproteins by the Liver

The classical work of Brown and Goldstein[47,48] established the role of LDL receptors in the uptake and regulation of cholesterol metabolism in the human fibroblast system. The apoprotein B-100, which is the major

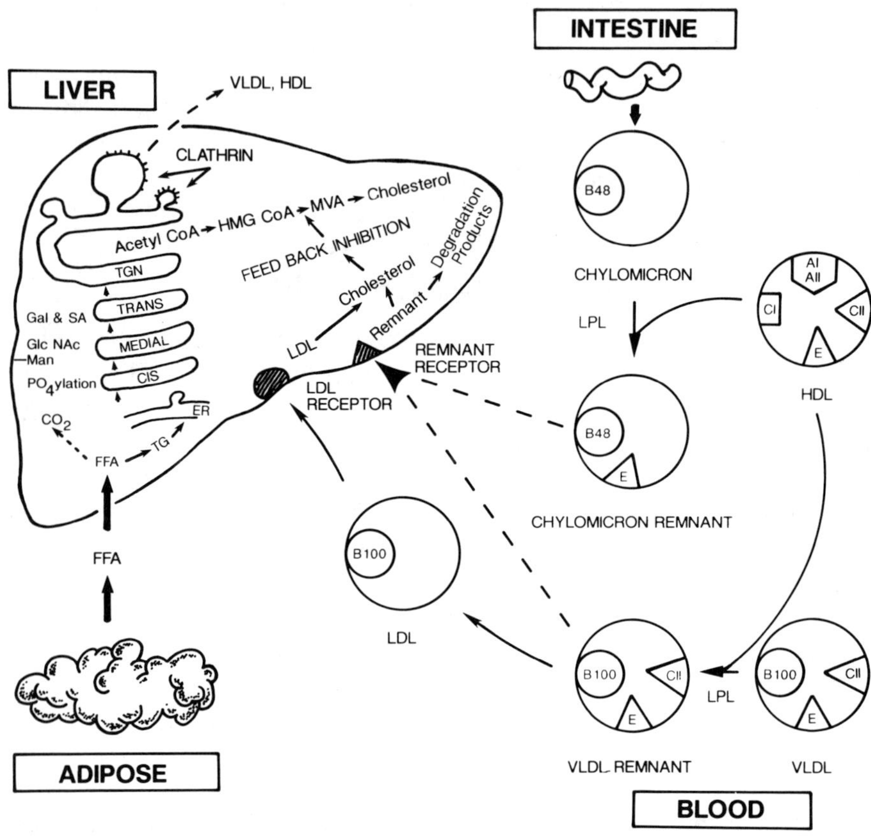

Fig. 1. Schematic overview of the current concepts in lipoprotein metabolism, their regulatory roles, and possible causes of alcoholic fatty liver. In this figure, "bold arrows" represent the metabolic pathways that are known to be stimulated by ethanol; "broken arrows" represent the ones that are inhibited by ethanol; and "thin arrows" represent those that are unaffected by ethanol. Abbreviations used are: B100, apo B-100; B48, apo B-48; AI, apo AI, AII, apo AII; CI, apo CI; CII, apo CII; E, apo E; LPL, lipoprotein lipase; ER, endoplasmic reticulum; TGN, *trans* Golgi Network; *Cis, Medial, Trans,* components of Golgi Apparatus; Gal, galactose; SA, sialic acid; Glc NAc, *N*-acetylglucosamine; Man, Mannose; PO4ylation, Phosphorylation; FFA, Free-fatty acids; HMG-CoA, 3-hydroxy 3-methylglutaryl Coenzyme A; MVA, mevalonic acid.

component of LDL and VLDL, is responsible for the interaction with these receptors, whereas apoprotein B-48, which is characteristic of chylomicrons does not interact.[49,50] However, apo E containing proteins, such as cholesterol-rich HDL (HDL$_c$), interact with these receptors. Therefore they are designated as apo B,E-receptors (LDL-receptors). These receptors of the liver are markedly induced after cholestyramine[51,52] or α-ethinyl estradiol[53] treatment. Apart from these LDL receptors, another class of high affinity receptors specific for apo E containing proteins has been described in the liver.[51,52] These are very likely the chylomicron remnant receptors. Thus, the metabolic fate of chylomicron remnants depends on their apo E content, whereas that of VLDL remnants depends on both apo B and apo E contents. The extent of remnant uptake and metabolism will also depend on the number and nature of apo B and apo E receptors on the hepatocyte membrane.

TGR-Lipoprotein Synthesis, Assembly, Transport, and Secretion

The intestine and the liver are the major sites for the synthesis of various apoproteins, the lipid components, and their assembly to form the TGR-lipoproteins. The enzymes responsible for the synthesis of triglycerides, cholesterol, and phospholipids are localized in the smooth endoplasmic reticulum (SER). Presumably, the newly synthesized lipid molecules are transported into the tubular channels of SER. Whether the assembly of the lipids and the newly synthesized apoproteins occurs at the junction of SER and the rough endoplasmic reticulum (RER) or in the Golgi is debatable. The *N*-glycosylation of the proteins occurs in the microsomes, whereas the *O*-glycosylation occurs in the Golgi apparatus. The smooth surfaced secretory vesicles containing the newly formed TGR-lipoprotein are secreted into the circulation by exocytosis. Excellent review articles[54,55] exist for the details of the structure and function of Golgi complex. As summarized in Fig. 1, the Golgi complex is a series of membrane compartments through which proteins destined for plasma membrane, vesicles, and lysosomes move sequentially. The Golgi stack consists of three functionally and compositionally distinct compartments that operate in succession to construct the oligosaccharide chains on the growing lipoprotein. The lipoproteins enter the Golgi stack at the *cis* (entry) face and exit at the *trans* (exit face).

The *cis* cisternae of the Golgi stack seems to be responsible for the phosphorylation of certain proteins, such as the lysosomal enzymes, and also for the proteolytic processing of proteins whenever required. The addition of *N*-acetyl glucosamine and removal of some of the mannose residues take place at the *medial* cisternae. Finally, the addition of galactose and sialic acid residues occurs at the *trans* cisternae. These are then sorted into different vesicles in the last Golgi compartment called *trans* Golgi network (TGN). Since chronic ethanol abuse alters membrane structure and function, it is possible that ethanol abuse could affect any of the aforementioned biosynthetic steps.

Intestine

Ethanol is known to produce pathological changes in intestinal structure and function, and to cause disturbances, such as diarrhea and malabsorption.[56,57] During ethanol ingestion the upper gastrointestinal tract is exposed to ethanol concentrations several times higher than that attained in other tissues. Ethanol can be entero-toxic whether ingested acutely or after chronic intake. Lieber's group[58,59] has shown that ethanol causes hemorrhagic erosions of the small intestinal villi accompanied by biochemical alterations, such as decreases in several intestinal enzyme activities. Several investigators[59–62] have shown that an acute dose of ethanol inhibits palmitate and acetate oxidation, whereas it increases esterification of available fatty acids to triglycerides. In contrast, chronic ethanol treatment causes increased fatty acid oxidation and triglyceride synthesis.

Liver

Ethanol is known to stimulate hepatic VLDL production after acute[63] as well as chronic intake.[64] However, ethanol markedly inhibits VLDL synthesis in the isolated hepatocyte system,[63] indicating that its stimulatory effect found in vivo is a complex process. The mechanism of ethanol action has been claimed to be the result of one or more of the following causes: (a) increased mobilization of fatty acids from the adipose tissue to the liver,[65–68] (b) decreased oxidation of fatty acids in the liver,[69,70] (c) increased esterification of the fatty acids in the liver,[71,72] and (d) impaired release of triglycerides by the liver.[73] There are conflicting reports regarding these various possibilities. Thus, ethanol has been shown to have no effect,[74,75] to increase[76] or to decrease[77] plasma free-fatty acids. Subsequent studies have shown an initial fall followed by a secondary rise in plasma free-fatty acids.[78]

Our recent studies[79] showed that the acute ethanol-mediated stimulation of hepatic VLDL synthesis is abolished in thyroidectomized rats. We further showed that thyroidectomy prevented the ethanol-mediated stimulation of (a) fatty acid mobilization from the adipose tissue and (b) hepatic esterification of free-fatty acids to neutral lipids. These results imply that thyroid hormones may play a permissive role in ethanol-mediated mobilization of fat. Thyroid hormones are known to amplify the catecholamine-mediated mobilization of depot fat. Subsequently, we also showed[80] that although chronic ethanol did not significantly affect the hepatic protein synthetic rate, leucine incorporation into the secretory protein fraction of the liver perfusate was inhibited by 36% ($p < 0.01$) in the ethanol-fed group. Specifically, the secretory rates of VLDL, apo A-I, apo E, and transferrin were inhibited by about 50%. In contrast, moderate ethanol feeding for 6 wk did not alter any of the aforementioned parameters. Thus, impaired secretion of VLDL and HDL could be the major cause for fatty liver after alcohol abuse. In order to explore whether this inhibitory effect of ethanol was owing to defective glycosylation of this glycoprotein, we have determined the effects of chronic ethanol on the synthesis, glycosylation, and secretion of apo E in vivo in the rat. The results showed a 45% decrease in mannose incorporation into hepatic apo E in the alcoholic group ($p < 0.0005$), whereas that of leucine was unaffected. A similar pattern was observed in the microsomal and Golgi fractions. Table 2 shows the mannose/leucine incorporation ratios of the precursors into the immunoprecipitable apo E in the liver, microsomes, and the Golgi fractions. The incorporation ratios also reflected the decreased glycosylation pattern (55%, $p < 0.05$) at the whole liver and microsomal level in the ethanol group. Thus, we conclude that it might be the under-glycosylation of apo E and not its synthesis that leads to its decreased hepatic secretion as a result of chronic ethanol feeding. Significantly, supplementation of fish oil (rich in ω-3 fatty acids) in the diet partially protected against these deleterious effects of ethanol. We have previously shown that the fish oil diet partially prevented the hyperlipidemic effects of chronic ethanol.[81]

Based on all the aforementioned studies, the mechanism of action of ethanol on TGR-lipoprotein synthesis and secretion can be summarized as follows:

1. Ethanol may increase the pool of incoming fatty acids to the liver by stimulating the mobilization of adipose fat possibly by promoting the release of catecholamines and thyroid hormones.

Table 2
Ratio of [3]H Mannose/[14]C Leucine Incorporation into Apo E of Liver, Microsomes,
and Golgi Apparatus of Rats Fed Chronic Ethanol and Fish Oil Diets

	[3]H/[14]C Ratio of apo E		
Groups	Liver	Microsomes	Golgi
CN	10.88 ± 1.27[a]	10.62 ± 1.29[a]	9.12 ± 1.34[a,b]
AN	5.05 ± 0.93[b]	4.76 ± 0 25[c]	5.37 ± 0.96[b]
CF	10.49 ± 1.05[a]	9.12 ± 0.56[a,b]	11.10 ± 1.83[a]
AF	7.54 ± 0.97[a,b]	5.96 ± 0.47[b,c]	5.49 ± 1.11[a,b]

Each rat was intraportally injected with a single dose of [U-^{14}C] leucine (0.2 µCi/g body wt) and/or [2-^{3}H] mannose (1.0 µCi/g body wt) and killed after 30 min. The incorporation of the precursors into the immunoprecipitable apo E was measured in the liver, microsomes, and the Golgi fractions. Values are mean ± SE from six rats in each group except in AF, where the number of animals is four. The statistical significance of each value of ethanol group is compared with the values in corresponding control group and crosscompared with the values in fish oil fed rats, using Tukey Contrasts method. Groups differing in superscripts are significantly different at $p < 0.05$ level.

2. As a result of hepatic mitochondrial injury, fatty acid oxidation is also inhibited.
3. At the same time hepatic esterification of fatty acids to triglycerides is enhanced.
4. Although acute ethanol stimulates the synthesis of apoprotein B for VLDL formation and secretion, chronic ethanol abuse inhibits VLDL synthesis and secretion. It may also affect the glycosylation, subsequent packaging of nascent VLDL, and the formation of secretory vesicles.
5. Finally, chronic ethanol abuse also disrupts the microtubular system, an obligatory step in the exocytosis of secretory proteins.

Extrahepatic and Hepatic Metabolism of TGR-Lipoproteins and Their Regulatory Role

Apart from its effects on the lipoprotein synthesis, alcohol abuse may also affect the subsequent metabolism and regulatory properties of the TGR-lipoproteins. In an attempt to resolve some of these issues, our laboratory has been elucidating the effects of chronic ethanol administration on the extrahepatic and hepatic metabolism of TGR-lipoproteins. Using lymph chylomicrons and VLDL labeled in their triglyceride, apoprotein, and cholesterol ester moieties we have looked at their catabolism both in vivo and

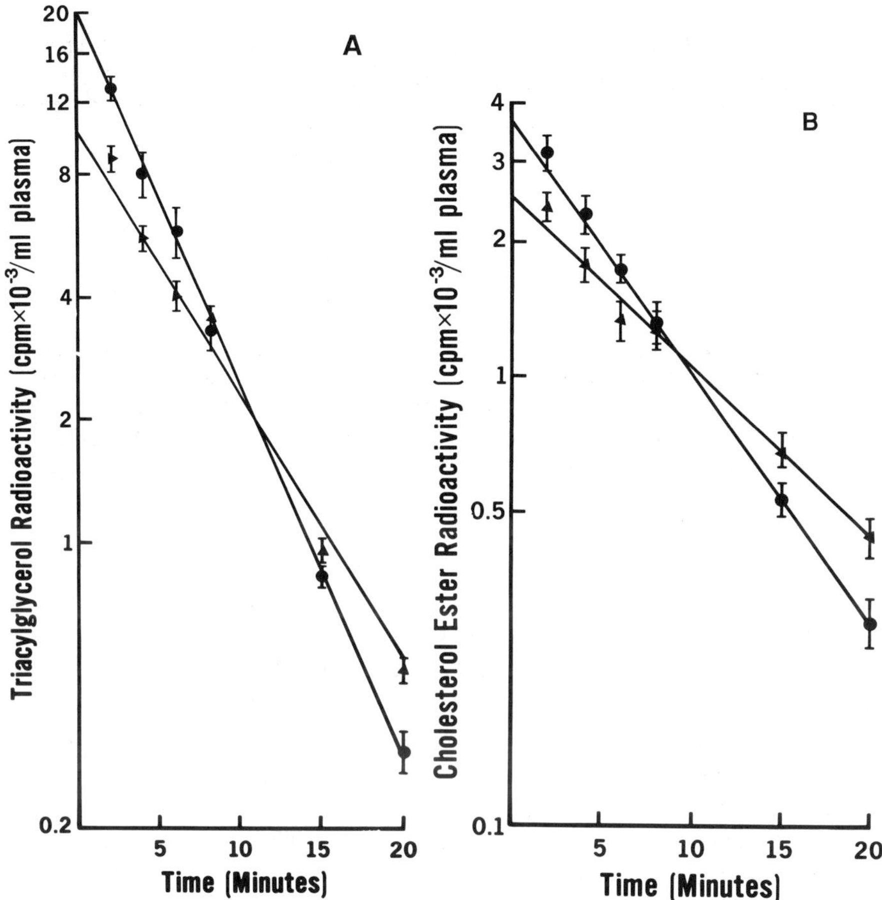

Fig. 2. Plasma turnover of [^{14}C]triglyceride (**A**) and [^{3}H]cholesterol ester (**B**) moieties of rat lymph chylomicrons in control and chronic ethanol-fed rats. The results are expressed as the amount of the radioactivity of the respective components remaining in the plasma compartment as a function of time. Each value is the mean ± SE of three independent determinations (●—●: Control and ▲—▲: Ethanol). The best fit lines were statistically computed by linear regression analysis (for details *see* ref. 82).

in the perfused heart system.[82,83] For example, based on the exponential decay curves for each moiety of lymph chylomicrons (Fig. 2), it has been found that chronic ethanol inhibited the catabolism of the triglyceride moiety of chylomicrons by 30%, whereas that of the cholesterol moiety was inhibited by 67%.[82] Similar results were observed for the catabolism of

Table 3

Effect of Chylomicron Remnants from Control and Chronic Ethanol-Fed Animals upon
Cholesterol Synthetic Rate in Isolated Hepatocytes from Normal Meal-Fed Rats[a]

Remnant type	Concentration in incubation medium, µg cholesterol/mL	Cholesterol synthetic rate, %	p
Control	73 ± 4.8	80 ± 3	<0.05
	145 ± 10.5	58 ± 6	
Ethanol	85 ± 7	95 ± 4	<0.05
	170 ± 15	87 ± 6	

[a]Rat lymph chylomicron remnants were isolated from supradiaphragmatic control and chronic ethanol-fed animals and their effect on hepatic cholesterol synthetic rate was determined. The results are expressed as % of synthetic activity observed in the absence of the remnant fraction. Each value is the mean ± SE for four independent respective remnant preparations.

VLDL.[83] Since the catabolism of the triglyceride moiety takes place essentially in the extrahepatic tissues, whereas that of the cholesterol moiety occurs in the liver, it is concluded that chronic ethanol abuse has a greater inhibitory effect on the catabolism of TGR-lipoproteins in the liver than in the extrahepatic tissues. Furthermore, we have found that chronic ethanol feeding leads to the plasma accumulation of abnormal remnants that are not as efficient as the normal remnants in the feedback regulation of *de novo* hepatic lipid synthesis (Table 3). In addition, the hepatocytes from chronic ethanol-fed animals exhibit defective feedback regulation of cholesterol synthesis by normal remnants (Table 4). We have extended these studies to show[84] that chronic ethanol significantly decreases the specific binding affinity of the hepatocytes for the remnants by 29% (Fig. 3), whereas their internalization is inhibited by 19% Also, chronic ethanol inhibits the catabolism of both triglyceride and cholesterol moieties of the remnants by 58 and 44%, respectively (Table 5). Thus, the net result of all these abnormalities is a delayed clearance of TGR-lipoproteins from circulation and their impaired catabolism by the liver.

Possible Mechanisms
of Accumulation of Hepatic Lipids

The development of fatty liver as a result of ethanol exposure may be a result of increased input into the liver of dietary lipids and depot fat as

Table 4

Effect of Chylomicron Remnants on Cholesterol Synthetic Rate
in Hepatocytes from Rats on Chronic Ethanol or Control Liquid Diet[a]

Remnant concentration,	Cholesterol synthetic rate, %		
µg cholesterol/mL	Ethanol group	Control group	p
0	100	100	
98	86 ± 5	72 ± 4	<0.1
196	69 ± 4	47 ± 6	<0.05

[a]Hepatocytes were isolated from control and chronic ethanol-fed animals and their cholesterol synthetic rates determined in the presence of indicated concentrations of normal chylomicron remnants. Each value is the mean $\pm$ SE for four independent respective hepatocyte preparations.

well as increased hepatic lipid synthesis. On the other hand, this may be the result of decreased disposal of the lipids from the liver because of defective (a) lipolysis, oxidation, and/or ketogenesis and (b) export as lipoproteins. The possible sites of action of ethanol on lipid and lipoprotein metabolism are also illustrated in Fig. 1.

Dietary Contribution

The accumulation of fat in the liver as a result of acute or chronic ethanol consumption is exacerbated by dietary fat. This accumulation of fat occurs in spite of lesser gain in body weight in the alcohol group compared to the pair-fed control group. Significantly, the manifestation of fatty liver persists even when adequate amounts of essential fatty acids are provided in the diet. However, it was reported that the supplementation of arachidonic acid in the diet prevented to some extent the accumulation of fat in the liver when the animals were fed *ad libitum*,[85] but not when they were pair-fed.[86] Ethanol exposure is known to inhibit the hepatic desaturase system, resulting in decreased formation of arachidonate from linoleate.[87–89] A more careful study[90] revealed that arachidonic supplementation even in *ad libitum* fed rats failed to prevent the fatty liver induced by chronic ethanol feeding. Our own studies[81] showed that a fish oil diet (rich in ϖ-3 fatty acids), but not a corn oil diet (rich in ϖ-6 fatty acids), was able to prevent hepatic steatosis partially. Thus, dietary fat plays an important role in the pathogenesis of ethanol-induced fatty liver.

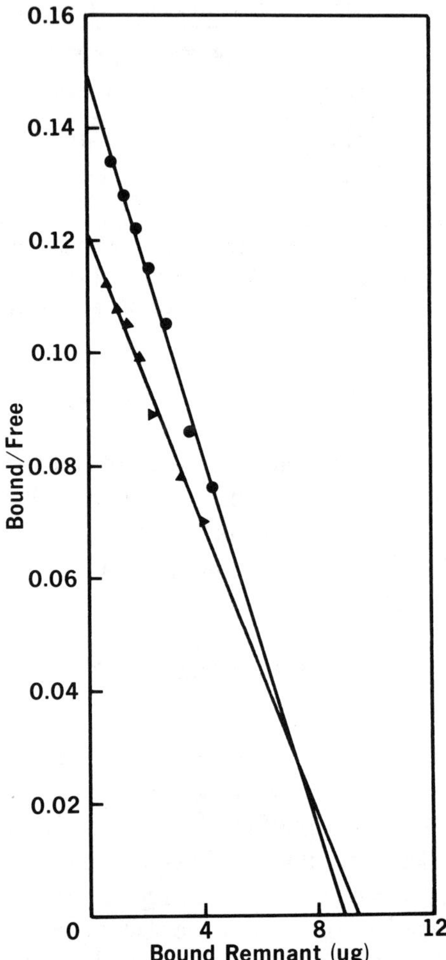

Fig. 3. Scatchard analysis of the data on specific binding of chylomicron remnants to hepatocytes from control and chronic ethanol-fed rats. Specific binding of [³H]retinyl ester labeled chylomicron remnants to hepatocytes from control (●—●) and chronic ethanol-fed (▲—▲) rats was determined and the best fit lines for Scatchard plots were statistically computed by linear regression analysis (for details *see* ref. 84).

Table 5
Catabolism of the Lipid Moieties of Remnants
by Hepatocytes from Control and Chronic Ethanol-Fed Rats[a]

| | $^{14}CO_2$ Produced owing to specific interaction | | | |
| | % Of label added | | % | |
Remnants labeled with	Control	Ethanol	Inhibition	*p*
Triacylglycerol[1-^{14}C]oleate	15.2 ± 0.72	6.3 ± 1.06	58	<0.001
Cholesterol[1-^{14}C]oleate	0.98 ± 0.29	0.55 ± 0.2	44	<0.01

[a]Five independent hepatocyte preparations (115 mg wet wt) from both chronic and control ethanol-fed rats were incubated with ~112 µg cholesterol equivalent of chylomicron remnants labeled in the indicated lipid moieties (20,340 dpm in triacylglycerol[1-^{14}C]oleate or 122,065 dpm in cholesterol [1-^{14}C]oleate) in 2 mL final volume for 90 min at 37°C both in the absence and presence of excess cold remnants, and the liberated $^{14}CO_2$ radioactivity was measured. The $^{14}CO_2$ liberated because of specific interaction is expressed as % of the total labeled remnant added to the incubation mixture. Each value is the mean ± SE.

Depot Fat

Ethanol-mediated fatty liver is characterized by the appearance of liver fatty acids closely resembling the adipose tissue fatty acids after acute intake,[65] whereas they resemble the dietary fatty acids after chronic ethanol ingestion.[91] However, a moderate single dose of ethanol (0.5–1.0 g/kg) tends to have an inhibitory effect on plasma free-fatty acid concentrations[77] and their turnover,[92] which presumably is mediated through acetate,[93] the hepatic oxidation product of ethanol.

Liver

Ethanol also increases the uptake of fatty acids by the liver.[94] Hepatic *de novo* fatty acid synthesis has been shown to be unaffected by acute or chronic ethanol exposure.[95–99] Hepatic esterification of fatty acids to triglycerides and phospholipids is markedly enhanced.[70,73] Because of the increased NAD/NADH ratio caused by ethanol oxidation a concomitant increase in hepatic α-glycerophosphate occurs.[74] Furthermore, acyltransferases including L-α glycerophosphate acyltransferase, involved in phospholipid synthesis, are stimulated.[71-73] At the same time, hepatic fatty acid oxidation is significantly inhibited by ethanol.[69,70,101,102] Thus, increased flux of dietary and depot fatty acids coupled with their increased esterification and decreased oxidation accounts for the accumulation of fat in the liver. Acute or chronic ethanol exposure does not significantly affect the hepatic *de novo* cholesterol synthesis.[103] However, hepatic degradation of cholesterol to bile acids is markedly depressed as a result of decreased activity of cholesterol 7α-hydroxylase, the rate limiting enzyme of this pathway.[103,104] This would explain the accumulation of cholesterol in the liver.

Alcoholic Fatty Liver and Fibrosis

The amount and the type of fat seem to play important roles in the development of alcoholic liver disease. Thus, diets high in linoleic acid promote the pathogenesis of alcoholic liver disease.[105] More recent studies by French and his coworkers[106] have shown that the greatest degree of fatty infiltration and subsequent development of necrosis, inflammation, and fibrosis was observed in the rats maintained on a high-fat, low-protein diet. In chronic alcoholic liver disease, the degree of fibrosis was inversely proportional to the amount of fat in the liver.[107] Current concepts[108] seem to support the view that the liver perisinusoidal cells, which are also known as stellate cells, become transformed into myofibroblasts as a result of alcohol abuse. These myofibroblasts actively synthesize collagen and proliferate into the adjoining parenchymal cells, and thereby lead to their necrosis. Thus, the fibrotic process continues until all the parenchymal cells are engulfed resulting in liver cirrhosis and total hepatic failure.

Ethanol, HDL, and Coronary Heart Disease (CHD)

Numerous cross-sectional and intervention studies have documented an increase in plasma high-density lipoprotein cholesterol (HDL_c) concentration as a result of chronic moderate ethanol consumption.[109–113] Correcting for smoking as another major risk factor, it has been found that a strong negative correlation still exists between moderate alcohol consumption and the incidence of CHD.[114–117] If it is true that the consumption of moderate amounts of ethanol protects against the development of CHD, then it would be very important to establish (a) which subfractions of HDL cholesterol are increased by alcohol consumption and (b) whether apo A-I and apo A-II, the major protein components of HDL, are also increased by alcohol consumption. There are conflicting reports[118–120] with regard to whether HDL_2 or HDL_3 cholesterol fraction is increased after alcohol intake. It is well known that it is HDL_2 that is positively correlated with the protective effects of HDL against CHD. It seems that relatively moderate doses tend to increase the HDL_3 subfraction, whereas large doses increased both the subfractions.[121] However, in severe alcohol-induced liver diseases the HDL fraction is markedly decreased.[122] On the other hand, plasma apo A-I and apo A-II increase in response to moderate alcohol consumption. Apo A-I is the activator of LCAT and, by virtue of increasing the cholesterol esterification, is beneficial in removing the cholesterol from peripheral tissues back to the liver for degradation and excretion.

Summary

Ethanol is a hepatotoxin. Total hepatic failure and death occur as a result of prolonged alcohol abuse. This pathogenic process manifests initially as fatty liver, which then develops into alcoholic liver disease. At some point, because of unknown reasons, the fibrotic process sets in as a result of the activation and transformation of stellate cells of the liver sinusoids into myofibroblasts. This leads to the necrosis of the liver parenchymal cells and hepatic failure. Alcohol-induced fatty liver is characterized by abnormal increases in lipids and lipoproteins in the liver and plasma. By serving as a preferential energy source to the fat in the diet, ethanol promotes lipid accumulation. Therefore the amount and the type of fat in the diet markedly affect the extent of fatty liver and hyperlipemia. Thus, diets rich in linoleic acid promote ethanol-induced fatty liver, whereas those rich in ϖ-3 fatty acids partially counteract the hyperlipidemic effects of ethanol. Furthermore, ethanol inhibits the endogenous oxidation of the fatty acids while enhancing their esterification. Part of the accumulated lipids is secreted out of the liver as lipoproteins leading to moderate hyperlipemia, which is accentuated in individuals with Type IV or Type V hyperlipidemia. Similarly, ethanol inhibits the hepatic degradation of cholesterol to bile acids without significantly affecting cholesterol synthesis. Our current work shows that one of the major effects of alcohol abuse is to cause an impaired hepatic secretion of triglyceride-rich lipoproteins. This seems to be caused by the defective glycosylation of apo E and possibly apo B. In addition, the extrahepatic and hepatic catabolism of these TGR lipoproteins is also impaired leading to the persistence of abnormal TGR lipoprotein particles in circulation. The inverse correlation between alcohol consumption and coronary heart disease is questionable and further studies are necessary to delineate the mechanism of action of ethanol consumption in altering the HDL subclasses.

Future Directions

In spite of considerable information on alcohol abuse and liver disease, many unresolved questions remain to be unraveled in order to delineate the mechanism of action of ethanol in causing abnormal lipoprotein metabolism and the subsequent transformation of the fatty liver to become fibrotic and cirrhotic. Some of these key questions are:

1. What is the exact step that is responsible for the defective glycosylation of apoproteins B and E, the key apoproteins of TGR lipoproteins?
2. Is this defect at the transcription or the posttranscriptional level?
3. If the defect is at the posttranscriptional level, what are the roles of Golgi and microsomes in contributing to this defect?
4. How does this defect affect the further metabolism and regulatory roles of these important apoproteins and their constituent lipid conjugates?
5. Is the deposition of lipids into parenchymal cells a prerequisite for them to undergo necrosis as a result of invasion by myofibroblasts?
6. What are the factors that trigger transformation of fat-storing stellate cells into myofibroblasts?
7. Is there a link between the proliferation of stellate cells and the susceptibility of fatty parenchymal cells to this process of fibrogenesis?

Intensive efforts from investigators around the world should see a burst of activities leading to our understanding of the pathogenesis of alcoholic fibrosis and cirrhosis.

References

[1] U. Harinasuta and H. J. Zimmerman (1971) Alcoholic steatonecrosis: Relationship between severity of hepatic disease and presence of Mallory bodies in the liver. *Gastroenterolgy* **60,** 1036–1046.

[2] J. T. Galambos (1972) Alcoholic hepatitis: Its therapy and prognosis, in *Progress in Liver Diseases*. H. Popper and F. Schaffner, eds. Grune & Stratton, New York, pp. 567–588.

[3] R. D. Hawkins and H. Kalant (1972) The metabolism of ethanol and its metabolic effects. *Pharmacol. Rev.* **24,** 67–157.

[4] E. Baraona and C. S. Lieber (1979) Effects of alcohol on lipid metabolism. *J. Lipid Res.* **20,** 289–306.

[5] C. S. Lieber and M. Savolainen (1979) Ethanol and lipids. *Alcohol. Clin. Exp. Res.* **8,** 409–423.

[6] R. W. Mahley, T. L. Innerarity, S. C. Rall, and K. H. Weisgraber (1984) Plasma lipoproteins; apolipoprotein structure and function. *J. Lipid Res.* **25,** 1277–1294.

[7] R. J. Havel (1988) Lowering cholesterol: Rationale, mechanisms, and means. *J. Clin. Invest.* **81,** 1653–1660.

[8] H. B. Brewer, R. E. Gregg, J. M. Hoeg, and S. F. Silvia (1988) Apolipoproteins and lipoproteins in human plasma: An overview. *Clin. Chem.* **34,** B4–B8.

[9] K. Higuchi, A. V. Hospattankar, S. W. Law, N. Meglin, J. Cortright, and H. B. Brewer (1988) Human apolipoprotein B (apoB) MRNA: Identification of two distinct apoB MRNAs, an MRNA with the apoB-100 sequence and an apoB MRNA containing a premature in-frame translational stop codon in both liver and intestine. *Proc. Natl. Acad. Sci. USA* **85,** 1772–1776.

[10] A. V. Hospattankar, K. Higuchi, S. W. Law, N. Meglin, and H. B. Brewer (1987) Identification of a novel in-frame translational stop codon in human intestinal apoB MRNA. *Biochem. Biophys. Res. Commun.* **148,** 279–285.

[11] S. H. Chen, G. Habib, C. Y. Yang, Z. W. Gu, B. R. Lee, S. A. Weng, S. R. Silberman, S. J. Cai, J. P. Deslypere, M. Rosseneu, A. M. Gotto, Jr., W. H. Li, and L. Chan (1987) Apolipoprotein B-48 is the product of a messenger RNA with an organ-specific in frame stop codon. *Science* **238,** 363–366.

[12] L. W. Powell, S. C. Wallis, R. J. Pease, Y. H. Edwards, T. J. Knott, and J. Scott (1987) A novel form of tissue-specific RNA processing produces apolipoprotein B-48 in intestine. *Cell* **50,** 831–840.

[13] J. Davignon, R. E. Gregg, and C. F. Sing (1988) Apolipoprotein E polymorphism and atherosclerosis. *Arteriosclerosis* **8,** 1–12.

[14] C. J. Fielding, V. G. Shore, and P. E. Fielding (1972) A protein cofactor of lecithin:cholesterol acyltransferase. *Biochem. Biophys. Res. Commun.* **298,** 1265–1273.

[15] J. C. LaRosa, R. I. Levy, P. Herbert, S. E. Lux, and D. S. Fredrickson (1970) A specific apoprotein activator for lipoprotein lipase. *Biochem. Biophys. Res. Commun.* **41,** 57–62.

[16] R. J. Havel, B. Shore, and D. M. Bier (1970) Role of specific glycopeptides of human serum lipoproteins in the activation of lipoprotein lipase. *Circ. Res.* **27,** 595–600.

[17] K. H. Weisgraber, S. C. Rall, and R. W. Mahley (1981) Human E apoprotein heterogeneity: Cysteine-arginine interchanges in the amino acid sequence of the apoE isoforms. *J. Biol. Chem.* **256,** 9077–9083.

[18] R. J. Havel, Y. S. Chao, E. E. Windler, L. Kolite, and L. S. S. Guo (1981) Isoprotein specificity in the hepatic uptake of apolipoprotein E and the patho-

genesis of familial dysbetalipoproteinemia. *Proc. Natl. Acad. Sci. USA* **77,** 4349–4353.

[19] R. E. Gregg, L. A. Zech, E. J. Schaefer, and H. B. Brewer (1981) Type III hyperlipoproteinemia: Defective metabolism of an abnormal apoprotein E. *Science* **211,** 584–586.

[20] P. Lee and W. C. Breckenridge (1976) The carbohydrate composition of human apo low density lipoprotein from normal and type II hyperlipoproteinemic subjects. *Can. J. Biochem.* **54,** 42–49.

[21] M. L. Blue, D. L. Williams, S. Zucker, S. A. Khan, and C. Blum (1983) Apolipoprotein E synthesis in human kidney, adrenal gland and liver. *Proc. Natl. Acad. Sci. USA* **80,** 283–287.

[22] N. A. Elshowerbagy, W. S. Liao, R. W. Mahley, and J. M. Taylor (1985) Apolipoprotein E MRNA is abundant in the brain and adrenals, as well as in the liver, and is present in other peripheral tissues of rats and marmasets. *Proc. Natl. Acad. Sci. USA* **82,** 203–207.

[23] T. C. Newman, P. A. Dawson, L. L. Rudel, and D. L. Williams (1985) Quantitation of apolipoprotein E MRNA in th liver and peripheral tissues of nonhuman primates. *J. Biol. Chem.* **260,** 2452–2457.

[24] S. H. Basu, Y. K. Ho, M. S. Brown, D. W. Bilheimer, R. G. W. Anderson, and J. L. Goldstein (1982) Biochemical and genetic studies of the apolipoprotein E secreted by mouse macrophages and monocytes. *J. Biol. Chem.* **257,** 9788–9795.

[25] J. K. Boyles, R. E. Pitas, E. Wilson, R. W. Mahley, and J. M. Taylor (1986) Apolipoprotein E associated with astrocytic glia of the central nervous system and with nonmyelinating glia of the peripheral nervous system. *J. Clin. Invest.* **76,** 1501.

[26] V. I. Zannis, J. McPherson, G. Goldberger, S. K. Karathanisis, and J. L. Breslow (1984) Synthesis, intracellular processing, and signal peptide of human apolipoprotein E. *J. Biol. Chem.* **259,** 5495–5499.

[27] M. E. Wernette-Hammond, S. J. Lauer, A. Corsini, D. Walker, J. M. Jaylor, and S. C. Rall, Jr. (1989) Glycosylation of human Apolipoprotein E. *J. Biol. Chem.* **264,** 9094–9101.

[28] V. I. Zannis, D. M. Kurnit, and J. L. Breslow (1982) Hepatic apoA-1 and apoE and intestinal apoA-1 are synthesized in precursor isoprotein forms by organ cultures of human fetal tissues. *J. Biol. Chem.* **257,** 536–544.

[29] T. G. Redgrave (1970) Formation of cholesteryl ester-rich particulate lipid during metabolism of chylomicrons. *J. Clin. Invest.* **49,** 465–471.

[30] E. N. Bergman, R. J. Havel, B. M. Wolfe, and T. Bohmer (1971) Quantitative studies of the metabolism of chylomicron triglycerides and cholesterol by liver and extrahepatic tissues of sheep and dogs. *J. Clin. Invest.* **50,** 1831–1839.

[31] O. D. Mjos, O. Faergeman, R. L. Hamilton, and R. J. Havel (1975) Characterization of remnants produced during the metabolism of triglyceride-rich

lipoproteins of blood plasma and intestinal lymph in the rat. *J. Clin. Invest.* **56,** 603–615.

[32] R. J. Havel (1978) Origin of HDL, in *High Density Lipoproteins and Atherosclerosis.* A. M. Gotto, N. E. Miller, and M. F. Oliver, eds. Elsevier, Amsterdam, pp. 21–25.

[33] T. Chajek and S. Eisenberg (1978) Very low density lipoprotein metabolism. Metabolism of phospholipid, cholesterol and apolipoprotein C in the isolated perfused rat heart. *J. Clin. Invest.* **61,** 1654–1665.

[34] J. R. Patsch, A. M. Gotto, T. Olivercrona, and S. Eisenberg (1978) Formation of high density lipoprotein-2-like particles during lipolysis of very low density lipoproteins in vitro. *Proc. Natl. Acad. Sci. USA* **75,** 4519–4523.

[35] D. S. Goodman (1962) The metabolism of chylomicron ester in the rat. *J. Clin. Invest.* **41,** 1886–1896.

[36] P. J. Nestel, R. J. Havel, and A. Bezman (1963) Metabolism of constituent lipids of dog chylomicrons. *J. Clin. Invest.* **42,** 1313–1321.

[37] D. W. Bilhemier, S. Eisenberg, and R. I. Levy (1972) The metabolism of very low density lipoproteins. I. Preliminary in vitro and in vivo observations. *Biochim. Biophys. Acta* **260,** 212–221.

[38] S. Noel, P. J. Dolphon, and D. Rubinstein (1975) An in vitro model for the catabolism of rat chylomicrons. *Biochem. Biophys. Res. Commun.* **63,** 764–772.

[39] J. M. Felts, H. Itakura, and R. T. Crane (1975) The mechanism of assimilation of constituents of chylomicrons, very low density lipoproteins and remnants—a new theory. *Biochem. Biophys. Res. Commun.* **66,** 1467–1475.

[40] C. H. Floren and A. Nilsson (1977) Binding, interiorization and degradation of cholesteryl ester-labeled chylomicron-remnant particles by rat hepatocyte monolayers. *Biochem. J.* **168,** 483–494.

[41] B. C. Sherrill and J. M. Dietschy (1978) Characterization of the sinusoidal transport process responsible for the uptake of chylomicrons by the liver. *J. Biol. Chem.* **253,** 1859–1867.

[42] B. C. Sherrill, T. L. Innerarity, and R. W. Mahley (1980) Rapid hepatic clearance of the canine lipoproteins containing only the E apoprotein by a high affinity receptor. *J. Biol. Chem.* **255,** 1804–1807.

[43] E. W. Windler, Y. Chao, and R. J. Havel (1980) Regulation of the hepatic uptake of triglyceride-rich lipoproteins in the rat. *J. Biol. Chem.* **255,** 8303–8307.

[44] F. Shelburne, J. Hanks, W. Myers, and S. Quartford (1980) Effects of apoproteins on uptake of triglyceride emulsions in the rat. *J. Clin. Invest.* **65,** 652–658.

[45] M. R. Lakshman, R. A. Muesing, and J. C. LaRosa (1981) Regulation of cholesterol biosynthesis and 3-hydroxy-3-methylglutaryl coenzyme A reductase activity by chylomicron remnants in isolated hepatocytes and perfused liver. *J. Biol. Chem.* **256,** 3037–3043.

[46] M. R. Lakshman, M. VanderMaten, R. A. Muesing, P. O'looney, and G. V. Vahouny (1983) Role of high density lipoproteins in regulation of hepatic fatty synthesis by chylomicron and very low density lipoprotein remnants. *J. Biol. Chem.* **258**, 4746–4749.

[47] J. L. Goldstein and M. S. Brown (1982) The LDL receptor in hypercholesterolemia. Implications for pathogenesis and therapy. *Med. Clin. North Am.* **66**, 335–362.

[48] J. L. Goldstein and M. S. Brown (1977) The low density lipoprotein pathway and its relation to atherosclerosis. *Ann. Rev. Biochem.* **46**, 897–930.

[49] J. P. Kane (1983) Apolipoprotein B: structural and metabolic heterogeneity. *Ann. Rev. Physiol.* **45**, 637–650.

[50] D. Y. Hui, T. L. Innerarity, R. W. Milne, Y. L. Marcel, and R. W. Mahley (1984) Binding of chylomicron remnants and beta very low density lipoproteins to hepatic and extrahepatic lipoprotein receptors. A process independent of apolipoprotein B-48. *J. Biol. Chem.* **259**, 15,060–15,068.

[51] D. Y. Hui, T. L. Innerarity, and R. W. Mahley (1981) Lipoprotein binding to canine hepatic membranes. Metabolically distinct apo-E and apo-B,E receptors. *J. Biol. Chem.* **256**, 5646–5655.

[52] R. W. Mahley, D. Y. Hui, T. L. Innerarity, and K. H. Weisgraber (1981) Two independent lipoprotein receptors on the hepatic membranes of dog, swine and man. Apo-B,E and apo-E receptors. *J. Clin. Invest.* **68**, 1197–1206.

[53] E. E. T. Windler, P. T. Kovanen, Y. S. Chao, M. S. Brown, R. J. Havel, and J. L. Goldstein (1980) The estradiol-stimulated lipoprotein receptor of rat liver. *J. Biol. Chem.* **255**, 10,464–10,471.

[54] W. G. Dunphy and J. E. Rothman (1985) Compartmental organization of the golgi stack. *Cell* **42**, 13–21.

[55] G. Griffiths and K. Simons (1986) The trans golgi network: sorting at the exit site of the golgi complex. *Science* **234**, 438–443.

[56] C. H. Halsted, E. A. Robles, and E. Mezey (1973) Distribution of ethanol in the human gastrointestinal tract. *Am. J. Clin. Nutr.* **26**, 831–834.

[57] O. Frank, A. Luisada-Opper, M. F. Sorrell, A. D. Thompson, and H. Baker (1971) Vitamin deficits in severe alcoholic fatty liver of man. *Exp. Mol. Biol.* **15**, 191–197.

[58] E. Baraona, R. C. Pirola, and C. S. Lieber (1974) Small intestinal damage and changes in cell population produced by ethanol ingestion in the rat. *Gastroenterology* **66**, 226–234.

[59] E. Baraona, R. C. Pirola, and C. S. Lieber (1975) Acute and chronic effects of ethanol on intestinal lipid metabolism. *Biochem. Biophys. Acta* **388**, 19–28.

[60] E. A. Carter, G. D. Drummey, and K. J. Isselbacher (1971) Ethanol stimulates triglyceride synthesis by the intestine. *Science* **174**, 1245–1247.

[61] J. B. Rodgers and R. J. O'Brien (1975) The effect of acute ethanol treatment

on lipid-reesterifying enzymes of the rat small bowel. *Am. J. Digest. Dis.* **20,** 354–358.

[62] A. Gangl and R. K. Ockner (1975) Intestinal metabolism of plasma free fatty acids. Intracellular compartmentation and mechanism of control. *J. Clin. Invest.* **55,** 803–813.

[63] M. R. Lakshman, M. E. Felver, and R. L. Veech (1980) Alcohol and VLDL synthesis and secretion by isolated hepatocytes. *Alcohol. Clin. Exp. Res.* **4,** 361–365.

[64] E. Baraona and C. S. Lieber (1970) Effects of chronic ethanol feeding on serum lipoprotein metabolism in the rat. *J. Clin. Invest.* **49,** 769–777.

[65] C. S. Lieber, N. Spritz, and M. Decarli (1966) Role of dietary, adipose, and endogenously synthesized fatty acids in the pathogenesis of alcoholic fatty liver. *J. Clin. Invest.* **45,** 51–62.

[66] E. A. Abramson and R. A. Arky (1968) Acute antilipolytic effects of ethyl alcohol and acetate in man. *J. Lab. Clin. Med.* **72,** 105–117.

[67] B. B. Brodie and R. P. Maichel (1962) Role of the sympathetic nervous system in drug induced fatty liver. *Ann. NY Acad. Sci.* **104,** 1049–1053.

[68] M. J. Savolanen, V. P. Jauhonen, and I. E. Hassinen (1977) Effects of clofibrate on ethanol induced modifications in liver and adipose tissue metabolism. *Biochem. Pharmacol.* **26,** 424–431.

[69] C. S. Lieber, N. Lefevre, L. Spritz, L. Feinsman, and M. Decarli (1979) Differences in hepatic metabolism of long and medium chain fatty acids. *J. Clin. Invest.* **63,** 14–20.

[70] J. A. Ontko (1973) Effects of ethanol on the metabolism of free fatty acids in isolated liver cells. *J. Lipid Res.* **14,** 78–86.

[71] J. G. Joly, L. Feinsman, H. Ishii, and C. S. Lieber (1973) Effect of chronic ethanol feeding on hepatic microsomal glycerophosphate acyltransferase activity. *J. Lipid Res.* **14,** 337–343.

[72] R. G. Lamb, C. E. Wood, and H. J. Fallon (1979) Effect of acute and chronic ethanol intake on hepatic glycerolipid biosynthesis in hamster. *J. Clin. Invest.* **63,** 14–20.

[73] C. L. Mendenhall, R. H. Bradford, and R. H. Furman (1969) Effects of ethanol on glycerolipid metabolism in rat liver. *Biochem. Biophys. Acta* **187,** 501–509.

[74] E. A. Nikkila and K. Ojala (1963) Role of hepatic L-alphaglycerophosphate and triglyceride synthesis in production of fatty liver by ethanol. *Proc. Soc. Exp. Biol. Med.* **113,** 814–817.

[75] E. E. Elko, W. R. Wooles, and N. R. Diluzio (1961) Alterations and mobilization of lipids in acute ethanol treated rats. *Am. J. Physiol.* **201,** 923–926.

[76] J. I. Kesler and S. Yalovsky-Mishkin (1966) Effect of ingestion of saline, glucose, and ethanol on mobilization and hepatic incorporation of epididymal pad palmitate-1-14C in rats. *J. Lipid Res.* **7,** 772–778.

[77] C. S. Lieber, C. M. Leevy, S. W. Stein, W. S. George, G. R. Cherrick, W. H. Abelmann, and C. S. Davidson (1962) Effects of ethanol on plasma free fatty acids in man. *J. Clin. Lab. Med.* **59,** 826–832.

[78] I. A. Bouchier and A. M. Dawson (1964) Effects of infusions of ethanol on the plasma free fatty acids in man. *Clin. Sci.* **26,** 47–54.

[79] M. R. Lakshman, M. E. Felver, and M. Ezekiel (1984) Relationship of endocrine status on the stimulatory effect of ethanol on hepatic very low density lipoprotein synthesis. *Alcohol. Clin. Exp. Res.* **8,** 359–361.

[80] M. R. Lakshman, S. J. Chirtel, L. C. Chambers, and B. S. Campbell (1989) Hepatic synthesis of apoproteins of very low density and high density lipoproteins in perfused rat liver: Influence of chronic heavy and moderate doses of ethanol. *Alcohol. Clin. Exp. Res.* **13,** 554–559.

[81] M. R. Lakshman, S. J. Chirtel, and L. L. Chambers (1988) Roles of omega 3 fatty acids and chronic ethanol in the regulation of plasma and liver lipids and plasma apoproteins Al and E in rats. *J. Nutr.* **118,** 1299–1303.

[82] M. R. Lakshman and M. Ezekiel (1982) Relationship of alcoholic hyperlipidemia to the feed-back regulation of hepatic cholesterol synthesis by chylomicron remnants. *Alcohol. Clin. Exp. Res.* **6,** 482–486.

[83] M. R. Lakshman and M. Ezekiel (1985) Effect of chronic ethanol feeding upon the catabolism of lipid and protein moieties of chylomicrons and very low density lipoproteins in vivo and in the perfused heart system. *Alcohol. Clin. Exp. Res.* **9,** 327–330.

[84] M. R. Lakshman, M. Ezekiel, B. S. Campbell, and R. A. Muesing (1986) Binding, uptake, and metabolism of chylomicron remnants by hepatocytes from control and chronic ethanol-fed rats. *Alcohol. Clin. Exp. Res.* **10,** 412–418.

[85] S. C. Goheen, E. C. Larkin, M. Manix, and G. A. Rao (1980) Dietary arachidonic acid reduces fatty liver, increases diet consumption and weight gain in ethanol-fed rats. *Lipids* **15,** 328–336.

[86] S. C. Goheen, E. E. Pearson, E. C. Larkin, and G. A. Rao (1981) The prevention of alcoholic fatty liver using dietary supplements: Dihydroxyacetone, pyruvate and riboflavin compared to arachidonic acid in pair-fed rats. *Lipids* **16,** 43–51.

[87] A. M. Nervi, R. O. Peluffo, R. R. Brenner, and A. L. Leikin (1980) Effect of ethanol administration on fatty acid desaturation. *Lipids* **15,** 263–268.

[88] D. L. Yang and R. C. Reitz (1983) Ethanol ingestion and polyunsaturated fatty acids: Effects of acyl-CoA desaturases. *Alcohol. Clin. Exp. Res.* **7,** 220–226.

[89] G. A. Rao, G. Lew, and E. C. Larkin (1984) Alcohol ingestion and levels of hepatic fatty acid synthetase and stearoyl-CoA desaturase activities in rats. *Lipids* **19,** 151–153.

[90] Z. Stern, M. A. Korsten, L. M. DeCarli, and C. S. Lieber (1990) Effects of arachidonic acid on hepatic lipids in ethanol-fed rats. *Alcohol. Clin. Exp. Res.* **14,** 127–129.

[91] B. B. Brodie, W. M. Butler, M. G. Horning, R. P. Maickel, and H. M. Maling (1961) Alcohol-induced triglyceride deposition in liver through derangement of fat transport. *Am. J. Clin. Nutr.* **9,** 432–435.

[92] D. P. Jones, E. S. Perman, and C. S. Lieber (1965) Free fatty acid turnover and triglyceride metabolism after ethanol ingestion in man. *J. Lab. Clin. Med.* **66,** 804–813.

[93] J. R. Crouse, C. D. Gerson, L. M. DeCarli, and C. S. Lieber (1968) Role of acetate in the reduction of plasma free fatty acids produced by ethanol in man. *J. Lipid Res.* **9,** 509–512.

[94] M. A. Abrams and C. Cooper (1976) Quantitative analysis of metabolism of hepatic triglyceride in ethanol treated rats. *Biochem. J.* **156,** 33–46.

[95] H. Brunengraber, M. Boutry, L. Lowenstein, and J. M. Lowenstein (1977) The effect of ethanol on lipogenesis by the perfused liver, in *Alcohol and Aldehyde Metabolizing Systems.* R. C. Thurman, T. Yonetani, J. R. Williamson, and B. Chance, eds. Academic, New York and London, pp. 329–337.

[96] R. W. Guynn, D. Veloso, R. L. Harris, J. W. R. Lawson, and R. L. Veech (1973) Ethanol administration and the relationship of malonyl-coenzyme A concentrations to the rate of fatty acid synthesis in rat liver. *Biochem. J.* **136,** 639–647.

[97] R. Scholz, A. Kaltstein, U. Schwabe, and R. G. Thurman (1977) Inhibition of fatty acid synthesis from carbohydrates in perfused rat liver by ethanol, in *Alcohol and Aldehyde Metabolizing Systems.* R. C. Thurman, T. Yonetani, J. R. Williamson, and B. Chance, eds. Academic, New York and London, pp. 315–328.

[98] M. J. Savolainen, J. K. Hiltunen, and I. E. Hassinen (1977) Effect of prolonged ethanol ingestion on hepatic lipogenesis and related enzyme activities. *Biochem. J.* **164,** 169–177.

[99] M. R. Lakshman and R. L. Veech (1977) Effect of an acute dose of ethanol upon the number of tritium atoms incorporated into sterol during its biosynthesis from mevalonate by rat liver *in vivo*, in *Alcohol and Aldehyde Metabolizing Systems.* R. C. Thurman, T. Yonetani, J. R. Williamson, and B. Chance, eds. Academic, New York and London, pp. 125–136.

[100] C. S. Lieber and R. Schmid (1961) The effect of ethanol on fatty acid metabolism: Stimulation of hepatic fatty acid synthesis in vitro. *J. Clin. Invest.* **40,** 394–399.

[101] R. Blomstrand, L. Kager, and O. Lantto (1973) Studies on the ethanol-induced decrease of fatty acid oxidation in rat and human liver slices. *Life Sci.* **13,** 1131–1141.

[102] R. Blomstrand and L. Kager (1973) The combustion of triolein-1-14C and its inhibition by alcohol in man. *Life Sci.* **13,** 113–123.

[103] M. R. Lakshman and R. L. Veech (1977) Short and long-term effects of ethanol administration *in vivo* upon rat liver HMG-CoA reductase and cholesterol 7α-hydroxylase activities. *J. Lipid Res.* **18,** 325–329.

[104] M. R. Lakshman, A. D. Gupta, and R. L. Veech (1978) Effect of chronic ethanol administration on cholesterol and bile acid synthesis *in vivo*. *Lipids* **13**, 134–136.

[105] A. A. Nanji and S. W. French (1986) Dietary factors and alcoholic cirrhosis. *Alcohol. Clin. Exp. Res.* **10**, 271–273.

[106] A. A. Nanji, C. L. Mendenhall, and S. W. French (1989) Beef fat prevents alcoholic liver disease in the rat. *Alcohol. Clin. Exp. Res.* **13**, 15–19.

[107] A. Maquedano, M. Guzman, and J. Castro (1988) Dependence with nutritional status of the ethanol effects on fatty acid metabolism in rat hepatocytes. *Int. J. Biochem.* **20**, 937–941.

[108] D. M. Bissell (1990) Cell-matrix interaction and hepatic fibrosis, in *Progress in Liver Diseases*. H. Popper and F. Schaffner, eds. W. B. Saunders, Philadelphia, pp. 143–155.

[109] B. G. Johansson and A. Medhus (1974) Increase in plasma alpha-lipoproteins in chronic alcoholics after acute abuse. *Acta Med. Scand.* **195**, 273.

[110] P. Belfrage, B. Berg, I. Hagerstrand, P. Nilsson-Ehle, H. Tornqvist, and T. Wiebe (1977) Alterations of lipid metabolism in healthy volunteers during long-term ethanol intake. *Eur. J. Clin. Invest.* **7**, 127.

[111] S. B. Hulley, R. Cohen, and G. Widdowson (1977) Plasma high density lipoprotein cholesterol level — Influence of risk factor intervention. *JAMA* **238**, 2269.

[112] W. P. Castelli, J. T. Doyle, T. Gordon, G. Hames, M. C. Hjortland, S. B. Hulley, A. Kagan, and W. J. Zukel (1977) Alcohol and blood lipids — The cooperative lipoprotein phenotyping study. *Lancet* **ii**, 153.

[113] A. Jacqueson, J. L. Richard, P. Ducimetiere, J. M. Warnet, and J. R. Claude (1983) High density lipoprotein cholesterol and alcohol consumption in a French male population. *Atherosclerosis* **48**, 131.

[114] A. L. Klatsky, G. D. Freidman, and A. B. Siegelaub (1974) Alcohol consumption before myocardial infarction: Results from the Kaiser-Permanente epidemiologic study of myocardial infarction. *Ann. Intern. Med.* **81**, 294–301.

[115] W. B. Stason, R. K. Neff, O. S. Miettinen, and H. Jick (1976) Alcohol consumption and non fatal myocardial infarction. *Am. J. Epidemiol.* **104**, 603–608.

[116] J. J. Barboriak, A. A. Rimm, A. J. Anderson, M. Schmidhoffer, and F. E. Tristani (1977) Coronary artery occlusion and alcohol intake. *Br. Heart J.* **39**, 289–293.

[117] J. R. L. Masarei, I. L. Puddey, W. J. Rouse, R. Lynch, R. Vandongen, and L. J. Beilin (1986) Effects of alcohol consumption on serum lipoprotein-lipid and apolipoprotein concentrations: Results from an international study in healthy subjects. *Atherosclerosis* **60**, 79–87.

[118] M.-R. Taskinen, M. Valimaki, E. A. Nikkila, T. Kuusi, C. Ehnholm, and R. Ylikahri (1982) High density lipoprotein subfractions and post-heparin plasma lipases in alcoholic men before and after ethanol withdrawal. *Metabolism* **31**, 1168–1174.

[119] W. L. Haskell, C. Camargo, Jr., P. T. Williams, K. M. Vranizan, R. M. Krauss, F. T. Lindgren, and P. D. Wood (1984) The effect of cessation and resumption of moderate alcohol intake on serum high-density lipoprotein subfractions: A controlled study. *N. Engl. J. Med.* **310,** 805–810.

[120] G. H. Hartung, J. P. Foreyt, R. E. Mitchell, J. G. Mitchell, R. S. Reeves, and A. M. Gotto (1983) Effect of alcohol intake on high-density lipoprotein cholesterol levels in runners and inactive men. *JAMA* **249,** 747–750.

[121] P. Cushman, J. Barboriak, and J. Kalbfleisch (1986) Alcohol: High density lipoproteins, apolipoproteins. *Alcohol. Clin. Exp. Res.* **10,** 154–157.

[122] C. S. Lieber (1984) To drink "moderately" or not to drink? *N. Engl. J. Med.* **310,** 846–848.

Effect of Ethanol
on Splanchnic Blood Flow

Edward T. Knych

Introduction

The splanchnic circulation is composed of six dissimilar vascular beds, arranged in parallel and in series. It supplies blood to the digestive organs, including the stomach, small and large intestines, pancreas, spleen, and liver. The splanchnic organs receive approx 25% of the cardiac output, extract 15–20% of the available oxygen in the blood stream, and contain 20–25% of the total blood volume.[1] In addition, splanchnic organs, such as the liver, are major regulators of metabolic homeostasis. It is not surprising that derangements in the hemodynamics of the splanchnic circulation lead to significant functional changes in individual organs of the splanchnic bed as well as to changes in overall cardiovascular and metabolic homeostasis.

Abusive ethanol consumption adversely affects many body organs, and prominent among these are the splanchnic organs.[2] Changes in blood flow play a critical role in the pathology induced by ethanol in these organs. For example, gastric mucosal injury induced by the instillation of ethanol into the stomach is characterized by stasis of gastric mucosal blood flow,[3,4] congestion,[5] platelet aggregation,[6] and endothelial damage.[7] Within 30 s of ethanol instillation, submucosal venoconstriction occurs.[8,9] Mucosal stasis follows during the first few minutes and histologic evidence of ischemic mucosal damage within 10 min.[4] Several possible mediators of

From: *Drug and Alcohol Abuse Reviews, Vol. 2: Liver Pathology and Alcohol*
Ed: R. R. Watson ©1991 The Humana Press Inc.

this pathologic response to ethanol have been suggested. One is leukotriene C_4. Intragastric administration of ethanol induces the mucosal release of leukotriene C_4,[10] which is a potent submucosal venoconstrictor.[11] However, although some inhibitors of leukotriene synthesis prevent ethanol-induced submucosal vasoconstriction and the development of mucosal lesions,[9,10,12] others do not.[12] A second possible mediator is suggested by the observation that ethanol-induced gastric injury can also be prevented by the administration of nitric oxide.[13] Nitric oxide has been shown to have actions that are identical to the endothelium-derived relaxing factor, EDRF.[14–17] In addition, EDRF and nitric oxide are both potent inhibitors of platelet aggregation and adhesion.[18] These observations are interesting in light of the recent observations that endothelium-dependent vasodilation in the perfused mesenteric bed is inhibited by the inhibitor of nitric oxide synthesis N^G-monomethyl-L-arginine[19] and also by ethanol.[20] Thus, ethanol may produce gastric injury by stimulating the release of the potent endogenous venoconstrictor leukotriene C_4 and by inhibiting the action of the endogenous vasodilator nitric oxide.

The pathologic effects of ethanol on the liver have occupied much attention. Since all forms of liver disease are accompanied by alterations in hepatic hemodynamics,[21] the remainder of this review will focus on the effect of ethanol on hepatic flow.

The hepatic vascular bed differs significantly in structure and regulation from most other organs, including the splanchnic organs. Rappaport defined the acinus as the microvascular unit of the liver.[22] It is composed of a group of hepatic parenchymal cells arranged in sinsusoidal array around a terminal hepatic arteriole, portal venule, and bile duct. Blood enters the center of the acinus by way of the hepatic arteriole and portal venule. Within this periportal zone (Rappaport Zone 1) the oxygen-rich arteriolar blood is mixed well with the oxygen-poor blood of the portal venule. Blood then flows concurrently through adjacent sinusoids and exits through hepatic venules located at the periphery of the acinus (Rappaport Zone 3). This one-way flow produces a gradient for oxygen and other substances that are added to or removed from the blood as it flows through the acinus.[23] The highest oxygen content is found in the periportal zone (Zone 1), and the lowest content is found in the perivenular zone (Zone 3).

Portal blood accounts for approx two-thirds of the hepatic blood flow; the remainder is provided by flow through the hepatic artery.[1] Three factors can, potentially, regulate hepatic flow: the intrahepatic vascular resistance;

the vascular resistance of the intestines, which regulates inflow into the portal vein; and the hepatic arterial resistance, which regulates hepatic-artery blood flow.[21,24] Intrahepatic pressure is essentially equal to portal pressure in the normal state and appears to be regulated by resistance sites located in the hepatic veins.[25,26] The principal function of these resistance sites appears to be the maintenance of constant portal and intrahepatic pressure.[25,26] Changes in intrahepatic resistance do not alter portal venous flow.[21] This flow fluctuates widely, depending on the metabolic activity of the splanchnic organs that drain into the portal vein, and is regulated by the resistance of these splanchnic vascular beds, in particular the superior mesenteric bed.[21,24] Therefore, hepatic control of flow through the liver is by way of the hepatic artery.

Arterial beds within most organs of the body are capable of altering flow through the organ in response to metabolic demands. This metabolic hypothesis regards tissue oxygen as the regulated variable. However, this intrinsic regulatory mechanism does not appear to operate within the hepatic circulation. Reduction of oxygen supply by isovolemic hemodilution increases flow through the mesenteric bed, but does not produce a dilation of the hepatic artery.[27] Administration of dinitrophenol increases the oxygen demand of both the intestines and the liver. However, although dinitrophenol administration increased flow through the mesenteric bed, it slightly reduced hepatic-artery conductance.[28] Lactic acidosis increases portal flow, but reduces hepatic arterial flow.[29] The increased hepatic oxygen consumption induced by ethanol administration does not lead to a dilation of the hepatic artery (*see discussion below*). Therefore, hepatic blood flow appears to be independent of the metabolic activity of the liver.

Other intrinsic regulatory mechanisms regulate flow through the hepatic circulation. The principal function of these mechanisms is to maintain a constant flow through the liver, rather than a constant oxygen supply. Two mechanisms have been described. The more important has been termed the hepatic arterial buffer response;[21,30,31] when portal blood flow increases, the hepatic artery constricts, and when portal blood flow decreases, the hepatic artery dilates. The buffer response has been observed in dogs, cats, rats, and humans.[21] It is not reciprocal, since changes in hepatic arterial flow do not alter portal flow or resistance.[26,32] The hepatic artery is maximally dilated at low portal flow and nearly maximally constricted at high portal flow.[33] It has been hypothesized that adenosine washout from the space of Mall, which surrounds the hepatic arterial resistance vessels and portal venules, is responsible for the buffer response.[31,34] When portal flow is reduced, less adenosine washes out and dilation of the hepatic artery occurs. When portal flow is increased, adenosine concentrations are reduced and constriction of the hepatic artery occurs. Several observations support this hypothesis. Adenosine dilates the hepatic artery when administered intraarterially.[34] Blockade of adenosine uptake with dipyridamole potentiates the effect of adenosine and the buffer response induced by reducing portal flow.[34] The adenosine antagonists 1-methyl-3-isobutyl xanthine and 8-phenyltheophylline reduce the effect of adenosine and also the buffer response.[34,35] In addition, the buffer response is not altered by atropine, propranolol, oubain, indomethacin, metiamide, or mepyramine.[36] Further, it is not altered by complete hepatic denervation.[32,37] The principal purpose of the hepatic arterial buffer system appears to be the maintenance of a constant flow through the liver, which ensures a steady portal and intrahepatic pressure, liver blood volume, and hepatic clearance of drugs and hormones.

Hepatic arterial flow also exhibits autoregulation. An increase in mean arterial pressure produces a constriction of the hepatic artery, which increases resistance and maintains a constant flow. Autoregulation of the hepatic artery appears to be relatively weak and is considered to be myogenic in origin.[38] However, recent studies suggest that adenosine may also play a role in the autoregulatory control of the hepatic artery.[39]

Extrinsic humoral control of the hepatic circulation is understood less well.[40] The hepatic artery responds in the same way as any other artery when a variety of endogenous vasoactive substances are administered intraarterially. However, when these substances are administered intravenously, the hepatic arterial buffer response may modify the response induced in the hepatic artery. Both the hepatic artery and the superior mesenteric artery dilate in response to direct intraarterial administration of adenosine, isoproterenol, and glucagon.[41] However, intravenous administration of these dilators produced dilation in the mesenteric bed, although the hepatic artery failed to dilate.[41] If flow through the mesenteric bed was clamped at a control level, intravenous administration of adenosine, isoproterenol, and glucagon produced dilation of the hepatic artery.[41] Similar differences between the responses induced by intraarterial vs intravenous administration have been reported for prostacyclin,[42] histamine,[43,44] dopamine,[45,46] and vasopressin.[43,47]

Alterations in hepatocyte function and changes in hepatic hemodynamics leading to portal hypertension are two major factors leading to mortality in ethanol-induced liver disease. Isreal and colleagues have proposed that liver-cell necrosis produced by abusive ethanol intake is attributable to hypoxia in the perivenular zone (Zone 3) of the liver.[48–52] This hypermetabolic theory states that liver-cell necrosis in Zone 3 occurs when the primary effect of ethanol, an increase in oxygen consumption, exceeds oxygen supply to this relatively hypoxic zone of the hepatic acinus. The simultaneous occurrence of these events is hypothesized to occur at random and to be independent of alcohol consumption.[53] Acute administration of ethanol induces an increase in hepatic oxygen consumption in several species.[54–62] The chronic consumption of alcohol increases oxygen consumption in isolated organs and tissues. Such an effect has been observed in several species, including humans.[48–50,53,63–70] In the rat chronically fed ethanol, the observed increase in hepatic oxygen consumption appears to be a function of active ethanol ingestion and is not related to blood ethanol levels.[61] Oxygen consumption returns to normal levels as animals are withdrawn from ethanol. Similarly, after an overnight fast, the splanchnic oxygen consumption in the baboon chronically fed ethanol was not statistically different from that in a pair-fed control animal.[54] However, a more recent study reported a significant increase in splanchnic oxygen consumption in the chronically ethanol-fed baboon fasted overnight.[62]

Increased hepatic oxygen consumption appears to be a common effect of ethanol ingestion, but most animal models do not develop liver necrosis after chronic ethanol administration.[71–74] Necrosis can be produced only when increased oxygen consumption is coupled with decreased oxygen availability.[48,50,74] Increased oxygen consumption is not sufficient, by itself, to produce necrosis. Two compensatory mechanisms might be expected to occur as a result of increased hepatic oxygen demand. The first involves the ability of the liver to extract more oxygen from hepatic blood when hepatic oxygen consumption increases.[30] The liver can effectively extract >90% of the oxygen delivered to it.[75] Yet, in most studies, oxygen tensions in the hepatic vein either are not reduced[54,57,58,61] or are increased[54,62] after acute ethanol administration. These observations suggest that hepatic oxygen extraction is not increased during ethanol-induced increases in oxygen consumption. The second mechanism for increasing oxygen supply to the liver would require an increase in oxygen delivery. This is the compensatory mechanism that apparently occurs most frequently. In both acute and chronic studies, the increased hepatic oxygen consumption observed following ethanol administration is fully compensated for by an increase in liver blood flow.[57,61,76] Yet, as discussed above, mechanisms controlling hepatic blood flow are considered to be independent of oxygen demand. They exist primarily to maintain a constant flow.[30] An understanding of the compensatory mechanism that operates following an ethanol-induced increase in hepatic oxygen consumption is important to our understanding of the ethanol-induced pathogenesis.

Early studies reported conflicting results regarding the effect of ethanol administration on hepatic blood flow. Castenfors et al.[77] infused low doses of ethanol into humans, resulting in blood alcohol levels of 2–14 mM, and reported no effect on hepatic blood flow. Mendelhoff,[78] on the other hand, reported an increase in hepatic blood flow after producing similar blood ethanol levels in sedated humans. Mendelhoff's subjects also all had peptic ulcers. Childset et al.[79] and Stein et al.,[80] using larger doses of ethanol, also reported increased hepatic blood flow. Using dogs anesthetized with pentobarbital, Smythe et al.[81] reported that the oral administration of 0.8–1.9 g/kg of ethanol produced no change in hepatic blood flow 30 and 60 min after ethanol administration. In contrast, an increase in hepatic blood flow was observed after the oral administration of 2 g/kg of ethanol to conscious, unrestrained dogs.[57] Similarly conflicting observations have been reported by others.[54,82–85] These inconsistencies have been attributed to a number of factors, including dose, route of administration, and anesthetic. McKaigney et al.[86] demonstrated that anesthetics reduced the effect of ethanol on hepatic blood flow. In the conscious, unrestrained rat, oral administration of 0.5 g/kg of ethanol induced a significant increase in hepatic blood flow, whereas 3.0 g/kg of ethanol, orally, was required to produce a similar increase in hepatic flow in an animal anesthetized with ketamine. Carmichael et al.[76] extended these observations and reported significant attenuation of ethanol-induced increases in hepatic blood flow in rats anesthetized with ketamine, fentanyl, and thiopental when compared to conscious, unrestrained control animals. Ketamine had the shortest duration of action and was recommended as the anesthetic of choice when the use of conscious animals was not practical.

Another possible source of inconsistency is found in the methods used to estimate hepatic blood flow. Most early studies estimated hepatic blood flow by measuring the clearance of a substance that is cleared from the circulation exclusively by the liver. Such dyes as sulfobromophtalein and indocyanine green are commonly used. However, clearance of these dyes reflects not only hepatic blood flow, but also hepatocyte and extrahepatic function. Hepatic extraction of indocyanine green decreases with liver disease in such a way that at low extraction rates small variations in measured blood levels can lead to large variations in estimated hepatic blood flow.[87] Sulfobromophtalein is cleared by extrahepatic phagocytes and other organs.[88,89] In addition, these methods estimate total hepatic blood flow. They do not allow separate estimates to be made of portal venous or hepatic arterial flow.

More recently, techniques that use radioactive microspheres[90–93] or electronic flow probes to measure cardiac output and organ blood flow have been used to estimate changes in hepatic blood flow induced by ethanol administration. They have also been used to estimate ethanol-induced changes in portal venous and hepatic arterial flow. Consistently, studies using these techniques have reported that acute ethanol administration induces an increase in hepatic blood flow[61,76,86,94–100] after the oral or intravenous administration of ethanol. In these studies, it has generally been observed that the increase in hepatic flow is attributable to an increase in portal-vein flow with little or no change in flow through the hepatic artery. The increased portal flow is accounted for by changes in the mesenteric flow through the small and large intestine.[61,95] McKaigney et al.[86] reported that the ethanol-induced increase in portal flow was accompanied by a decrease in flow through the hepatic artery. In contrast, using dogs[96] and cats[100] anesthetized with pentobarbital, increases in hepatic blood flow following acute ethanol administration were caused by increases in hepatic-artery flow with no change in portal-vein flow. The increase in hepatic flow produced by the acute administration of ethanol is also observed in animals chronically administered ethanol, suggesting that tolerance to this effect does not develop.[61,95] The increase in portal blood flow induced by ethanol is not dose-dependent. Ethanol concentrations >3.4 mM produce changes in portal blood flow that are not altered by increasing the ethanol concentration.[86,101] The affinity constant (K_m) of the hepatic alcohol dehydrogenase is 0.5–2.0 mM,[102] suggesting an association between the ethanol-induced hemodynamic effects and ethanol metabolism. Supporting the hypothesis that changes in hepatic flow are the result of ethanol metabolism is the observation that pretreatment with alcohol dehydrogenase inhibitor 4-methylpyrazole completely blocks the acute increase in blood flow induced by ethanol.[86] Further, the effect of acute ethanol administration persists until blood ethanol concentrations decrease below 4 mM, the saturation level for alcohol dehydrogenase.[101] The effects of ethanol do not appear to be caused directly by ethanol; rather they appear to be mediated by the metabolism of ethanol.

The effect of ethanol on hepatic flow could be caused by either of the principal metabolic products of ethanol metabolism, acetaldehyde or acetate. Early studies of the effect of acetaldehyde have been contradictory. Intravenous injection of acetaldehyde produced a pressor response.[103] Administration of ethanol to animals pretreated with disulfiram or nitrefazole produced vasodilation.[104,105] Altura et al.[106] demonstrated that acetaldehyde inhibited spontaneous activity in isolated rat aorta and portal vein, and lowered resting tension. In addition, they observed that ethanol dose-dependently attenuated the contractions caused by epinephrine, angiotensin, vasopressin, serotonin, potassium, and calcium. However, acetaldehyde applied locally, intravenously, or intraarterially caused dose-dependent contractions of mesenteric arterioles and venuoles.[107,108] Pretreatment with the aldehyde dehydrogenase inhibitor cyanamide completely blocked the increase in portal flow induced by ethanol.[95] Further, infusion of acetaldehyde into the left ventricle or the portal vein did not alter the portal blood flow and did not alter ethanol-induced increase in portal flow.[95] Carmichael[95] has argued that the ability of cyanamide to inhibit the ethanol-induced increase in portal flow is not the result of an inhibition of ethanol metabolism, but of a presently undetermined effect of cyanamide on splanchnic hemodynamics.

The second metabolite of ethanol, acetate, has also been investigated as a possible mediator of ethanol-induced changes in portal blood flow. Altura and Gebrewold[107] observed no change in the diameter of mesenteric terminal arterioles and venules after the administration of acetate (0.025–250 m*M*) locally, intravenously, or intraarterially. *M*ore recently, the intravenous infusion of acetate (7–250 µ*M*/kg/min) was observed to produce a dose-dependent increase in portal blood flow. The infusion rates of acetate were chosen to mimic the rate of acetate release observed during the metabolism of ethanol.[82] The observed increase in hepatic flow following acetate infusion was primarily attributable to an increase in mesenteric flow and mimics the effect of ethanol administration.[109] Since acetate can be metabolized to adenosine, the effect of adenosine was also studied. Adenosine dose-dependently increased portal flow by increasing mesenteric flow.[97] Furthermore, ethanol administration resulted in a fourfold increase in adenosine blood levels. The A2-adenosine receptor agonist 5'-*N*-ethylcaboxamido adenosine (NECA) was capable of inducing an increase in portal flow. However, the A1-adenosine receptor agonist *N*-6-cyclohexyl adenosine (CHA) had no effect.[109] Therefore, the effects of adenosine appear to be mediated via A2-adenosine receptors, which mediate activation of adenylate cyclase and increase intracellular cAMP. The actions of acetate and adenosine are blocked by 8-phenyltheophylline, an A1- and A2-adenosine receptor antagonist.[97,109] In addition, 8-phenyltheophylline blocked the increase in portal blood flow induced by ethanol administration.[97] These investigators have noted that adenosine concentrations produced by ethanol were only one-half of those required to produce an effect on the mesenteric circulation.[110] Further, infusions of adenosine that increased the portal circulation also increased coronary- and hepatic-artery flow.[97] However, increases in coronary- or hepatic-artery flow are not observed following ethanol administration. It therefore appears that an increase in circulating adenosine is not capable of explaining the effect of ethanol on hepatic flow. Alternatively, the effect of ethanol might be accounted for by the conversion of acetate to adenosine within a selective vascular bed. The activity of 5'-nucleotidase, which converts AMP to adenosine, is high in the small intestine.[111] Another possible mechanism is suggested by the recently reported inhibitory effect of ethanol on adenosine uptake.[112] Inhibition of the uptake mechanism for adenosine would lead to an increased extracellular level of adenosine. It remains to be established if the nucleoside transporter exhibits differential sensitivities to ethanol in various vascular beds.

The results discussed above have tried to link the production of a hepatic ethanol metabolite with a selective effect on mesenteric blood flow, but little attention has been paid to the direct effect of ethanol or its metabolites on mesenteric flow. Altura and colleagues[107,108] have reported that alcohol will induce an increase in the diameter of resistance vessels in the mesenteric bed. They have further reported the development of tolerance to this effect following 6 wk of ethanol feeding.[108] Thus ethanol administration may stimulate an increase in portal flow by directly altering flow through the mesenteric bed. This action would be independent of the stimulation of oxygen consumption or metabolite production by the liver. Further, flow through the mesentery is extremely sensitive to the oxygen demands of the tissue. Increased oxygen consumption is accompanied by an increased flow through the bed. Alcohol dehydrogenase activity is present in many tissues, including the gastrointestinal tract. Recently it has been demonstrated that a sex-related difference in gastric alcohol dehydrogenase activity accounts for the higher blood alcohol observed in women compared to that observed in men after consumption of comparable amounts of alcohol.[113] It is therefore conceivable that ethanol metabolism could increase oxygen consumption by these splanchnic organs and thereby increase flow. It may not be necessary to invoke a hepatic mechanism to account for the increase in hepatic flow that appears to accompany increased oxygen consumption by the liver.

The development of portal hypertension as a consequence of liver disease is a major factor in mortality in alcoholics.[114] Increases in portal pressure could be in consequence of an increase in hepatic vascular resistance and/or an increase in portal blood flow. These two possibilities are incorporated into two theories that have been proposed for the development and maintenance of portal hypertension. Whipple[115] proposed that an increased hepatic vascular resistance accounted for the development of portal hypertension. The "forward flow" theory, in contrast, states that the maintenance of the portal hypertension is the result of an increased portal flow. The initiating factor in portal hypertension is an increased vascular resistance. The increased pressure results in the opening of portal venous collaterals, which reduce the elevated portal resistance.

Groszmann and colleagues[116–118] have developed a rat model in which chronic portal-vein stenosis produces a portal hypertension characterized by the development of portal-systemic shunts and an increase in portal-vein flow. In the cirrhotic rat with portal hypertension, a similar increase in portal flow has been described.[116] Using this model it has been estimated that 60% of the increase in portal pressure is attributable to an increased vascular resistance and 40% is attributable to increased portal flow.[117] More importantly, the initiation of the portal hypertension is attributable to an increase in hepatic portal resistance.[117] Pressure decreased rapidly after removal of constriction; however, changes in splanchnic flow were maintained.[119] In the stenotic portal hypertensive rat, ethanol induces a further increase in portal flow; however, there is no increase in portal pressure.[120] Although 8-phenyltheophylline blocks the increase in portal flow induced by ethanol, it has no effect on the increase caused by constriction of the portal vein, nor does it alter the elevated portal pressure. Finally, in the absence of circulating ethanol, hepatic blood flow is significantly decreased in alcoholic cirrhosis[121] and unchanged in the cirrhotic baboon.[99] It appears that portal hypertension may in part be sustained by an increase in splanchnic flow, but it does not appear to be the major factor initiating or maintaining the hypertension.

Changes in vascular resistance play a major role in initiating and maintaining portal hypertension. The site of this increased hepatic resistance is of some controversy. In the normal animal, the major site of hepatic resistance appears to be in the postsinusoidal veins.[122,123] In the cat, hepatic resistance is localized to a small segment of the hepatic vein, and in the dog it is localized to a segment of the hepatic vein just proximal to its entry into the vena cava. In the alcohol-fed baboon, fibrous tissue deposition around the terminal hepatic venules and adjacent sinusoids increases, and the degree of fibrosis correlates to the degree of portal hypertension.[25] Animals with fatty livers, but no thickening of the perivenular rims, did not exhibit portal hypertension. Hepatic-cell size increased significantly and to a similar degree in animals with and without portal hypertension when compared to control animals. Thus, in this model, portal hypertension appears to develop along with the appearance of fibrosis in the perivenular portion of the acinus.

A second anatomical site, the intrahepatic portal vein and sinusoids, has been postulated as the site of increased hepatic resistance producing portal hypertension. Direct measurement of pressure at various sites in hepatic vasculature of the normal and cirrhotic rat suggested that the intrahepatic portal vein and sinusoids were the sight of increased resistance in cirrhosis.[26] This hypothesis is also supported by the prevalence of hepatomegaly in alcoholic liver disease.[123,124] The hepatomegaly is the result of an increased hepatocyte size, rather than an increase in number of hepatocytes.[125–127] A major factor in the increased size is the osmotic effect exerted by an increased intracellular potassium concentration.[128] There is a strong correlation between hepatocyte size and the magnitude of portal hypertension.[129] A critical expansion in the size of the hepatocyte, approx 40%, appears to be required before portal pressure increases.[131] Expansion beyond this limit exceeds the capacity of the liver capsule to expand, and any further increase in hepatocyte size begins to decrease the extravascular space, causing an increased resistance. Infusion of hypotonic solutions produces an increased perfusion pressure, which is correlated to the expansion of hepatocytes.[130] The increased pressure and the increased hepatocyte size are rapidly reversed by perfusion with isotonic solutions.

In summary, the acute administration of ethanol leads to an increase in hepatic oxygen consumption. An increased flow from the portal vein to the liver compensates for the increase in oxygen demand. Chronic treatment with ethanol, in the absence of liver injury, does not alter this acute response, nor does it appear to alter hepatic flow. The increased portal flow is accounted for by a decreased vascular resistance and increased flow in the mesenteric bed perfusing the small intestine. This increased flow is dependent on the metabolism of ethanol, and recent evidence suggests that it is attributable to the production of adenosine formed within the splanchnic bed from acetate released by the liver. Perivenular hepatic necrosis is postulated to occur when the delivery of oxygen does not meet the demand. In the presence of hepatocyte injury, increased hepatic resistance occurs and initiates portal hypertension. This portal hypertension is maintained by both an increase in hepatic resistance and an increased portal flow. The site of this increased resistance has been suggested to be pre- and postsinusoidal, and may depend on the species under investigation.

References

[1] D. E. Donald (1983) Splanchnic circulation, in *Handbook of Physiology. Section 2: The Cardiovascular System,* vol. III: *Peripheral Circulation,* Part 1. J. T. Shepherd and F. M. Abboud, eds. American Physiological Society, Bethesda, MD, pp. 219–240.

[2] Secretary of Health and Human Services, Seventh special report to the U.S. Congress on alcohol and health. January 1990. National Institute on Alcohol Abuse and Alcoholism, Rockville, MD (DHHS publication [ADM] 90-1656). 1990.

[3] G. Pihan, D. Majzoulin, G. Haudenschied, J. S. Trier, and S. Szabo (1986) Early microcirculatory stasis in acute gastric mucosal injury in the rat and prevention by 16,16-dimethyl prostaglandin E_2 or sodium thiosulfate. *Gastroenterology* **91,** 1415–1426.

[4] C. F. Bou-Abboud, H. Wayland, G. Paulsen, and P. H. Guth (1988) Microcirculatory stasis precedes tissue necrosis in ethanol-induced gastric mucosal injury in the rat. *Dig. Dis. Sci.* **33,** 872–877.

[5] P. H. Guth, G. Paulsen, and H. Nagata (1984) Histologic and microcirculatory changes in alcohol-induced gastric lesions in the rat: Effect of prostaglandin cytoprotection. *Gastroenterology* **87,** 1083–1090.

[6] G. P. Morris and J. L. Wallace (1981) The role of ethanol and of acid in production of gastric mucosal erosions in the rat. *Virchows Arch. [Cell Pathol.]* **38,** 23–38.

[7] S. Szabo, J. S. Trier, A. Brown, and J. Schnoor (1985) Early vascular injury and increased permeability in gastric mucosal injury caused by ethanol in the rat. *Gastroenterology* **88,** 228–236.

[8] P. J. Oates and J. P. Hakkinen (1988) Studies on the mechanism of ethanol-induced gastric damage in rats. *Gastroenterology* **94,** 10–21.

[9] Y. Yonei and P. H. Guth (1989) Lipoxygenase metabolites in the rat gastric microvascular response to intragastric ethanol. *Gastroenterology* **97,** 304–312.

[10] B. M. Peskar, K. Lange, U. Hoppe, and B. A. Peskar (1986) Ethanol stimulates formation of leukotriene C_4 in rat gastric mucosa. *Prostaglandins* **31,** 283–293.

[11] B. J. R. Whittle, N. Oren-Wolman, and P. H. Guth (1985) Gastric vasoconstrictor actions of leukotriene C_4, $PGF_{2\alpha}$, and thromboxane mimetic U-46619 on rat submucosal microcirculation in vivo. *Am. J. Physiol.* **248,** G580–G586.

[12] J. L. Wallace, P. L. Beck, and G. P. Morris (1988) Is there a role for the leukotrienes as a mediator of ethanol-induced gastric mucosal damage? *Am. J. Physiol.* **254,** G117–G123.

[13] W. K. MacNaughton, G. Cirino, and J. L. Wallace (1989) Endothelium-derived relaxing factor (nitric oxide) has protective actions in the stomach. *Life Sci.* **45,** 1869–1876.

[14] M. T. Khan and R. F. Furchgott (1987) Similarities of behavior of nitric oxide (NO) and endothelium-derived relaxing factor in a perfusion cascade bioassay system. *Fed. Proc.* **46,** 385.

[15] L. T. Ignarro, R. E. Byrns, G. M. Buga, and K. S. Wood (1987) Endothelium-derived relaxing factor (EDRF) released from artery and vein appears to be nitric oxide or a closely related radical species. *Fed. Proc.* **46,** 644.

[16] R. M. Palmer, A. G. Ferrige and S. Moncada, S (1987) Nitric oxide release accounts for the biologic activity of endothelium-derived relaxing factor. *Nature* **327,** 524–526.

[17] L. T. Ignarro, R. E. Byrns, G. M. Buga, and K. S. Wood (1987) Endothelium-derived relaxing factor from pulmonary artery and vein possesses pharmacologic and chemical properties identical to those of nitric oxide radical. *Circ. Res.* **61,** 866–879.

[18] M. W. Radomski, R. M. Palmer, and S. Moncada (1987) The anti-aggregating properties of vascular endothelium: Interaction between prostacyclin and nitric oxide. *Br. J. Pharmacol.* **92,** 639–646.

[19] A. B. Ebeigbe, F. Cressier, M. K. Konneh, T. D. Luu, and L. Criscione (1990) Influence of N^G-monomethyl-L-arginine on endothelium-dependent relaxations in the perfused mesenteric vascular bed of the rat. *Biochem. Biophys. Res. Commun.* **169,** 873–879.

[20] L. Criscione, J. R. Powell, R. Burdet, S. Engesser, F. Schlager, and A. Schoepfer (1989) Alcohol suppresses endothelium-dependent relaxation in rat mesenteric vascular beds. *Hypertension* **13,** 964–967.

[21] W. W. Lautt and C. V. Greenway (1987) Conceptual review of the hepatic vascular bed. *Hepatology* **7,** 952–963.

[22] A. M. Rappaport (1973) The microcirculatory hepatic unit. *Microvasc. Res.* **6,** 212–228.

[23] C. A. Goresky (1981) Tracer behavior in the hepatic microcirculation, in *Hepatic Circulation in Health and Disease.* W. W. Lautt, ed. Raven, New York, pp. 25–38.

[24] P. D. I. Richardson and P. G. Withrington (1981) Liver blood flow. I. Intrinsic and nervous control of liver blood flow. *Gastroenterology* **81,** 159–173.

[25] W. W. Lautt, C. V. Greenway, D. J. Legare, and H. Weisman (1986) Localization of intrahepatic portal vascular resistance. *Am. J. Physiol.* **251,** G375–G381.

[26] D. J. Legare and W. W. Lautt (1987) Hepatic venous resistance site in the dog: Localization and validation of intrahepatic pressure measurements. *Can. J. Physiol. Pharmacol.* **65,** 352–359.

[27] W. W. Lautt (1977) Control of hepatic and intestinal blood flow: Effect of isovolemic haemodilution on blood flow and oxygen uptake in the intact liver and intestines. *J. Physiol.* **265,** 313–326.

[28] W. W. Lautt (1980) Control of hepatic arterial blood flow: Independence from liver metabolic activity. *Am. J. Physiol.* **239,** H559–H564.

[29] R. L. Huges, R. T. Mathie, W. Fitch, and D. Campbell (1980) Liver blood flow and oxygen consumption during metabolic acidosis and alkalosis in the greyhound. *Clin. Sci.* **60,** 355–361.

[30] W. W. Lautt (1977) The hepatic artery: Subservient to hepatic metabolism or guardian of normal hepatic clearance rates of humoral substances. *Gen. Pharmacol.* **8,** 73–78.

[31] W. W. Lautt (1985) Mechanism and role of intrinsic regulation of hepatic arterial blood flow: Hepatic arterial buffer response. *Am. J. Physiol.* **249,** G549–G556.

[32] W. W. Lautt (1981) Role and control of the hepatic artery, in *Hepatic Circulation in Health and Disease.* W. W. Lautt, ed. Raven, New York, pp. 203–220.

[33] W. W. Lautt, D. J. Legare, and W. R. Ezzat (1990) Quantitation of the hepatic arterial buffer response to graded changes in portal blood flow. *Gastroenterology* **98,** 1024–1028.

[34] W. W. Lautt, D. J. Legare, and M. S. D'Almedida (1985) Adenosine as putative regulator of hepatic arterial flow (the buffer response). *Am. J. Physiol.* **248,** H331–H338.

[35] W. W. Lautt and D. J. Legare (1985) The use of 8-phenyltheophylline as a competitive antagonist of adenosine and an inhibitor of the intrinsic regulatory mechanism of the hepatic artery. *Can. J. Physiol. Pharmacol.* **63,** 717–722.

[36] W. W. Lautt (1983) Relationship between hepatic blood flow and overall metabolism: The hepatic arterial buffer response. *Fed. Proc.* **42,** 1662–1666.

[37] R. T. Mathie, P. H. M. Lam, A. M. Harper, and L. H. Blumgart (1980) The hepatic arterial blood flow response to portal vein occlusion in the dog: Effect of hepatic denervation. *Pflugers Arch.* **386,** 77–83.

[38] P. D. I. Richardson (1982) Physiological regulation of the hepatic circulation. *Fed. Proc.* **41,** 2111–2116.

[39] W. R. Ezzat and W. W. Lautt (1986) Hepatic arterial pressure-flow regulation is adenosine mediated. *Am. J. Physiol.* **252,** H836–H845.

[40] P. D. I. Richardson and P. G. Withrington (1981) Liver blood flow. 2. Effects of drugs and hormones on liver blood flow. *Gastroenterology* **81,** 356–375.

[41] W. W. Lautt, M. S. D'Almeida, J. McQuaker, and L. D'Aleo (1988) Impact of hepatic arterial buffer response on splanchnic vascular responses to intravenous adenosine, isoproterenol and glucagon. *Can. J. Physiol. Pharmacol.* **66,** 807–813.

[42] S. Einzig, G. H. R. Rao, and J. G. White (1980) Differential sensitivity of regional vascular beds in the dog to low-dose prostacyclin infusion. *Can. J. Physiol. Pharmacol.* **58,** 940–946.

[43] N. Krarup (1975) Effects of histamine, vasopressin, and angiotensin II on hepatosplanchnic hemodynamics, liver function, and hepatic metabolism in cats. *Acta Physiol. Scand.* **95,** 311–317.

[44] P. D. I. Richardson and P. G. Withrington (1978) Responses of the simultaneously-perfused hepatic arterial and intra-portal venous vascular beds of the dog to histamine and 5-hydroxytryptamine. *Br. J. Pharmacol.* **64,** 581–588.

[45] L. L. Shanbour and L. B. Hinshaw (1969) Effects of dopamine on the liver before and following administration of endotoxin. *Can. J. Physiol. Pharmacol.* **47,** 923–928.

[46] R. Kullmann, W. R. Bruell, K. Wassermann, and A. Konopatzki (1983) Blood flow redistribution by dopamine in the feline gastrointestinal tract. *Naunyn-Schmiedebergs Arch. Pharmacol.* **323,** 145–148.

[47] P. D. I. Richardson and P. G. Withrington (1978) The effects of intro-arterial and intra-portal injections of vasopressin on the simultaneously perfused hepatic arterial and portal venous vascular beds of the dog. *Circ. Res.* **43,** 496–503.

[48] Y. Israel, H. Kalant, H. Orrego, J. M. Khanna, L. Videla, and J. M. Phillips (1975) Experimental alcohol-induced hepatic necrosis: Suppression by propylthiouracil. *Proc. Natl. Acad. Sci. USA* **72,** 1137–1141.

[49] Y. Israel, L. Videla, and J. Bernstein (1975) Hypermetabolic state after chronic ethanol consumption. Hormonal interrelations and pathogenic implications. *Fed. Proc.* **34,** 2052–2059.

[50] Y. Israel, H. Kalant, H. Orrego, J. M. Khanna, M. J. Phillips, and D. J. Stewart (1979) Hypermetabolic state: Oxygen availability and alcohol-induced liver damage, in *Biochemistry and Pharmacology of Ethanol.* E. Majchrowicz and E. P. Noble, eds. Plenum, New York, pp. 433–444.

[51] Y. Israel and H. Orrego (1981) Hepatocyte demand and substrate supply as factors in the susceptibility to alcoholic liver injury: Pathogenesis and prevention. *Clin. Gastroenterol.* **10,** 355–373.

[52] Y. Israel and H. Orrego (1987) Hypermetabolic state, hepatocyte expansion,

and liver blood flow: An interaction triad in alcoholic liver injury. *Ann. NY Acad. Sci.* **492,** 303–323.

[53] Y. Israel and H. Orrego (1984) Hypermetabolic state and hypoxic liver damage, in *Recent Developments in Alcoholism.* M. Galanter, ed. Plenum, New York, pp. 119–133.

[54] S. Shaw, E. A. Heller, H. S. Friedman, E. Baraona, and C. S. Lieber (1977) Increased hepatic oxygenation following ethanol administration in the baboon. *Proc. Soc. Exp. Biol. Med.* **156,** 509–513.

[55] N. Sato, T. Kamada, T. Schichiri, T. Matsumura, H. Abe, and B. Hagihara (1980) Effect of ethanol on hemoperfusion and oxygen sufficiency in livers in vivo. *Adv. Exp. Med. Biol.* **132,** 355–362.

[56] T. Yuki and R. G. Thurman (1980) The swift increase in alcohol metabolism: Time course for the increase in hepatic oxygen uptake and the involvement of glycolysis. *Biochem. J.* **186,** 119–126.

[57] J. P. Villeneuve, G. Pomier, and P. M. Huet (1981) Effect of ethanol on hepatic blood flow in unanesthetized dogs with chronic portal and hepatic vein catheterization. *Can. J. Physiol. Pharmacol.* **59,** 598–603.

[58] P. Jauhonen, E. Baraona, H. Miyakawa, and C. S. Lieber (1982) Mechanism for selective perivenular hepatoxicity of ethanol. *Alcohol. Clin. Exp. Res.* **6,** 350–357.

[59] T. Yuki, Y. Israel, and R. G. Thurman (1982) The swift increase in alcohol metabolism: Inhibition by propylthiouracil. *Biochem. Pharmacol.* **31,** 2403–2407.

[60] N. Sato, T. Kamada, S. Kawano, N. Hayashi, Y. Kishida, H. Meren, H. Yoshihara, and H. Abe (1983) Effect of acute and chronic ethanol consumption on hepatic tissue oxygen tension in rats. *Pharmacol. Biochem. Behav.* **18,** 443–447.

[61] J. E. Bredfeldt, E. M. Riley, and R. J. Groszmann (1985) Compensatory mechanisms in response to an elevated hepatic oxygen consumption in chronically ethanol-fed rats. *Am. J. Physiol.* **248,** G507–G511.

[62] C. S. Lieber, E. Baraona, R. Hernadez-Munoz, S. Kubota, N. Sato, S. Kawano, T. Matsumura, and N. Inatomi (1989) Impaired oxygen utilization. A new mechanism for the hepatotoxicity of ethanol in sub-human primates. *J. Clin. Invest.* **83,** 1682–1690.

[63] B. J. Kessler, J. B. Leibler, G. J. Bronfin, and M. Sass (1954) The hepatic blood flow and splanchnic oxygen consumption in alcoholic fatty liver. *J. Clin. Invest.* **33,** 1338–1345.

[64] L. Videla and Y. Israel (1970) Factors that modify the mechanism of ethanol in rat liver and adaptive changes produced by its chronic administration. *Biochem. J.* **118,** 275–281.

[65] L. Videla, J. Bernstein, and Y. Israel (1973) Metabolic alterations produced in the liver by chronic ethanol administration: Increased oxidative capacity. *Biochem. J.* **134,** 507–514.

[66] H. Iturriaga, G. Urgarte, and Y. Israel (1980) Hepatic vein oxygenation, liver blood flow and the rate of ethanol metabolism in recently abstinent patients. *J. Clin. Invest.* **10,** 211–218.

[67] S. Ji, J. J. Lemasters, V. Christenson, and R. G. Thurman (1982) Periportal and pericentral pyridine nucleotide fluorescence from the surface of the perfused liver: Evaluation of the hypothesis that chronic treatment with ethanol produces pericentral hypotoxia. *Proc. Natl. Acad. Sci. USA* **79,** 5415–5419.

[68] S. Ji, J. J. Lemasters, V. Christenson, and R. G. Thurman (1983) Selective increase in precentral oxygen gradient in perfused rat liver following ethanol treatment. *Pharmacol. Biochem. Behav.* **18,** 439–442.

[69] H. Orrego, J. E. Blake, A. Medline, and Y. Israel (1985) Interrelation of the hypermetabolic state, necrosis, anemia and cell enlargement as determinants of severity of alcoholic liver disease. *Acta Med. Scand.* **218,** 81–95.

[70] A. Hadengue, R. Moreau, S. S. Lee, C. Gaudin, B. Rueff, and D. Lebrec (1988) Liver hypermetabolism during alcohol withdrawal in human. *Gastroenterology* **94,** 1047–1052.

[71] C. S. Lieber and L. M. DeCarli (1976) Animal models of ethanol dependence and liver injury in rats and baboons. *Fed. Proc.* **35,** 1232–1236.

[72] H. Popper and C. S. Lieber (1980) Histogenesis of alcoholic fibrosis and cirrhosis in the baboon. *Am. J. Pathol.* **98,** 695–710.

[73] A. E. Rodgers, J. G. Fox, and L. S. Gottlieb (1981) Effects of ethanol and malnutrition on non-human primate liver, in *Frontiers of Liver Disease.* P. D. Berk and T. C. Chalmers, eds. Thieme–Stratton Inc., New York, pp. 165–175.

[74] S. W. French, N. C. Benson, and P. S. Sun (1984) Centrilobular liver necrosis induced by hypoxia in chronic ethanol fed rats. *Hepatology* **4,** 912–917.

[75] J. Lutz, H. Henrich, and E. Bauereisen (1975) Oxygen supply and uptake in the liver and intestine. *Pflugers Arch.* **360,** 7–15.

[76] F. J. Carmichael, V. Saldivia, Y. Israel, J. P. McKaigney, and H. Orrego (1987) Ethanol-induced increase in portal hepatic blood flow: Interference by anesthetic agents. *Hepatology* **7,** 89–94.

[77] H. Castenfors, E. Hultman, and B. Josephson (1960) Effect of intravenous infusions of ethyl alcohol on estimated hepatic blood flow in man. *J. Clin. Invest.* **39,** 776–781.

[78] A. I. Mendeloff (1954) Effect of intravenous infusions of ethanol upon estimated hepatic blood flow in man. *J. Clin. Invest.* **33,** 1298–1302.

[79] A. W. Childs, R. M. Kinel, and A. Lieberman (1963) Effect of ethyl alcohol on hepatic circulation, sulfobromophtalein clearance and hepatic glutamic-oxaloacetic transaminase production in man. *Gastroenterology* **45,** 176–180.

[80] S. W. Stein, C. S. Lieber, C. Leevy, G. R. Cherrick, and W. H. Abelman (1963) The effect of ethanol upon systemic and hepatic blood flow in man. *Am. J. Clin. Nutr.* **13,** 68–74.

[81] C. M. Smythe, H. O. Heinemann, and S. E. Bradely (1953) Estimated hepatic blood flow in the dog. Effect of ethyl alcohol on it, renal blood flow, cardiac output and arterial pressure. *Am. J. Physiol.* **172,** 737–742.

[82] F. Lundquist, N. Tygstrup, K. Winkler, H. Mellengaard, and S. Munck-Peterson (1962) Ethanol metabolism and production of free acetate in the human liver. *J. Clin. Invest.* **41,** 955–961.

[83] L. Jorfeldt and A. Juklin-Dannfeldt (1976) The influence of ethanol on splanchnic and skeletal muscle metabolism in man. *Metabolism* **27,** 97–106.

[84] I. R. Bravo, C. G. Acevedo, and V. Gallardo (1980) Acute effects of ethanol on liver blood circulation in the anesthetized dog. *Alcohol. Clin. Exp. Res.* **4,** 248–253.

[85] H. Iturriaga, D. Bunout, M. Petermann, G. Ugarte, and Y. Israel (1981) Effect of ethanol on hepatic blood flow in the rat. *Alcohol. Clin. Exp. Res.* **5,** 221–224.

[86] J. P. McKaigney, F. J. Charmichael, V. Saldivia, Y. Israel, and H. Orrego (1986) Role of ethanol metabolism in the ethanol-induced increase in splanchnic circulation. *Am. J. Physiol.* **250,** G518–G523.

[87] P. M. Huet, C. A. Goresky, J. P. Villeneuve, D. Marleau, and J. O. Lough (1982) Assessment of liver microcirculation in human cirrhosis. *J. Clin. Invest.* **70,** 1234–1244.

[88] C. M. Leevy, M. Silverberg, and J. Naylor (1963) Physiology of dye extraction by the liver: Comparative studies of sulfobromophthalin and indocyamine green. *Ann. NY Acad. Sci.* **111,** 161–175.

[89] K. Winkler, J. A. Larson, T. Munkner, and N. Tygstrup (1965) Determination of hepatic blood flow in man by the simultaneous use of five test substances measured in two parts of the liver. *Scand. J. Clin. Lab. Invest.* **17,** 423–432.

[90] J. Bartrum, D. M. Berkowitz, and N. K. Hollenberg (1974) A simple radioactive microsphere method for measuring regional flow and cardiac output. *Invest. Radiol.* **9,** 126–132.

[91] A. G. Malik, J. E. Kaplan, and T. M. Sabre (1976) Reference sample method for cardiac output and regional blood flow determinations in the rat. *J. Appl. Physiol.* **40,** 472–475.

[92] K. Nishiyama, A. Nishiyama, and E. Frolich (1976) Regional blood flow in normotensive and spontaneously hypertensive rats. *Am. J. Physiol.* **230,** 691–698.

[93] S. Ishise, B. I. Pegram, J. Yamamoto, Y. Kitamura, and E. D. Frolich (1980) Reference sample microsphere method: Cardiac output and blood flows in conscious rats. *Am. J. Physiol.* **239,** H443–H449.

[94] S. A. Jenkins, J. N. Baxter, P. Devitt, I. Taylor, and R. Shields (1986) Effects of alcohol on hepatic hemodynamics in the rat. *Digestion* **34,** 236–242.

[95] F. J. Carmichael, Y. Israel, V. Saldivia, H. G. Giles, S. Meggiorini, and H. Orrego (1987) Blood acetaldehyde and the ethanol-induced increase in splanchnic circulation. *Biochem. Pharmacol.* **36,** 2673–2678.

[96] M. Kogire, K. Inoue, R. Doi, S. Sumi, K. Takadori, M. Yun, T. Suzuki, and T. Tobe (1988) Effects of intravenous ethanol on hepatic and pancreatic blood flow in dogs. *Dig. Dis. Sci.* **33**, 592–597.

[97] H. Orrego, F. J. Carmichael, V. Saldivia, H. G. Giles, S. Sandrin, and Y. Israel (1988) Ethanol-induced increase in portal blood flow: Role of adenosine. *Am. J. Physiol.* **254**, G495–G501.

[98] A. Gulati, R. C. Srimal, and H. N. Bhargava (1989) Effect of varying concentration of ethanol on systemic hemodynamics and regional circulation. *Alcoholism* **6**, 9–15.

[99] B. Verma-Ansil, F. J. Carmichael, V. Saldivia, G. Varghese and H. Orrego (1989) Effect of ethanol on splanchnic hemodynamics in awake and unrestrained rats with portal hypertension. *Hepatology* **10**, 946–952.

[100] C. V. Greenway and W. W. Lautt (1990) Acute and chronic ethanol on hepatic oxygen ethanol and lactate metabolism in cats. *Am. J. Physiol.* **258**, G411–G418.

[101] H. Orrego, F. J. Carmichael, and Y. Israel (1988) New insights on the mechanism of the alcohol-induced increase in portal blood flow. *Can. J. Physiol. Pharmacol.* **66**, 1–9.

[102] J. M. Khanna and Y. Israel (1980) Ethanol metabolism. *Int. Rev. Physiol.* **21**, 275–315.

[103] J. L. Egle, P. M. Hudgins, and F. M. Lai (1973) Cardiovascular effects of intravenous acetaldehyde and propionaldehyde in the anesthetized rat. *Toxicol. Appl. Pharmacol.* **24**, 636–644.

[104] J. Nakano, A. G. Gin, and S. K. Nakano (1974) Effects of disulfiram on cardiovascular responses to acetaldehyde and ethanol in dogs. *Q. J. Stud. Alcohol.* **35**, 620–634.

[105] L. Y. Koda, S. G. Madamba, and F. E. Bloom (1984) Hypotensive response of ethanol in rats pretreated with disulfiram or nitrefazole. *Life Sci.* **35**, 1659–1665.

[106] B. M. Altura, A. Carella, and B. T. Altura (1978) Acetaldehyde on vascular smooth muscle: Possible role in vasodilator action of ethanol. *Eur. J. Pharmacol.* **52**, 73–83.

[107] B. M. Altura and A. Gebrewold (1981) Failure of acetaldehyde or acetate to mimic the splanchnic arteriolar or venular dilator actions of ethanol: Direct *in situ* studies on the microcirculation. *Br. J. Pharmacol.* **73**, 580–582.

[108] B. M. Altura and B. T. Altura (1982) Microvascular and vascular smooth muscle actions of ethanol, acetaldehyde, and acetate. *Fed. Proc.* **41**, 2447–2451.

[109] F. J. Carmichael, V. Saldivia, G. A. Varghese, Y. Israel, and H. Orrego (1988) Ethanol induced increase in portal blood flow: Role of acetate and A1- and A2-adenosine receptors. *Am. J. Physiol.* **255**, G417–G423.

[110] D. N. Granger, J. D. Valleau, R. E. Parker, R. S. Lane, and A. E. Taylor (1978) Effects of adenosine on intestinal hemodynamics, oxygen delivery and capillary fluid exchange. *Am. J. Physiol.* **235**, H707–H719.

[111] R. M. Burger and J. M. Lowenstein (1970) Preparation and properties of 5'-nucleotidases from smooth muscle of small intestine. *J. Biol. Chem.* **245,** 6274–6280.

[112] L. E. Nagy, I. Diamond, D. J. Casso, C. Franklin, and A. S. Gordon (1990) Ethanol increases extracellular adenosine by inhibiting adenosine uptake via the nucleoside transporter. *J. Biol. Chem.* **265,** 1946–1951.

[113] M. Frezza, C. diPadova, G. Pozzato, M. Terpin, E. Baraona, and C. S. Lieber (1990) High blood alcohol levels in women. The role of decreased gastric alcohol dehydrogenase activity and first-pass metabolism. *N. Engl. J. Med.* **322,** 95–99.

[114] H. O. Conn and R. J. Groszmann (1982) The pathophysiology of portal hypertension, in *The Liver: Biology and Pathobiology.* I. M. Arias, H. Popper, D. Schicter, and D. A. Shafritz, eds. Raven, New York, pp. 821–848.

[115] A. O. Whipple (1945) The problem of portal hypertension in relation to the hepatosplenopathies. *Ann. Surg.* **122,** 449–475.

[116] J. Vorobioff, J. E. Bredfeldt, and R. J. Groszmann (1983) Hyperdynamic circulation in portal-hypertensive rat model: A primary factor for maintenance of chronic portal hypertension. *Am. J. Physiol.* **244,** G52–G57.

[117] J. Vorobioff, J. E. Bredfeldt, and R. J. Groszmann (1984) Increased blood flow through the portal system in cirrhotic rats. *Gastroenterology* **87,** 1120–1126.

[118] R. J. Groszmann, J. Vorobioff, and E. Riley (1982) Splanchnic hemodynamics in portal-hypertensive rats: Measurement with γ-labeled microspheres. *Am. J. Physiol.* **242,** G156–G160.

[119] J. N. Benoit, W. A. Womack, L. Hernandez, and D. N. Granger (1985) "Forward" and "backward" flow mechanisms of portal hypertension. Relative contributions in the rat model of portal vein stenosis. *Gastroenterology* **89,** 1092–1096.

[120] E. Sikuler, D. Kravetz, and R. J. Groszmann (1985) Evolution of portal hypertension and mechanisms involved in its maintenance in a rat model. *Am. J. Physiol.* **248,** G618–G625.

[121] E. Sikuler and R. J. Groszmann (1986) Interaction of flow and resistance in maintenance of portal hypertension in a rat model. *Am. J. Physiol.* **250,** G205–G212.

[122] J. Caesar, S. Shaldon, L. Chiandussi, L. Guevara, and S. Sherlock (1961) The use of indocyamine green in the measurement of hepatic blood flow and as a test of hepatic function. *Clin. Sci.* **21,** 43–57.

[123] H. Miyakawa, S. Iida, M. A. Leo, R. J. Greenstein, D. S. Zimmon, and C. S. Lieber (1985) Pathogenesis of precirrhotic portal hypertension in alcohol-fed baboons. *Gastroenterology* **88,** 143–150.

[124] Y. Shibayama and K. Nakata (1985) Localization of increased hepatic vascular resistance in liver cirrhosis. *Hepatology* **5,** 643–648.

[125] H. J. Fallon (1975) Alcoholic liver disease, in *Abnormal Protein Biosynthesis: Biochemical and Clinical.* M. A. Rothschild, M. Oratz, and S. S. Schreiber, eds. Pergamon, New York, pp. 473–490.

[126] J. G. D. Rankin, H. Orrego-Matte, J. Deschenes, A. Medline, J. E. Findlay, and A. I. M. Armstrong (1978) Alcoholic liver disease: The problem of diagnosis. *Alcohol. Clin. Exp. Res.* **4,** 327–338.

[127] E. Baraona, M. A. Leo, S. A. Borowsky, and C. S. Lieber (1975) Alcoholic hepatomegaly: Accumulation of protein in the liver. *Science* **190,** 794,795.

[128] Y. Israel, J. M. Khanna, H. Orrego, G. Rachamin, S. Wahid, R. Britton, A. Macdonald, and H. Kalant (1979) Studies on metabolic tolerance to alcohol, hepatomegaly and alcoholic liver disease. *Drug Alcohol Depend.* **4,** 109–118.

[129] H. Orrego, L. M. Blendis, I. R. Crossley, A. Medline, A. Macdonald, S. Ritchie, and Y. Israel (1981) Correlation of intrahepatic pressure with collagen in the Disse space and hepatomegaly in humans and in the rat. *Gastroenterology* **80,** 546–556.

[130] Y. Israel, H. Orrego, J. C. Colman, and R. S. Britton (1981) Alcohol-induced hepatomegaly: Pathogenesis and role in the production of portal hypertension. *Fed. Proc.* **41,** 2472–2477.

[131] L. M. Blendis, H. Orrego, I. R. Crossley, J. E. Blanke, A. Medline, and Y. Israel (1982) The role of hepatocyte enlargement in hepatic pressure in cirrhotic and noncirrhotic alcoholic liver disease. *Hepatology* **2,** 539–546.

Interaction of Ethanol and the Glucocorticoids

Effects on Hepatic Gene Expression

Rolf F. Kletzien

Introduction

The liver is the central warehouse and processing center for nutrients and, as such, is subject to control by a variety of hormones. In addition, it is the organ that first encounters drugs carried in by the portal blood. For these reasons, ingestion of alcohol can result in changes in hepatic metabolism leading to alcohol-induced liver disorders. Prominent among these is that of alcoholic fatty liver, a syndrome seen in 90–100% of heavy drinkers[1] and to some extent in others following modest intake of ethanol. This syndrome, which may result from increased synthesis of fatty acids or a defect in packaging or secretion of lipoproteins, represents a change in the phenotype of the hepatocyte. Underlying this phenotypic change is an alteration of gene expression. It has been the goal of our research program to attempt to understand at a molecular level how alcohol causes these changes in gene expression.

We have employed adult rat liver parenchymal cells in primary culture as the model cell system to carry out our studies. In this system, the cells exhibit the terminally differentiated phenotype and are maintained in a serum-free, chemically defined medium.[2,3] Thus, it is possible to define

From: *Drug and Alcohol Abuse Reviews, Vol. 2: Liver Pathology and Alcohol*
Ed: R. R. Watson ©1991 The Humana Press Inc.

precisely effects of nutrients, hormones, or drugs (ethanol), individually or in combination, on metabolism and gene expression. Using this system, we have demonstrated that ethanol enhances the expression of a lipogenic enzyme, glucose-6-phosphate dehydrogenase (G6PDH; EC1.1.1.49) during induction of hepatic lipogenesis by the glucocorticoids and insulin. We have demonstrated that ethanol, in combination with the glucocorticoids and insulin, induced G6PDH activity,[4] relative rate of G6PDH protein synthesis,[5] functional mRNA encoding G6PDH,[5,6] and hybridizable mRNA encoding G6PDH.[7,8]

Ethanol is a commonly ingested drug that has numerous metabolic consequences, some of which are dependent on diet and nutritional status.[9] In addition, ethanol consumption can affect the secretion of several hormones including the glucocorticoids,[10,11] which then secondarily alter hepatic metabolism. The synthesis of fatty acids in liver is known to be regulated by the glucocorticoids in addition to insulin[12,13] and the development of alcoholic fatty liver appears to depend to some extent on the glucocorticoids.[14,15] Therefore, understanding the mechanism by which ethanol and the glucocorticoids regulate G6PDH may illuminate some of the underlying, fundamental molecular mechanisms by which ethanol can alter hepatic gene expression and influence the development of alcoholic fatty liver.

It is clear from the literature[12] and our studies on G6PDH that the ethanol-mediated increase in glucocorticoid secretion coupled with direct effects of ethanol on liver, results in inappropriate enhancement of insulin action in liver, specifically, exaggeration of insulin-stimulated lipogenesis. I will first review what is known about how ethanol causes increased glucocorticoid secretion and, subsequently, lipogenesis. Second, I will review what is known about metabolite regulation of hepatic metabolism at the level of gene expression, since it is likely that ethanol or a metabolite of ethanol is exerting influence at this level. The final sections of this review will deal with our model cell system and the results we have obtained with it.

Ethanol and the
Hypothalamic-Pituitary-Adrenal Axis

Ethanol consumption elicits corticotropin releasing factor (CRF) secretion in humans and experimental animals, which ultimately results in secretion of the adrenal glucocorticoids.[11,16–18] Clinical studies have established that acute or chronic consumption of ethanol causes hypercortisolemia,[11,16] occasionally to the extent that pseudo-Cushing's syndrome is apparent.[18,19] In rats, acute administration of ethanol results in dose-related increases in corticosterone levels[17] and this effect can be blocked by removal of the pituitary gland.[10]

Increased glucocorticoid concentrations in humans and experimental animals have been shown to be associated with elevated rates of hepatic lipogenesis and increased concentrations of hepatic and plasma lipids.[13,20–22] Physiological concentrations of the glucocorticoids in conjunction with insulin are required to observe the enhanced lipogenesis associated with refeeding rats a high carbohydrate diet following a 24-h fast.[23,24] Studies employing primary cultures of hepatocytes in a chemically defined medium have shown that the glucocorticoids amplified the effect of insulin on hepatic lipogenesis.[12] Thus, the hepatic stearatosis and hyperlipidemia observed in situations of glucocorticoid excess, seem to be the result of glucocorticoid enhancement of insulin-stimulated lipogenesis.

Considering that ethanol consumption increases glucocorticoid secretion and that the glucocorticoids enhance insulin-stimulated hepatic lipogenesis, it is likely that the glucocorticoids are involved in the development of alcoholic fatty liver. Indeed, early studies revealed that adrenalectomy in rats blocked the appearance of fat accumulation in liver caused by ethanol.[14] Additionally, it was shown that the degree of hepatic fat accumulation was a function of the ethanol dose and that chronic ethanol consumption caused hypertrophy of the adrenals.[14] This study has been confirmed under somewhat different experimental conditions[15] and strongly suggests involvement of the glucocorticoids in the development of alcoholic fatty liver.

Metabolite Regulation
of Hepatic Gene Expression:
The Metabolite Response System

Recent studies have shown that nutrients, such as D-glucose, D-fructose, fatty acids, and sterols, can affect the expression of hepatic genes. Earlier studies had revealed that feeding animals high levels of either carbohydrates or lipid[23,25] could affect the levels of certain enzymes. The problem with results from intact animals was that one could not be certain that the effect was directly that of the nutrient or that of some hormone or other factor that could not be appropriately controlled. With the advent of defined culture systems it has been possible to demonstrate with a high degree of precision that nutrients or their metabolites inhibit or activate the expression of hepatic genes. We have called this control mechanism the metabolite response system and suggest that ethanol effects on gene expression are, to some extent, mediated through this system.

Carbohydrate regulation of Type L pyruvate kinase has been explored in detail. Kahn et al. have demonstrated that carbohydrate refeeding transiently increases transcription of the pyruvate kinase gene in liver.[26,27] Differences were apparent in the kinetics of the increase depending on whether the carbohydrate was glucose or fructose. Earlier work from our laboratory demonstrated that the level of D-glucose in the culture medium could affect the level of G6PDH expression.[4] We have subsequently demonstrated in animals that transcription of the gene is transiently activated following carbohydrate refeeding.[28] Other examples of carbohydrate regulation of gene expression are known[29] and there is likely some unifying theme in terms of molecular mechanism.

Lipid metabolites or nutrients are also known to regulate gene expression. For example, expression of several enzymes that are involved in lipid metabolism appear to be repressed by feeding animals a high fat diet or by incubating cells in tissue culture with high levels of fatty acids.[25,30–32] In some cases, this appears to be the result of inhibition of transcription.[32] Indeed, genes that encode enzymes involved in cholesterol metabolism can be repressed by the presence of the end product of the pathway. The *cis*-elements (sterol response elements) that mediate this regulation have been cloned and their activity in chimeric plasmid constructs characterized.[33]

The molecular details of a metabolite response system for regulation of hepatic gene expression are not known. However, it is clear that this system in combination with hormonal regulation modulates the flow of carbon through the pathways of lipid and carbohydrate metabolism. Ethanol could potentially influence both aspects of metabolic control since it increases glucocorticoid levels[11,16-18] and, secondly, we will demonstrate here that ethanol influences the metabolite response system. We speculate that it is the sum of these two effects that cause metabolic abnormalities to occur in liver following alcohol ingestion.

Primary Cultures of Hepatocytes: A Model for Ethanol Studies

The study of ethanol/nutrient/hormonal regulation of hepatic metabolism is facilitated by the use of a system in which the effects of ethanol and hormones added singly, simultaneously, or sequentially can be studied on the target cell. Studies involving hormonal regulation of liver cell metabolism have employed several different liver preparations. The parenchymal cells constitute less than 80% of the cells present in liver and, therefore, it is difficult to relate data specifically to the parenchymal cell when studying the intact liver in vivo or in vitro as perfused liver or liver slices. In addition, the effects of the endogenous substrates present during the experiment or immediately prior to the time the liver was excised have to be considered. This is particularly important with the glucocorticoids since they generally produce responses of long duration. Although hormonal regulation can be conveniently studied in tissue culture, established lines of liver cells have lost certain differentiated functions, such as the ability to carry out gluconeogenesis, glycogenesis, and glycogenolysis. Therefore, the established liver cell lines are often inadequate for carrying out studies involving hormonal or metabolite control of metabolism.

For short-term studies, suspensions of liver parenchymal cells isolated by the Berry and Friend technique[34] and freed of nonparenchymal cells by centrifugation, are adequate when incubation times are not longer than a few hours. However, this system has two shortcomings. First, the cells are in suspension and evidence does exist to show that cells that are normally in an attached matrix must be attached to a substrate to carry out complex functions.[35] Second, treatments that require several hours to elicit a response are impossible since the cells do not remain viable during this time frame. Prior treatment of animals is an option, but one is left with the uncertainty of precisely which factor is responsible for the effect on the cells.

The aforementioned problems are overcome by plating the parechymal cells onto a collagen coated dish or into a three-dimensional mesh of collagen and connective tissue fibers. Inoculation of the freshly isolated hepatocytes onto collagen coated dishes results in attachment of cells within 2–4 h.[2,3] The cells are then stable as nonreplicating, monolayer cultures for up to 2 wk and much longer times are possible if cells are in a three-dimensional network.[36] The cells can be maintained in serum-free chemically defined medium or in medium containing fetal calf or calf serum. For longer term maintenance in the serum-free medium, one must supplement the medium with factors to preserve viability and differentiated function. In our hands the most important factor is epidermal growth factor (EGF), but we do not add nicotinic acid, which is often added with EGF.[37] When the cells are maintained in the EGF containing medium, they are not exposed to many of the hormones, growth factors, and nutrients present in serum-containing culture medium or in vivo. Furthermore, any compensatory changes that might occur in vivo after hormone injection or surgical treatment (e.g., adrenalectomy) that affect liver function are avoided. This approach allows cells time to repair injuries incurred during isolation. Experiments lasting several days can be carried out in a medium that is completely defined as to what hormones/nutrients are present. This method was initially developed for rat hepatocytes but has been adapted for use with primate hepatocytes including humans.[38] Hormonal responsiveness of primate hepatocytes appears to be similar to rat when maintained in culture under the aforementioned conditions.[39]

The accumulation of fat in the liver is one of the earliest and most common disturbances of lipid metabolism that is observed resulting from ethanol intake.[1] The mechanisms by which ethanol causes the accumulation of fat in liver are undoubtedly multifocal and involve an interplay of hormones, nutrients, and ethanol. Dissecting complex interactions such as this in an experimental animal is difficult since one cannot be certain that a specific experimental manipulation results in direct effects on liver vs indirect effects owing to the action of another organ or metabolic process in response to the experimental manipulation. Thus, use of the primary cultures of hepatocytes maintained in a well-controlled, chemically defined environment presents an experimental stage for understanding how the combinations of ethanol with nutrients and hormones can elicit changes in hepatic gene expression.

Ethanol Regulation of Glucose-6-Phosphate Dehydrogenase: Experimental Studies in Rat Hepatocytes

Glucose-6-phosphate dehydrogenase (G6PDH) is the key rate-limiting enzyme in the pentose phosphate pathway. This hepatic enzyme is at the interface of carbohydrate and lipid metabolism in that the enzyme obviously metabolizes carbohydrate, but it is induced at a time when the liver is synthesizing fatty acids from excess dietary carbohydrate. The NADPH produced in the pentose phosphate pathway is utilized for the biosynthesis of fatty acids and cholesterol. It is considered to be in the constellation of lipogenic enzymes, since it is induced during times of elevated lipogenesis. Indeed, studies with livers from intact animals have shown that the four key, lipogenic enzymes (acetyl CoA carboxylase, fatty acid synthase, malic enzyme, G6PDH) are induced by insulin and the glucocorticoids during normal hepatic lipogenesis,[23,24,40] although only G6PDH exhibits the large "overshoot" induction after refeeding fasted animals a high carbohydrate diet.[24]

Regulation of Enzyme Activity and Relative Rate of Synthesis

Our initial interest in G6PDH regulation in primary cultures of hepatocytes was to determine how the glucocorticoids and insulin interacted to regulate the expression of the enzyme. As noted earlier,[23,24,40] it had been known for some time from studies with intact animals that both insulin and the glucocorticoids were involved in regulation of hepatic lipogenesis and induction of the lipogenic enzymes. Our goal was to ascertain whether the effect of the glucocorticoids and insulin was a direct effect on liver or an indirect effect involving other factors. The primary culture of rat hepatocytes is a system ideally suited to use in answering this type of question.

Our initial results demonstrated that the glucocorticoids by themselves did not influence G6PDH activity. They did, however, enhance the induction of the enzyme by insulin.[4] The maximum effect of the glucocorticoids was observed at 100 nM, but no effect on the enzyme was observed at concentrations above this unless insulin was also present. During the course of these studies we found that the level of D-glucose in the culture medium influenced the level of G6PDH activity observed in the presence or absence of the hormones.[4] Thus, one could incubate the cells in a culture medium, such as S-77, which contains 5 mM glucose, and supplement it with higher glucose concentrations to obtain higher levels of activity. This was our first indication that a metabolite response system participated in the regulation of G6PDH.

While the preceding studies were in progress, we tested several glucocorticoid analogs for their ability to enhance insulin's induction of G6PDH. Some of the analogs were dissolved in DMSO and others in ethanol. We

Table 1
Regulation of G6PDH Activity and mRNA in Primary Cultures
of Hepatocytes Treated with Hormones, Glucose, and Ethanol[a]

Condition	Activity, mU/mg	mRNA, relative U
Control	7.25 ± 0.35	2.9 ± 0.15
Ethanol (eth)	7.45 ± 0.22	3.1 ± 0.10
High glucose (HG)	12.10 ± 0.91	5.2 ± 0.35
Eth $\pm$ HG	17.35 ± 1.05	7.5 ± 0.55
Dex, ins, HG	24.70 ± 1.33	10.1 ± 0.67
Dex, ins, HG, eth	32.65 ± 1.10	13.4 ± 0.78

[a]Primary cultures of rat hepatocytes were incubated for 48 h in S-77 medium containing either 5.5 mM D-glucose or 27.5 mM (designated high glucose). Ethanol (30 mM), dexamethasone (1 μM), and Insulin (45 mU/mL) when present were incubated with the cultures for 48 h. G6PDH activity and G6PDH mRNA were assayed as described previously.[4,5] Each value represents the mean $\pm$ SE for four (activity) or five (mRNA) determinations.

realized that the large degree of variability that we were observing in these studies was the result of ethanol enhancing the effect of the glucocorticoids, whereas the solvent DMSO did not exhibit this effect. We then carried out studies on the time course and ethanol dose response of this effect.[4] We found that the maximum effect of ethanol was observed at a dose of 30 mM (liver would be expected actually to see higher doses during alcohol ingestion) and that the effect of ethanol required several hours of incubation to be observed, a result consistent with a requirement for induction of G6PDH gene expression. Thus, none of the effects that we examined were the result of post-translational activation of the enzyme; rather, these were increases mediated by changes in either transcription or translation.

The first indication that the ethanol enhancement of G6PDH activity was related to the metabolite response system came in experiments published earlier. We reported that no effect of ethanol on G6PDH was noted if cells were incubated in medium containing 5 mM glucose.[4] In the experiments shown in Table 1, ethanol did not enhance G6PDH activity unless elevated glucose concentration was present in the medium. Thus, ethanol and glucose directly affect the expression of G6PDH, but the precise details of how this occurs is not understood. Ethanol can also be considered to enhance G6PDH activity indirectly since ethanol would cause glucocorticoid levels to increase, which then enhances insulin induction of G6PDH.

To establish that the increased enzyme activity was in fact the result of increased enzyme protein and not activation of preexisting enzyme, we carried out a series of studies on the relative rate of G6PDH synthesis.[5] Using a monospecific G6PDH antibody, we demonstrated that increased synthesis of G6PDH followed increased G6PDH activity.[5] Thus, the interaction of ethanol, D-glucose, insulin, and the glucocorticoids resulted in increased synthesis of G6PDH. Ethanol and high glucose were sufficient to elevate synthesis 1.8-fold, whereas simultaneous incubation of ethanol, insulin, and glucocorticoid increased it 5.5-fold. Our next goal was to determine if these hormones, nutrients, and ethanol increased the amount of mRNA encoding G6PDH or if they increased the rate of translation of a constant amount of mRNA.

Molecular Studies on G6PDH mRNA

Our early studies on G6PDH mRNA employed in vitro translation systems and utilized a G6PDH antibody to identify nascent G6PDH synthesized from mRNA added to the system. These studies demonstrated that insulin and the glucocorticoids elevated G6PDH mRNA, but insulin appeared to be required for translation.[5,41] Ethanol also elevated mRNA encoding G6PDH,[5,6] and the effect was additive with that of the glucocorticoids and insulin. In order to explore these issues in greater depth we needed to utilize molecular probes for G6PDH. However, only one laboratory had reported the successful cloning of G6PDH from any source,[42] and this was later retracted.[43] Therefore, we had to carry out the molecular cloning of G6PDH mRNA from liver.

We utilized the G6PDH antibody to immuno-enrich polysomes with nascent G6PDH from livers of rats fed a high carbohydrate diet. Several cDNA clones were obtained and were used to demonstrate that G6PDH mRNA in livers of intact animals could be regulated by diet.[7] This was the first reported cloned G6PDH cDNA from any source.[7] The major portions of the rat G6PDH gene and pseudogene have also been isolated using these probes.[28,44]

The effect of insulin and the glucocorticoids on G6PDH mRNA has been studied in primary cultures of rat hepatocytes using the molecular probes. We demonstrated that G6PDH mRNA levels were increased by both hormones and that simultaneous incubation caused an additive increase.[8] A result that confirmed earlier findings was that the glucocorticoids increased G6PDH mRNA but not the relative rate of synthesis or enzyme activity.[5] Thus, insulin appears to be required for increased translation and can increase the level of G6PDH mRNA as well. The glucocorticoids elevate the level of mRNA, but that is not sufficient for expression of G6PDH at the level of the protein. We have recently extended this work to demonstrate that ethanol and D-glucose also exert effects on G6PDH mRNA (Table 1). There is the suggestion that both are working through the same system (metabolite response system) and that ethanol can directly affect the level of mRNA for this enzyme if the cells are in a medium containing high glucose concentrations.

The aforementioned studies demonstrated that mRNA levels encoding G6PDH can be elevated within the cell following ethanol/nutrient/hormone treatment. The increased mRNA could be the result of increased transcription or a change in the stability of the mRNA. Therefore, a series of studies were carried out to look at transcriptional activity of the gene and stability of the G6PDH mRNA. A prerequisite of these studies was to isolate a genomic G6PDH fragment that would contain enough sequence such that sufficient amounts of the nascent G6PDH would hybridize to it and detection would be carried out in a reliable fashion.[28] Initial studies were carried out in intact animals subjected to a high carbohydrate diet. We found that refeeding previously fasted animals a high carbohydrate diet resulted in a transient activation of the G6PDH gene.[28] This increased transcription occurred approx 5–10 h after refeeding, and the level decreased back to nearly control levels after 48–72 h. However, increased transcription did not account for all of the increase in mRNA. The G6PDH mRNA stability clearly increased also during this time frame (2 h vs 9–11 h).[28] Thus, both increased transcription and increased mRNA stability accounted for the increase in the livers of intact animals fed a high carbohydrate diet.

We have recently carried out a similar study in primary cultures of hepatocytes (Table 2). Our results demonstrate that both insulin and the glucocorticoids are responsible for transcriptional increases in the G6PDH gene and appear to do very little with respect to mRNA stability, although insulin displays a modest effect. Ethanol and D-glucose exhibit quite a different effect. Neither causes any increase in the transcription assay, but both influence the stability of G6PDH mRNA. Note that the ethanol effect is really dependent on the presence of glucose (higher than 5 m*M*). Thus, ethanol and glucose appear to exert influence through the metabolite response system, whereas the primary effect of the hormones is at transcription.

Table 2
Regulation of G6PDH Transcription and mRNA Stability
in Primary Cultures of Hepatocytes[a]

Condition	Transcription, ppm	mRNA half-life, h
Control	5.5 ± 0.45	14.0
Ethanol (eth)	5.3 ± 0.50	14.2
High glucose (HG)	5.5 ± 0.37	26.4
Eth, HG	5.7 ± 0.42	38.9
Ins	7.7 ± 0.65	18.3
Dex	8.9 ± 0.71	14.4
Dex, ins	13.9 ± 0.96	14.4
Dex, ins, eth	14.1 ± 1.10	14.6
Dex, ins, eth, HG	13.7 ± 0.76	37.5

[a]Primary cultures of rat hepatocytes were incubated for 48 h in S-77 medium containing 5.5 mM D-glucose or 27.5 mM (designated high glucose). Also included in the 48 h incubation where indicated were ethanol (30 mM), dexamethasone (1 μM), and insulin (45 mU/mL). G6PDH "run off" transcription rate and G6PDH mRNA half-life were determined as described previously.[28] Each value for the transcription rate represents the mean ± SE for six determinations. Each mRNA half-life value was determined from five time points with duplicate culture dishes per point.

Future Molecular Studies

The goal of our future studies will be to identify the sequences in the G6PDH gene and mRNA responsible for regulation of G6PDH mRNA production. With respect to hormone regulation, transcription appears to be the primary site of control. Plasmid constructs utilizing the G6PDH promoter fused to a reporter will be transfected into cells and the transcriptional activity analyzed. With respect to the direct effects of ethanol regulation of G6PDH, there are two facets to the problem. First, the interaction of ethanol and glucose in the metabolite response system is not understood. Experiments will need to be carried out to define this system and to dissect its components. Second, the sequences in the G6PDH mRNA that are important for stability will need to be identified. In this regard, recent work has suggested that the 3' flank of mRNA contains important sequence elements that are involved in mRNA stability.[45,46] Thus, we have replaced the 3' flank of the pSV2CAT construct with the 3' flank of the G6PDH gene and have successfully expressed this construct in primary cultures of rat hepatocytes.

Preliminary indications are that this construct contains sufficient information to increase mRNA levels. Work is in progress to define more precisely the sequences involved.

Conclusions

Our studies employing adult rat liver parenchymal cells in primary culture have demonstrated that ethanol can regulate the level of expression of a key lipogenic enzyme. Ethanol has both direct and indirect effects in this system. The direct effect is mediated through the metabolite response system and results in increasing the stability of the mRNA encoding G6PDH. The indirect effect is mediated through the ethanol-induced release of CRF, which results in elevated glucocorticoid levels. Our studies have demonstrated that the glucocorticoids enhance the action of insulin. This causes an increase in G6PDH transcription. We speculate that other key lipogenic enzymes are similarly increased and that alcoholic fatty liver development is related to these changes in gene expression.

Acknowledgments

This study was supported by Grant AA06728 from the N.I.A.A.A.

References

[1] B. F. Grant, M. C. DuFour, and T. C. Harford. (1988) Epidemiology of alcoholic liver disease. *Semin. Liver Dis.* **8,** 12–25.

[2] R. F. Kletzien, M. W. Pariza, J. E. Becker, V. R. Potter, and F. R. Butcher (1976) Induction of amino acid transport in primary cultures of adult rat liver parenchymal cells by insulin. *J. Biol. Chem.* **251,** 3014–3020.

[3] R. F. Kletzien, C. A. Weber, F. R. Butcher, and D. J. Stumpo (1982) Glucagon and choleragen stimulation of glycogenolysis in primary cultures of adult rat liver parenchymal cells: Lack of involvement of the glucocorticoids. *J. Cell. Physiol.* **110,** 304–310.

[4] D. S. Kelley and R. F. Kletzien (1984) Ethanol modulation of the hormonal and nutritional regulation of glucose 6-phosphate dehydrogenase activity in primary cultures of rat hepatocytes. *Biochem. J.* **217,** 543–549.

[5] D. J. Stumpo and R. F. Kletzien (1985) The effect of ethanol, alone and in combination with the glucocorticoids and insulin, on glucose-6-phosphate dehydrogenase synthesis and mRNA in primary cultures of hepatocytes. *Biochem. J.* **226,** 123-130.

[6] D. J. Stumpo, C. R. Prostko, and R. F. Kletzien (1985) Ethanol and gluco-corticoid regulation of glucose 6-phosphate dehydrogenase. *Alcohol. Clin. Exp. Res.* **2,** 169–172.

[7] R. F. Kletzien, C. R. Prostko, D. J. Stumpo, J. K. McClung, and K. L. Dreher (1985) Molecular cloning of DNA sequences complementary to rat liver glucose 6-phosphate dehydrogenase mRNA: Nutritional regulation of mRNA levels. *J. Biol. Chem.* **260,** 5621–5624.

[8] R. S. Fritz, D. S. Stumpo, and R. F. Kletzien (1986) Glucose 6-phosphate dehydrogenase mRNA sequence abundance in primary cultures of rat hepatocytes: Effect of insulin and dexamethasone. *Biochem. J.* **237,** 617–619.

[9] E. Mezey (1985) Metabolic effects of alcohol. *Fed. Proc.* **44,** 134–138.

[10] J. C. Crabbe and H. Rigter (1980) Hormones, peptides, and ethanol response, in *Alcohol Tolerance and Dependence.* H. Rigter and J. C. Crabbe, eds. Elsevier, Amsterdam, pp. 293–316.

[11] R. Kakihana and J. A. Moore (1976) Circadian rhythm of corticosterone in mice: The effect of chronic consumption of alcohol. *Psychopharmacology* **46,** 301–307.

[12] J. M. Amatruda, S. A. Danahy, and C. L. Chang (1983) The effect of the glucocorticoids on insulin-stimulated lipogenesis in primary cultures of rat hepatocytes. *Biochem. J.* **212,** 135–139.

[13] E. P. Reaven, O. G. Kolterman, and G. M. Reaven (1974) Ultrastructural and physiological evidence for corticosteroid-induced alterations in hepatic production of very low density lipoprotein particles. *J. Lipid Res.* **15,** 74–81.

[14] S. Mallov and J. L. Bloch (1956) Role of hypophysis and adrenals in fatty infiltration of liver resulting from acute ethanol intoxication. *Am. J. Physiol.* **184,** 29–51.

[15] R. P. Maickel and B. B. Brodie (1963) Interaction of drugs with the pituitary-adreno-cortical system in the production of the fatty liver. *Ann. NY Acad. Sci.* **104,** 1059–1065.

[16] J. S. Jenkins and J. Connolly (1968) Adrenocortical response to ethanol in man. *Br. Med. J.* **2,** 804–806.

[17] C. Rivier, T. Bruhn, and W. Vale (1984) Effect of ethanol on the Hypothalamic-pituitary-adrenal axis in the rat: Role of corticotropin releasing factor (CRF). *J. Pharm. Exp. Ther.* **229,** 127–134.

[18] S. W. J. Lamberts, J. G. M. Klign, and J. C. DeJong (1979) Hormonal secretion in alcohol-induced Pseudo-Cushing's syndrome. *J. Am. Med. Assoc.* **242,** 1640–1646.

[19] L. H. Rees, G. M. Besser, W. J. Jeffcoate, D. J. Goldie, and V. Marks (1977) Alcohol-induced Pseudo-Cushing's syndrome. *Lancet* **412,** 726–728.

[20] C. J. Kirk, T. R. Vecrinder, and D. A. Hems (1976) Fatty acid synthesis in the perfused liver of adrenalectomized rats. *Biochem. J.* **156,** 593–601.

[21] J. D. Bagdade, E. Yess, J. Albers, and O. J. Pykalalisto (1976) Glucocorticoids and triglyceride transport. *Metab. Clin. Exp.* **25**, 533–538.

[22] S. Diamont and E. Shafrir (1975) Modulation of the activity of insulin-dependent enzymes of lipogenesis by glucocorticoids. *Eur. J. Biochem.* **53**, 541–548.

[23] C. D. Berdanier and D. Shubeck (1979) Interaction of glucocorticoids and insulin in the responses of rats to starvation-refeeding. *J. Nutr.* **109**, 1766–1772.

[24] D. J. Bouillon and C. D. Berdanier (1980) Role of glucocorticoids in adaptive hyperlipogenesis in the rat. *J. Nutr.* **110**, 286–291.

[25] D. S. Kelley, J. J. Watson, D. O. Mack, and B. C. Johnson (1975) Repression of lipogenic enzymes by dietary fat. *Nutr. Rep. Int.* **12**, 121–129.

[26] S. Vaulont, A. Munnich, J. Decaux, and A. Kahn (1986) Transcriptional and post-transcriptional regulation of L-type pyruvate kinase gene expression in rat liver. *J. Biol. Chem.* **261**, 7621–7625.

[27] A. Munnich, S. Lyonnet, D. Chauvet, E. Van Schaftingen, and A. Kahn (1987) Differential effects of glucose and fructose on liver L-type pyruvate kinase gene expression in vivo. *J. Biol. Chem.* **262**, 17,065–17,071.

[28] C. R. Prostko, R. S. Fritz, and R. F. Kletzien (1989) Nutritional regulation of hepatic glucose 6-phosphate dehydrogenase: Transient activation of transcription. *Biochem. J.* **258**, 295–299.

[29] F. M. Matschinsky (1990) Glucokinase as glucose sensor and metabolic signal generator in pancreatic B-cells and hepatocytes. *Diabetes* **39**, 647–652.

[30] P. S. Hamblin, Y. Ozawa, A. Jefferds, and C. N. Mariash (1989) Interaction between fructose and glucose on the regulation of the nuclear precursor for mRNA-S14. *J. Biol. Chem.* **264**, 21,646–21,651.

[31] L. M. Salati, B. Adkins-Finke, and S. D. Clarke (1988) Free fatty acid inhibition of the insulin induction of glucose 6-phosphate dehydrogenase in rat hepatocyte monolayers. *Lipids* **23**, 36–41.

[32] S. D. Clarke, M. K. Armstrong, and D. B. Jump (1990) Dietary polyunsaturated fats uniquely suppress rat liver fatty acid synthase and S14 mRNA content. *J. Nutr.* **120**, 225–231.

[33] J. R. Smith, T. F. Osborne, M. S. Brown, G. L. Goldstein, and G. Gil (1988) Multiple sterol regulatory elements in promoter for hamster 3-hydroxy-3-methylglutaryl-coenzyme A synthase. *J. Biol. Chem.* **263**, 18,480–18,487.

[34] M. N. Berry and D. S. Friend (1969) High yield preparation of isolated rat liver parenchymal cells. A biochemical and fine structure study. *J. Cell Biol.* **43**, 506–520.

[35] G. Schreiber and M. Schreiber (1973) The preparation of single cell suspensions from liver and their use for the study of protein synthesis. *Subcell. Biochem.* **2**, 321–367.

[36] J. C. Y. Dunn, M. L. Yarmush, H. G. Koebe, and R. G. Tompkins (1989) Hepatocyte function and extracellular matrix geometry: Long-term culture in a sandwich configuration. *Fed. Proc.* **3**, 174–177.

[37] C. Inoue, H. Yamamoto, T. Nakamura, A. Ichihara, and H. Okamoto (1989) Nicotinamide prolongs survival of primary cultured hepatocytes without involving loss of hepatocyte-specific functions. *J. Biol. Chem.* **264**, 4747–4750.

[38] C. Guguen-Guillouzo, J. P. Campion, P. Brissot, D. Glaise, B. Launois, M. Bourel, and A. Guillouzo (1982) High yield preparation of isolated human adult hepatocytes by enzymatic perfusion of the liver. *Cell Biol. Int. Rep.* **6**, 625–628.

[39] R. G. Ulrich, D. G. Aspar, C. T. Cramer, R. F. Kletzien, and L. C. Ginsberg (1990) Isolation and culture of hepatocytes from the Cynomologous monkey *in vitro*. *Cell. Dev. Biol.* **26**, 815–823.

[40] R. Wurdeman, C. D. Berdanier, and R. B. Tobin (1978) Enzyme overshoot in starved-refed rats: Role of the adrenal glucocorticoids. *J. Nutr.* **108**, 1457–1463.

[41] D. J. Stumpo and R. F. Kletzien (1984) Regulation of glucose 6-phosphate dehydrogenase mRNA by insulin and the glucocorticoids in primary cultures of rat hepatocytes. *Eur. J. Biochem.* **144**, 497–502.

[42] M. G. Persico, D. Toniolo, C. Nobile, M. D'Urso, and L. Luzzato (1981) Molecular cloning of human glucose 6-phosphate dehydrogenase from erythrocytes. *Nature* **294**, 778–780.

[43] G. Martini, D. Toniolo, T. Vulliamy, L. Luzzatto, R. Dono, G. Viglietto, G. Paonessa, M. D'Urso, and M. G. Persico (1986) Structural analysis of the X-linked gene encoding human glucose 6-phosphate dehydrogenase. *EMBO J.* **5**, 1849–1855.

[44] R. S. Fritz, K. D. Dreher, E. A. Jones, and R. F. Kletzien (1991) Analysis of the glucose 6-phosphate dehydrogenase gene, pseudogene, and cDNA. *Nuc. Acids Res.* In press.

[45] J. Ross and G. Kobs (1986) H4 histone messenger RNA decay in a cell-free extract initiates at or near the 3' terminus and proceeds 3' to 5'. *J. Mol. Biol.* **188**, 579–593.

[46] E. W. Mullner and L. Kuhn (1988) A stem-loop in the 3' untranslated region mediates iron-dependent regulation of transferrin receptor mRNA stability in the cytoplasm. *Cell* **53**, 815–825.

Genetic and Dietary Control of Alcohol Degradation in *Drosophila*

Role in Cell Damage

Billy W. Geer, Robert R. Miller, Jr., and Pieter W. H. Heinstra

Introduction

Because of the consumption of ethanol-containing beverages by humans, information about the metabolism of ethanol is important. To be an alcoholic, a person need only consume enough ethanol to interfere with one of his or her important activities within our society. The decrease in efficiency of workers, the loss of life in alcohol-related accidents, and the personal grief are the result of the physiological and biochemical effects of ethanol. Chronic alcoholism is a health hazard to many individuals and, as such, poses a variety of social and economic problems.

Ethanol is detoxified in humans mainly by alcohol dehydrogenase (ADH, EC 1.1.1.1) in the liver, but secondary ethanol-degrading (MEOS) pathways involving catalase and the microsomal ethanol-oxidizing system have been speculated to be of varied importance.[1] Chronic alcohol consumption can lead to defects in lipid metabolism and transport in the human

From: *Drug and Alcohol Abuse Reviews, Vol. 2: Liver Pathology and Alcohol*
Ed: R. R. Watson ©1991 The Humana Press Inc.

liver.[2] The elucidation of the genetic and dietary factors that control alcohol degradation is of prime importance to understanding the biochemical basis of alcohol toxicity and alcohol-abuse-related pharmacological consequences.

Drosophila melanogaster is a logical experimental subject for studies of the biochemical basis of ethanol tolerance. *D. melanogaster* is an established laboratory organism and can be subjected to controlled and defined conditions over many generations, and there is a wealth of information on its genetics, biochemistry, physiology, and ecology. *D. melanogaster* feeds on fermenting plant materials, in which ethanol is the most abundant of several short-chain alcohols in the natural environment.[3–5] *D. melanogaster* is quite tolerant to the toxic effects of ethanol and efficiently uses ethanol as a food.[6–9]

We have chosen *D. melanogaster* as a model system in which to study the metabolic adaptations to ethanol. Consequently, the purpose of this chapter is to review the information about the dietary and genetic control of alcohol degradation in *D. melanogaster* and to relate it to cell damage.

The Metabolic Role
of the Larval Fat Body

During its life cycle, *D. melanogaster* undergoes complete metamorphosis (*see* Fig. 1 for some examples). Embryonic development is completed within 24 h after the egg is oviposited, and the larva emerges to begin a period of feeding and rapid growth. Under optimal environmental conditions, the larva increases in size and completes its growth in about 6 d. The larval fat body is a key to the metabolism of this growth period. The fat body is located between the viscera and the musculature of the body wall and extends bilaterally from the anterior region of the body to the most posterior segment.[10] Because it is the center of metabolism, the insect fat body has been compared to the vertebrate liver. Protein, lipid, and glycogen stores are deposited in the fat body during the larval period and are used during pupal development. When growth is completed, the larva attaches to a firm, dry substrate and forms a pupal case around its body. During the next 6 d, almost all the larval tissues are replaced by adult tissues. When pupal development is complete, the adult ecloses and becomes sexually mature within 12 h. Most of the activities of the adult flies are devoted to reproduction.

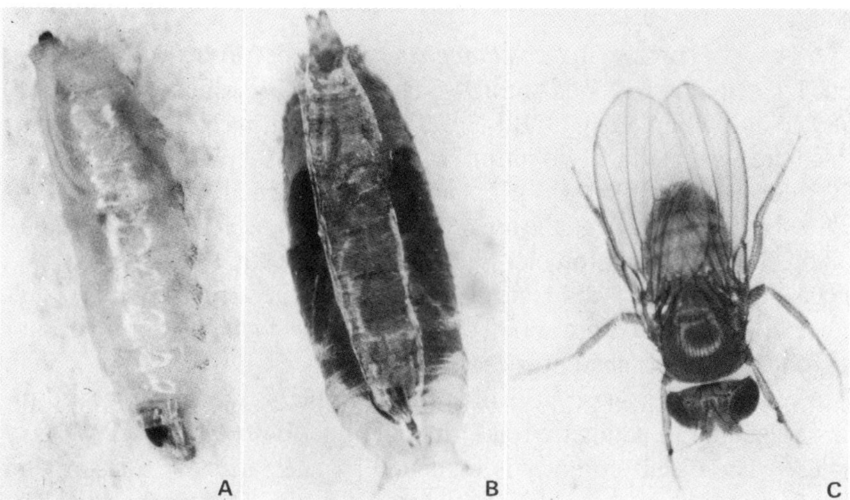

Fig. 1. Some life stages of the fruit fly *D. melanogaster* are shown. **A** is a third-instar larva, **B** is a pupa, and **C** is an adult male.

The eggs of *D. melanogaster* are typically deposited on fermenting plant materials. As a result, the capacity of the relatively immobile larva to detoxify and utilize environmental alcohols is crucial for survival and growth. To this end, ADH, the initial enzyme of the major pathway for ethanol degradation, is concentrated in the larval gut and fat body. Consequently, ethanol is efficiently converted into lipid in the larval fat body.[11,12]

The Genetics, Evolution, and Biochemistry of the *Drosophila* ADH Gene–Enzyme System

Since ADH plays a prominent role in alcohol degradation, a concise overview of the regulation of *Adh* expression, ADH properties, and a possible evolutionary history follow. For detailed information, one is referred to two recent reviews.[13,14]

The Adh *Gene*

The ADH protein in *D. melanogaster* is encoded by a single structural gene located on the second chromosome at 50.1 U,[15] which is cytogenetically found within bands 35B2–3.[16] The *Adh* gene includes three exons, which are separated by two introns of 65 bp and 70 bp in length (Fig. 2). The three exons are 96 bp, 405 bp, and 264 bp in length, respectively.[17–19] *Adh* is transcribed through the use of two promoters, which are separated by 708 bp. The proximal promoter is active during the three larval instars, and the distal promoter is active during the late, third larval instar and the adult stage.[20,21] Sequences from –5000 to +2510 relative to the transcription start site of the distal promoter are necessary to produce wild-type expression in all developmental stages.[22] The proximal promoter is repressed in third-instar larvae and in adults by transcriptional interference of the distal promoter.[23] The distal promoter is regulated by stage-specific transcription factors that bind to the distal promoter and to the adult enhancer.[24] The temporal expression of the *Adh* gene is regulated in a complex manner. Two upstream enhancer modules,[22,23,25] as well as stage-specific protein factors that bind to specific DNA sequence motifs, are upstream from the promoters. Two of these protein factors have been identified: Adf-1, a 34 kDa protein, and Adf-2[13,24,26–28] (*see* Fig. 2).

A variety of putative 5' regulatory transcriptional activation sites was also identified by means of footprinting methods in which certain DNA sequences are protected upon torsional stress.[29] In short, *cis*- and *trans*-acting regulatory elements functioning on short-genetic distance are involved in the temporal and tissue-specific expression of the *Adh* gene. Transposable genetic elements with sizes up to 5.2 kilobases inserted 400 bp or 3 kilobases 5' of the distal promoter have been suggested to affect the stage-specific expression of the *Adh* gene.[30,31] Long-distance modifiers were localized on the X- and third chromosome by conventional genetic methods.[32–35] However, their mode of action on the expression remains unknown.

The Evolution
of Drosophila Alcohol Dehydrogenase

Although the evolutionary history of *Drosophila* ADH is still not well understood, some novel aspects have recently emerged. Through analysis of primary sequences, it has become apparent that *Drosophila* ADH bears

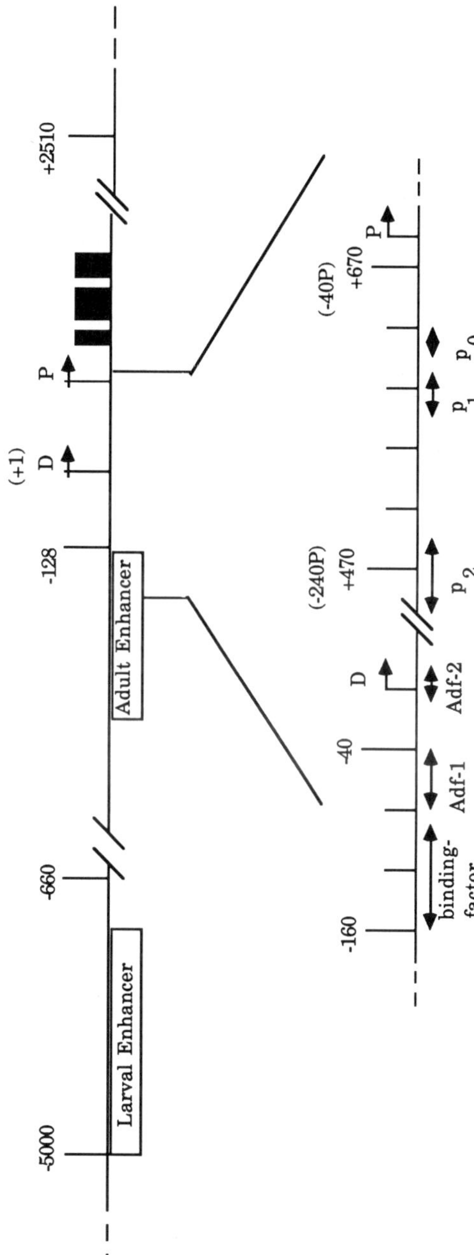

Fig. 2. General organization of the *Adh* gene of *D. melanogaster* (compiled from refs. 19–28). The enhancer regions (open boxes), promoters (distal and proximal), and the three exons (black boxes) are indicated. Footprint regions are represented by p0, p1, and p2, whereas Adf-1 and Adf-2 are transcription factors (for details, *see text*).

little homology with its yeast and mammalian counterparts.[36] However, within the NAD-binding region, small similarities exist. This suggests a common ancestor for several dehydrogenases and kinases.[37–39] *Drosophila* ADH specifically belongs to the "shortchain" type of dehydrogenases that are not dependent on metals as cofactors. As a result, *Drosophila* ADH is distantly related to bacterial sugar dehydrogenases[40] and to mammalian steroid/prostaglandin dehydrogenases.[41] The first 140 *N*-terminal residues within *Drosophila* ADH may be involved in coenzyme binding and exhibit some homology with corresponding C-terminal regions of ADH isolated from other sources.[19]

Residues 140–185 of *Drosophila* ADH show strong similarity to the *act*III gene product from several Streptomyces species.[42] In *Streptomyces*, the *act*III product is known to be involved in polyketide biosynthesis and is related to the β-ketoacyl reductase portion of the multifunctional enzyme complex, fatty acid synthetase.[43,44] C-terminal residues 231–255 show homology with rabbit phosphorylase residues 344–368.[19] Although the functional relationship of these regions is not yet known, the primary sequence similarities between these proteins are intriguing and certainly deserve further biochemical exploration.

Natural populations of *D. melanogaster* are polymorphic for two common alleloenzymes, ADH-F and ADH-S. These two ADHs differ by a single amino acid, and ADH-F is thought to be the most recently evolved protein.[14]

The Biochemistry of Drosophila *Alcohol Dehydrogenase*

The 255 total amino acid residues of the *Drosophila* ADH protein form a homodimer that has a mol wt of approx 54,800 daltons.[45] Exon 1 codes for the residues 1–32, exon 2 codes for residues 33–167, and exon 3 codes for residues 168–255.[19] *Drosophila* ADH requires NAD^+, but enzymatic activity is not dependent on metal ions.[46,47] Site-directed mutagenesis has recently shown that mutation of the N-terminal glycine at position 14 strongly affects coenzyme binding,[39] whereas the cysteine residue at position 218 is close to the catalytic domain. Mutation of lysine-192 affects the dissociation of the ADH:NADH binary complex.[48–50] N- and C-terminal amino acids at positions 1,82, 192, and 214 are distinguishing residues for some naturally occurring genetic variants of *Drosophila* ADH. Replacements at these residues have dramatic effects on the inhibition constants toward NADH and/or acetaldehyde,[51,52] so the whole tertiary structure seems to be quite important for catalysis.

The ADH of *D. melanogaster* displays different catalytic mechanisms when different substrates are used. There is a large kinetic isotope effect in vitro that has been noted when deuterated ethanol was compared to protonated ethanol at pH 9.5[50] and at pH 7.4.[51] This indicates that there is a rate-limiting conversion of ternary complexes when primary alcohols are used as substrates and that the mechanism is "rapid equilibrium." Product-inhibition patterns at pH 7.4 when NADH and acetaldehyde were employed under varying NAD^+ and ethanol concentrations suggested a "rapid-equilibrium random" mechanism concurrent with multiple dead-end inhibition and/or allosteric effects by acetaldehyde.[51,52] The prevalence of a "rapid-equilibrium ordered" mechanism at pH 9.5 was suggested mainly by inhibition studies with trifluoroethanol as an alternate inhibitor.[53] The dissociation of the ADH:NADH binary complex is then also rate-limiting. The reason for the discrepancy in the deduction of the mechanism remains unknown and cannot be explained by the effect of different pHs.[53] However, it should be borne in mind that *Drosophila* ADH is able to dehydrogenate acetaldehyde into acetate in vitro[11,47,54–56] as well as in vivo (ref. 56; *see also below*), and this makes it difficult to infer the catalytic mechanism reliably. With secondary alcohols, a Theorell-Chance type of mechanism predominates because the dissociation of the binary ADH:NADH complex solely is rate-limiting.[48–50]

At pH 7, the activity of *Drosophila* ADH is approximately eight times higher with secondary alcohols as substrates than with primary alcohols.[53,55] Ketones produced from secondary-alcohol oxidation form abortive ADH:NAD–ketone ternary complexes.[57–60] Each subunit of *Drosophila* ADH contains a coenzyme binding site and a catalytic region.[48,49] When one subunit of *Drosophila* ADH is occupied with the NAD–ketone complex, the ADH is identified as isoenzyme ADH-3. When associated with two complexed subunits, the ADH is identified as isozyme ADH-1. Uncomplexed ADH is referred to as the ADH-5 isoenzyme.[55,59] ADH-1 is the least active, but most stable, form, whereas ADH-5 is the most active isoenzyme, but is the least stable.[59] When moderate amounts of ethanol are consumed, the relative concentrations of ADH-3 and ADH-5 increase in wild-type *D. melanogaster* larvae.[8] These changes may constitute a relatively rapid mode for the adaptation of larvae to environmental ethanol.

Whether *Drosophila* ADH catalyzes the second step of ethanol degradation has been debated. According to one viewpoint, aldehyde dehydrogenase (ALDH, EC 1.2.1.3.) is responsible for the conversion of acetaldehyde to acetate.[61,62] Meanwhile, others claim that *Drosophila* ADH catalyzes the conversion of acetaldehyde into acetate.[11,47,54,63,64] This putative dual function of *Drosophila* ADH was recently analyzed by means of in vivo tracer studies.[56] The ALDH-enzyme activity was almost completely inhibited in vivo by prefeeding larvae cyanamide, whereas the ADH activity was only mildly affected. Under these conditions the in vivo flux from ethanol into lipid was only mildly decreased, indicating that ADH catalyzes the first two steps of ethanol degradation.

Control of the Ethanol-Degrading Pathway in Drosophila

Several lines of evidence indicate that wild-type *D. melanogaster* larvae metabolize approx 90% of ingested ethanol by the ADH pathway. In vivo studies supporting this stance include the incorporation of ^{14}C-ethanol into lipid,[11,56,65] alcohol accumulation patterns as analyzed by gas-liquid chromatography,[12,55,60,66,67] and ^{13}C nuclear magnetic resonance spectroscopy studies.[68] *In situ* studies indicate that the larval fat body handles approx 60% of ADH-mediated metabolism, whereas the alimentary tract handles approx 30%.[56,69,70]

Other studies suggest that the ADH system exerts major control over the ethanol catabolic pathways, at least in third-instar larvae. Kapoun et al.[67] observed in vivo a kinetic isotope effect of about a factor of three in wild-type third-instar larvae. This suggests that a similar "rapid equilibrium" mechanism prevails in vivo, and that the pro-S transfer of hydrogen from ethanol to NAD$^+$ [14] represents a significant rate-determining step. Through the use of six different wild-type strains of *D. melanogaster*, ADH activity in larvae was correlated to the in vivo flux of label from ^{14}C-ethanol into lipid, and a correlation coefficient of 0.92 was observed.[71] Other tracer studies, using cyanamide-treated wild-type larvae of *D. melanogaster* and *D. simulans,* have correlated ADH activity and aldehyde dehydrogenase activity (ALDH, EC 1.2.1.3.) to the flux of label from ^{14}C-ethanol into lipid. These studies produced a "flux control coefficient" (as defined in ref. 65) of 0.86 ± 0.12 when comparing ADH activity, and of 0.02 ± 0.07 when comparing ALDH activity, to lipid flux (*see* Fig. 3, ref. 72). However, similar studies performed with adult *D. melanogaster* of different strains produced

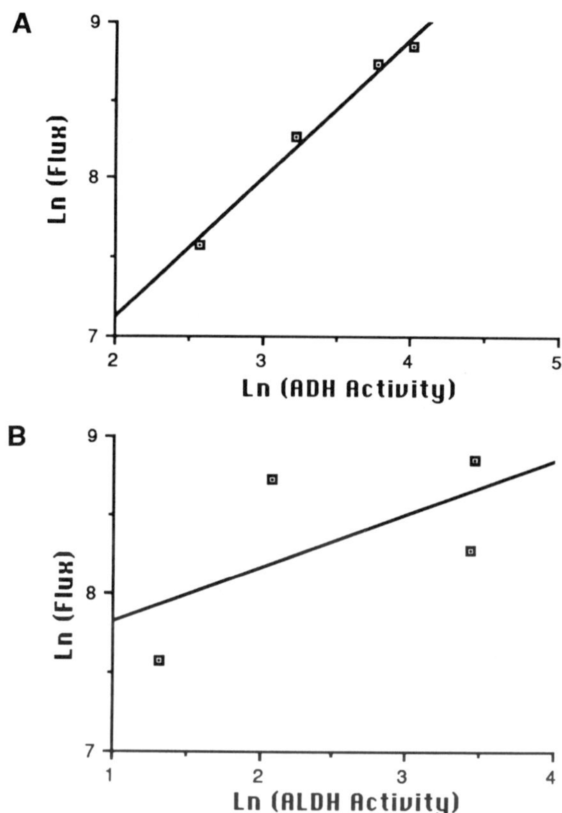

Fig. 3. Relationships between ^{14}C-ethanol-into-lipid fluxes and **(A)** alcohol dehydrogenase (ADH) and **(B)** aldehyde dehydrogenase (ALDH) activities. The slope of the plots determines the "flux control coefficient" as defined in ref. 65.

conflicting results. When ADH activity was correlated to the flux of label from ^{14}C-ethanol into lipid and carbon dioxide, a flux control coefficient of only 0.04 ± 0.10 was found.[65] It can be anticipated that the general metabolic physiology in larvae is different from that of the adult, providing a plausible explanation for the aforementioned differences in metabolic control.

Dietary Modulation of the ADH Pathway

Ethanol, methanol, *n*-propanol, isopropanol, and *n*-butanol all are commonly found in areas in which *D. melanogaster* larvae are present.[4] ADH activity increases in mid-third instar larvae of *D. melanogaster* within 5 h after exposure to ethanols, and the larval (proximal) *Adh* transcript increases within 2 h.[73] Presumably, this represents a mode of adaptation of larvae to environmental ethanol, because the flux from ethanol to lipid is also increased when ADH is induced by ethanol.[73] This may also explain why adults who, as larvae, have been administered relatively low concentrations of ethanol in a defined diet are heavier than adults who were fed an ethanol-free diet as larvae.[71] Consequently, the conversion of ethanol to nontoxic products, such as lipid, appears to be an important means of detoxifying ethanol for larvae.

McKechnie and Geer[8] found that ADH activity was increased in both the fat body and the gut of wild-type larvae that were fed a moderate concentration (2.5% v/v) of ethanol. Wild-type larvae can survive up to 6% dietary ethanol. ADH was induced by ethanol in cultured larval fat body and larval gut, establishing that ADH induction occurs in isolated organs.[74] The observation that the proximal *Adh* transcript increased in <2 h in isolated fat body after the initial ethanol exposure, whereas the amplification of ADH activity occurred in <3 h was expected. The in vitro penetration of ethanol into intact cells is most likely more rapid than the in vivo entrance of ethanol into cells of larvae that are fed alcohol. In either case, the induction of ADH activity is relatively rapid and may be important when the alcohol content of the environment changes.

In order to determine which DNA sequences are required for the induction of *Adh*, P-element-transformed strains of *D. melanogaster*, which possess deletions 5' to the *Adh* gene, have been tested.[67] A sequence between −110 and −187 of the proximal promoter start site (p_1 in Fig. 2) was found to be essential for the induction of Adh by ethanol. A DNA sequence between −660 and about −5000 of the distal transcript start site was also found to be important for the down-regulation of the induction response. It is likely that these sequences bind regulatory proteins that function as "second messengers."

Trivinos and Geer[74] noted that all primary alcohols of four carbons or less were effective inducers of ADH. Although the capacities of different alcohols for induction appeared to differ in isolated larval fat body and larval gut, the spectrum of alcohols that exerted an inducing action on the *Adh* of the two tissues were the same.

Dietary alcohols exert at least three biochemical effects on *D. melanogaster* larvae. First, elevated concentrations of alcohols are toxic and inhibit growth. Second, alcohols may be substrates for the ADH pathway and may be converted to beneficial end products.[11] Third, alcohols may be inducers of ADH and increase the capacity of the ADH pathway for alcohol degradation. The mechanism for tolerance to the toxic effects of alcohols seems to be relatively specific. That is, *D. melanogaster* larvae can tolerate a much higher level of dietary ethanol than the other shortchain, primary alcohols. This may be the product of a selective process that is based on the fact that ethanol is usually the most concentrated alcohol in the environment.[4]

The capacities of alcohols to serve as substrates for ADH or as inducers of ADH are similar, but possess some marked differences. An inducer of ADH does not have to be a substrate. Although methanol is an in vivo *Adh* inducer, it is not a substrate. Nonetheless, methanol is a competitive inhibitor of ADH in vitro.[14] On the other hand, isopropanol is a substrate for ADH and is converted into acetone, a compound that inactivates ADH.[55] Furthermore, isopropanol induces the proximal (larval) *Adh* transcript.

Most likely, it is beneficial for *D. melanogaster* to be subject to a broad spectrum of ADH inducers. *Drosophila* encounters a number of alcohols in its environment and must be capable of adapting. The species accomplishes this by degrading the alcohols to nontoxic substrates. The presence of a variety of inducing alcohols allows ADH, with its broad substrate specificity, to amplify in order to degrade the alcohols that are in the environment.

The Metabolic Profile of Ethanol Degradation

As in humans,[75] the metabolism of ethanol in *D. melanogaster* occurs mainly through oxidative pathways.[66] In order to understand the general dietary and genetic control of alcohol degradation, the routes of carbon flow of ethanol to products must be established. Two methods have been employed for *D. melanogaster*. These include ^{14}C-ethanol tracer studies.[11,65] and studies utilizing ^{13}C nuclear magnetic resonance (NMR).[68] The ^{14}C-ethanol tracer studies indicate that dietary ethanol is an excellent substrate for the *de novo* synthesis of lipid in both third-instar larvae and adults. In the ^{13}C NMR studies, the following enrichment patterns were observed when [2-^{13}C]-ethanol was fed to wild-type *D. melanogaster* larvae: citrate-C(2),4; succinate-C2,3; glutamate-C2,3,4; glutamine-C2,3,4; proline-C2,3,4; lactate-C2,3; alanine-C2,3; and all six carbon atoms of trehalose (Fig. 4). This indicates significant carbon flow from ethanol into these compounds.

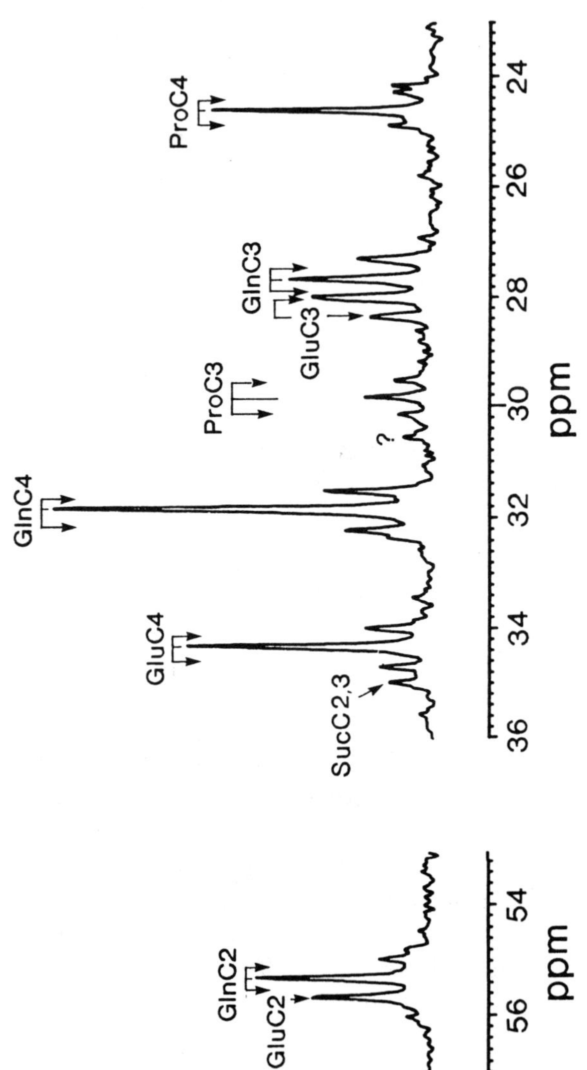
ProC4
GlnC3
GluC3
ProC3
GlnC4
GluC4
SucC 2,3
?
ppm
24
26
28
30
32
34
36
GlnC2
GluC2
ppm
54
56

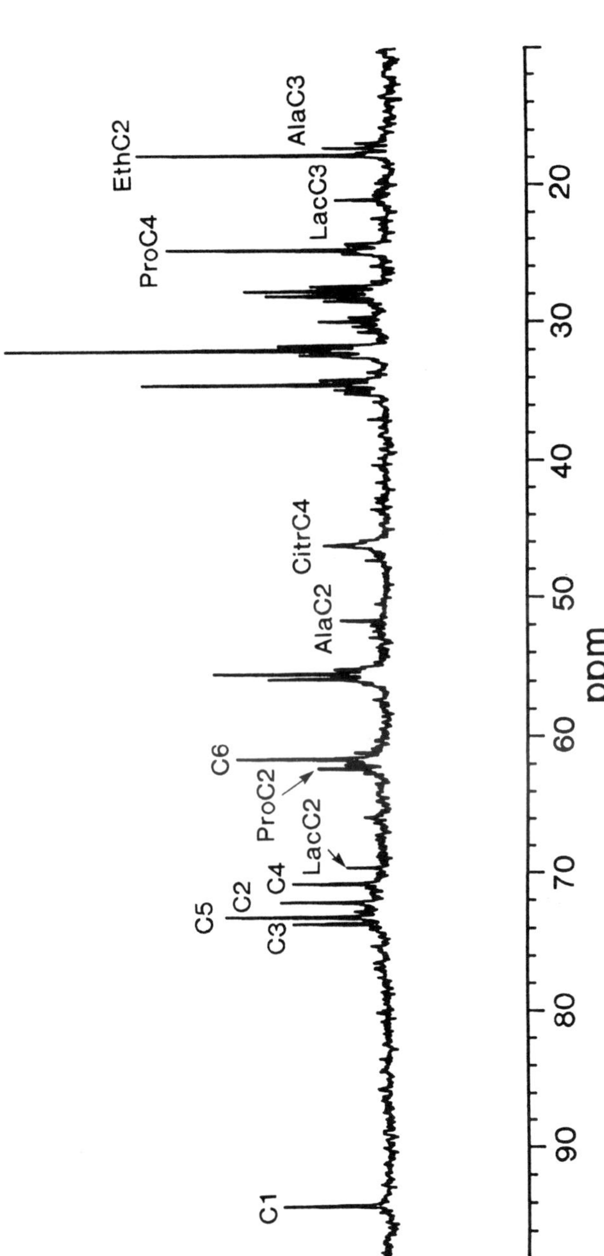

Fig. 4. ^{13}C NMR spectrum of a perchloric acid extract from whole third-instar larvae of *D. melanogaster* that were homozygous for the *Adh*^{S} allele. The larvae were exposed to 5% (v/v) [2-^{13}C]-ethanol for 8 h (A. Freriksen and P. Heinstra, unpublished; *see* ref. 68 for further details). Ala, alanine; Eth, ethanol; Lac, lactate; Pro, proline; Gln, glutamine; Glu, glutamate; Suc, succinate; Citr, citrate. The atoms C1–C6, as shown in the region between 61 and 94 parts per million (ppm), belong to the carbohydrate α,α-trehalose. The upper parts of the figure show important regions where spin–spin scalar coupling can be observed within the same compound as a result of multiple tricarboxylic acid cycle turns in which ^{13}C2,3-oxaloacetate condenses with ^{13}C2-acetyl-CoA forming ^{13}C2,3,4-citrate, and so on.

From these ^{13}C NMR studies, we have postulated a scheme for the intermediary metabolism of ethanol degradation in larvae (Fig. 5). During the first hours after ethanol ingestion, most of the ethanol enters the tricarboxylic acid (TCA) cycle as 2-^{13}C-acetyl-CoA. In the TCA cycle, a branchpoint exists; α-ketoglutarate may be converted either to glutamate or to succinyl-CoA. Glutamate may serve as a precursor for the biosynthesis of glutamine and proline. Since the two glutamine synthetase (EC 6.3.1.2.) isoenzymes present in *Drosophila* are located in different subcellular fractions,[76] it is not known whether glutamine is synthesized in the cytoplasm and/or in the mitochondrion. If *Drosophila* proline dehydrogenase is located in the cytoplasm,[77,78] then a novel NADH reoxidation system may be present. Such a system would provide cells with NAD$^+$ and drive the ADH pathway. The succinyl-CoA can be converted into malate in the TCA cycle. Malate may then cross the mitochondrial membranes to enter the cytoplasm (Fig. 5). There the malate may fuel the synthesis of alanine and lactate, or it may be used for the synthesis of trehalose.

Lactate is prevalent in *D. melanogaster* larvae (Fig. 4) and lactate dehydrogenase (LDH, EC 1.1.1.27.) may provide another cytosolic mechanism for the reoxidation of NADH into NAD$^+$. Such a system may also help drive the ADH-mediated reaction(s). In trehalogenesis, malic enzyme (EC 1.1.1.40) may function and provide NADPH for lipid synthesis.[79] That the pentose phosphate shunt pathway was operating during ethanol degradation was evidenced by a loss of C_2 into C_5-enriched trehalose (Fig. 4; ref. 68). This pathway may also provide NADPH for fatty acid biosynthesis. *De novo* synthesis of saturated fatty acids was also observed after a lag period of initial exposure to [2-^{13}C]-ethanol. The enrichment of label into mono-unsaturated fatty acids was approximately three times slower than the incorporation of label into saturated fatty acids.

Minor Metabolic Pathways

Minor systems for the degradation of alcohols exist in *D. melanogaster* larvae.[80] These presumably include MEOS, the glutathione transferase (EC 2.5.1.18) system, and the catalase system (EC 1.11.1.6). Knowledge of these minor pathways may be important to understanding the mechanisms that underlie alcohol-induced cellular damage, for alcohol tolerance in *Drosophila* may not only be attributed to an active ADH pathway, but may also be a result of selection pressure that operates against the minor metabolic pathways.

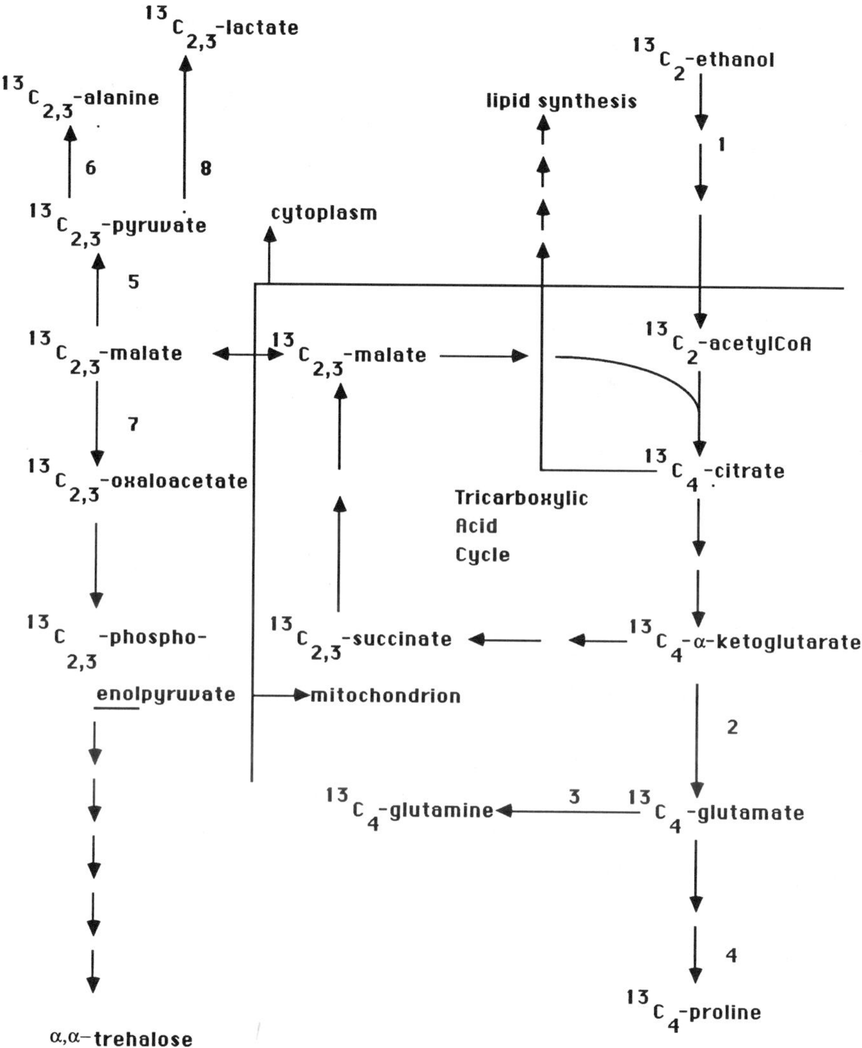

Fig. 5. A simplified scheme of the intermediary metabolism of ethanol degradation as based on NMR data (*see* Fig. 4; from ref. 68, and A. Freriksen and P. Heinstra, unpublished). Enzymes: 1, Alcohol dehydrogenase; 2, glutamate dehydrogenase and/or glutamate-oxaloacate transaminase; 3, glutamine synthetase; 4, proline dehydrogenase; 5, malic enzyme; 6, alanine dehydrogenase and/or glutamate-pyruvate transaminase; 7, cytosolic malate dehydrogenase; and 8, lactate dehydrogenase.

The Catalase System in Drosophila

Degradation of ethanol by the catalase system in *D. melanogaster* was originally proposed.[81] The *Drosophila* catalase system has been found to metabolize only methanol and ethanol.[80] In the catalase system, ethanol is degraded in a two-step fashion that is dependent on hydrogen peroxide. These reactions are outlined below.

$$\text{catalase} + H_2O_2 \longrightarrow \text{catalase} - H_2O_2 \text{ (compound 1)} \tag{1}$$

$$\text{catalase} - H_2O_2 + C_2H_5OH \longrightarrow \text{catalase} + CH_3CHO + H_2O \tag{2}$$

Although ADH activity in *Drosophila* is largely restricted to the larval gut, Malpighian tubules, and fat body,[56,69,70] catalase activity has a more widespread tissue distribution.[82] Despite the wide tissue-distribution pattern in *Drosophila* larvae, catalase does not have a major involvement in ethanol degradation. Through observations of Adh^{n2} larvae that were fed the catalase inhibitor 3-amino-1,2,4-triazole, it was determined that only 3–5% of the label from ^{14}C-ethanol was incorporated into lipids.[83]

There may be a price to pay at the cellular level for the use of the ADH and catalase pathways to provide protection from methanol and ethanol. Formaldehyde and acetaldehyde are produced. In vertebrates, hepatotoxicity has been linked to alterations of cell membranes[84,85] and has been attributed to an accumulation of acetaldehyde.[86] Acetaldehyde is capable of covalently bonding to a wide variety of hepatic macromolecules[87] and hepatic cell membranes,[88] as well as bonding to hemoglobin,[89] erythrocyte membranes,[90] human serum albumin,[91] and tubulin.[92] In chronic cases of alcohol abuse, the covalent bonding of acetaldehyde to macromolecules apparently generates autoimmune responses in mice[93] and humans.[94] In both studies,[93,94] antibodies directed at acetaldehyde adducts were found.

Cytochrome P-450

Although it is unclear whether or not *Drosophila* undergo acetaldehyde-directed autoimmune responses, membrane alteration may result from the peroxidation of membrane lipids as the result of cytochrome P-450. The bonding of acetaldehyde to hepatic microsomes correlates to increased MEOS activity.[84,86] Therefore, the ethanol induction of cytochrome P-450 in vertebrates may be the result of the complexing of acetaldehyde to microsomal membranes.[84,86] In turn, elevated MEOS activity may be quite important in cell damage. In humans who abuse alcohol, ADH activity may be normal[95] while cytochrome P-450 activity is elevated.[96] The ethanol-inducible protein that is associated with increased MEOS activity has been identified as cytochrome 450IIIEI.[97] However, Nebert and Gonzalez[98] indicate that two ethanol-inducible cytochromes reside within the P-450IIE family. The genes of the ethanol-inducible P-450s that are found in humans, rat,[99] and rabbit[100,101] have been sequenced.

Though ethanol-inducible forms of cytochrome P-450 have not yet been isolated in *Drosophila*, a number of cytochrome P-450s have been reported and reviewed.[102,103] In *Drosophila*, cytochrome P-450 activity in the metabolism of carcinogenic or precarcinogenic products[104–109] and for the metabolism of insecticides[110,111] has been detected. At present our laboratory is attempting to establish whether an ethanol-inducible form of cytochrome P-450 exists within *Drosophila* larvae. The existence of alcohol-inducible forms of cytochrome P-450 may provide *Drosophila* larvae with a source of hydrogen peroxide. Such a source may not only drive the catalase system, but also lead to the peroxidation of membrane lipids.

Glutathione Transferase

It has been demonstrated in vertebrates that increased intercellular levels of acetaldehyde stimulate the peroxidation of lipids.[112] Elevated levels of peroxidation can be caused by two different mechanisms. In the first mechanism, increased levels of oxygen radicals can be generated by low levels of catalase activity,[113] coupled with high activities for aldehyde oxidase[114] and xanthine oxidase.[115,116] In the second mechanism, H_2O_2 may accumulate within tissue as a result of a loss of reduced glutathione (GSH).[117,118] In this mechanism, the reduction of H_2O_2 along with lipid peroxides is catalyzed by glutathione transferase (GSH peroxidase system).[119,120] Lipid peroxides and H_2O_2 are converted by this pathway to less-reactive lipid alcohols (hydroxylated fatty acids) and water by the oxidation of GSH (reduced glutathione) to GSSH (oxidized glutathione). Any depletion of the GSH pool would slow down the GSH peroxidase system and the repair of peroxidated lipids. The exhibition of abnormally high levels of serum and hepatic lipid peroxides in alcohol abusers is consistent with this viewpoint.[121,122]

Besides catalyzing the repair of lipid peroxides,[121,122] glutathione transferases have also been shown to possess fatty acid esterase activity.[123] In the presence of ethanol, glutathione transferase can catalyze the formation of fatty acid ethyl esters while converting GSH to GSSH.[123] In acutely intoxicated subjects, high levels of fatty acid ethyl esters have been found in adipose, pancreatic, liver, and heart tissue.[124]

Although the formation of ethanol–lipid conjugates have been demonstrated in vertebrates, ethanol–lipid conjugates have yet to be demonstrated in *Drosophila*. However, our laboratory has recently discovered that wild-type Canton-S and *Adh^{n2}* larvae possess glutathione transferase activity that is enhanced by dietary ethanol.[125] Since the less tolerant *Adh^{n2}* strain possessed higher levels of glutathione transferase activity than Canton-S, glutathione transferase activity appears to correlate to alcohol toxicity in *Drosophila*. We are currently focusing our attentions on whether or not glutathione transferase is an ethanol-inducible enzyme and whether or not fatty acid ethyl esters can be detected within *Drosophila* larval tissues.

Lipid Metabolism and Cell Damage

In *D. melanogaster* larvae, one of the major routes of carbon flow from ethanol is into lipids. The effects of ethanol on lipid metabolism have recently been reviewed,[125–127] but these articles deal almost exclusively with lipid metabolism in vertebrates. Alcohol-related effects on lipid metabolism and, subsequently, on cell structure in *Drosophila* and vertebrates are dealt with in the remainder of this chapter.

Although the genetic regulation of ADH is well documented,[13,14] very little information exists concerning the cellular damage inflicted on *Drosophila* by alcohols. Cell damage may occur when the capacities of the ADH system and the secondary routes for ethanol metabolism are exceeded. Like anesthetics, ethanol and other alcohols can influence cell membranes. Alcohols penetrate into membranes and cause the membranes to swell.[128–131] In vertebrate systems, alcohols have been demonstrated to alter the activity of a number of membrane-bound enzymes, presumably by altering lipid–protein relationships within hydrophobic domains.[128–131] Sun and Sun[129] reported that chronic ethanol exposure is known to alter voltage-sensitive sodium channels, calcium uptake, and adenylate cyclase as well as impair receptors for γ-amino butyric acid (GABA), glutamate, opiates, dopamine, muscarine cholinergic compounds, and α-adrenergic compounds.[129]

Exposure to ethanol has been shown to destabilize membrane order in vertebrate cells, which in turn promotes increased fluidity within membranes.[130–133] This phenomenon has been demonstrated in rat and mouse synaptic membranes;[132–135] rat mitochondrial membranes;[135,136] rat liver microsomal membranes;[135–138] rat liver plasma membranes;[139,140] and rat, mouse, and quail erythrocyte membranes.[133,136,141] In these systems, ethanol causes an immediate increase in membrane disorder in animals not tolerant of alcohol. Nonetheless, membranes isolated from alcohol-tolerant animals resist the membrane-disordering effects of ethanol.[133–141]

We suspect that *Drosophila* may also exhibit ethanol-induced alterations in membrane fluidity. A comparison of alcohol-induced damage in *Drosophila* and vertebrate cells follows.

The Effect of Alcohol
on Vertebrate Organ and Tissue Damage

Several recent reviews have dealt with organ pathogenesis in vertebrates[142–147] and may be consulted for a more complete view of alcohol-related pathogenesis. The earliest and most common response to ethanol in vertebrates is fatty infiltration of the liver.[148–151] Chronic ingestion of ethanol in humans has been reported to increase triacylglycerol levels in biopsied liver cells four- to 10-fold.[152–155] In extreme cases of prolonged ethanol ingestion, as much as 50% of the wet weight of the liver is attributed to triacylglycerol.[152,156] This response is not considered to be a dangerous response and is reversible.[157] Despite the potential for reversibility, the appearance of lipogranulomas, necrosis of hepatocytes, and resulting immunological responses during acute fatty infiltration of the liver are thought to be a prerequisite for alcoholic hepatitis[158,159] and alcoholic cirrhosis of the liver.[160] Alcoholic hepatitis in turn precedes the development of cirrhosis in humans[158] and baboons.[159] Fatty infiltration of the liver is an almost-immediate response to drinking.[160–162] As a result, some investigators indicated that fatty infiltration of the liver is a causal prerequisite to alcoholic cirrhosis,[158] whereas others have argued against this stance.[163–166]

Although 90–100% of all heavy drinkers develop fatty infiltration of the liver, only 10–35% develop alcoholic hepatitis and 8–20% develop alcoholic cirrhosis.[167–169] Based on these statistics, it is questionable whether or not fatty infiltration of the liver predisposes the liver for ensuing hepatitis or cirrhosis.[163–166] This stance is supported by several observations. First, few humans actually die from fatty infiltration of the liver as a result of chronic alcohol abuse.[162] Second, the functional capabilities of the liver remain essentially normal during fatty infiltration, and the morphological signs of fatty infiltration of the liver reverse during a few days of absti-nence.[160,161,170] Third, human and animal studies suggest that alcohol-induced cirrhosis may develop in the absence of hepatitis.[84,171–173] Thus, liver damage may not be caused by fatty infiltration of the liver in verte-brates. Necrosis appears to correlate best to alterations in cell membranes, alterations of the mitochondria, and the inducement of fibrinogenesis.

The origin of the fatty acids of the triacylglycerol that accumulates in the liver is subject to debate. As shown in perfused liver, freshly isolated hepatocytes, cultured hepatocytes, and in vivo studies,[174–178] the ingestion of ethanol does not stimulate an immediate round of fatty acid synthesis within liver tissue. Thus, the ethanol-induced accumulation of triacylglycerol within hepatocytes is either caused by a decrease in fatty acid degradation or the stimulation of fatty acid synthesis in peripheral tissues accompanied by increased fatty acid uptake by hepatocytes.

When ethanol is consumed chronically, the β-oxidation of fatty acids in liver is low because of the limited oxygen supply[179,180,181] and limited NAD^+ pool.[171,182,183] Also, the elevated levels of acetyl-CoA may inhibit β-oxidation by allosterically inhibiting acyl CoA thiolase.[184] Such inhibi-tion would increase the concentration of 3-oxyacyl CoA intermediates, which are known to inhibit longchain acyl CoA dehydrogenase.[185] Because fatty acid levels increase in the form of triacylglycerol when β-oxidation is inhibited in perfused rat liver,[186,187] an inhibition of β-oxidation could partially explain the accumulation of triacylglycerol.

The increased lipid content of the liver could also be attributed to the enhancement of fatty acid uptake by liver cells by ethanol. In rats, injections of ethanol were found to increase the hepatic uptake of fatty acids.[188,189] Kondrup et al.[190] reported that ethanol exposure increased the uptake of fatty acids into perfused rat liver by 15% and reduced the secretion of low-density lipoprotein (VLDL).[191] This effect was not inhibited by 4-methylpyrazole in hepatocytes,[191,192] indicating that ethanol, not a derivative, stimulates fatty acid uptake in hepatocytes.

Finally, the fatty acids that accumulate in the liver in response to etha-nol may be derived from the diet rather than from *de novo* synthesis. Lieber and Spritz[150] reported that the fatty acid composition of triacylglycerol iso-lated from human hepatocytes was closely related to the fatty acid composi-tion of ingested food. Also, in rats, approx 90% of the fatty acids found in the triacylglycerol of hepatocytes were derived from the diet.[193]

The Effect of Alcohol
on Fat Body Cell Morphology in Drosophila

Like vertebrates, wild-type *D. melanogaster* larvae use ethanol as a substrate for lipid synthesis.[56] It has been demonstrated that the activities of ADH, fatty acid synthetase, and *sn*-glycerol-3-phosphate dehydrogenase (EC 1.1.1.8) all positively correlate to dietary concentrations of ethanol.[8,194] Besides increasing fatty acid synthetase activity, dietary ethanol also stimulates the synthesis of triacylglycerols of third-instar *D. melanogaster* larvae.[8,194] The major site for diacylglycerol, triacylglycerol, and phospholipid synthesis in insects is the fat body;[195–197] consequently, the ethanol-induced lipid-filled vacuoles of third-instar fat-body cells[12] are thought to be primarily triacylglycerol. This is reminiscent of fatty infiltration of the vertebrate liver. As in fatty infiltration of the liver, fatty infiltration of fat body cells may not necessarily be detrimental. Lipids are stored during the larval period and provide energy for pupal development.[198] Thus, differences in the ability of larvae to convert ethanol into lipids may be of adaptive significance.[80]

Dietary fatty acids and the newly synthesized fatty acids are transported through the hemolymph to the fat body of the larva via fatty acid binding proteins. As in vertebrates, ethanol may stimulate the uptake of fatty acids into fat body cells, which in turn stimulates the synthesis of diacylglycerol, triacylglycerol, and phospholipid. To test this model in *Drosophila, in situ* hybridization studies must be performed on larval tissues, utilizing probes and/or antibodies for fatty acid synthetase and fatty acid binding proteins.

The effects of ethanol and isopropanol on morphology of fat body cell in third-instar *D. melanogaster* larvae have been examined by feeding third-instar larvae of the Canton-S and *Adh^{n2}* strains low-sucrose diets with and without alcohol supplements.[12,80] Then fat bodies were removed and processed for light and transmission electron microscopy. Larvae of the *Adh^{n2}* strain have <5% of normal ADH-protein; larvae of the Canton-S wild-type strain are homozygous for the *Adh^F* allele.[199] Wild-type Canton-S larvae can tolerate up to 6% ethanol; *ADH^{n2}* larvae 2% ethanol.

In *Adh^{n2}* larvae, high intracellular concentrations of ethanol caused a decrease in lipid droplets and glycogen deposits (Fig. 6A,C, and E) and promoted a decrease in cell-membrane infoldings of fat body cells (Fig. 6B and D), indicating that the ability to absorb and release molecules may be

 Geer, Miller, and Heinstra

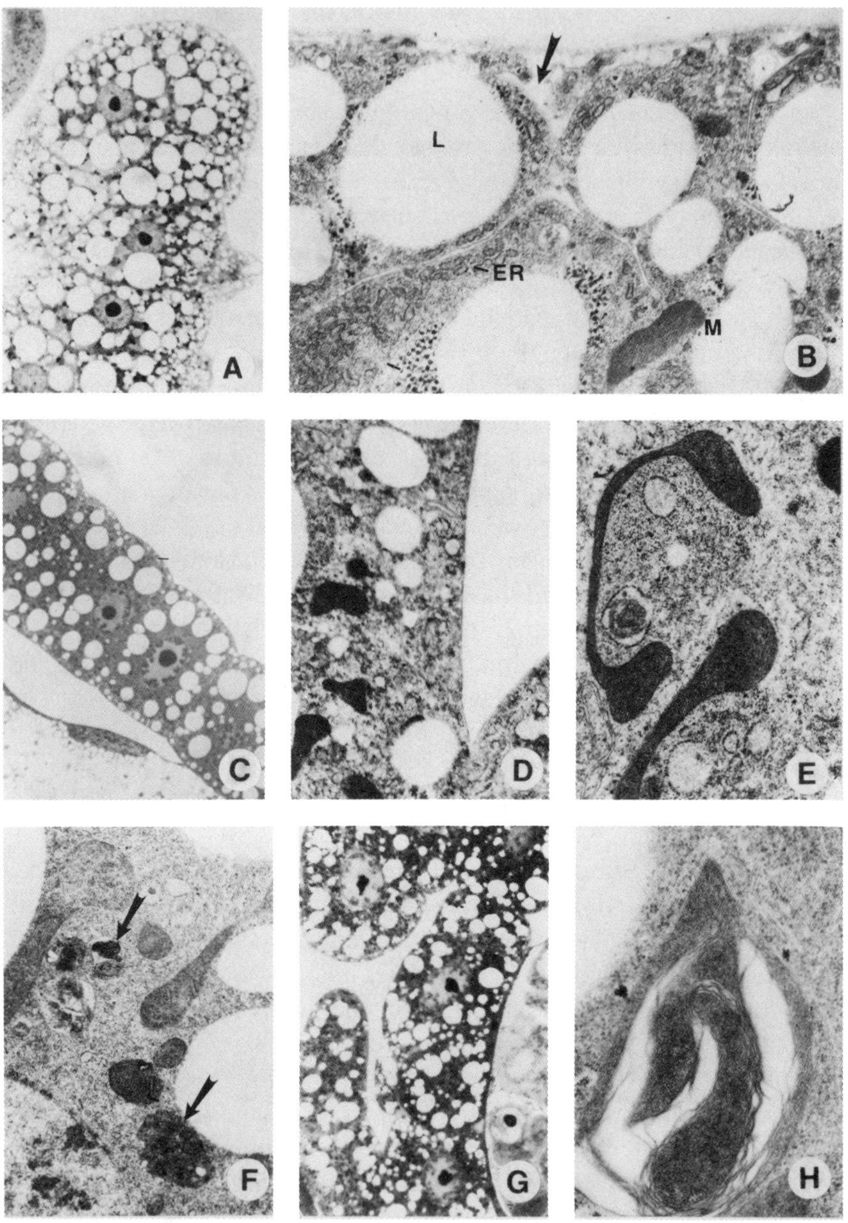

Fig. 6. Micrographs that show some of the effects of alcohols on the structure of fat body cells of *D. melanogaster*.[12] **A** is a light-micrograph overview of fat-

impaired.[12] Ethanol-stimulated alterations to the mitochondria and endoplasmic reticulum were also found (Fig. 6E and F). Mitochondria appeared swollen and often possessed bizarre shapes, whereas the rough endoplasmic reticulum appeared dilated. Numerous autophagosomes were also evident in the fat body cells of Adh^{n2} larvae that were fed ethanol (Fig. 6F), suggesting that protein granules were being degraded. Large lipid droplets were common throughout the cytoplasm. The large lipid droplets seen in the fat body cells of *D. melanogaster* larvae[12,80] are reminiscent of fat droplets seen in fatty infiltrated liver cells.[142,157,160]

The enlargement of mitochondria in vertebrate cells in response to ethanol has been noted.[200–202] Cells of human liver biopsies of chronic alcoholics also had abnormally shaped mitochondria.[200–202] French[203] indicated

---

body cells of a 7-d-old Adh^{n2} larva cultured on the alcohol-free control diet. The fat body cells have a high concentration of lipid droplets. Semithin section, toluidine blue stain ×120. **B** is an electron micrograph that depicts a region beneath the basement membrane of a 7-d-old Adh^{n2} larva cultured on the alcohol-free control diet. The alternating cytoplasmic strands and hemolymph spaces (arrow) are evident. Organelles, such as the mitochondria (M), rough endoplasmic reticulum (ER), lipid droplets (L), and glycogen (G), are evident, × 18,000. **C** is a light-micrograph overview of fat body cells of a 7-d-old Adh^{n2} larva fed a diet supplemented with 1.25% ethanol. Compared to the fat body cells of the larva fed the ethanol-free control diet (shown in **A**), the fat-body cells are smaller and there are fewer lipid droplets. Semithin section, toluidine blue stain, × 115. **D** is an electron micrograph of a fat body cell of a 7-d-old Adh^{n2} larva fed a diet containing 1.25% ethanol. There is a marked reduction in the amount of alternating interdigitating cytoplasmic strands and hemolymph spaces compared to the cell periphery of Adh^{n2} larvae fed the ethanol-free diet (shown in **B**). **E** is an electron micrograph of a fat body cell of a 7-d-old Adh^{n2} larva fed a diet supplemented with 1.25% ethanol. Mitochondria with abnormal shapes and an absence of glycogen deposits are evident, × 25,000. **F** is an electron micrograph of a fat body cell of a 7-d-old Adh^{n2} larva fed a diet containing 1.25% ethanol. Numerous autophagosomes (arrows) were observed along with mitochondria with abnormal shapes, × 18,300. **G** is a light micrograph of fat body cells of a 6-d-old Canton-S larva cultured on a diet supplemented with 1.5% isopropanol (v/v). The number of lipid droplets is less than that observed in larvae fed a control, alcohol-free diet. Semithin section, toluidine blue stain, × 110. **H** is an electron micrograph of a fat body cell of a 7-d-old Canton-S larva cultured on a diet containing 1.5% isopropanol. Myelin figures, such as depicted here, were frequently observed, × 55,000.

that in vertebrates the exposure to ethanol increased the permeability of the mitochondrial membrane, which increased the uptake and storage of Ca^{2+}. In rats chronically fed ethanol, disrupted mitochondrial cristae were observed, along with a dilation of the sarcoplasmic reticulum.[204] These mitochondrial alterations were correlated to decreased activities of cytochrome a_3, cytochrome b, and cytochrome oxidase,[205–207] and a reduction in ATP synthesis was reported.[204] The uncoupling of oxidative phosphorylation by increased Ca^{2+} influx may, presumably, be caused by increased phospholipase activity.[208] At the present, it is uncertain whether ethanol treatments alter mitochondrial membrane fluidity and uncouple the respiratory chain of *D. melanogaster.*

Quantification of the inclusions of fat body cells of *D. melanogaster* by cytometric analysis[12,80] revealed ethanol-stimulated reductions in glycogen, lipid, and protein stores in *Adh^{n2}* larvae. In the Canton-S wild-type strain, which is more tolerant of alcohol, ethanol consumption decreased glycogen and protein deposits and increased lipid deposits. Consequently, the fatty infiltration of fat body cells in larvae was associated with the degradation of ethanol by ADH. When fed ethanol as larvae, the Canton-S individuals that eclose had greater adult body weights than individuals fed an ethanol-free diet. This suggests that Canton-S larvae use the ADH pathway to degrade ethanol into acetate for triacylglycerol synthesis. The stored triacylglycerols may act as energy reserves in fat body cells.[12] This view was further supported by the observation that isopropanol exposure failed to increase cytoplasmic lipid reserves (ref. 12, Fig. 6G) and caused the formation of myelin figures (Fig. 6H). This alcohol also decreased membrane infoldings and depleted glycogen reserves within the fat body cells of Canton-S larvae.[12] Thus, as in vertebrates, alcohol toxicity causes alterations of membranes.

Fatty infiltration of fat body cells may be a beneficial response to ethanol ingestion. The triacylglycerol that is synthesized from ethanol may be used as an energy source during pupal development. The lipids that are stored during the larval period serve as the primary energy source for developing pupa.[209]

Alcohol-Induced Alterations
in Drosophila Fatty Acids

The reasons why we suspect that the membranes of fat body cells of *D. melanogaster* are altered by ethanol are (1) alcohol exposure alters the relative concentration of phospholipids and (2) exposure to alcohol induces alterations within fatty acids, ostensibly altering membrane fluidity. Unsaturated, shortchain fatty acids disorganize membranes and increase membrane fluidity, whereas longchain, saturated fatty acids stabilize membrane bilayers and decrease membrane fluidity.[209]

In wild-type third-instar *D. melanogaster* larvae, a moderate concentration of dietary ethanol (2.5% v/v) reduced the chain length of total fatty acids and increased the desaturation of shortchain fatty acids.[210] The reduction in fatty acid chain length by ethanol was ADH-dependent, whereas the effect on desaturation was not.[210] Since the ethanol-induced reduction in chain length of desaturated fatty acids was blocked by exogenous supplies of linoleic acid (18:3) in *D. melanogaster*,[210] the ethanol stimulation of desaturation was thought to involve the Δ9-desaturase system. However, Keith[236] reported that there is a Δ3-desaturase in *D. melanogaster* that has a preference for shorter-chained fatty acids and proposed the following pathways:

$$10:0 \longrightarrow \Delta^3 10:1 \longrightarrow \Delta^5 12:1 \longrightarrow \Delta^7 14:1 \longrightarrow \Delta^9 16:1 \qquad (3)$$

$$12:0 \longrightarrow \Delta^3 12:1 \longrightarrow \Delta^5 14:1 \longrightarrow \Delta^7 16:1 \longrightarrow \Delta^9 18:1 \qquad (4)$$

Regardless of which desaturase is involved, the induction of shortchain, unsaturated fatty acids by ethanol would decrease membrane organization and, thus, increase the membrane fluidity of fat body cells. Other alcohols were found to affect the total fatty acid composition of Canton-S larvae in our laboratory.[237] Shortchain, unsaturated fatty acids were more prevalent when 1.5% (v/v) isopropanol, *n*-propanol, or *n*-butanol was fed.

Alcohol-Induced Changes in Fatty Acid Composition in Other Systems

Studies on the effect of ethanol on membrane fatty acid composition in primarily vertebrate systems are reviewed elsewhere[129,130] and provide a body of conflicting literature. To add clarity, the results of other studies are presented in Tables 1 and 2. These tables attempt to classify studies on the following basis: studies that demonstrate that ethanol promotes an increase in shortchain and/or unsaturated fatty acids (Table 1) and studies that demonstrate that ethanol stimulates an increase in longchain and/or saturated fatty acids (Table 2). The rationale for this classification is that Table 1

Table 1
Studies Indicating that Ethanol Promotes
the Emergence of Shortchain and/or Unsaturated Fatty Acids

Ref.	System	Data summary		
211	*E. coli*	More unsaturated fatty acids		
212	*Clostridium thermocellum*	More unsaturated fatty acids		
213, 214	*Saccharomyces cerivisiae*	More unsaturated fatty acids		
210	*Drosophila melanogaster*	Shorter, more unsaturated fatty acids.		
			Increase	Decrease
215	Mouse liver mitochondria and microsomes		16:1	16:0
216	Rat liver mitochondria and microsomal PE and PC fractions		18:1	16:0
215	Mouse liver		18:2	20:4 and 20:6
217	Rat liver		18:2	20:4 and 20:6
218	Rat liver mitochondria		18:2	20:4 and 20:6
219	Rat hepatocytes		18:2	20:4 and 20:6
220	Rat liver plasma membrane		22:6	–
221	Mouse synaptosomal membranes		18:0	20:4
222	Guinea pig synaptosomal membranes		22:4 and 22:6, in PE fraction	–
223	Guinea pig adrenal gland mitochondria		18:2	20:4, in PC and PE fractions
224	Rat heart		18:2	20:4
225	Monkey myocardial mitochondria		18:2	20:4
226	Mouse myocardial phospholipids		18:1 and 18:2	22:6
227	Rat erythrocyte phospholipids		18:2	20:4

supports the view that ethanol promotes a disordering of membranes that increases membrane fluidity. The observations reported in Table 2 provide evidence that chronic alcohol exposure promotes a reorganization of the membrane, which may in turn increase resistance to the disordering effects of ethanol.

As one can see, some studies fit both categories. These discrepancies may in part be explained by varied periods of exposure to different quantities of ethanol. These differences, along with variable rates of metabolism,

Table 2
Studies Indicating that Ethanol Promotes the Emergence
of Longer-Chain and/or More Saturated Fatty Acids

Ref.	System	Data summary	
		Increase	Decrease
216	Rat liver mitochondria and microsomal PE and PC fractions	18:1	16:0
215	Mouse liver	–	18:2, 20:4 and 20:6
217	Rat liver	18:2	20:4 and 20:6
218	Rat liver mitochondria	18:2	20:4 and 20:6
219	Rat hepatocytes	18:2	20:4 and 20:6
228	Rat liver phospholipids	–	20:4
229	Rat liver mitochondrial phospholipids	–	20:4
216	Rat liver cardiolipin	–	18:2
220	Rat liver plasma membrane	22:6	–
230	Human liver	–	18:2, 20:4
221	Mouse synaptosomal membranes	18:0	20:4
231	Mouse synaptosome membranes	–	22:6 in PS fractions
222	Guinea pig synaptosomal membranes	22:4, 22:6 in PE fraction	
223	Guinea pig adrenal gland mitochondria	18:2	20:4 in PC and PE fractions
224	Rat heart	18:2	20:4
225	Monkey myocardial mitochondria	18:2	20:4
221	Mouse myocardial phospholipids	18:1, 18:2	22:6
232, 233	Human serum	–	18:2 and/or polyunsaturated fatty acids
234	Pig serum	–	18:2, PC
227	Rat erythrocyte phospholipids	18:2	20:4
235	Mouse erythrocyte membranes	–	18:2, PC

may provide evidence that some organisms make the transition from membrane damage to membrane repair more rapidly than other organisms. Early exposure to ethanol may stimulate a disorganization of membranes by increasing the quantities of shortchain and/or unsaturated fatty acids. Meanwhile, chronic exposure to ethanol may promote the synthesis of longer fatty acid chains and/or more-saturated fatty acids that restabilize and reorganize membranes. The studies reported in Tables 1 and 2 may simply indicate that the organisms are in transition from damage to repair and tolerance.

The observations of Tables 1 and 2 may also reflect differences in the induction of fatty acid synthesis by ethanol. The fatty acid profile seen during fatty infiltration of the liver in vertebrates closely resembles the fatty acid composition of the diet.[151,193] As a result, vertebrates may, at first, utilize dietary fatty acids before they are induced by ethanol to synthesize fatty acids.[126] This problem would be less pronounced in studies conducted on lower organisms, such as *Drosophila*, because these organisms may be cultured on sterile, defined media without a source of fatty acids. Since the modified Sang's media[210] used in our laboratory do not contain fatty acids, larvae are dependent on *de novo* fatty acid synthesis to form membranes. Consequently, the effects of ethanol on fatty acid profiles are clearly evident.

Ethanol-Induced Alterations in Vertebrate Phospholipids

Ethanol-induced changes within fatty acid profiles may in part explain ethanol-induced alterations in membrane organization, but other mechanisms also appear to be at work. One such mechanism acts through alterations in phospholipid profiles. The effects of phospholipid composition on membrane organization have been reviewed previously[129,130] and will only be summarized here. Membranes that are rich in phosphatidylcholine (PC), phosphatidylserine (PS), and phosphatidylglycerol exist in highly organized bilayers that exhibit low fluidity. Conversely, membranes rich in lysophospholipids, cardiolipin, phosphatidic acid, and/or unsaturated phosphatidylethanolamine (PE) easily fall out of their bilayer configurations and adopt either micellar or hexagonal (H_{II}) configurations (Fig. 7). Such membranes are less organized and more fluid.

Ethanol-induced membrane damage associated with a decrease in PC levels is evident in vertebrates. In the study by Alling et al.,[238] 80% of all alcoholics studied possessed abnormally low levels of PC. This observation was also made in a number of vertebrate systems. Decreases in the levels of PC and linoleic acid (18:2) have also been observed in human serum,[233,235] pig serum,[234] and the membranes of mouse erythrocytes.[235] Such losses in PC could disorganize membranes[129,209] and contribute to the necrosis seen within the vertebrate liver and insect fat body.

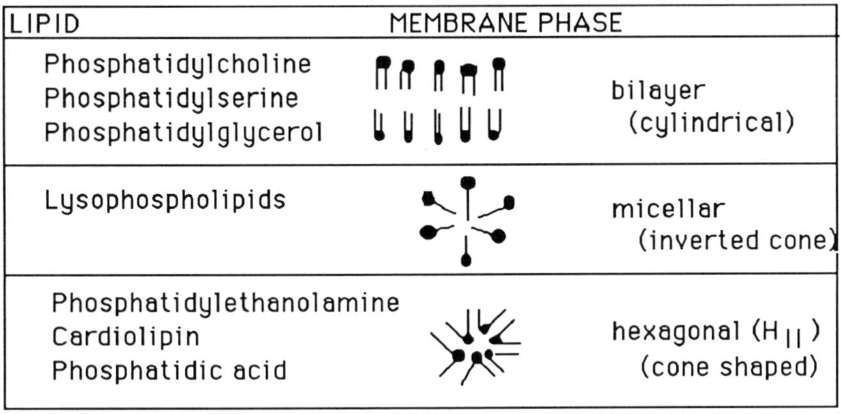

LIPID		MEMBRANE PHASE
Phosphatidylcholine Phosphatidylserine Phosphatidylglycerol		bilayer (cylindrical)
Lysophospholipids		micellar (inverted cone)
Phosphatidylethanolamine Cardiolipin Phosphatidic acid		hexagonal (H_{II}) (cone shaped)

Fig. 7. The effects of phospholipid composition on membrane structure.

Although ethanol-induced decreases in PC can be correlated to the disorganization effects of ethanol on membranes, other phospholipids may also be affected. In rat liver microsomes, Taraschi et al.[136] demonstrated that membrane tolerance is correlated to changes in phosphatidylinositol (PI) content. Although PI-conveyed tolerance is rapidly lost after ethanol withdrawal,[239] Hoek and Taraschi[240] have reported a model whereby membrane tolerance may be associated with the effects of ethanol on G proteins.

PI-conveyed tolerance may not be caused by inositol. Since resistance to the disorganizing effects of ethanol was observed in reconstructed liposomes only when PI was isolated from chronically exposed rats, the PI-conveyed tolerance reported by Taraschi et al.[138] may be dependent on ethanol-induced alterations within PI residues. Reconstructed liposomes that contained PI that was isolated from control animals failed to resist ethanol-induced membrane disorganization.[241] Therefore, it appears that PI-conveyed tolerance is not conveyed by the inositol head group, but rather by the fatty acid tails.

The Effects of Alcohols
on Drosophila *Phospholipid Composition*

Because *D. melanogaster* has a strict dietary requirement for choline,[241,242] the relative amount of PE is greater than that of PC.[243,244] By tracing [U-^{14}C]-glucose into phospholipids when third-instar *D. melano-*

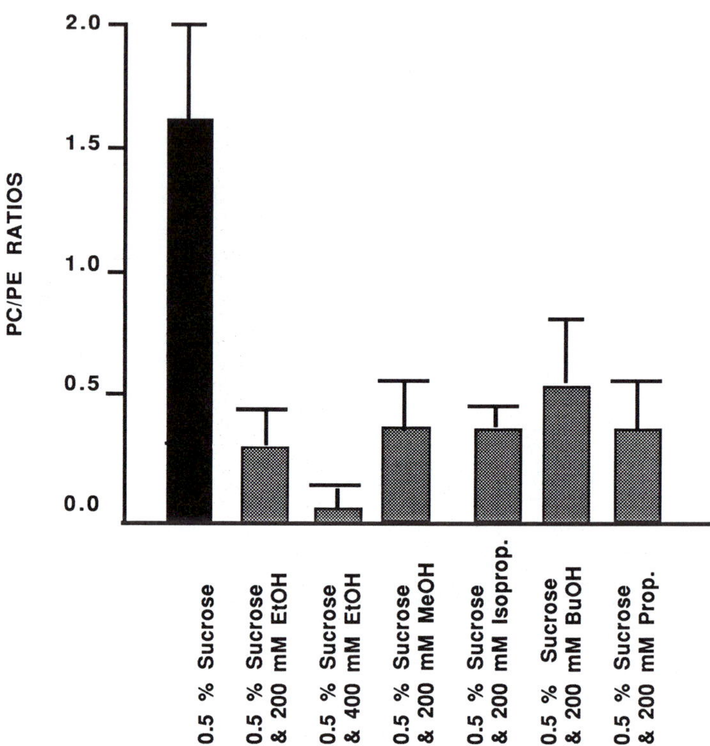

Fig. 8. The effects of alcohols on PC/PE ratios in third-instar Canton-S larvae. All experimental groups (▒) differ from the control group (■) in statistically significant manners ($p < 0.001$).

gaster were fed various concentrations of dietary ethanol, Geer et al.[210] observed an increased incorporation of label into PE and a decrease in the amount of label incorporated into PC. To investigate whether the enhanced incorporation of label into PE was a result of the stimulation of PE synthesis, our laboratory recently exposed third-instar Canton-S larvae to various concentrations of dietary ethanol and/or isopropanol for a limited feeding period. By measuring the phosphorus content of phospholipids, ethanol (2.5% v/v) was found to promote nearly a fourfold increase in PE levels, whereas PC levels dropped by nearly threefold (Fig. 8).[237] Since ethanol, as well as other, more toxic alcohols, caused increases in PE,[237] the change in the PE/PC ratio may be a result of alcohol-induced damage of *Drosophila* membranes.

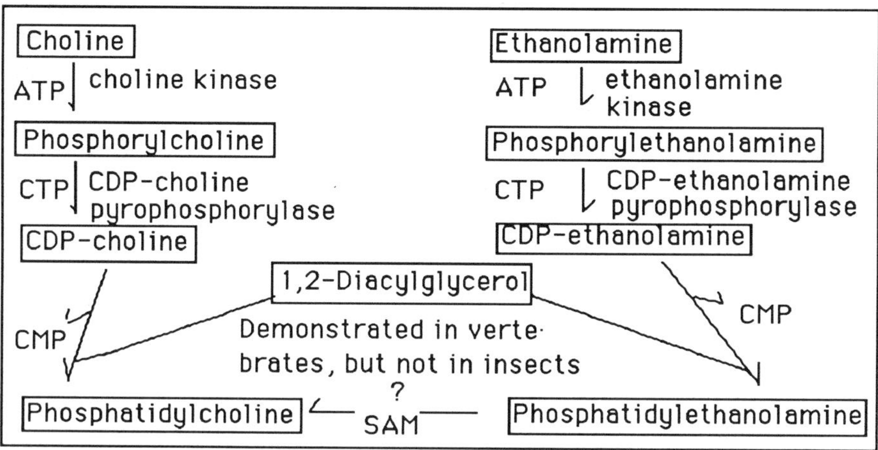

Fig. 9. The pathways for phosphatidylcholine and phosphatidylethanolamine synthesis.[197]

The observation that PE increases and PC decreases in response to alcohols is consistent with the concept that alcohols disorganize *Drosophila* membranes and make the membranes more fluid. *Drosophila* cells may compensate for the loss of PC from membranes by incorporating other phospholipids. Because of the inability to synthesize choline for phospholipid synthesis, *D. melanogaster* may form from ethanolamine more PE for membrane synthesis (Fig. 9), resulting in membranes with a diminished bilayer organization and greater fluidity.

Wild-type *D. melanogaster* larvae that contained only 10% of the normal level of PC because of a dietary deficiency of choline were much less tolerant to the toxic influence of ethanol than larvae fed an optimum concentration of choline.[245] Susceptibility to the toxic effects of ethanol also has a strong genetic basis in *D. melanogaster*.[71] In a recent study, a number of biochemical traits of seven isochromosomal lines of *D. melanogaster* with different second chromosomes were compared. Each line had a heritable level of ethanol tolerance, and differences could be attributed to the differences in genes carried by the second chromosomes. The lines with the greatest tolerance to ethanol as larvae had the largest proportion of longchain (18-carbons) and unsaturated fatty acids.[71] Since *Drosophila* phospholipids contain more longchain fatty acids than triacylglycerols[246] and since phospholipids are concentrated in membranes, the observations suggest that the fatty acid compositions of cell membranes may be important to the determination of the degree of ethanol tolerance for *D. melanogaster*. Membranes with longchain, unsaturated fatty acids may be less subject to the damaging effects of ethanol. Therefore, the impact of the toxic effects of alcohols on *D. melanogaster* larvae may be a function of the phospholipid content of the cell membranes.

Retrospective

Although some differences exist, many of the consequences of ethanol exposure in vertebrates are also seen in the larvae of *D. melanogaster*. Since it can be readily manipulated by nutritional and genetic means, one can use *D. melanogaster* to study whether alcohol effects on cell structure are dependent on the ADH pathway or on one of the minor pathways. Furthermore, the genetic and dietary mechanisms that underlie the regulation of alcohol degradation can be established more easily in *D. melanogaster*. From the use of *Drosophila*, it should be possible to verify which mechanisms are also operating in vertebrates. In this way, *D. melanogaster* may provide shortcuts to important information about the metabolic and genetic bases of liver damage.

Acknowledgments

We would especially like to thank the many Knox College students who helped perform the research projects that were the foundation for this review. We are especially grateful to Marilyn Langevin, Christine Baumgardner, and Rajeev Dadoo, who provided leadership in our laboratory during the time that our research on alcohol metabolism was performed. Special acknowledgments go to Stephen McKechnie, who sparked our initial interest in alcohol dehydrogenase, and to Linda Dybas, whose interpretations of fat body cell structure were critical to this review. We would like to thank Wim Scharloo, Astrid Freriksen, and Barbara de Ruiter for their moral and scientific support. We also thank Dick Smit for preparing Figs. 1 and 4 and Robert Miller for his assistance in photography. Finally, we are grateful for the support of National Institutes of Health Grant AA06702.

References

[1] R. Rognstad and N. Grunnet (1979) Enzymatic pathways of ethanol metabolism, in *Biochemistry and Pharmacology of Ethanol,* vol. 1. E. Majchrowicz and E. P. Nobel, eds. Plenum, New York, pp. 65–87.

[2] L. G. Gelrud, D. H. Gregory, Z. R. Vlahcevic, C. C. Schwartz, and L. Swell (1979) Effect of ethanol and ethanol-related diseases on biliary lipid metabolism, in *Biochemistry and Pharmacology of Ethanol,* vol. 1. E. Majchrowicz and E. P. Nobel, eds. Plenum, New York, pp. 445–458.

[3] J. B. Gibson, T. W. May, and A. V. Wilks (1981) Genetic variation at the alcohol dehydrogenase locus in *Drosophila melanogaster* in relation to environmental variation: Ethanol levels in breeding sites and allozyme frequencies. *Oecologia* **51,** 191–198.

[4] S. W. McKechnie and P. Morgan (1982) Alcohol dehydrogenase polymorphism of *Drosophila melanogaster.* Aspects of alcohol and temperature variation in the larval environment. *Aust. J. Biol. Sci.* **35,** 85–93.

[5] J. A. McKenzie and P. A. Parsons (1972) Alcohol tolerance: An ecological parameter in the relative success of *Drosophila melanogaster* and *Drosophila simulans. Oecologia* **10,** 373–388.

[6] J. David, C. Bocquet, M. Arens, and P. Fouillet (1976) Biological role of alcohol dehydrogenase in the tolerance of *Drosophila melanogaster* to aliphatic alcohols: Utilization of an ADH-null mutant. *Biochem. Genet.* **14,** 989–997.

[7] S. S. Chawla, J. M. Perron, and C. Radouco-Thomas (1981) Effect of ingested ethanol on adult *Drosophila melanogaster* (Diptera; Drosophilidae). *Can. Entomol.* **113,** 315–323.

[8] S. W. McKechnie and B. W. Geer (1984) Regulation of alcohol dehydrogenase in *Drosophila melanogaster* by dietary alcohol and carbohydrate. *Insect Biochem.* **14,** 231–242.

[9] J. Van Herrewege and J. R. David (1984) Extension of life duration by dietary ethanol in *Drosophila melanogaster*: Response to selection in two strains of different origins. *Genetica* **63,** 61–70.

[10] T. M. Rizki (1978) Fat body, in *The Genetics and Biology of* Drosophila, vol. 2b. M. Ashburner and T. Wright, eds. Academic, New York, pp. 561–601.

[11] B. W. Geer, M. L. Langevin, and S. W. McKechnie (1985) Dietary ethanol and lipid synthesis in *Drosophila melanogaster. Biochem. Genet.* **23,** 607–622.

[12] B. W. Geer, L. Dybas, and L. Shanner (1989) Alcohol dehydrogenase and ethanol tolerance at the cellular level in *Drosophila melanogaster. J. Exp. Zool.* **250,** 22–39.

[13] W. Sofer and P. F. Martin (1987) Analysis of alcohol dehydrogenase gene expression in *Drosophila. Annu. Rev. Genet.* **21,** 203–235.

[14] G. K. Chambers (1988) The *Drosophila* alcohol dehydrogenase gene–enzyme system. *Adv. Genet.* **25,** 40–107.

[15] E. H. Grell, K. B. Jacobson, and J. B. Murphy (1968) Alterations of genetic material for analysis of alcohol dehydrogenase isozymes of *Drosophila melanogaster. Ann. NY Acad. Sci.* **51,** 441–455.

[16] J. O'Donnell, H. C. Mandel, M. Krauss, and W. Sofer (1977) Genetic and cytogenetic analysis of the *Adh* region in *Drosophila melanogaster. Genetics* **86,** 553–566.

[17] D. A. Goldberg (1980) Isolation and partial characterization of the *Drosophila* alcohol dehydrogenase gene. *Proc. Natl. Acad. Sci. USA* **77,** 5794–5798.

[18] C. Benyajati, N. Wang, A. Reddy, E. Weinberg, and W. Sofer (1980) Alcohol dehydrogenase in *Drosophila*; isolation and characterization of messenger RNA and cDNA clone. *Nucleic Acids Res.* **8,** 5649–5667.

[19] C. Benyajati, A. R. Place, D. A. Powers, and W. Sofer (1981) Alcohol dehydrogenase gene of Drosophila melanogaster: Relationship of intervening sequences to functional domains in the protein. *Proc. Natl. Acad. Sci. USA* **78,** 2717–2721.

[20] C. Benyajati, N. Spoerel, H. Haymerle, and M. Ashburner (1983) The messenger RNA for alcohol dehydrogenase in *Drosophila melanogaster* differs in its 5' end in different developmental stages. *Cell* **33,** 125–133.

[21] C. Savakis, M. Ashburner, and J. Willis (1986) The expression of the gene coding for alcohol dehydrogenase during the development of *Drosophila melanogaster. Dev. Biol.* **114,** 194–207.

[22] V. Corbin and T. Maniatis (1989) The role of specific enhancer-promotor interactions in *Drosophila Adh* promotor switch. *Genes Dev.* **3,** 2191–2201.

[23] V. Corbin and T. Maniatis (1989) Role of transcriptional interference in the *Drosophila melanogaster Adh* promotor switch. *Nature* **337,** 279–282.

[24] U. Heberlein, B. England, and R. Tjian (1988) Temporal pattern of alcohol dehydrogenase gene transcription reproduced by *Drosophila* stage-specific extracts. *Nature* **331,** 410–415.

[25] V. Corbin and T. Maniatis (1990) Identification of *cis*-regulatory elements required for larval expression of the *Drosophila* alcohol dehydrogenase gene. *Genetics* **124,** 637–646.

[26] U. Heberlein, B. England, and R. Tjian (1985) Characterization of *Drosophila* transcription factors that activate the tandem promotors of the alcohol dehydrogenase gene. *Cell* **41,** 965–977.

[27] B. England, U. Heberlein, and R. Tjian (1990) Purified *Drosophila* transcription factor *Adf-1* binds to sites in several *Drosophila* promotors and activates transcription. *J. Biol. Chem.* **265,** 5086–5094.

[28] A. Ewel, J. R. Jackson, and C. Benyajati (1990) Alternative DNA–protein interactions in variable-length internucleosomal regions associated with *Drosophila* distal promotor expression. *Nucleic Acids Res.* **18,** 1771–1781.

[29] K. Miyahara and H. Naora (1989) Plasticity of DNA conformation around the *Drosophila melanogaster* alcohol dehydrogenase gene under torsional stress. *J. Mol. Biol.* **206,** 281–293.

[30] C. F. Aquadro, S. F. Desse, M. M. Bland, C. H. Langley, and C. C. Laurie-Ahlberg (1986) Molecular population genetics of the alcohol dehydrogenase gene region of *Drosophila melanogaster. Genetics* **114,** 1165–1190.

[31] D. R. Schoot, P. D. East, and K. Paigen (1988) Characterization of the *Adh^{SL}* regulatory mutation in *Drosophila melanogaster. Genetics* **119,** 631–637.

[32] R. D. Ward (1975) Alcohol dehydrogenase activity in *Drosophila melanogaster*: A quantitative trait. *Genet. Res.* **26,** 81–93.

[33] B. W. Barnes and A. J. Birley (1978) Genetic variation for enzyme activity in a population of *Drosophila melanogaster.* IV. Analysis of alcohol dehydrogenase activity in chromosomal substitution lines.*Heredity* **40,** 51–57.

[34] C. C. Laurie-Ahlberg, G. Maroni, C. Bewley, J. C. Lucchesi, and B. S. Weir (1980) Quantitative genetic variation of enzyme activities in natural populations of *Drosophila melanogaster. Proc. Natl. Acad. Sci. USA* **77,** 1073–1077.

[35] J. J. King and J. F. McDonald (1987) Post-translational control of alcohol dehydrogenase levels in *Drosophila melanogaster. Genetics* **115,** 693–699.

[36] H. Jörnvall, M. Persson, and J. Jeffrey (1980) Alcohol and polyol dehydrogenase are both divided into protein types, and structural properties cross-relate the different enzyme activities into each type. *Proc. Natl. Acad. Sci. USA* **78,** 4226–4230.

[37] G. Duester, H. Jörnvall, and G. W. Hatfield (1986) Intron-dependent evolution of the nucleotide-binding domains within alcohol dehydrogenases and related enzymes. *Nucleic Acids Res.* **14,** 1931–1941.

[38] P. M. Rougraff, B. Zhang, M. J. Kuntz, K. R. A. Harris, and D. A. Crabb (1989) Cloning and sequence analysis of a cDNA for 3-hydroxyisobutyrate dehydrogenase. *J. Biol. Chem.* **264,** 5899–5903.

[39] Z. Chen, L. Lu, M. Shirley, W. R. Lee, and S. H. Chang (1990) Site-directed mutagenesis of glycine-14 and two "critical" cysteinyl residues in *Drosophila* alcohol dehydrogenase. *Biochemistry* **29,** 1112–1118.

[40] H. Jörnvall, H. von Bahr-Lindstrom, D. D. Jang, W. Ulmer, and M. Fröschle (1984) Extended superfamily of short alcohol-polyol-sugar dehydrogenases: Structural similarities between glucose and ribitol dehydrogenase. *FEBS Lett.* **165,** 190–195.

[41] M. Krook, L. Marekov, and H. Jörnvall (1990) Purification and structural characterization of placental NAD$^+$-linked 15-hydroxyprostaglandin dehydrogenase. *Biochemistry* **29,** 738–743.

[42] S. E. Hallam, F. Malpartida, and D. A. Hopwood (1988) Nucleotide sequence, transcription and deduced function of a gene involved in polyketide antibiotic synthesis in *Streptomyces coelicolor. Gene* **74,** 305–320.

[43] D. H. Sherman, F. Malpartida, M. J. Bibb, H. M. Kieser, and D. A. Hopwood

(1989) Structure and deduced function of the granaticin-producing polyketide synthetase gene cluster of *Streptomyces violaceoruber* Tü22. *EMBO J.* **8,** 2717–2725.

[44] S. J. Wakil, J. H. Stoops, and V. C. Joshi (1983) Fatty acid synthesis and its regulation. *Annu. Rev. Biochem.* **52,** 537–579.

[45] D. R. Thatcher (1980) The complete amino acid sequence of three alcohol dehydrogenase alleloenzymes from the fruit fly, *Drosophila. Biochem. J.* **187,** 875–883.

[46] A. R. Place, D. A. Powers, and W. Sofer (1980) *Drosophila melanogaster* alcohol dehydrogenase does not require metals for catalysis. *Fed. Proc.* **39,** 1640.

[47] K. N. Moxom, R. S. Holmes, P. A. Parsons, M. G. Irving, and D. M. Doddrell (1985) Purification and molecular properties of alcohol dehydrogenase from *Drosophila melanogaster*: Evidence from NMR and kinetic studies for function as an aldehyde dehydrogenase. *Comp. Biochem. Physiol.* **80B,** 525–535.

[48] J.-O. Winberg, D. R. Thatcher, and J. S. McKinley-McKee (1982) Alcohol dehydrogenase from the fruit fly Drosophila melanogaster: Substrate specificity of the alleloenzymes ADH-^{S} and ADH-^{F}. *Biochim. Biophys. Acta* **704,** 7–16.

[49] J.-O. Winberg, D. R. Thatcher, and J. S. McKinley-McKee (1982) Alcohol dehydrogenase from the fruit fly *Drosophila melanogaster*: Inhibition studies of the alleloenzymes ADH-^{S} and ADH-^{F}. *Biochim. Biophys. Acta* **704,** 17–25.

[50] R. Hovik, J.-O. Winberg, and J. S. McKinley-McKee (1984) *Drosophila melanogaster* alcohol dehydrogenase: Substrate specificity of the ADH-F alleloenzyme. *Insect Biochem.* **14,** 345–351.

[51] P. W. H. Heinstra, G. E. W. Thörig, W. Scharloo, W. Drenth, and R. J. M. Nolte (1988) Kinetics and thermodynamics of ethanol oxidation catalyzed by genetic variants of the alcohol dehydrogenase from *Drosophila melanogaster* and *D. simulans. Biochim. Biophys. Acta* **967,** 224–233.

[52] P. W. H. Heinstra, W. Scharloo, and G. E. W. Thörig (1988) Alcohol dehydrogenase polymorphism in *Drosophila*: Enzyme kinetics of product inhibition. *J. Mol. Evol.* **28,** 145–150.

[53] J.-O. Winberg and J. S. McKinley-McKee (1989) The ADH-S alleloenzyme of alcohol dehydrogenase from *Drosophila melanogaster*: Variation of kinetic parameters with pH. *Biochem. J.* **255,** 589–599.

[54] P. W. H. Heinstra, K. T. Eisses, W. Schoonen, W. Aben, A. de Winter, D. van der Horst, W. van Marrewijk, A. M. T. Beenakkers, W. Scharloo, and G. E. W. Thörig (1983) A dual function of alcohol dehydrogenase in *Drosophila. Genetica* **60,** 129–137.

[55] P. W. H. Heinstra, K. T. Eisses, W. Scharloo, and G. E. W. Thörig (1986) Metabolism of secondary alcohols in *Drosophila melanogaster*: Effects on alcohol dehydrogenase. *Comp. Biochem. Physiol.* **83B,** 403–408.

[56] P. W. H. Heinstra, B. W. Geer, D. Seykens, and M. L. Langevin (1989) The metabolism of ethanol-derived acetaldehyde by alcohol dehydrogenase (EC 1.1.1.1.) and aldehyde dehydrogenase (EC 1.2.1.3.) in *Drosophila melanogaster* larvae. *Biochem. J.* **259**, 791–797.

[57] M. Schwartz and W. Sofer (1976) Diet-induced alterations in distribution of multiple forms of alcohol dehydrogenase in *Drosophila*. *Nature* **263**, 129–131.

[58] J. Papel, M. Henderson, J. van Herrewege, J. David, and W. Sofer (1979) *Drosophila* alcohol dehydrogenase activity *in vitro* and *in vivo*: Effects of acetone feeding. *Biochem. Genet.* **17**, 553–564.

[59] P. W. H. Heinstra, W. Scharloo, and G. E. W. Thörig (1986) Alcohol dehydrogenase of *Drosophila*: Conversion and retroconversion of isozyme patterns. *Comp. Biochem. Physiol.* **83B**, 409–414.

[60] P. W. H. Heinstra, W. Aben, W. Scharloo, and G. E. W. Thörig (1986) Alcohol dehydrogenase of *Drosophila melanogaster*: Metabolic differences mediated through cryptic allozymes. *Heredity* **57**, 23–29.

[61] F. J. Garcin, G. L. Y. Hin, J. Cote, S. Radouco-Thomas, S. Chawla, and C. Radouco-Thomas (1985) Aldehyde dehydrogenase in *Drosophila*: Developmental and functional aspects. *Alcohol* **2**, 85–89.

[62] J. R. David, K. Daly, and J. van Herrewege (1984) Acetaldehyde utilization and toxicity in adults lacking alcohol dehydrogenase and aldehyde oxidase. *Biochem. Genet.* **22**, 1015–1029.

[63] K. T. Eisses, W. Schoonen, W. Aben, W. Scharloo, and G. E. W. Thörig (1985) Dual function of the alcohol dehydrogenase of Drosophila melanogaster: Ethanol and acetaldehyde oxidation by two allozymes ADH-71k and ADH-F. *Mol. Gen. Genet.* **199**, 76–81.

[64] K. T. Eisses (1989) On the oxidation of aldehydes by alcohol dehydrogenase of *Drosophila melanogaster*: Evidence for the gem-diol as the reacting substrate. *Bioorg. Chem.* **17**, 268–274.

[65] R. J. Middleton and H. Kacser (1983) Enzyme variation, metabolic flux and fitness: Alcohol dehydrogenase in *Drosophila melanogaster*. *Genetics* **105**, 633–650.

[66] P. W. H. Heinstra, W. Scharloo, and G. E. W. Thörig (1987) Physiological significance of the alcohol dehydrogenase polymorphism in larvae of *Drosophila*. *Genetics* **117**, 75–84.

[67] A. M. Kapoun, B. W. Geer, P. W. H. Heinstra, V. Corbin, and S. W. McKechnie (1990) Molecular control of the induction of alcohol dehydrogenase by ethanol in *Drosophila melanogaster* larvae. *Genetics* **124**, 881–888.

[68] P. W. H. Heinstra, D. Seykens, A. Freriksen, and B. W. Geer (1990) Metabolic physiology of alcohol degradation and adaptation in *Drosophila* larvae as studied by means of carbon-13 nuclear magnetic resonance spectroscopy. *Insect Biochem.* **20**, 343–348.

[69] H. Ursprung, W. Sofer, and N. Burroughs (1970) Ontogeny and tissue distribution of alcohol dehydrogenase in *Drosophila melanogaster*. *Wilhelm Roux Arch.* **164**, 201–208.

[70] G. Maroni and S. C. Stamey (1983) Developmental profile and tissue distribution of alcohol dehydrogenase. *Drosophila Information Serv.* **59**, 77–79.

[71] B. W. Geer, S. W. McKechnie, M. J. Pyka, and P. W. H. Heinstra (1991) Heritable variation in ethanol tolerance and its association with biochemical traits in *Drosophila melanogaster*. *Evolution*, **45**.

[72] P. W. H. Heinstra and B. W. Geer (1991) Metabolic control analysis and enzyme variation: Nutritional manipulation of the flux from ethanol to lipids in *Drosophila*. *Mol. Biol. Evol.* **8**.

[73] B. W. Geer, S. W. McKechnie, M. M. Bentley, J. G. Oakeshott, E. M. Quinn, and M. L. Langevin (1988) Induction of alcohol dehydrogenase by ethanol in *Drosophila melanogaster*. *J. Nutr.* **118**, 398–407.

[74] L. Trivinos and B. W. Geer (1991) The induction of alcohol dehydrogenase by primary alcohols in the fat body of *Drosophila melanogaster*, in preparation.

[75] S.-J. Yin and T.-K. Li (1989) Genetic polymorphism and properties of human alcohol and aldehyde dehydrogenase: Implications for ethanol metabolism and toxicity, in *Molecular Mechanisms of Alcohol*. G. Y. Sun, P. K. Rudeen, W. G. Wood, Y. H. Wei, and A. Y. Sun, eds. Humana, Clifton, NJ, pp. 227–247.

[76] R. Caizzi, M. P. Bozzetti, C. Caggese, and F. Ritossa (1990) Homologous nuclear genes encode cytoplasmic and mitochondrial glutamine synthetase in *Drosophila melanogaster*. *J. Mol. Biol.* **212**, 17–26.

[77] E. Balboni (1978) A proline shuttle in insect flight muscle. *Biochem. Biophys. Res. Commun.* **85**, 1090–1096.

[78] J. Farrès, P. Julià, and X. Parés (1988) Aldehyde oxidation in human placenta: Purification and properties of 1-pyrroline-5-carboxylate dehydrogenase. *Biochem. J.* **256**, 461–467.

[79] B. W. Geer, C. G. Woodward, and S. D. Marshall (1978) Regulation of the oxidative NADP-enzyme tissue levels in *Drosophila melanogaster*. II. The biochemical basis of dietary carbohydrate and D-glycerate modulation. *J. Exp. Zool.* **203**, 391–402.

[80] B. W. Geer, P. W. H. Heinstra, A. M. Kapoun, and A. van der Zel (1990) Alcohol dehydrogenase and alcohol tolerance in *Drosophila melanogaster*, in *Ecological and Evolutionary Genetics of* Drosophila. J. S. F. Barker and W. T. Starmer, eds. Plenum, New York, pp. 231–252.

[81] M. C. Deltombe-Lietaert, J. Delcour, N. Lenelle-Monfort, and A. Elens (1979) Ethanol metabolism in *Drosophila melanogaster*. *Experientia* **35**, 579–581.

[82] G. C. Bewley, J. A. Nahmias, and J. L. Cook (1983) Developmental and tissue specific control of catalase expression in *Drosophila melanogaster*. *Dev. Genet.* **4**, 49–60.

[83] A. van der Zel, R. Dadoo, B. W. Geer, and P. W. H. Heinstra (1991) The involvement of catalase in alcohol metabolism in *Drosophila melanogaster* larvae. *Arch. Biochem. Biophys.* **287,** 121–127.

[84] L. Sullivan (1990) Medical consequences, in *Seventh Special Report to the U. S. Congress on Alcohol and Health.* US Department of Health and Human Services, Washington, DC, pp.107–138.

[85] T. M. Donohue, Jr., D. J. Tuma, and M. F. Sorrell (1983) Binding of metabolically derived acetaldehyde to hepatic proteins *in vivo. Lab. Invest.* **49,** 226–229.

[86] C. S. Lieber (1989) Toxic and metabolic changes induced by ethanol, in *Alcoholism: Biomedical and Genetic Aspects.* H. Goedde and D. P. Agarwal, eds. Pergamon, New York, pp. 57–83.

[87] T. J. Mauch, T. M. Donohue, R. K. Zetterman, M. F. Sorrell, and D. J. Tuma (1986) Covalent binding of acetaldehyde selectively inhibits the catalytic activity of lysine-dependent enzymes. *Hepatology* **6,** 263–269.

[88] R. E. Barry and J. D. McGivan (1985) Acetaldehyde alone may initiate hepatocellular damage in acute alcoholic liver disease. *Gut* **26,** 1065–1069.

[89] V. J. Stevens, W. J. Fantl, C. B. Newman, R. V. Sims, A. Cerami, and C. M. Peterson (1981) Acetaldehyde adducts with hemoglobin. *J. Clin. Invest.* **67,** 361–369.

[90] K. C. Gaines, J. M. Salhany, D. J. Tuma, and M. F. Sorell (1977) Reaction of acetaldehyde with human erythrocyte membrane proteins. *FEBS Lett.* **75,** 115–117.

[91] T. M. Donohue, Jr., D. J. Tuma, and M. F. Sorrell (1983) Binding of metabolically derived acetaldehyde to hepatic proteins *in vitro. Lab. Invest.* **49,** 226–229.

[92] E. Baraona and C. S. Lieber (1983) Effects of ethanol on hepatic protein metabolism, in *Alcohol and Protein Synthesis: Ethanol, Nucleic Acids, and Protein Synthesis in Brain and Other Organs,* NIAAA Research Monogram No. 10 (DHHS Publication No. [ADM] 83-1198), pp. 75–95.

[93] Y. Israel, E. Hurwitz, O. Niemela, and R. Arnon (1986) Monoclonal and polyclonal antibodies against acetaldehyde-containing epitopes in acetaldehyde-protein adducts. *Proc. Natl. Acad. Sci. USA* **83,** 7923–7927.

[94] M. Hoerner, U. J. Behrens, T. M. Worner, and C. S. Lieber (1986) Humoral immune response to acetaldehyde adducts in alcoholic patients. *Res. Commun. Chem. Pathol. Pharmacol.* **54,** 3–12.

[95] A. Zorzano, L. R. del Arbol, and E. Herrera (1989) Effect of liver disorders on ethanol elimination and alcohol and aldehyde dehydrogenase activities in liver and erythrocytes. *Clin. Sci.* **76,** 51–57.

[96] H. P. Hoensch, I. Schreier, and E. E. Ohnhaus (1986) Inducing efficacy of ethanol on hepatic drug metabolizing enzymes in patients. *Eur. J. Clin. Invest.* **16,** 284–291.

[97] U. J. Behrens, M. Hoerner, J. M. Lasker, and C. S. Lieber (1988) Formation of acetaldehyde adducts with ethanol-inducible P450IIE1 *in vivo*. *Biochem. Biophys. Res. Commun.* **154,** 584–590.

[98] D. W. Nebert and F. J. Gonzalez (1987) P450 genes: Structure, evolution, and regulation. *Annu. Rev. Biochem.* **56,** 945–993.

[99] B. J. Song, H. V. Gelboin, S. S. Park, C. S. Yang, and F. J. Gonzalez (1986) Complementary DNA and protein sequences of ethanol-inducible rat and human P-450s. *J. Biol. Chem.* **261,** 16,689–16,697.

[100] D. R. Koop, E. T. Morgan, G. E. Tarr, and M. J. Coon (1982) Purification and characterization of a unique isozyme of cytochrome P-450 from liver microsomes of ethanol-treated rabbits. *J. Biol. Chem.* **257,** 8472–8480.

[101] D. R. Koop, and M. J. Coon (1984) Purification of liver cytochrome P-450 isozymes 3a and 6 from imidazole-treated rabbits. *Mol. Pharmacol.* **25,** 494–501.

[102] C. F. Wilkenson and L. B. Brattsten (1972) Microsomal drug metabolizing enzymes in insects. *Drug Metab. Rev.* **1,** 153–228.

[103] J. A. Zijlstra, E. W. Vogel, and D. D. Breimer (1986) Pharmacological and toxicological aspects of mutagenicity research in *Drosophila melanogaster,* in *Reviews in Biochemical Toxicology,* vol. 8. E. Hodgson, J. R. Bend, and R. M. Philpot, eds. Elsevier, New York, pp. 123–153.

[104] A. J. Baars, J. A. Zijlstra, E. Vogel, and D. D. Breimer (1977) The occurrence of cytochrome P-450 and aryl hydrocarbon hydroxylase activity in *Drosophila microsomes,* and the importance of this metabolizing capacity for the screening of mutagenic properties of foreign compounds. *Mutat. Res.* **44,** 257–268.

[105] I. Hallstrom and R. Grafstrom (1981) The metabolism of drugs and carcinogens in isolated subcellular fractions of *Drosophila melanogaster.* II. Enzyme induction and metabolism of benzo[a]pyrene. *Chem. Biol. Interact.* **34,** 145–159.

[106] L. C. Waters, C. E. Nix, and J. L. Epler (1982) Dimethylnitrosamine demethylase activity in *Drosophila melanogaster. Biochem. Biophys. Res. Commun.* **106,** 779–785.

[107] L. C. Waters, C. E. Nix, and J. L. Epler (1983) Studies on the relationship between dimethylnitrosamine-demethylase activity and dimethylnitrosamine-dependent mutagenesis in *Drosophila melanogaster. Chem. Biol. Interact.* **46,** 55–66.

[108] L. C. Waters, S. I. Simms, and C. E. Nix (1984) Natural variation in the expression of cytochrome P-450 and dimethylnitrosamine demethylase in *Drosophila. Biochem. Biophys. Res. Commun.* **123,** 907–913.

[109] L. C. Waters, C. E. Nix, K. M. Solden, and J. L. Epler (1984) Effects of genotype and age on mixed-function oxidase activities in adult *Drosophila melanogaster. Mutat. Res.* **139,** 51–55.

[110] D. R. Houpt, J. C. Pursey, and R. A. Morton (1988) Genes controlling malathion resistance in a laboratory-selected population of *Drosophila melanogaster. Genome* **30,** 844–853.

[111] S. S. Sundseth, C. E. Nix, and L. C. Waters (1990) Isolation of insecticide resistance-related forms of cytochrome P-450 from *Drosophila melanogaster. Biochem. J.* **265,** 213–217.

[112] D. L. Tribble, T. Y. Aw, and D. P. Jones (1987) The pathophysiological significance of lipid peroxidation in oxidative cell injury. *Hepatology* **7,** 377–387.

[113] J. A. Handler, B. U. Bradford, E. B. Glassman, D. T. Forman, and R. G. Thurman (1987) Inhibition of catalase-dependent ethanol metabolism in alcohol dehydrogenase-deficient deermice by fructose. *Biochem. J.* **248,** 415–421.

[114] V. Massey, S. Strickland, and S. G. Mayhew (1969) The production of superoxide anion radicals in the reaction of reduced flavin and flavoproteins with molecular oxygen. *Biophys. Res. Commun.* **36,** 891–897.

[115] E. W. Kellogg and I. Fridovich (1975) Superoxide hydrogen peroxide and singlet oxygen in lipid peroxidation by a xantine oxidase system. *J. Biol. Chem.* **250,** 8812–8817.

[116] M. Younes and O. Strubelt (1987) Enhancement of hypoxic liver damage by ethanol. *Biochem. Pharmacol.* **36,** 2973–2977.

[117] J. Vina, J. M. Estrela, C. Guerri, and F. J. Romero (1980) Effect of ethanol on glutathione concentration in isolated hepatocytes. *Biochem. J.* **188,** 549–552.

[118] S. Shaw, K. P. Rubin, and C. S. Lieber (1983) Depressed hepatic glutathione and increased diene conjugates in alcoholic liver disease. *Dig. Dis. Sci.* **28,** 585–589.

[119] S. Orrenius, K. Ormstad, H. Thor, and S. A. Jewell (1983) Turnover and functions of glutathione studied in isolated hepatic and renal cells. *Fed. Proc.* **42,** 3177–3188.

[120] H. Speisky, H. Orrego, and Y. Israel (1990) Hepatic glutathione metabolism: Alterations induced by alcohol consumption, in *Human Metabolism of Ethanol,* vol. III. K. E. Crow and R. D. Batt, eds. CRC, Boca Raton, FL, pp. 125–139.

[121] T. Suematsu, T. Matsumura, N. Sato, T. Miyamoto, T. Ooka, T. Kamada, and H. Abe (1981) Lipid peroxidation in alcoholic liver disease in humans. *Alcohol. Clin. Exp. Res.* **5,** 427–430.

[122] P. S. Bora, C. A. Spilburg, and L. G. Lange (1989) Metabolism of ethanol and carcinogens by glutathione transferases. *Proc. Natl. Acad. Sci. USA* **86,** 4470–4473.

[123] E. A. Laposata and L. G. Lange (1986) Presence of nonoxidative ethanol metabolism in human organs commonly damaged by ethanol abuse. *Science* **231,** 497–499.

[124] C. Beelman, R. R. Miller, Jr., and B. W. Geer (1991) Unpublished data.

[125] J. Kondrup, N. Grunnert, and J. Dich (1990) Interactions of ethanol and lipid

metabolism, in *Human Metabolism of Ethanol,* vol. III. K. E. Crow and R. D. Batt, eds. CRC, Boca Raton, FL, pp. 97–113.

[126] C. S. Lieber and M. Savolainen (1984) Ethanol and lipids. *Alcohol. Clin. Exp. Res.* **8,** 409–423.

[127] J. Kondrup (1984) The *in vitro* effect of ethanol on the synthesis of triacylglycerol in hepatic cytoplasmic lipid droplets. *Dan. Med. Bull.* **31,** 109–120.

[128] J. H. Chin and D. B. Goldstein (1985) Effects of alcohols on membrane fluidity and lipid composition, in *Membrane Fluidity in Biology,* vol. 3. R. C. Aloia, ed. Academic, New York, pp. 1–37.

[129] G. Y. Sun and A. Y. Sun (1985) Ethanol and membrane lipids. *Alcohol. Clin. Exp. Res.* **9,** 164–180.

[130] T. F. Taraschi and E. Rubin (1985) Effects of ethanol on the chemical and structural properties of biologic membranes. *Lab. Invest.* **52,** 120–131.

[131] D. B. Goldstein (1989) Alcohol and biological membranes, in *Alcoholism: Biomedical and Genetic Aspects.* H. Goedde and D. P. Agarwal, eds. Pergamon, New York, pp. 87–98.

[132] B. LeBourhis, F. Beauge, and G. Aufrere (1986) Membrane fluidity and alcohol dependence. *Alcohol. Clin. Exp. Res.* **10,** 337–341.

[133] J. H. Chin and D. B. Goldstein (1977) Drug tolerance in biomembranes: A spin label study of the effects of ethanol. *Science* **196,** 684,685.

[134] W. G. Wood, C. Gorka, and F. Schroeder (1989) Acute and chronic effects of ethanol on transbilayer membrane domains. *J. Neurochem.* **52,** 1925–1930.

[135] H. Rottenberg, D. Robertson, and E. Rubin (1980) The effect of ethanol on the temperature dependence of respiration and ATPase activities of rat liver mitochondria. *Lab. Invest.* **42,** 318–326.

[136] T. F. Taraschi, A. Wu, and E. Rubin (1985) Phospholipid spin probes measure the effects of ethanol on the molecular order of liver microsomes. *Biochemistry* **24,** 7096–7101.

[137] H. Rottenberg, A. Waring, and E. Rubin (1981) Tolerance and cross-tolerance in chronic alcoholics: Reduced membrane binding of ethanol and other drugs. *Science* **213,** 583,584.

[138] T. F. Taraschi, J. S. Ellingson, A. Wu, R. Zimmerman, and E. Rubin (1986) Phosphatidylinositol from ethanol-fed rats convers membrane tolerance to ethanol. *Proc. Natl. Acad. Sci. USA* **83,** 9398–9402.

[139] M. A. Polokof, T. J. Simon, A. Harris, F. R. Simon, and M. Iwahashi (1985) Chronic ethanol increases liver plasma membrane fluidity. *Biochemistry* **24,** 3114–3120.

[140] F. Koszo, L. I. Horvath, N. Simon, C. Ciklosi, and M. Kiss (1982) The role of possible membrane damage in porphyria cutanea tarda: A spin label study of rat liver cell membranes. *Biochem. Pharmacol.* **31,** 11–17.

[141] J. H. Chin and D. B. Goldstein (1984) Cholesterol blocks the disordering effects of ethanol in biomembranes. *Lipids* **19,** 929–935.

[142] M. Salaspuro (1989) The organ pathogenesis of alcoholism: Liver and gastrointestinal tract, in *Alcoholism: Biomedical and Genetic Aspects.* H. W. Goedde and D. P. Agarwal, eds. Pergamon, New York, pp. 133–166.

[143] B. M. Altura and B. T. Altura (1989) Cardiovascular functions in alcoholism and after acute administration of alcohol: Heart and blood vessels., in *Alcoholism: Biomedical and Genetic Aspects.* H. W. Goedde and D. P. Agarwal, eds. Pergamon, New York, pp. 167–215.

[144] K. E. Crow and R. M. Greenway (1990) The effects of alcohol on the liver, in *Human Metabolism of Alcohol,* vol. III. K. E. Crow and R. D. Batt, eds. CRC, Boca Raton, FL, pp. 4–18.

[145] J. N. Santamaria (1990) The effects of ethanol and its metabolism on the brain, in *Human Metabolism of Alcohol,* vol. III. K. E. Crow and R. D. Batt, eds. CRC, Boca Raton, FL, pp. 36–60.

[146] L. O. Simpson and R. J. Olds (1990) Ethanol and the flow properties of blood, in *Human Metabolism of Alcohol,* vol. III. K. E. Crow and R. D. Batt, eds. CRC, Boca Raton, FL, pp. 62–79.

[147] J. S. Gavaler and D. H. Van Thiel (1990) Alcohol interactions with the reproductive system, in *Human Metabolism of Alcohol,* vol. III. K. E. Crow and R. D. Batt, eds. CRC, Boca Raton, FL, pp. 82–94.

[148] C. M. Leevy (1968) Cirrhosis in alcoholics. *Med. Clin. North Am.* **52,** 1445–1451.

[149] P. W. Brunt, M. C. Kew, P. J. Scheuer, and S. Sherlock (1974) Studies of alcoholic liver disease in Britain. I. Clinical and pathological patterns related to natural history. *Gut* **15,** 52–58.

[150] C. S. Lieber and N. Spritz (1966) Effects of prolonged ethanol intake in man: Role of dietary, adipose, and endogenously synthesized fatty acids in the pathogenesis of alcoholic fatty liver. *J. Clin. Invest.* **45,** 1400–1411.

[151] C. S. Lieber, N. Spritz, and L. M. De Carli (1966) Role of dietary, adipose, and endogenously synthesized fatty acids in the pathogenesis of alcoholic fatty liver. *J. Clin. Invest.* **45,** 51–62.

[152] J. Kondrup (1984) *In vitro* effects of ethanol on the synthesis of triacylglycerol in hepatic cytoplasmic lipid droplets. *Dan. Med. Bull.* **31,** 109–120.

[153] S. Laurell and A. Lundquist (1971) Lipid composition of human liver biopsy specimens. *Acta Med. Scand.* **189,** 65–68.

[154] P. G. Mavrelis, H. V. Ammon, J. J. Glysteen, R. A. Komorowski, and U. K. Charaf (1983) Hepatic free fatty acids in alcoholic liver disease and morbid obesity. *Hepatology* **3,** 226–231.

[155] S. R. Cairns and T. J. Peters (1983) Biochemical analysis of hepatic lipid content in alcoholics. *Clin. Sci.* **65,** 645–652.

[156] A. Lundquist, T. Weibe, and P. Belfrage (1973) Liver lipid content in alcoholics. *Acta Med. Scand.* **194,** 501–504.

[157] R. Fraser (1990) Structural changes in liver caused by ethanol, in *Human Metabolism of Alcohol,* vol. III. K. E. Crow and R. D. Batt, eds. CRC, Boca Raton, FL, pp. 20–33.

[158] R. A. Helman, M. H. Temko, S. W. Nye, and H. J. Fallon (1971) Alcoholic hepatitis: Natural history and evaluation of prednisolone therapy. *Ann. Intern. Med.* **74,** 311–321.

[159] E. Rubin and C. S. Lieber (1968) Alcohol-induced hepatic injury in non-alcoholic volunteers. *N. Engl. J. Med.* **278,** 869–876.

[160] K. A. Fleming and J. O.-D. McGee (1984) Alcoholic liver disease. *J. Clin. Pathol.* **37,** 721–733.

[161] E. Rubin and C. S. Lieber (1968) Alcohol-induced hepatic injury in nonalcoholic volunteers. *N. Eng. J. Med.* **290,** 128-135.

[162] N. R. Primstone and S. W. French (1984) Alcoholic liver disease. *Med. Clin. North Am.* **68,** 39–56.

[163] T. A. Sorenson, M. Orholm, K. D. Bentsen, G. Hoyby, K. Eghoje, and P. Christofferson (1984) Prospective evaluation of alcohol abuse and alcoholic liver injury in man as predictors of development of cirrhosis. *Lancet* **ii,** 241–244.

[164] E. Mezey (1974) Ethanol and hepatic fibrogenesis, in *Biochemistry and Pharmacology of Ethanol.* E. Majchrowicz and E. P. Noble, eds. Plenum, New York, pp. 459–478.

[165] H. Popper, S. Thung, and N. Gerber (1981) Pathology of alcoholic liver disease. *Semin. Liv. Dis.* **1,** 203–216.

[166] R. G. Shorter and A. H. Baggenstoss (1959) Observations on the histogenesis of cirrhosis of the liver in chronic alcoholism. *Am. J. Clin. Pathol.* **32,** 422–429.

[167] G. Klatskin (1961) Alcohol and its relation to liver damage. *Gastroenterology* **41,** 443–451.

[168] C. M. Leevy and W. tenHove (1967), in *Biochemical Factors in Alcoholism.* R. P. Maickel, ed. Pergamon, Oxford, pp. 151–165.

[169] B. F. Grant, M. C. Dufour, and T. C. Harford (1988) Epidemeology of alcoholic liver disease. *Semin. Liv. Dis.* **8(1),** 12–25.

[170] Y. Israel, R. S. Britton, and H. Orrego (1982) Liver cell enlargement induced by chronic alcohol consumption: Studies on its causes and consequences. *Clin. Biochem.* **15,** 189–192.

[171] C. S. Lieber (1984) Alcohol and the liver: 1984 update. *Hepatology* **4,** 1243–1260.

[172] W. C. Maddrey (1988) Alcoholic hepatitis: Clinicopathologic features and therapy. *Semin. Liv. Dis.* **8(1),** 91–102.

[173] H. Popper and C. S. Lieber (1980) Histogenesis of alcoholic fibrosis and cirrhosis in baboon. *Am. J. Pathol.* **98,** 695–715.

[174] H. Brunengraber, M. Boutry, L. Lowenstein, and J. M. Lowenstein (1974) The effect of ethanol on lipogenesis by the perfused liver., in *Alcohol and Aldehyde Metabolizing Systems*. R. G. Thurman, T. Yonetani, J. R. Williamson, and B. Chance, eds. Academic, New York, pp 329.

[175] J. Selmer and N. Grunnet (1976) Ethanol metabolism and lipid synthesis by isolated liver cells from fed rats. *Biochim. Biophys. Acta* **428**, 123–137.

[176] N. Grunnet, F. Jensen, J. Kondrup, and J. Dich (1985) Effect of ethanol on fatty acid metabolism in cultured hepatocytes: Dependency on incubation time and fatty acid composition. *Alcohol* **2**, 157–161.

[177] M. J. Savolainen, J. K. Hiltunen, and I. E. Hassinen (1977) Effect of prolonged ethanol ingestion on hepatic lipogenesis and related enzyme activities. *Biochem. J.* **164**, 169–177.

[178] S. Venkatesan, N. W. Y. Leung, and T. J. Peters (1986) Fatty acid synthesis *in vitro* by liver tissue from control subjects and patients with alcoholic liver disease. *Clin. Sci.* **71**, 723–728.

[179] E. Majchrowicz and J. H. Quastel (1961) Effects of aliphatic alcohols and fatty acids on the metabolism of acetate by rat liver slices. *Can. J. Biochem. Physiol.* **39**, 1895–1909.

[180] O. A. Forsander (1970) in *International Encyclopedia of Pharmacology and Therapeutics*, Section 20. J. Tremolieres, ed. Pergamon, New York, pp. 117–135.

[181] Y. Israel, H. Kalant, H. Orrego, J. M. Khanna, M. J. Phillips, and D. J. Stewart (1979) Hypermetabolic state, oxygen avaliability, and alcohol-induced liver damage, in *Biochemistry and Pharmacology of Ethanol*. E. Majchrowicz and E. P. Noble, eds. Plenum, New York, pp. 433–443.

[182] C. S. Lieber (1988) Metabolic effects of ethanol and its interaction with other drugs, hepatotoxic agents, vitamins, and carcinogens (1988 update). *Sem. Liv. Dis.* **8(1)**, 47–68.

[183] Y. Israel and H. Orrego (1987) Hypermetabolic state, hepatocyte expansion, and liver blood flow: An interaction triad in alcoholic liver injury. *Ann. NY Acad. Sci.* **492**, 303–323.

[184] Y. Olowe and H. Schultz (1980) Regulation of thiolases from pig heart. *Eur. J. Biochem.* **109**, 425–430.

[185] B. Davidson and H. Schultz (1982) Separation, properties, and regulation of acyl coenzyme A dehydrogenases from bovine heart and liver. *Arch. Biochem. Biophys.* **213**, 155–162.

[186] J. D. McGarry and D. W. Foster (1971) The regulation of ketogenesis from oleic acid and the influence of antiketogenic agents. *J. Biol. Chem.* **246**, 6247–6253.

[187] T. Ide and J. A. Ontko (1981) Increased secretion of very low density lipoprotein triglyceride following inhibition of long chain fatty acid oxidation in isolated rat liver. *J. Biol. Chem.* **256**, 10,247–10,255.

[188] B. M. Wolfe, J. R. Havel, E. B. Marliss, J. P. Kane, J. Seymour, and S. P. Ahuja (1976) Effects of a 3-day fast and of ethanol on splancnic metabolism of FFA, amino acids, and carbohydrates in healthy young men. *J. Clin. Invest.* **57,** 329–340.

[189] L. Jorfeldt and A. Juhlin-Dannfelt (1978) The influence of ethanol on splancnic and skeletal muscle metabolism in man. *Metabolism* **27,** 97–106.

[190] J. Kondrup, F. Lundquist, and S. E. Damgaard (1979) Metabolism of palmitate in perfused rat liver. Effect of low and high ethanol concentrations at various concentrations of palmitate in the perfusion medium. *Biochem. J.* **184,** 83–95.

[191] N. Grunnet, J. Kondrup, and J. Dich (1985) Effect of ethanol on lipid metabolism in cultured hepatocytes. *Biochem. J.* **228,** 673–681.

[192] N. Grunnet, J. Kondrup, and J. Dich (1987) Ethanol-induced accumulation of triacylglycerol in cultured hepatocytes: Dependency on ethanol metabolism. *Alcohol Alcohol.* **(Suppl. 1),** 257.

[193] C. L. Mendenhall (1972) Origin of hepatic triglyceride fatty acids: Quantitative estimation of the relative contributions of linoleic acid by diet and adipose tissue in normal and ethanol-fed rats. *J. Lipid. Res.* **13,** 177–183.

[194] B. W. Geer, S. W. McKechnie, and M. L. Langevin (1983) Regulation of sn-glycerol 3-phosphate dehydrogenase in *Drosophila melanogaster* larvae by dietary ethanol and sucrose. *J. Nutr.* **113,** 1632–1642.

[195] A. Tietz, H. Weintraub, and Y. Peled (1975) Utilization of 2-acyl-sn-glycerol by locust fat body microsomes. *Biochim. Biophys. Acta* **388,** 165–170.

[196] M. L. Williams, F. L. Bygrave, and L. M. Birt (1974) Phospholipid synthesis in developing flight muscle of *Lucilia*. *Insect Biochem.* **4,** 161–172.

[197] R. G. H. Downer (1978) Functional role of lipids in insects, in *Biochemistry of Insects*. M. Rockenstein, ed. Academic, New York, pp. 57–92.

[198] P. R. Green and B. W. Geer (1979) Changes in the fatty acid composition of *Drosophila melanogaster* during development and ageing. *Arch. Int. Physiol. Biochim.* **87,** 485–493.

[199] H. Hollocher and A. R. Place (1987) Reexamination of alcohol dehydrogenase structural mutants in *Drosophila* using protein blotting. *Genetics* **116,** 253–263.

[200] F. Schaffner, A. Loebel, A. Weiner, and T. Barka (1963) Hepato-cellular cytoplasmic changes in acute alcoholic hepatitis. *JAMA* **183,** 343–346.

[201] F. M. Klion and F. Schaffner (1968) Ultrastructural studies in alcoholic liver disease. *Digest* **1,** 2–14.

[202] O. A. Iseri and L. S. Gottlieb (1971) Alcoholic hyalin and megamitochondria as separate and distinct entities in liver disease associated with alcoholism. *Gastroenterology* **60,** 1027–1046.

[203] S. W. French (1979) Role of mitochondrial damage in alcoholic liver disease., in *Biochemistry and Pharmacology of Ethanol*. E. Majchrowicz and E. P. Noble, eds. Plenum, New York, pp. 409–432.

[204] A. Lundquist, T. Weibe, and P. Belfrage (1973) Liver lipid content in alcoholics. *Acta Med. Scand.* **194,** 501–504.

[205] D. S. Rubin, S. Beattie, and C. S. Lieber (1970) Effects of ethanol on the biogenesis of mitochondrial membranes and associated mitochondrial functions *Lab Invest.* **23,** 620–627.

[206] J. D. Bernstein and R. Penniall (1978) Effect of chronic ethanol treatment upon rat liver mitochondria. *Biochem. Pharmacol.* **27,** 2337–2341.

[207] A. I. Cederbaum, C. S. Lieber, and E. Rubin (1974) The effect of acetaldehyde on mitochondrial function. *Arch. Biochem. Biophys.* **161,** 26–39.

[208] P. M. Vignais, J. Nachbaur, and P. V. Vignais (1969) Incorpration of fatty acids into the outer and inner membranes of isolated rat liver mitochondria. *FEBS Lett.* **3,** 121–124.

[209] M. Jain (1972) *The Bimolecular Lipid Membrane.* Van Nostrand Reinhold, New York, pp. 1–51, 383–408.

[210] B. W. Geer, S. W. McKechnie, and M. L. Langevin (1986) The effect of dietary ethanol on the composition of lipids of *Drosophila melanogaster* larvae. *Biochem. Genet.* **24,** 51–69.

[211] L. O. Ingram, B. F. Dickens, and T. M. Butke (1980) Reversible effects of ethanol on *E. coli.,* in *Biological Effects of Alcohol.* H. Begleitter, ed. Plenum, New York, pp. 299–337.

[212] A. A. Herrero, R. Gomez, and M. F. Roberts (1982) Ethanol-induced changes in the membrane lipid composition of *Clostridium thermocellum. Biochim. Biophys. Acta* **693,** 195–204.

[213] S. Hayashida, D. D. Feng, and M. Hongo (1974) Function of the high concentration of alcohol-producing factor. *Agr. Biol. Chem.* **38,** 2001–2006.

[214] D. S. Thomas, J. A. Hossack, and A. H. Rose (1978) Plasma membrane lipid composition and ethanol tolerance in *Sacchromyces cerivisiae. Arch. Microbiol.* **117,** 239–246.

[215] J. N. Miceli and W. J. Ferrell (1974) Effects of ethanol on membrane lipids. III. Quantitative changes in lipid and fatty acid composition of nonpolar and polar lipids of mouse total liver mitochondria and microsomes following ethanol feeding. *Lipids* **8,** 722–727.

[216] C. C. Cunningham, S. Filus, R. E. Bottenus, and P. I. Spach (1982) Effect of ethanol consumption on the phospholipid composition of rat liver microsomes and mitochondria. *Biochim. Biophys. Acta* **712,** 225–233.

[217] R. G. Reitz (1979) The effects of ethanol ingestion of lipid. *Prog. Lipid Res.* **18,** 87–115.

[218] J. A. Thompson and R. C. Reitz (1978) Effects of ethanol ingestion and dietary fat levels on mitochondrial lipids in male and female rats. *Lipids* **13,** 540–550.

[219] T. L. Smith, A. E. Vickers, K. Brendel, and M. J. Gerhart (1982) Effects of

ethanol diets on cholesterol content and phospholipid acyl composition of rat hepatocytes. *Lipids* **17,** 124–128.

[220] B. Rovinski and E. A. Hosein (1983) Adaptive changes in lipid composition of rat liver plasma membrane during postnatal development following ethanol ingestion. *Biochim. Biophys. Acta* **735,** 407–417.

[221] J. M. Littleton, S. J. Grieve, P. J. Griffiths, and J. R. John (1980) Ethanol-induced alteration in membrane phospholipid composition: Possible relationship to development of cellular tolerance to ethanol, in *Biological Effects of Alcohol.* Begleitter, H., ed. Plenum, New York, pp 7–19.

[222] G. Y. Sun and A. Y. Sun (1979) Effect of chronic ethanol administration on phospholipid acyl groups of synaptic plasma membrane isolated from guinea pig brain. *Res. Commun. Chem. Path. Pharmacol.* **24,** 405–408.

[223] G. Y. Sun and A. Y. Sun (1978) The effects of chronic ethanol administration on acyl group composition of mitochondrial phospholipids from guinea pig adrenal. *Res. Commun. Chem. Path. Pharmacol.* **21,** 355–358.

[224] R. G. Reitz, E. Helsabeck, and D. P. Mason (1973) Effects of chronic ethanol ingestion on the fatty acid composition of the heart. *Lipids* **8,** 80–84.

[225] M. Arai, E. R. Gordon, and C. S. Lieber (1984) Decreased cytochrome oxidase activity in hepatic mitochondria after chronic ethanol consumption and the possible role of decreased cytochrome aa_3 content and changes in phospholipids. *Biochim. Biophys. Acta* **797,** 320–327.

[226] J. M. Littleton and G. John (1979) Alterations in phospholipid composition in ethanol tolerance and dependence. *Alcohol. Clin. Exp. Res.* **3,** 50–56.

[227] G. A. Rao, S. C. Goheen, M. Manix, and E. C. Larkin (1980) Enhanced ratio of linoleic acid to arachidonic acid in erythrocyte phosphatidyl-choline in rats during withdrawal from ethanol. *Toxicol. Lett.* **7,** 37–40.

[228] H. Tsukamoto, G. Lew, E. C. Larkin, C. Largman, and G. A. Rao (1984) Hepatic origin of triglycerides in fatty livers produced by the continuous intragastric infusion of an ethanol diet. *Lipids* **19,** 419–422.

[229] A. J. Waring, H. Rottenberg, T. Ohnishi, and E. Rubin (1981) Membranes and phospholipids of liver mitochondria from chronic alcoholic rats are resistant to membrane disordering by ethanol. *Proc. Natl. Acad. Sci. USA* **78,** 2582–2586.

[230] S. R. Cairns and T. J. Peters (1983) Biochemical analysis of hepatic lipid in alcoholic and diabetic and control subjects. *Clin. Sci.* **65,** 645–652.

[231] R. A. Harris, M. A. Mitchell, and R. J. Hitzemann (1984) Physical properties of brain membrane from ethanol tolerant-dependent mice. *Mol. Pharmacol.* **25,** 401–409.

[232] C. Alling, S. J. Dencker, L. Svennerholm, and J. Tichy (1969) Serum fatty acid pattern in chronic alcoholics after acute abuse. *Acta Med.* **185,** 99–105.

[233] R. T. Holman and S. Johnson (1982) Changes in essential fatty acid profile of serum phospholipids in human disease. *Prog. Lipid. Res.* **20,** 67–73.

[234] L. Foudin, M. E. Tumbleson, A. Y. Sun, R. W. Geisler, and G. Y. Sun (1984) Ethanol consumption and serum lipid profiles in Sinclair (S-1) minature swine. *Life Sci.* **38,** 819–826.

[235] D. R. Wing, D. J. Harvey, J. Hughes, P. G. Dunbar, K. A. McPherson, and W. D. M. Paton (1982) Effects of chronic ethanol administration on the composition of membrane lipids in mouse. *Biochem. Pharmacol.* **31,** 3431–3439.

[236] A. D. Keith (1967) Fatty acid metabolism in D. melanogaster: Formation of palmitoleate. *Comp. Biochem. Physiol.* **21,** 587-600.

[237] R. R. Miller, Jr., J. Yates, and B. W. Geer (1991) The effects of ethanol on phospholipid composition, Ca^{+2} distribution, and the activities of phospholipases C and D in *Drosophila melanogaster* larvae. *Biochim. Biophys. Acta,* submitted.

[238] C. Alling, J. Balldin, K. Kahlson, and R. Olsson (1980) Decreased linoleic acid in serum lecithin after ethanol abuse. *Subst. Alcohol. Act/Mis.* **1,** 557–563.

[239] T. F. Taraschi, J. S. Ellingson, A. Wu., R. Zimmerman, and E. Rubin (1986) Membrane tolerance to ethanol is rapidly lost after withdrawal: A model for studies of membrane adaptation. *Proc. Natl. Acad. Sci. USA* **83,** 3669–3673.

[240] J. B. Hoek and T. F. Taraschi (1988) Cellular adaptations to ethanol. *TIBS* **13,** 269–274.

[241] B. W. Geer and G. F. Vovis (1965) The effects of choline and related compounds on the growth and development of *Drosophila melanogaster. J. Exp. Zool.* **158,** 223–236.

[242] B. W. Geer, G. F. Vovis, and M. A. Yund (1968) Choline activity during the development of *Drosophila melanogaster. Physiol. Zool.* **41,** 280–292.

[243] P. G. Fast (1966) A comparative study of phospholipids and fatty acids of some insects. *Lipids* **1,** 201–215.

[244] B. W. Geer, W. W. Dolph, J. A. Maquire, and R. J. Dates (1971) The metabolism of dietary carnitine in *Drosphila melanogaster. J. Exp. Zool.* **176,** 445–460.

[245] J. A. Tilghman and B. W. Geer (1988) The effects of a choline deficiency on the lipid composition and ethanol tolerance of *Drosophila melanogaster. Comp. Biochem. Physiol.* **90C,** 439–444.

[246] B. W. Geer and T. T. Perille (1977) Effects of dietary sucrose and environmental temperature on fatty acid synthesis in *Drosophila melanogaster. Insect Biochem.* **7,** 371–379.

Human Liver Alcohol Dehydrogenase Gene Expression

Retinoic Acid Homeostasis and Fetal Alcohol Syndrome

Gregg Duester

Alcohol Dehydrogenases in Human Liver and Other Tissues

Multiple Genes Encode Alcohol Dehydrogenase

Alcohol dehydrogenase (ADH; alcohol:NAD$^+$ oxidoreductase, EC 1.1.1.1) is a well-characterized enzyme present in all organisms analyzed, which catalyzes numerous alcohol/aldehyde interconversions. Human and rodent ADH exists as a heterogeneous group of isozymes that can be placed into three classes based on structural and functional distinctions.[1,2] All isozymes are dimeric, each monomer having a mol wt of about 40,000.[3] The human class I ADH isozymes include homodimers and heterodimers of the closely related α, β, and γ protein chains, which are encoded by *ADH1*, *ADH2*, and *ADH3*, respectively.[4] Human class II ADH is composed of homodimers of the π protein chain encoded by *ADH4*,[5] and human class III ADH is composed of homodimers of the χ protein chain encoded by *ADH5*.[6]

From: *Drug and Alcohol Abuse Reviews, Vol. 2: Liver Pathology and Alcohol*
Ed: R. R. Watson ©1991 The Humana Press Inc.

The structures of the human class I ADH protein chains have been determined from amino acid sequencing of the purified homodimeric isoenzymes and from nucleotide sequencing of cDNA clones encoding *ADH1*, *ADH2*, and *ADH3*.[7–10] From these studies it was learned that the α, β, and γ ADH isozymes share 93–94% amino acid sequence identity. In addition to their high degree of structural similarity, these isozymes also have very similar substrate specificities.[11] Thus, the existence of three genes for class I ADH in humans, instead of one, as in rodents,[12,13] may not be simply to catalyze different reactions, but to "fine tune" the expression of ADH in the developing human. Indeed, the three human class I ADH genes differ markedly in their patterns of expression, as discussed below.

Structures for human class II and III ADH have also been determined, and comparisons of the amino acid sequences of all three ADH classes indicate that they share about 58–62% sequence identity.[14] The extensive sequence homology indicates that the three ADH classes evolved from a common ancestor. Further studies on the function of ADH and the patterns of ADH gene expression may determine why mammals have selected and maintained three classes of ADH.

Function of ADH

Human class I ADH catalyzes the reversible oxidation/reduction of a wide variety of alcohols and aldehydes,[11,15,16] including the rate-limiting step in ethanol metabolism.[3,17] Human ADH classes II and III are very inefficient in oxidizing ethanol, and appear to have substrate specificities that are significantly different than that of class I.[18] For all human ADH classes, long-chain aliphatic and aromatic alcohols or aldehydes are much better substrates than ethanol or acetaldehyde.[11] Human class I ADH catalyzes the interconversion of alcohols and aldehydes in bile acid synthesis,[19] norepinephrine and dopamine metabolism,[20,21] and retinol metabolism.[22] The γ subunit of class I ADH has been shown to catalyze the oxidation of 3β-hydroxy-5β-steroids in testosterone metabolism.[23] Human class II ADH reduces an aldehyde intermediate in norepinephrine metabolism.[24] Mouse and rat class II ADH has been shown to function in retinol oxidation.[25,26] Human class III ADH catalyzes an ω-oxidation step in leukotriene B_4 synthesis in neutrophils.[27] Also, class III ADH has been identified as the glutathione-dependent formaldehyde dehydrogenase that is involved in elimination of formaldehyde produced as a byproduct of some metabolic reactions.[28] Thus, the ethanol/acetaldehyde interconversion is not the main function of ADH in mammals as it is for ADH in bacteria,[29] yeast,[30] *Drosophila*,[31] and maize.[32] During anaerobic fermentation in bacteria, yeast, and plant roots, ADH uses the reducing power of NADH to catalyze the reduction of acetaldehyde to form the byproduct ethanol, thus regenerating NAD^+ from NADH in the absence of respiration. In *Drosophila*, ethanol is used as a food source, since eggs are often laid in rotting fruit that is undergoing alcoholic fermentation by microbes; in this case, ADH catalyzes the oxidation of ethanol to form acetaldehyde that can subsequently be converted into acetyl-CoA and lipids. ADH in higher animals can certainly oxidize ethanol, but this compound is not a normal food source. As suggested by Krebs and Perkins,[17] the ethanol-oxidizing ability of mammalian ADH may facilitate the elimination of ethanol produced by alcoholic fermentation of normal intestinal microbes. Thus, ADH may play a physiologically significant role in eliminating endogenous ethanol from the body, but it certainly has several additional functions that are unique to higher animals.

Tissue and Developmental Regulation of ADH Gene Expression

All classes of ADH are expressed in the human liver, where the highest amount of ADH is seen. ADH accounts for about 2–3% of the soluble protein in adult human liver, most of this being class I ADH.[33,34] Differential regulation of the class I genes *ADH1*, *ADH2*, and *ADH3* is observed in liver. Starch gel analysis of human liver extracts from several stages of development indicates that a low level of α-ADH is produced during early fetal development, with additional low-level production of β-ADH during late fetal development and of γ-ADH several months postnatally.[4,35] The total amount of α, β, and γ ADH activity in the human liver increases by more than an order of magnitude postnatally between birth and five years of age, when adult levels of all three are achieved.[4,36,37] Hepatomas in human adults often revert to production of primarily α-ADH,[38] suggesting that there is a reversion to the type of ADH gene expression seen in early fetuses. A cDNA encoding human *ADH2*[7] was used as a hybridization probe in RNA blot experiments, and it was observed that there is a 50-fold increase in the level of human liver class I ADH mRNA between the 20-wk fetal stage and adulthood.[39] Also, gene-specific oligonucleotide probes have been used to show that the mRNAs for all three ADH species (α, β, and γ) undergo developmental increases in liver.[40] This suggests that there is increased transcription of the class I ADH genes as development proceeds, or increased mRNA stability, or both. The single class I ADH present in the mouse[41] and the rat[42] is also subject to a large increase in production during postnatal liver development.

Human class I ADH is also produced in other tissues, such as intestine, stomach, kidney, lung, and skin, at a level that is at least an order of magnitude less than that observed in liver.[4,35,38] In intestine, stomach, and kidney, γ-ADH is produced prenatally and postnatally, with additional production of β-ADH postnatally in kidney, and an absence of α-ADH.[4] In lung and skin, only β-ADH has been detected.[4,38] Thus, the tissue and developmental regulation of the three class I ADH genes is quite different in liver compared to other tissues. In rodents, class I ADH is expressed in intestine, kidney, lung, and skin, but is noticeably absent from stomach.[43,44]

The nucleotide sequences for the human *ADH1*, *ADH2*, and *ADH3* promoters, as well as their transcription start points, have been determined.[45,46] Also, the promoters for the mouse class I gene, *Adh-1*,[12,13] and the rat class I ADH gene[47] have been characterized.[9,10] These promoters are now being analyzed to dissect the transcriptional mechanisms controlling class I ADH gene expression in liver and other tissues.

Regulation of human class II and III ADH production differs from that of class I. Human class II ADH has been dectected only in adult liver,[34] whereas class III ADH is detected in almost all tissues analyzed.[48] In mice and rats, the class III enzyme is widely distributed in much the same tissues as in humans.[43,44] However, the rodent class II ADH enzyme is distributed much differently than its human counterpart, being absent in liver and present in stomach and sexual organs of the mouse,[43] and in stomach, intestine, lungs, skin, and sexual organs of the rat.[44] The different tissue distribution of class II ADH in rodents and humans may be a result of the presence of only one class I ADH gene in rodents, instead of three. Thus, rodent class II ADH may be present in some tissues to perform functions that class I ADH performs in homologous human tissues. For instance, since class II ADH is the major stomach isozyme in rodents, it may be the functional homolog of class I γ-ADH, which is the major stomach isozyme in humans.

Role of Alcohol Dehydrogenase in Retinoic Acid Homeostasis

Metabolism of Retinol to Form Retinoic Acid

One of the most interesting features of ADH is that it participates in the conversion of retinol (vitamin A) into retinoic acid, a known control molecule (morphogen) for vertebrate growth and development.[49,50] Retinol is reversibly oxidized to retinal by a cytosolic retinol dehydrogenase that is identical to liver class I ADH derived from the horse,[51] rat,[52–54] deermouse,[55] and human.[22] Rat testes have also been reported to contain a retinol dehydrogenase activity that is very similar to class I ADH, exhibiting a K_m for ethanol of about 1.0 mM and inhibition by low levels of 4-methylpyrazole.[56,57] Also, class II ADH has been reported to convert retinol to retinal in mouse epidermis[25] and rat ocular tissues.[26] Retinal is irreversibly oxidized to retinoic acid by an aldehyde dehydrogenase,[58–61] but the reversible retinol/retinal interconversion is the rate-limiting step in retinoic acid synthesis under most conditions.[60,61] Retinoic acid synthesis must occur in many tissues during embryonic and fetal development to program pattern formation,[49,50] and retinoic acid synthesis must be maintained in the adult for differentiation of epithelial tissues in liver, kidney, lung, intestine, stomach, skin, and reproductive organs.[62] Interestingly, these adult epithelial tissues are the locations where the highest class I and/or II ADH activity is found in humans and rodents.[4,35,43,44]

In addition to class I ADH, retinol dehydrogenase activities distinct from class I ADH exist in cytosol[52,55] and microsomes[54] of rodents. It has been difficult to determine the relative importance of the various enzymes in retinol metabolism and retinoic acid synthesis. A mutant deermouse exists that completely lacks class I ADH activity or immunologically crossreactive material[63] because of a deletion of the gene (M. Felder, personal communication). Compared to the wild-type deermouse, the ADH⁻ deermouse has retinoic acid synthetic activity that is greatly reduced in liver and kidney, but maintains most or all of its retinoic acid synthetic activity in testes, lung, and intestine.[55] Since the mutant deermouse appears to develop and reproduce normally, this indicates that this non-class-I ADH cytosolic retinol dehydrogenase provides enough retinol oxidation to maintain retinoic acid synthesis in the deermouse. It has been reported that the ADH activity missing in the ADH⁻ deermouse is equivalent to ethanol dehydrogenase or class I ADH, but it was not made clear whether the deermouse contains class II or III ADH.[55] This is important, since class II ADH from the laboratory mouse and rat has been reported to oxidize retinol.[25,26] ADH-inhibitor studies using 4-methylpyrazole were performed on the remaining retinol dehydrogenase activity present in the ADH- deermouse, and it was concluded that the activity was fairly insensitive to the inhibitor at 10 mM.[55] Rat and mouse class II ADHs are sensitive to the inhibitor 4-methylpyrazole with K_i values in the 0.5–1.5 mM range when assayed at pH 10, but this sensitivity has a large pH dependence, since at pH 7.5 rat class II ADH has a much lower sensitivity with a K_i value of 33 mM.[44] Since the ADH⁻ deermouse studies described above were performed at pH 7 with 10 mM 4-methylpyrazole,[55] it is unlikely that these conditions would have led to a significant inhibition of any potential class II ADH activity. Recent studies have indicated that the ADH⁻ deermouse does indeed have ADH species that correspond to laboratory mouse class II and III ADHs according to starch gel mobility assays and differential utilization of various types of alcohols (M. Felder, personal communication). Thus, the mutant deermouse should formally be termed the class I ADH⁻ deermouse to indicate clearly that it is not totally devoid of all ADH species. Furthermore, class II ADH in the deermouse (or other rodent species) should not be ruled out as a source of retinol dehydrogenase activity, especially in extrahepatic tissues, such as stomach, lung, skin, and some reproductive organs, in which class II ADH activity exceeds class I ADH activity.[43,44]

In humans, class II ADH is unlikely to play a role in extrahepatic retinol oxidation, since it has only been detected in adult liver.[34] However, since the human class I γ ADH isozyme has been detected in many extrahepatic tissues,[35] it may serve as the primary retinol dehydrogenase in humans. This difference between rodents and humans may be a consequence of human class I ADH being encoded by three genes (encoding α, β, and γ ADH) whereas rodent class I ADH being encoded by a single gene. Evolutionary divergence of the three class I ADH genes in humans may have led to the differential tissue distribution of human class I ADH isozymes that we see today, and may have allowed the divergence of human and rodent class II ADH genes to produce forms expressed in totally different tissues. Recent studies performed in our laboratory indicate that the human class I γ ADH isozyme encoded by the *ADH3* gene is likely to play a major physiological role in the control of human retinoic acid synthesis. Our studies indicate that *ADH3* is regulated transcriptionally by retinoic acid,[64] suggesting that a feedback-induction mechanism controls the level of retinol dehydrogenase (i.e., γ ADH) in humans (*see below*).

Retinoic Acid Controls Vertebrate Morphogenesis at the Transcriptional Level

Retinoic acid has profound effects on vertebrate limb[65] and nervous system[66] morphogenesis, as well as epithelial cell differentiation.[62] The effects of retinoic acid are transduced by binding to a nuclear retinoic acid receptor (RAR), which, in the presence of ligand, is transformed into a transcription factor.[67–69] Recently, an RAR gene family (RARα, β, and γ) has been discovered,[70,71] and differential expression of these receptors is undoubtedly important for correct transduction of the retinoic acid signal in various target tissues.[72] Also, another nuclear receptor has been uncovered, termed the retinoid X receptor (RXRα), which responds to retinoic acid as well as other retinoids, and which is expressed highly in the liver, unlike the RAR family.[73] Retinoic acid probably initiates a cascade of events that regulate the transcription of many key genes. Retinoic acid has been shown to induce several genes encoding homeobox-containing proteins that probably regulate transcription of the next set of genes in a morphogenetic cascade.[74–78] Genes encoding structural proteins needed for differentiation of many cells, such as laminin B1 and collagen IV(α1), are also induced by retinoic acid.[79,80] The RARβ gene (but not the RARα or γ genes) is induced by retinoic acid in teratocarcinoma and hepatoma cell lines,[81,82] suggesting that the selective induction of this RAR species is crucial to differentiation. Another indication of the major impact of retinoic acid on differentiation has come from the finding that this compound induces expression of the transcription factor AP-2 in a human teratocarcinoma cell line.[83]

The signal that dictates the release of retinoic acid is not yet known. In the developing limb bud, retinoic acid is produced by the zone of polarizing activity located in a posterior location, and diffuses out to form a local concentration gradient of between 20 and 50 n*M*, with the highest concentration being in the posterior tissue.[49,65] Studies proving that the limb-bud tissue can itself synthesize retinoic acid from retinol have been reported,[84,85] but the enzymatic activity responsible has not been elucidated. It is intriguing to speculate that this activity may be produced by ADH in the zone of polarizing activity. Since the substrate retinol is evenly distributed throughout the entire limb bud at 600 n*M*,[84] selective expression of ADH in the posterior tissue could possibly establish such a gradient of retinoic acid.

It has been noted that the shallowness of the retinoic acid concentration gradient in the limb bud may make differential gene expression in the anteroposterior axis unlikely. However, recent studies on cytoplasmic retinoic acid binding protein (CRABP) have made this issue more clear. CRABP avidly binds retinoic acid in the cytoplasm, thus modulating binding of retinoic acid to the nuclear RAR.[50,86] *In situ* studies of developing limb-bud tissue indicate that CRABP is also present in an anteroposterior concentration gradient, but with the high end being on the anterior side.[87] It has been proposed that by selectively binding retinoic acid, which is diffusing out to the anterior tissue from its site of synthesis in the posterior tissue, CRABP steepens the gradient of free retinoic acid across the anteroposterior axis.[86–88] Thus, even though there is 20 n*M* retinoic acid on the anterior side, much of it may be complexed with CRABP and unable to reach the nucleus to effect transcription. According to this model, a level of free retinoic acid appropriate for the differential regulation of transcription in the anteroposterior axis is established, resulting in the appropriate development of the tissues destined to form a limb.

A similar scenario appears to occur in the developing nervous system. Retinoic acid transforms developing anterior neural tissue into a posterior specification,[66] suggesting that this molecule helps to determine the anteroposterior positioning of neural cells. Also, CRABP is produced in a dorsal–ventral concentration gradient in the developing nervous system, with the high end being on the dorsal side.[89] This suggests that in the nervous system, as in the limb bud, CRABP selectively sequesters retinoic acid during development to produce a steepened retinoic acid gradient and, thus, differential regulation of gene expression.

Regulation of Retinoic Acid Synthesis by Feedback Induction of Alcohol Dehydrogenase

Understanding the mechanism that regulates synthesis of retinoic acid from retinol (vitamin A) is the key to understanding the physiological process whereby retinoic acid regulates morphogenesis. The controlled synthesis of retinoic acid in the correct embryonic location at the correct time is what triggers the morphogenetic cascade. A hypothesis is presented that suggests that class I ADH plays a major role in regulating the synthesis of retinoic acid needed for correct morphogenesis.

In support of this hypothesis, recent experiments in this laboratory have indicated that expression of the human *ADH3* gene is regulated transcriptionally by retinoic acid.[64] Various lengths of *ADH3* promoter DNA have been fused to the *E. coli* gene encoding chloramphenicol acetyltransferase (*cat*). The *ADH3–cat* fusions were individually introduced into hepatoma and teratocarcinoma cell lines by transfection, and *cat* expression was monitored in the presence and absence of added retinoic acid. These deletion-mapping experiments have identified a retinoic acid response element in the *ADH3* promoter located between –328 and –272 bp (relative to the transcription start point, designated +1) that functions in transfected Hep3B human hepatoma and F9 mouse teratocarcinoma cell lines (M. L. Shean and G. Duester, unpublished results). The 5'-flanking nucleotide sequence of the *ADH3* gene contains two copies of the sequence 5'-TGACC-3', previously noticed as an essential sequence for the retinoic acid response elements present in the control regions for the laminin B1[79] and RARβ[82] genes. In human *ADH3*, these sequences are located at –318 and –289 bp, both within the DNA fragment shown to impart retinoic acid responsiveness on *cat* expression.[64]

Since human class I ADH is known to function as a retinol dehydrogenase in retinoic acid synthesis,[22] this new finding indicates that retinoic acid can potentially stimulate its own synthesis via a positive-feedback loop effecting *ADH3* transcription in liver and nonliver cells. The very existence of such a feedback loop argues strongly that class I ADH activity plays a physiologically significant role in retinoic acid synthesis.

To achieve homeostasis of retinoic acid levels using a positive-feedback mechanism for stimulating synthesis, it would be necessary to couple this to a mechanism for degrading excess retinoic acid. Indeed, liver and other tissues possess an enzymatic activity, induced by retinoic acid, that oxidizes retinoic acid ($K_m = 10^{-6}M$) to the inactive 4-oxo-derivative.[90] Thus, retinoic acid feedback induces its degradation as well as its synthesis. A scheme for achieving retinoic acid homeostasis is presented in Fig. 1. The scheme combines previous knowledge of retinoid metabolism[22,53,58–60,90–92] with recent findings from this laboratory concerning positive feedback regulation of *ADH* gene expression.[64]

It is important to note that retinoic acid is likely to function as an intracrine hormone to self-regulate retinoic acid levels in liver and other tissues. Intracrine regulation is defined as a mechanism whereby hormones are synthesized and act within a cell without the need for exit and reentry, as

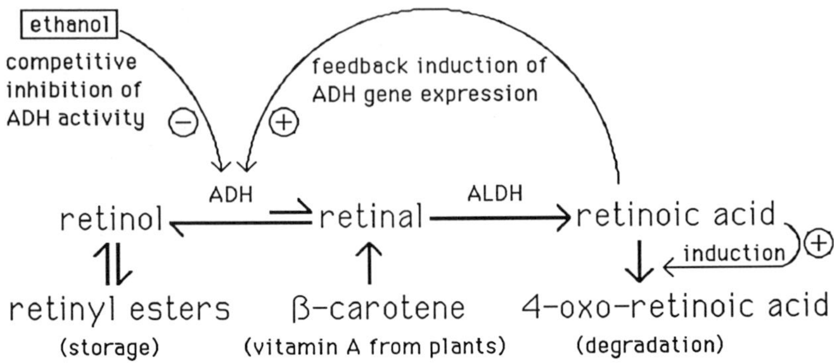

Fig.1. Retinoic acid homeostasis. β-Carotene, the ultimate source of vitamin A from plants, is oxidized to form retinal in the intestine and liver by β-carotene-15,15'-oxygenase. Intestinal retinaldehyde reductase efficiently converts retinal to retinol. Retinol is transported to the liver for storage as retinyl esters, and the liver releases retinol to the serum in a controlled fashion to keep the concentration constant. Retinol in the liver, or retinol taken up by many other tissues, can be converted to retinoic acid via a two-step oxidation in which ADH produces retinal and aldehyde dehydrogenase (ALDH) produces retinoic acid. Since the equilibrium of the ADH step is in the opposite direction, it is the high NAD$^+$/NADH ratio that pulls the retinol towards retinoic acid. Retinoic acid can be further oxidized to 4-oxo-retinoic acid as part of a degradation pathway for excretion, and the enzyme catalyzing this reaction is induced by retinoic acid. Our studies now indicate that retinoic acid can also feedback-induce *ADH* gene expression, indicating that retinoic acid synthesis is autoregulated. The effect of ethanol as a competitive inhibitor of ADH retinol oxidation is also indicated.

is the case for hormones that act by endocrine, paracrine, or autocrine mechanisms.[93] It is likely that retinoic acid also functions in a paracrine fashion (affecting cells closely neighboring the cells that synthesize the hormone), as predicted by the model in which a gradient of retinoic acid acts as a morphogen specifying the anteroposterior axis of the developing limb bud.[49] In this model, the zone of polarizing activity located in the posterior portion of the limb bud acts as the paracrine supplier of retinoic acid, which then diffuses to anterior tissues as a result of its ability to pass easily through cell membranes. A prediction that can be made from our findings is that the zone of polarizing activity may possess more ADH activity than tissue in the anterior portion of the limb bud, thus enabling it to serve as the paracrine supplier of retinoic acid.

As mentioned above, the limb bud has been shown to convert retinol to retinoic acid.[84] Also, F9 teratocarcinoma cells, which are analogous to cells in early embryonic tissue, can convert retinol to retinoic acid,[94] thus explaining why many of the well-known effects of retinoic acid can also be accomplished by retinol treatment.[95] Since our studies indicate that mouse F9 cells can support retinoic acid-induced transcription of a transfected human *ADH3* promoter, we suggest that these cells may be expressing an endogenous mouse ADH gene (either class I or II ADH), which is the source of the retinol dehydrogenase activity previously seen in F9 cells.[94]

Retinol and Ethanol Metabolism: Connection with Fetal Alcohol Syndrome

We propose that class I ADH is a very good candidate for the enzyme that regulates retinoic acid synthesis during embryonic development, as well as during adult life in many target tissues. The positive-feedback mechanism proposed for ADH expression would provide a very efficient method for creating localized synthesis of retinoic acid, thus establishing the morphogenetic gradient known to be necessary for correct development. Studies on the pathogenesis of fetal alcohol syndrome, as well as studies on the effects of ethanol on retinol metabolism, lend further support to the hypothesis that class I ADH is a major regulator of retinoic acid synthesis.

Ethanol acts as a competitive inhibitor of the retinol dehydrogenase activity attributed to human class I ADH,[22] but not other retinol dehydrogenase activities.[54,55] Ethanol also acts as a teratogen, causing brain, craniofacial, and limb abnormalities in those suffering from fetal alcohol syndrome.[96,97] Interestingly, these tissues are very sensitive to retinoic acid levels during fetal development.[65,66] Thus, many of the abnormalities observed in fetal alcohol syndrome could be caused by high levels of ethanol acting as a competitive inhibitor of class I ADH retinol oxidation, resulting in a reduction of retinoic acid synthesis in tissues that require critical levels of this molecule to specify spatial patterns. One would predict that, by lowering the rate of retinoic acid synthesis, chronic ethanol ingestion would also cause a decrease in the feedback induction of ADH expression that we have described.[64] In short, excess ethanol would be predicted to upset fetal retinoic acid homeostasis severely.

The connection between ethanol and retinoid metabolism is made even more apparent when one reviews the teratogenic effects that either compound exhibits when taken in excess. There are many similarities between the birth defects that occur in those suffering from fetal alcohol syndrome and those suffering from retinoid overdose. The latter problem often leads to teratogenesis and has been seen in some individuals who have taken the antiacne medicine Accutane (Roche, Basel, Switzerland; isotretinoin; 13-*cis*-retinoic acid) or other retinoids during pregnancy.[98,99] Retinol (vitamin A) ingested in large amounts leads to hypervitaminosis A, which has also been linked to birth defects.[99] In teratogenesis induced by hypervitaminosis A, it is believed that excessive retinoic acid derived from the excess retinol is at blame. Retinoic acid has been shown to be transported in the serum bound to albumin,[100] and both all-*trans*-retinoic acid and 13-*cis*-retinoic acid can be delivered to the fetus via placental transfer.[101] Malformations of human and animal offspring induced by retinoic acid occur to an extent that depends on the concentration and the stage of gestation at exposure. The major damages can be classified as defects of the neural tube, the facial cranium, and the bones of the spinal column, and include such abnormalities as microcephaly, hydrocephaly, spina bifida, club foot, and other limb defects.[99] This list of abnormalities makes sense, because it is now realized that there is an optimum concentration of retinoic acid needed to direct morphogenesis of the central nervous system and the limb bud. Presumably, retinoic acid present at high levels in the serum enters cells and upsets the delicate balance of retinoic acid homeostasis in target tissues, thus leading to birth defects. Perhaps many target tissues of retinoic acid normally respond only to the retinoic acid that they synthesize locally from retinol, and not to retinoic acid that they receive from the serum, which normally has low levels (i.e., 1.32 ng/mL [4.7 nM] all-*trans*-retinoic acid and 1.63 ng/mL [5.8 nM] 13-*cis*-retinoic acid in human serum[102]).

Ethanol taken during pregnancy is delivered to the fetus, and excessive ethanol ingestion can be teratogenic. The birth defects noticed in fetal alcohol syndrome are very similar to those described above for retinoid toxicity. Defects include abnormalities of the central nervous system, such as microcephaly, mental retardation, cleft palate, spinal stenosis, polydactyly, and many other limb abnormalities.[96,97] The defects vary in severity, depending on the amount of ethanol ingested and the stage of gestation. When enough ethanol is ingested to reach a blood-alcohol level of 0.1%, at which level one is designated legally intoxicated, the blood contains about 17 mM ethanol. Human liver class I ADH isozymes exhibit a range of K_m values for ethanol of 0.16–1.1 mM,[20] and ethanol inhibits human liver retinol oxidation with a K_i of 0.36 mM.[22] Thus, most of the class I ADH activity will be tied up in ethanol oxidation during alcohol intoxication and will not be available for retinol oxidation, even though the K_m for retinol (0.028 mM) is much lower than that for ethanol.[22]

Fetal alcohol syndrome has recently been recognized as a major public health problem and is one of the leading causes of mental retardation.[97] A single molecular mechanism that helps explain the multiple defects noticed in fetal alcohol syndrome has not been described.[103] Based on the information presented above concerning the role of ADH in the metabolism of retinol and ethanol, and the role of retinoic acid in fetal development, it seems reasonable to propose that fetal alcohol syndrome is primarily a disease caused by an imbalance in retinoic acid homeostasis. As opposed to retinoid teratogenesis, however, it appears that fetal alcohol syndrome may be the result of too little retinoic acid produced during critical stages of fetal development. This may not explain all of the defects seen in cases of fetal alcohol syndrome, but should be considered as playing a major role in its pathogenesis.

Developmental Control
of Alcohol Dehydrogenase Gene Expression

Developmental Regulation of Liver ADH
by CCAAT/Enhancer Binding Protein

Since ADH production is subject to developmental regulation, a particular interest of our laboratory is the question of why it is important to increase the level of liver ADH postnatally. The abundance of ADH correlates with the knowledge that it catalyzes not only ethanol oxidation, but the reversible oxidation/reduction of numerous alcohols and aldehydes, including the retinol/retinal interconversion discussed above. A postnatal developmental increase in liver ADH production may complete the establishment of retinoic acid metabolism in the neonate who can no longer rely on maternal retinoid metabolism. Since expression of the three closely related members of the human class I ADH gene family increases during liver development,[4,36,37,104] it is informative to determine the mechanism of this induction and how this relates to liver development as well as to metabolism of alcohol and retinol in the fetus and adult.

Previous studies have shown that liver-specific gene expression is controlled primarily at the level of transcription.[105] The study of liver-specific gene expression is now focusing on the transcription factors that make possible this tissue specificity. A protein that has been implicated in liver-specific transcriptional regulation is CCAAT/enhancer binding protein (C/EBP).[106,107] C/EBP binds the promoter and/or enhancer regions of several genes expressed highly in liver, such as those encoding albumin and α1-antitrypsin,[108] and has been proven to function as a positively acting transcription factor in cultured hepatoma cells.[109] Expression of C/EBP is noticed in liver, fat, intestine, and lung tissue; in liver and intestine from either rat or mouse, C/EBP levels increase severalfold a few days before birth, and then return to the baseline level a few days after birth.[110] It has been suggested that the increase in liver C/EBP at birth stimulates the post-natal expression of other genes in liver, thus acting as a major regulator of liver development. Studies in this laboratory indicate that class I ADH falls into this category of genes.

Initial studies on the human *ADH2* promoter indicated that purified C/EBP could bind at several locations, in particular at two sites (–40 and –15 bp relative to the transcription start point) that flank a DNA sequence called the TATA box, located at –30 bp.[46] Since the TATA box normally plays a major role in assembly of RNA polymerase II into a transcription complex,[111] the presence of C/EBP molecules bound in such close proximity hint that they may be playing a significant role in regulation of the *ADH2* transcription initiation process. Transfection studies on human hepatoma cells have indicated that C/EBP does have a major positive effect on *ADH2* transcription and smaller effects on *ADH1* and *ADH3* transcription.[112] Mutations of either C/EBP binding site flanking the *ADH2* TATA box eliminates both binding and transcriptional activation.[112] The major conclusion from these studies is that C/EBP provides a liver-specific cue for human class I ADH gene expression, and facilitates differential regulation of the *ADH1*, *ADH2*, and *ADH3* genes during liver development. Also, the mechanism by which C/EBP acts on the *ADH2* promoter may be novel in that it requires binding sites on both sides of the TATA box to function.

Hormone-Induced and Basal-Level Expression of ADH Genes

In addition to C/EBP regulation, class I ADH gene expression is regulated by glucocorticoids, androgens, and retinoic acid. Each of these hormones functions via a specific member of a family of evolutionarily related transcription factors referred to as the nuclear receptors.[113] Glucocorticoids have been shown to regulate transcription via a hormone-dependent interaction of the glucocorticoid receptor with a discrete DNA sequence, termed a glucocorticoid response element, that acts as an enhancer for a nearby gene promoter.[114] All steroid hormones, as well as thyroid hormone, vitamin D, and vitamin A (retinoic acid), are now known to exert their effects via binding to specific nuclear receptors. Upon binding a particular ligand, the receptor is transformed into an active nuclear transcription factor that seeks out and binds to genes containing a specific hormone-response element.[113,115]

It has been observed that ADH activity and mRNA levels are induced by glucocorticoid treatment of rat hepatoma cells.[116,117] Also, liver ADH induction has been demonstrated by feeding rodents excessive ethanol, and glucocorticoids play a permissive role in this induction.[118] When the human *ADH2* gene was cloned and sequenced, it was noticed that the promoter region contained two sequences (at −215 and −180 bp) that have homology to previously characterized glucocorticoid response elements.[45] Further analysis of the *ADH2* gene revealed that these putative elements were functional in transfected hepatoma and nonhepatoma cells, and DNA-binding studies with purified glucocorticoid receptor indicated that there are three (instead of two) tandem binding sites that compose the *ADH2* glucocorticoid response element.[119] This indicates that human *ADH2*, like the rodent class I ADH gene, is regulated by glucocorticoids. Preliminary studies on human *ADH1* and *ADH3* genes have not revealed a significant effect of glucocorticoids on transcriptional activity (M. L. Shean and G. Duester, unpublished results). Several liver enzymes, such as tyrosine aminotransferase and tryptophan oxygenase, undergo postnatal inductions in which glucocorticoids play a major role.[120,121] Perhaps liver *ADH2* is subject to glucocorticoid control during its postnatal induction. The further induction of adult liver ADH by excessive ethanol ingestion may be considered a nonphysiological anomaly that operates via the glucocorticoid pathway.

ADH in mouse kidney, but not in liver, is inducible by androgens.[122] The mechanism of this induction appears to involve a combination of transcriptional and posttranscriptional events.[123,124] This response is part of a major effect that androgens exert on kidney tissue, involving the induction of several enzymes, such as β-glucuronidase, ADH, and ornithine decar boxylase.[125] The DNA sequences responsible for androgen induction of class I ADH have not been elucidated, but one can speculate that they may be similar or identical to those that compose the glucocorticoid response element. This is because recent findings have indicated that the androgen receptor can bind the mouse mammary tumor virus glucocorticoid response element and activate transcription.[126]

As mentioned above, this laboratory has recently provided evidence for regulation of human *ADH3* by retinoic acid,[64] another member of the class of hormones that operate through nuclear receptors. Unlike receptors for glucocorticoid and androgen hormones, the retinoic acid receptor binds a much different type of hormone response element, i.e., the retinoic acid response element.[113,115] Our studies have concentrated on two sequences in the *ADH3* gene (5'-TGACC-3') that resemble other known retinoic acid response elements. Studies on the *ADH1* and *ADH2* genes indicate that retinoic acid has no effect on transcription, contrary to what is observed for *ADH3*.[64] Thus, retinoic acid may be providing a signal to *ADH3* specifically, perhaps helping to determine its unique pattern of tissue and developmental expression.

Transfection studies on cultured cells, as discussed above, have allowed the elucidation of human ADH gene regulatory factors, such as C/EBP, glucocorticoids, and retinoic acid. In vitro transcription studies on the human *ADH2* gene have provided additional information. Two DNA sequences critical for in vitro transcription of the *ADH2* gene have been located between −94 and −84 bp, and between −72 and −64 bp.[127] These sequences correspond to two sites that exhibit binding (in a DNA footprinting assay) to protein factors present in a rat-liver nuclear extract.[46,112] The homologous DNA sites in the mouse *Adh-1* gene also bind proteins derived from a liver nuclear extract.[128] The site at −94 to −84 bp appears to have homology with the binding site for a common transcription factor called Sp1, or stimulatory protein 1.[129] Competition studies indicate that Sp1 is likely to be involved in *ADH2* transcription.[127] The other site important for in vitro transcription, located at −72 to −64 bp, has homology to the binding site for yet another common transcription factor, called USF, or upstream stimulatory factor.[130] Since Sp1 and USF are involved in the basal-level transcription of many genes in many types of cells, it is possible that they help regulate the basal-level expression of *ADH2* observed in many tissues.

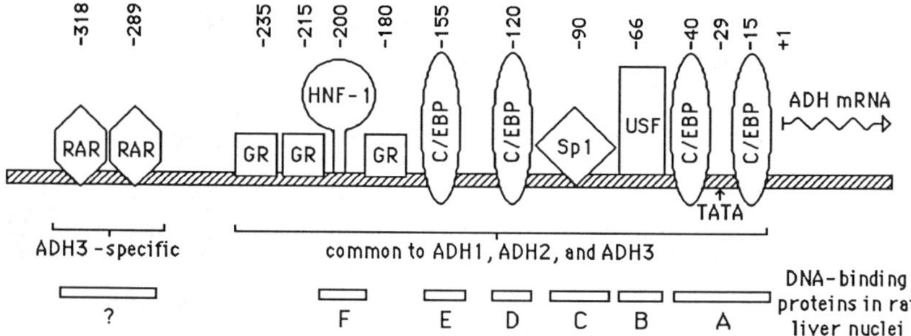

Fig. 2. ADH transcription factors. Structural and functional studies performed on the human *ADH1*, *ADH2*, and *ADH3* genes have identified several binding sites for potential regulatory proteins. Shown is a composite of binding sites for the three genes. The numbering is in base pairs upstream of the transcription start points for the three genes, which are in approximately equivalent positions relative to the structural genes.[46] All three genes possess six regions (designated A through F) that bind proteins present in a rat liver nuclear extract.[46,112] Sites A, D, and E in *ADH1*, *ADH2*, and *ADH3* have been confirmed to be C/EBP binding sites through the use of purified C/EBP in a DNA footprinting assay.[112] Site C is implied to bind Sp1 based on competition experiments using a synthetic Sp1-binding site oligonucleotide.[127] Site B has homology to USF binding sites,[130] and site F has homology to HNF-1 (hepatocyte nuclear factor 1) binding sites, the latter being a transcription factor present at high levels in liver and kidney.[133] Even though all three genes possess DNA sequences that resemble putative glucocorticoid receptor (GR) binding sites between –240 and –170 bp, only *ADH2* has been demonstrated to both bind purified GR and respond to the hormone.[119] The DNA sequences of the three genes diverge greatly upstream of –250 bp, and the *ADH3* gene possesses two putative RAR binding sites at –289 and –318 bp.[64] DNA sequences upstream of –350 bp in *ADH1*, *ADH2*, or *ADH3* have not been closely analyzed for the presence of transcription-factor binding sites.

Model for Transcriptional Regulation of Human Class I ADH Genes

A model summarizing the transcriptional regulation of human class I ADH is presented in Fig. 2. The various transcription factors that bind the ADH genes are presumed to operate by facilitating the formation of an active RNA polymerase II transcription initiation complex. Eukaryotic RNA polymerase is a relatively weak DNA-binding protein compared to bacterial RNA polymerase, and relatively nonspecific as to what DNA sequence it requires for binding. The tight binding and sequence specificity of many eukaryotic transcription factors allows them to assemble first onto the promoter at specific locations and then to await a random collision with the polymerase. It is believed that protein–protein interactions between eukaryotic RNA polymerase and various transcription factors, rather than the DNA itself, actually directs binding of the polymerase to the site of transcription initiation.[131,132] Possibly, the more transcription factors that can bind to the promoter, the better, since this will increase the chances for productive polymerase binding.

Undoubtedly, the large number of factors regulating class I ADH gene expression is a result of the need for several mechanisms to establish the levels of expression seen in many different tissues and at many different times during development. Since there is now good evidence that class I ADH is a major regulator of retinoic acid synthesis, this provides another reason for the complexity of regulation of ADH gene expression. Hopefully, future studies will shed further light on the connections among ADH gene expression, retinoic acid homeostasis, and vertebrate growth and development.

Acknowledgments

I would like to acknowledge the enlightening and lively discussions of the members of the Duester laboratory: M. L. Shean, M. J. Stewart, M. S. McBride, B. W. Paeper, P. P. Harding, and C. Vanooij. The work performed in this laboratory was supported by Public Health Service grant AA07261 from the National Institute on Alcohol Abuse and Alcoholism, as well as by Research Scientist Development Award K02 AA00119 to G. Duester.

References

[1] D. J. Strydom and B. L. Vallee (1982) Characterization of human alcohol dehydrogenase isoenzymes by high-performance liquid chromatographic peptide mapping. *Anal. Biochem* **123**, 422–429.

[2] E. M. Algar, T.-L. Seeley, and R. S. Holmes (1983) Purification and molecular properties of mouse alcohol dehydrogenase isozymes. *Eur. J. Biochem.* **137**, 139–147.

[3] T.-K. Li (1977) Enzymology of human alcohol metabolism. *Adv. Enzymol.* **45**, 427–483.

[4] M. Smith., D. A. Hopkinson, and H. Harris (1971) Developmental changes

and polymorphism in human alcohol dehydrogenase. *Ann. Hum. Genet.* **34,** 251–271.

[5] T.-K. Li and L. J. Magnes (1975) Identification of a distinctive molecular form of alcohol dehydrogenase in human livers with high activity. *Biochem. Biophys. Res. Commun.* **63,** 202–208.

[6] X. Parés and B. L. Vallee (1981) New human liver alcohol dehydrogenase forms with unique kinetic characteristics. *Biochem. Biophys. Res. Commun.* **98,** 122–130.

[7] G. Duester, G. W. Hatfield, R. Buhler, J. Hempel, H. Jornvall, and M. Smith (1984) Molecular cloning and characterization of a cDNA for the β subunit of human alcohol dehydrogenase. *Proc. Natl. Acad. Sci. USA* **81,** 4055–4059.

[8] H. von Bahr-Lindstrom, J.-O. Hoog, L.-O. Heden, R. Kaiser, L. Fleetwood, K. Larsson, M. Lake, B. Holmquist, A. Holmgren, J. Hempel, B. L. Vallee, and H. Jornvall (1986) cDNA and protein structure for the alpha subunit of human liver alcohol dehydrogenase. *Biochemistry* **25,** 2465–2470.

[9] L.-O. Heden, J.-O. Hoog, K. Larsson, M. Lake, E. Lagerholm, A. Holmgren, B. L. Vallee, H. Jornvall, and H. von Bahr-Lindstrom (1986) cDNA clones coding for the β subunit of human liver alcohol dehydrogenase have differently sized 3'-noncoding regions. *FEBS Lett.* **194,** 327–332.

[10] J.-O. Hoog, L.-O. Heden, K. Larsson, H. Jörnvall, and H. von Bahr-Lindstrom (1986) The gamma-1 and gamma-2 subunits of human liver alcohol dehydrogenase: cDNA structures, two amino acid replacements, and compatibility with changes in the enzymatic properties. *Eur. J. Biochem.* **159,** 215–218.

[11] F. W. Wagner, A. R. Burger, and B. L. Vallee (1983) Kinetic properties of human liver alcohol dehydrogenase: Oxidation of alcohols by class I isoenzymes. *Biochemistry* **22,** 1857–1863.

[12] J. D. Ceci, Y.-W. Zheng, and M. R. Felder (1987) Molecular analysis of mouse alcohol dehydrogenase: Nucleotide sequence of the *Adh-1* gene and genetic mapping of a related nucleotide sequence to chromosome 3. *Gene* **59,** 171–182.

[13] K. Zhang, W. F. Bosron, and H. J. Edenberg (1987) Structure of the mouse *Adh-1* gene and identification of a deletion in a long alternating purine–pyrimidine sequence in the first intron of strains expressing low alcohol dehydrogenase activity. *Gene* **57,** 27–36.

[14] R. Kaiser, B. Holmquist, J. Hempel, B. L. Vallee, and H. Jörnvall (1988) Class III human liver alcohol dehydrogenase: A novel structural type equidistantly related to the class I and class II enzymes. *Biochemistry* **27,** 1132–1140.

[15] A. H. Blair and B. L. Vallee (1966) Some catalytic properties of human liver alcohol dehydrogenase. *Biochemistry* **5,** 2026–2034.

[16] M. Smith, D. A. Hopkinson, and H. Harris (1973) Studies on the properties of the human alcohol dehydrogenase isozymes determined by the different loci *ADH1, ADH2, ADH3. Ann. Hum. Genet.* **37,** 49–67.

[17] H. A. Krebs and J. R. Perkins (1970) The physiological role of liver alcohol dehydrogenase. *Biochem. J.* **118,** 635–644.

[18] B. L. Vallee and T. J. Bazzone (1983) Isozymes of human liver alcohol dehydrogenase, in *Isozymes,* vol. 8: *Cellular Localization, Metabolism, and Physiology.* M. C. Rattazzi, J. G. Scandalios, and G. S. Whitt, eds. Alan R. Liss, New York, pp. 219–244.

[19] A. Okuda and K. Okuda (1983) Physiological function and kinetic mechanism of human liver alcohol dehydrogenase as 5β-cholestane-3a,7a,12a,26-tetrol dehydrogenase. *J. Biol. Chem.* **258,** 2899–2905.

[20] G. Mårdh and B. L. Vallee (1986) Human class I alcohol dehydrogenases catalyze the interconversion of alcohols and aldehydes in the metabolism of dopamine. *Biochemistry* **25,** 7279–7282.

[21] G. Mårdh, C. A. Luehr, and B. L. Vallee (1985) Human class I alcohol dehydrogenases catalyze the oxidation of glycols in the metabolism of norepinephrine. *Proc. Natl. Acad. Sci. USA* **82,** 4979–4982.

[22] E. Mezey and P. R. Holt (1971) The inhibitory effect of ethanol on retinol oxidation by human liver and cattle retina. *Exp. Mol. Pathol.* **15,** 148–156.

[23] A. J. McEvily, B. Holmquist, D. S. Auld, and B. L. Vallee (1988) 3β-hydroxy-5β-steroid dehydrogenase activity of human liver alcohol dehydrogenase is specific to gamma-subunits. *Biochemistry* **27,** 4284–4288.

[24] G. Mårdh, A. L. Dingley, D. S. Auld, and B. L. Vallee (1986) Human class II (π) alcohol dehydrogenase has a redox-specific function in norepinephrine metabolism. *Proc. Natl. Acad. Sci. USA* **83,** 8908–8912.

[25] M. J. Connor and M. H. Smit (1987) Terminal-group oxidation of retinol by mouse epidermis: Inhibition *in vitro* and *in vivo. Biochem. J.* **244,** 489–492.

[26] P. Julià, J. Farrés, and X. Parés (1986) Ocular alcohol dehydrogenase in the rat: Regional distribution and kinetics of the ADH-1 isoenzyme with retinol and retinal. *Exp. Eye Res.* **42,** 305–314.

[27] Y. Gotoh, H. Sumimoto, and S. Minakami (1990) Formation of 20-oxoleukotriene B$_4$ by an alcohol dehydrogenase isolated from human neutrophils. *Biochim. Biophys. Acta Lipids Lipid Metab.* **1043,** 52–56.

[28] M. Koivusalo, M. Baumann, and L. Uotila (1989) Evidence for the identity of glutathione-dependent formaldehyde dehydrogenase and class III alcohol dehydrogenase. *FEBS Lett.* **257,** 105–109.

[29] E. A. Dawes and S. M. Foster (1956) The formation of ethanol by *Escherichia coli. Biochim. Biophys. Acta* **22,** 253–265.

[30] V. Lutsdorf and R. Megnet (1968) Multiple forms of alcohol dehydrogenase in *Saccharomyces cerevisiae. Arch. Biochem. Biophys.* **126,** 933–944.

[31] A. M. Kapoun, B. W. Geer, P. W. H. Heinstra, V. Corbin, and S. W. McKechnie (1990) Molecular control of the induction of alcohol dehydrogenase by ethanol in *Drosophila melanogaster* larvae. *Genetics* **124,** 881–888.

[32] R. H. Hageman and D. Flesher (1960) The effect of an anaerobic environment on the activity of alcohol dehydrogenase and other enzymes of corn seedlings. *Arch. Biochem. Biophys.* **87,** 203–209.

[33] L. G. Lange, A. J. Sytkowski, and B. L. Vallee (1976) Human liver alcohol dehydrogenase: Purification, composition, and catalytic features. *Biochemistry* **15,** 4687–4693.

[34] C. C. Ditlow, B. Holmquist, M. M. Morelock, and B. L. Vallee (1984) Physical and enzymatic properties of a class II alcohol dehydrogenase isozyme of human liver: π-ADH. *Biochemistry* **23,** 6363–6368.

[35] M. Smith, D. A. Hopkinson, and H. Harris. (1972) Alcohol dehydrogenase isozymes in adult human stomach and liver: Evidence for activity of the *ADH3* locus. *Ann. Hum. Genet.* **35,** 243–253.

[36] R. F. Murray, Jr. and A. G. Motulsky (1971) Developmental variation in the isoenzymes of human liver and gastric alcohol dehydrogenase. *Science* **171,** 71–73.

[37] P. H. Pikkarainen and N. C. R. Raiha (1967) Development of alcohol dehydrogenase activity in the human liver. *Pediat. Res.* **1,** 165–168.

[38] M. Smith (1986) Genetics of human alcohol and aldehyde dehydrogenases. *Adv. Hum. Genet.* **15,** 249–290.

[39] V. Bilanchone, G. Duester, Y. Edwards, and M. Smith (1986) Multiple mRNAs for human alcohol dehydrogenase (ADH): Developmental and tissue-specific differences. *Nucleic Acids Res.* **14,** 3911–3926.

[40] T. Ikuta and A. Yoshida (1986) mRNA for the three human alcohol dehydrogenase subunits: Size heterogeneity and developmental changes. *Biochem. Biophys. Res. Commun.* **140,** 1020–1027.

[41] K. J. Balak, R. H. Keith, and M. R. Felder (1982) Genetic and developmental regulation of mouse liver alcohol dehydrogenase. *J. Biol. Chem.* **257,** 15,000–15,007.

[42] N. C. R. Raiha, M. Koskinen, and P. H. Pikkarainen (1967) Developmental changes in alcohol dehydrogenase activity in rat and guinea pig liver. *Biochem. J.* **103,** 623–626.

[43] R. S. Holmes, J. A. Duley, and J. N. Burnell (1983) The alcohol dehydrogenase gene complex on chromosome 3 of the mouse, in *Isozymes,* vol. 8: *Cellular Localization, Metabolism, and Physiology.* M. C. Rattazzi, J. G. Scandalios, and G. S. Whitt, eds. Alan R. Liss, New York, pp. 155–174.

[44] M. D. Boleda, P. Julià, A. Moreno, and X. Parés (1989) Role of extrahepatic alcohol dehydrogenase in rat ethanol metabolism. *Arch. Biochem. Biophys.* **274,** 74–81.

[45] G. Duester, M. Smith, V. Bilanchone, and G. W. Hatfield (1986) Molecular analysis of the human class I alcohol dehydrogenase gene family and nucleotide sequence of the gene encoding the β subunit. *J. Biol. Chem.* **261,** 2027–2033.

[46] M. J. Stewart, M. S. McBride, L. A. Winter, and G. Duester (1990) Promoters for the human alcohol dehydrogenase genes *ADH1*, *ADH2*, and *ADH3*: Interaction of CCAAT/enhancer binding protein with elements flanking the *ADH2* TATA box. *Gene* **90,** 271–279.

[47] D. W. Crabb, P. M. Stein, K. M. Dipple, J. B. Hittle, R. Sidhu, M. Qulali, K. Zhang, and H. J. Edenberg (1989) Structure and expression of the rat class I alcohol dehydrogenase gene. *Genomics* **5,** 906–914.

[48] A. Adinolfi, M. Adinolfi, and D. A. Hopkinson (1984) Immunological and biochemical characterization of the human alcohol dehydrogenase chi-ADH isozyme. *Ann. Hum. Genet.* **48,** 1–10.

[49] G. Eichele (1989) Retinoids and vertebrate limb pattern formation. *Trends Genet.* **5,** 246–251.

[50] D. Summerbell and M. Maden (1990) Retinoic acid, a developmental signalling molecule. *Trends Neurosci.* **13,** 142–147.

[51] A. F. Bliss (1951) The equilibrium between vitamin A alcohol and aldehyde in the presence of alcohol dehydrogenase. *Arch. Biochem.* **31,** 197–204.

[52] J. L. Napoli and K. R. Race (1987) The biosynthesis of retinoic acid from retinol by rat tissues in vitro. *Arch. Biochem. Biophys.* **255,** 95–101.

[53] R. D. Zachman and J. A. Olson (1961) A comparison of retinene reductase and alcohol dehydrogenase of rat liver. *J. Biol. Chem.* **236,** 2309–2313.

[54] M. A. Leo, C. Kim, and C. S. Lieber (1987) NAD^+-dependent retinol dehydrogenase in liver microsomes. *Arch. Biochem. Biophys.* **259,** 241–249.

[55] K. C. Posch, W. J. Enright, and J. L. Napoli (1989) Retinoic acid synthesis by cytosol from the alcohol dehydrogenase negative deermouse. *Arch. Biochem. Biophys.* **274,** 171–178.

[56] D. H. Van Thiel, J. Gavaler, and R. Lester (1974) Ethanol inhibition of vitamin A metabolism in the testes: Possible mechanism for sterility in alcoholics. *Science* **186,** 941,942.

[57] Y.-B. Chiao and D. H. Van Thiel (1986) Characterization of rat testicular alcohol dehydrogenase. *Alcohol Alcoholism* **21,** 9–15.

[58] S. Futterman (1962) Enzymatic oxidation of vitamin A aldehyde to vitamin A acid. *J. Biol. Chem.* **237,** 677–680.

[59] T. D. Elder and Y. J. Topper (1962) The oxidation of retinene (vitamin A aldehyde) to vitamin A acid by mammalian steroid-sensitive aldehyde dehydrogenase. *Biochim. Biophys. Acta* **64,** 430–437.

[60] M. A. Leo, C. Kim, N. Lowe, and C. S. Lieber (1989) Increased hepatic retinal dehydrogenase activity after phenobarbital and ethanol administration. *Biochem. Pharmacol.* **38,** 97–103.

[61] J. L. Napoli (1986) Retinol metabolism in LLC-PK1 cells: Characterization of retinoic acid synthesis by an established mammalian cell line. *J. Biol. Chem.* **261,** 13,592–13,597.

[62] A. B. Roberts and M. B. Sporn (1984) Cellular biology and biochemistry of the retinoids, in *The Retinoids,* vol. 2. M. B. Sporn, A. B. Roberts, and D. S. Goodman, eds. Academic, Orlando, pp. 209–286.

[63] K. G. Burnett and M. R. Felder (1978) *Peromyscus* alcohol dehydrogenase: Lack of cross-reacting material in enzyme-negative animals. *Biochem. Genet.* **16,** 1093–1105.

[64] G. Duester, M. L. Shean, M. S. McBride, and M. J. Stewart (1991) Retinoic acid response element in the human alcohol dehydrogenase gene *ADH3:* Implications for regulation of retinoic acid synthesis. *Mol. Cell Biol.* **11,** 1638–1646.

[65] C. Thaller and G. Eichele (1987) Identification and spatial distribution of retinoids in the developing chick limb bud. *Nature* **327,** 625–628.

[66] A. J. Durston, J. P. M. Timmermans, W. J. Hage, H. F. J. Hendriks, N. J. De Vries, M. Heideveld, and P. D. Nieuwkoop (1989) Retinoic acid causes an anteroposterior transformation in the developing central nervous system. *Nature* **340,** 140–144.

[67] M. Petkovich, N. J. Brand, A. Krust, and P. Chambon (1987) A human retinoic acid receptor which belongs to the family of nuclear receptors. *Nature* **330,** 444–450.

[68] V. Giguere, E. S. Ong, P. Segui, and R. M. Evans (1987) Identification of a receptor for the morphogen retinoic acid. *Nature* **330,** 624–629.

[69] H. De Thé, A. Marchio, P. Tiollais, and A. Dejean (1987) A novel steroid thyroid hormone receptor-related gene inappropriately expressed in human hepatocellular carcinoma. *Nature* **330,** 667–670.

[70] N. Brand, M. Petkovich, A. Krust, P. Chambon, H. De Thé, A. Marchio, P. Tiollais, and A. Dejean (1988) Identification of a second human retinoic acid receptor. *Nature* **332,** 850–853.

[71] A. Zelent, A. Krust, M. Petkovich, P. Kastner, and P. Chambon (1989) Cloning of murine α and β retinoic acid receptors and a novel receptor gamma predominantly expressed in skin. *Nature* **339,** 714–721.

[72] P. Dollé, E. Ruberte, P. Kastner, M. Petkovich, C. M. Stoner, L. J. Gudas, and P. Chambon (1989) Differential expression of genes encoding α, β and gamma retinoic acid receptors and CRABP in the developing limbs of the mouse. *Nature* **343,** 702–705.

[73] D. J. Mangelsdorf, E. S. Ong, J. A. Dyck, and R. M. Evans (1990) Nuclear receptor that identifies a novel retinoic acid response pathway. *Nature* **345,** 224–229.

[74] G. J. LaRosa and L. J. Gudas (1988) Early retinoic acid-induced F9 teratocarcinoma stem cell gene ERA-1: Alternate splicing creates transcripts for a homeobox-containing protein and one lacking the homeobox. *Mol. Cell Biol.* **8,** 3906–3917.

[75] S. P. Murphy, J. Garbern, W. F. Odenwald, R. A. Lazzarini, and E. Linney (1988) Differential expression of the homeobox gene Hox-1.3 in F9 embryonal carcinoma cells. *Proc. Natl. Acad. Sci. USA* **85**, 5587–5591.

[76] A. Simeone, D. Acampora, L. Arcioni, P. W. Andrews, E. Boncinelli, and F. Mavilio (1990) Sequential activation of *HOX2* homeobox genes by retinoic acid in human embryonal carcinoma cells. *Nature* **346**, 763–766.

[77] A. Stornaiuolo, D. Acampora, M. Pannese, M. D'Esposito, F. Morelli, E. Migliaccio, M. Rambaldi, A. Faiella, V. Nigro, A. Simeone, and E. Boncinelli (1990) Human HOX genes are differentially activated by retinoic acid in embryonal carcinoma cells according to their position within the four loci. *Cell Differ. Dev.* **31**, 119–127.

[78] G. Oliver, E. M. De Robertis, L. Wolpert, and C. Tickle (1990) Expression of a homeobox gene in the chick wing bud following application of retinoic acid and grafts of polarizing region tissue. *EMBO J.* **9**, 3093–3099.

[79] G. W. Vasios, J. D. Gold, M. Petkovich, P. Chambon, and L. J. Gudas (1989) A retinoic acid-responsive element is present in the 5' flanking region of the laminin B1 gene. *Proc. Natl. Acad. Sci. USA* **86**, 9099–9103.

[80] S.-Y. Wang, G. J. LaRosa, and L. J. Gudas (1985) Molecular cloning of gene sequences transcriptionally regulated by retinoic acid and dibutyryl cyclic AMP in cultured mouse teratocarcinoma cells. *Dev. Biol.* **107**, 75–86.

[81] L. Hu and L. J. Gudas (1990) Cyclic AMP analogs and retinoic acid influence the expression of retinoic acid receptor α, β, and γ mRNAs in F9 teratocarcinoma cells. *Mol. Cell Biol.* **10**, 391–396.

[82] H. De Thé, M. D. M. Vivanco-Ruiz, P. Tiollais, H. Stunnenberg, and A. Dejean (1990) Identification of a retinoic acid responsive element in the retinoic acid receptor β gene. *Nature* **343**, 177–180.

[83] B. Lüscher, P. J. Mitchell, T. Williams, and R. Tjian (1989) Regulation of transcription factor AP-2 by the morphogen retinoic acid and by second messengers. *Genes Dev.* **3**, 1507–1517.

[84] C. Thaller and G. Eichele (1988) Characterization of retinoid metabolism in the developing chick limb bud. *Development* **103**, 473–483.

[85] M. A. Satre and D. M. Kochhar (1989) Elevations in the endogenous levels of the putative morphogen retinoic acid in embryonic mouse limb-buds associated with limb dysmorphogenesis. *Dev. Biol.* **133**, 529–536.

[86] M. Maden, D. E. Ong, D. Summerbell, and F. Chytil (1989) The role of retinoid-binding proteins in the generation of pattern in the developing limb, the regenerating limb and the nervous system. *Development* **107(Suppl.)**, 109–119.

[87] M. Maden, D. E. Ong, D. Summerbell, and F. Chytil (1988) Spatial distribution of cellular protein binding to retinoic acid in the chick limb bud. *Nature* **335**, 733–735.

[88] S. M. Smith, K. Pang, O. Sundin, S. E. Wedden, C. Thaller, and G. Eichele (1989) Molecular approaches to vertebrate limb morphogenesis. *Development* **107(Suppl.),** 121–131.

[89] A. V. Perez-Castro, L. E. Toth-Rogler, L. Wei, and M. C. Nguyen-Huu (1989) Spatial and temporal pattern of expression of the cellular retinoic acid-binding protein and the cellular retinol-binding protein during mouse embryogenesis. *Proc. Natl. Acad. Sci. USA* **86,** 8813–8817.

[90] A. B. Roberts, M. D. Nichols, D. L. Newton, and M. B. Sporn (1979) In vitro metabolism of retinoic acid in hamster intestine and liver. *J. Biol. Chem.* **254,** 6296–6302.

[91] G. Wolf (1984) Multiple functions of vitamin A. *Physiol. Rev.* **64,** 873–937.

[92] C. A. Frolik (1984) Metabolism of retinoids, in *The Retinoids,* vol. 2. M. B. Sporn, A. B. Roberts, and D. S. Goodman, eds. Academic, Orlando, pp. 177–208.

[93] B. W. O'Malley (1989) Editorial: Did eukaryotic steroid receptors evolve from intracrine gene regulators? *Endocrinology* **125,** 1119,1120.

[94] J. B. Williams and J. L. Napoli (1985) Metabolism of retinoic acid and retinol during differentiation of F9 embryonal carcinoma cells. *Proc. Natl. Acad. Sci. USA* **82,** 4658–4662.

[95] S. Strickland and V. Mahdavi (1978) The induction of differentiation in teratocarcinoma stem cells by retinoic acid. *Cell* **15,** 393–403.

[96] A. P. Streissguth, S. Landesman-Dwyer, J. C. Martin, and D. W. Smith (1980) Teratogenic effects of alcohol in humans and laboratory animals. *Science* **209,** 353–361.

[97] L. Burd and J. T. Martsolf (1989) Fetal alcohol syndrome: Diagnosis and syndromal variability. *Physiol. Behav.* **46,** 39–43.

[98] F. W. Rosa (1983) Teratogenicity of isotretinoin. *Lancet* **ii,** 513.

[99] H. K. Biesalski (1989) Comparative assessment of the toxicology of vitamin A and retinoids in man. *Toxicology* **57,** 117–161.

[100] J. E. Smith, P. O. Milch, Y. Muto, and D. S. Goodman (1973) The plasma transport and metabolism of retinoic acid in the rat. *Biochem. J.* **132,** 821–827.

[101] J. C. Kraft, B. Löfberg, I. Chahoud, G. Bochert, and H. Nau (1989) Teratogenicity and placental transfer of all-*trans*-, 13-*cis*-, 4-oxo-all-*trans*-, and 4-oxo-13-*cis*-retinoic acid after administration of a low oral dose during organogenesis in mice. *Toxicol. Appl. Pharmacol.* **100,** 162–176.

[102] C. Eckhoff and H. Nau (1990) Identification and quantitation of all-*trans*- and 13-*cis*-retinoic acid and 13-*cis*-4-oxoretinoic acid in human plasma. *J. Lipid Res.* **31,** 1445–1454.

[103] S. Schenker, H. C. Becker, C. L. Randall, D. K. Phillips, G. S. Baskin, and G. I. Henderson (1990) Fetal alcohol syndrome: Current status of pathogenesis. *Alcohol Clin. Exp. Res.* **14,** 635–647.

[104] P. H. Pikkarainen and N. C. R. Raiha (1969) Change in alcohol dehydrogenase isoenzyme pattern during development of human liver. *Nature* **222**, 563,564.

[105] E. Derman, K. Krauter, L. Walling, C. Weinberger, M. Ray, and J. E. Darnell, Jr. (1981) Transcriptional control in the production of liver-specific mRNAs. *Cell* **23**, 731–739.

[106] W. H. Landschulz, P. F. Johnson, and S. L. McKnight (1989) The DNA binding domain of the rat liver nuclear protein C/EBP is bipartite. *Science* **243**, 1681–1688.

[107] W. H. Landschulz, P. F. Johnson, E. Y. Adashi, B. J. Graves, and S. L. McKnight (1988) Isolation of a recombinant copy of the gene encoding C/EBP. *Genes Dev.* **2**, 786–800.

[108] R. H. Costa, D. R. Grayson, K. G. Xanthopoulos, and J. E. Darnell, Jr. (1988) A liver-specific DNA-binding protein recognizes multiple nucleotide sites in regulatory regions of transthyretin, α_{-1}-antitrypsin, albumin, and simian virus 40 genes. *Proc. Natl. Acad. Sci. USA* **85**, 3840–3844.

[109] A. D. Friedman, W. H. Landschulz, and S. L. McKnight (1989) CCAAT/ enhancer binding protein activates the promoter of the serum albumin gene in cultured hepatoma cells. *Genes Dev.* **3**, 1314–1322.

[110] E. H. Birkenmeier, B. Gwynn, S. Howard, J. Jerry, J. I. Gordon, W. H. Landschulz, and S. L. McKnight (1989) Tissue-specific expression, developmental regulation, and genetic mapping of the gene encoding CCAAT/enhancer binding protein. *Genes Dev.* **3**, 1146–1156.

[111] N. Nakajima, M. Horikoshi, and R. G. Roeder (1988) Factors involved in specific transcription by mammalian RNA polymerase II: purification, genetic specificity, and TATA box-promoter interactions of TFIID. *Mol. Cell Biol.* **8**, 4028–4040.

[112] M. J. Stewart, M. L. Shean, and G. Duester (1990) *Trans*-activation of human alcohol dehydrogenase gene expression in hepatoma cells by C/EBP molecules bound in a novel arrangement just 5' and 3' to the TATA box. *Mol. Cell Biol.* **10**, 5007–5010.

[113] R. M. Evans (1988) The steroid and thyroid hormone receptor superfamily. *Science* **240**, 889–895.

[114] K. R. Yamamoto (1985) Steroid receptor regulated transcription of specific genes and gene networks. *Annu. Rev. Genet.* **19**, 209–252.

[115] B. M. Forman and H. H. Samuels (1990) Interactions among a subfamily of nuclear hormone receptors: The regulatory zipper model. *Mol. Endocrinol.* **4**, 1293–1301.

[116] C. E. Wolfla, R. A. Ross, and D. W. Crabb (1988) Induction of alcohol dehydrogenase activity and mRNA in hepatoma cells by dexamethasone. *Arch. Biochem. Biophys.* **263**, 69–76.

117 Y. Dong, L. Poellinger, S. Okret, J.-O. Hoog, H. von Bahr-Lindstrom, H. Jornvall, and J.-Å.Gustafsson (1988) Regulation of gene expression of class I alcohol dehydrogenase by glucocorticoids. *Proc. Natl. Acad. Sci. USA* **85,** 767–771.

118 P. Y. Sze (1975) The permissive effect of glucocorticoids in the induction of liver alcohol dehydrogenase by ethanol. *Biochem. Med.* **14,** 156–161.

119 L. A. Winter, M. J. Stewart, M. L. Shean, Y. Dong, L. Poellinger, S. Okret, J.-Å. Gustafsson, and G. Duester (1990) A hormone response element upstream of the human alcohol dehydrogenase gene *ADH2* consists of three tandem glucocorticoid receptor binding sites. *Gene* **91,** 233–240.

120 H.-M. Jantzen, U. Strahle, B. Gloss, F. Stewart, W. Schmid, M. Boshart, R. Miksicek, and G. Schütz (1987) Cooperativity of glucocorticoid response elements located far upstream of the tyrosine aminotransferase gene. *Cell* **49,** 29–38.

121 U. Danesch, B. Gloss, W. Schmid, G. Schütz, R. Schüle, and R. Renkawitz (1987) Glucocorticoid induction of the rat tryptophan oxygenase gene is mediated by two widely separated glucocorticoid-responsive elements. *EMBO J.* **6,** 625–630.

122 J. D. Ceci, R. Lawther, G. Duester, G. W. Hatfield, M. Smith, M. P. O'Malley, and M. R. Felder (1986) Androgen induction of alcohol dehydrogenase in mouse kidney: Studies with a cDNA probe confirmed by nucleotide sequence analysis. *Gene* **41,** 217–224.

123 M. R. Felder, G. Watson, M. O. Huff, and J. D. Ceci (1988) Mechanism of induction of mouse kidney alcohol dehydrogenase by androgen: Androgen-induced stimulation of transcription of the *Adh-1* gene. *J. Biol. Chem.* **263,** 14,531–14,537.

124 L. Tussey and M. R. Felder (1989) Tissue-specific genetic variation in the level of mouse alcohol dehydrogenase is controlled transcriptionally in kidney and posttranscriptionally in liver. *Proc. Natl. Acad. Sci. USA* **86,** 5903–5907.

125 R. T. Swank, K. Paigen, R. Davey, V. Chapman, C. Labarca, G. Watson, R. Ganschow, E. J. Brandt, and E. Novak (1978) Genetic regulation of mammalian glucuronidase. *Recent Prog. Horm. Res.* **34,** 401–436.

126 M. Beato, G. Chalepakis, M. Schauer, and E. P. Slater (1989) DNA regulatory elements for steroid hormones. *J. Steroid Biochem.* **32,** 737–748.

127 L. G. Carr and H. J. Edenberg (1990) *cis*-Acting sequences involved in protein binding and *in vitro* transcription of the human alcohol dehydrogenase gene *ADH2*. *J. Biol. Chem.* **265,** 1658–1664.

128 L. G. Carr, K. Zhang, and H. J. Edenberg (1989) Protein-DNA interactions in the 5' region of the mouse alcohol dehydrogenase gene *Adh-1*. *Gene* **78,** 277–285.

129 J. T. Kadonaga, A. J. Courey, J. Ladika, and R. Tjian (1988) Distinct regions of Sp1 modulate DNA binding and transcriptional activation. *Science* **242,** 1566–1570.

130 M. Sawadogo and R. G. Roeder (1985) Interaction of a gene-specific

transcription factor with the adenovirus major late promoter upstream of the TATA box region. *Cell* **43,** 165–175.

[131] M. R. Paule (1990) Transcription initiation: In search of the single factor. *Nature* **344,** 819,820.

[132] M. Sawadogo and A. Sentenac (1990) RNA polymerase B (II) and general transcription factors. *Annu. Rev. Biochem.* **59,** 711–754.

[133] S. Baumhueter, D. B. Mendel, P. B. Conley, C. J. Kuo, C. Turk, M. K. Graves, C. A. Edwards, G. Courtois, and G. R. Crabtree (1990) HNF-1 shares three sequence motifs with the POU domain proteins and is identical to LF-B1 and APF. *Genes Dev.* **4,** 372–379.

Influence of Ethanol on Functional and Biochemical Characteristics of Skeletal Muscle

William E. Sonntag,
Rhonda L. Boyd, Anselm D'Costa,
and Charles R. Breese

Introduction

The functional disturbances induced in skeletal muscle in response to chronic alcoholism are well known.[1-8] There is marked muscle weakness, tenderness, and muscle atrophy, which may be accompanied by muscle necrosis, edema, hemorrhage, and acute inflammation of affected tissues. Although the incidence and severity of muscle disease vary widely in chronic alcoholics, it is estimated that at least 50% of these individuals suffer from some type of myopathy.[9] Since skeletal muscle comprises approx 40% of body weight, alterations in the metabolic function of this tissue are likely to have profound implications on the health and well-being of the individual and may be indicative of pathological changes that occur in other tissues with alcohol abuse.

From: *Drug and Alcohol Abuse Reviews, Vol. 2: Liver Pathology and Alcohol*
Ed: R. R. Watson ©1991 The Humana Press Inc.

A

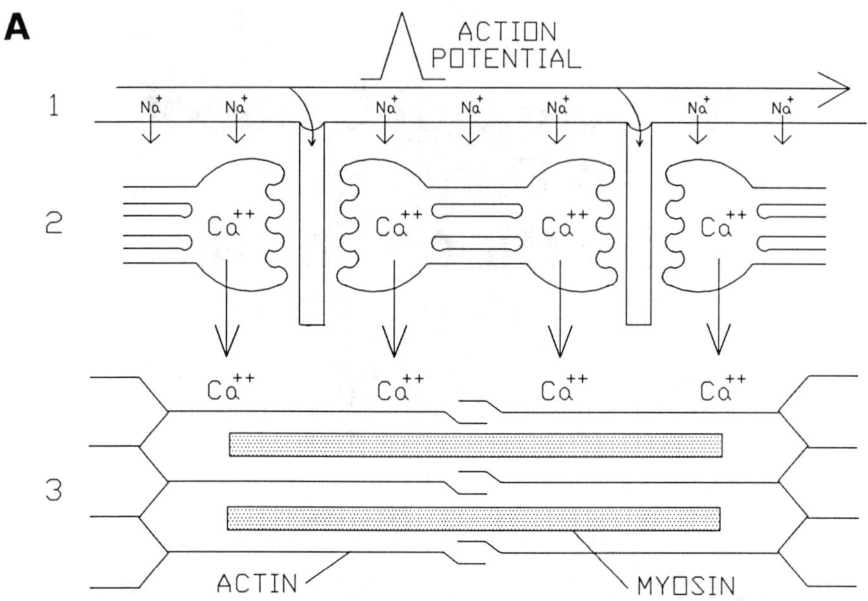

Fig. 1. **(A)** Schematic diagram of the mechanics of skeletal muscle contraction. (1) The action potential travels along the transverse tubule system and depolarizes the membrane resulting in increased Na^+ conductance, (2) membrane depolarization releases Ca^{2+} from the longitudinal tubules and terminal cisterns of the sarcoplasmic reticulum, and (3) free intracellular calcium facilitates the interaction between actin and myosin filaments.

Although the specific mechanisms responsible for the decline in muscle mass and strength in response to ethanol are unknown, a cursory review of skeletal muscle contraction clearly indicates that ethanol has the potential of interacting at a number of levels, including neurotransmitter release, receptor binding, ion transport, calcium storage and release, protein synthesis, metabolism, and conformation.[10] For example, during a normal contraction cycle (Fig. 1), acetylcholine is released from neurons into the myoneural junction and binds to receptors on the membrane of the sarcolemma, resulting in increased conductance and the generation of an end plate potential. The current spreads along the transverse tubule (T) system, depolarizes the membrane, and releases calcium from the terminal cisterns

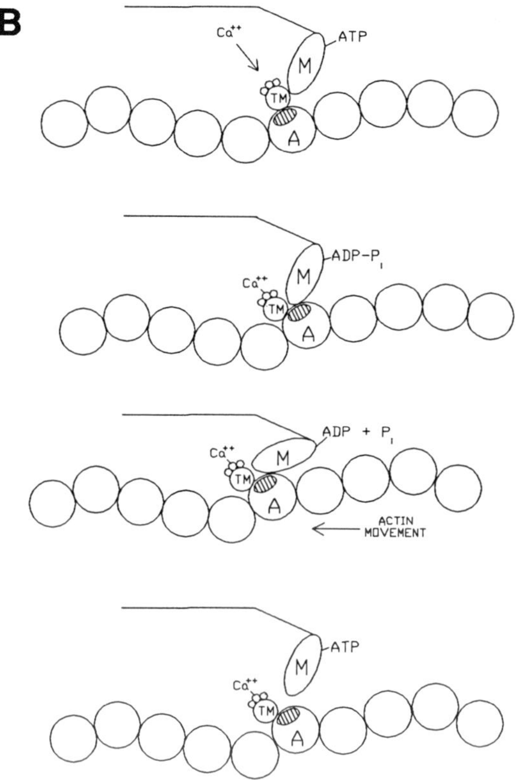

Fig. 1. **(B)** Magnification of the interactions between actin (A) and myosin (M) filaments in response to Ca^{2+}. Calcium binds to the troponin molecule (TM), which alters the configuration of the protein allowing myosin to bind actin. The hydrolysis of ATP with the release of P_i results in movement of the myosin head along the actin filament. The contraction cycle continues as long as Ca^{2+} is present and energy is available for production of ATP.

and longitudinal tubules of the sarcoplasmic reticulum. The free intracellular calcium binds to troponin-C resulting in the removal of tropomyosin inhibition, and the exposure of binding sites between actin and myosin. Energy is released from ATP and the myosin head contracts. The contraction cycle continues as long as ATP is present or until the free calcium is pumped back into the sarcoplasmic reticulum resulting in muscle relaxation.

In addition, to the mechanical properties that govern skeletal muscle contraction, anabolic hormones, such as testosterone, and insulin-like growth factors also contribute to skeletal muscle function by increasing the rate of protein synthesis. Since ethanol induced alterations at any level of skeletal muscle function would have important implications for this tissue, it is probable that a single mechanism alone would not be adequate to account for the actions of the drug.

The current chapter does not attempt to be all-inclusive in an approach to understanding the specific mechanisms for the decline in skeletal muscle mass and function in response to alcoholism. Rather, an attempt has been made to provide a broad background to develop an understanding of the range of factors that impact skeletal muscle and to delineate potential interactions between ethanol induced myopathies and skeletal muscle metabolism.

Morphological Changes
in Skeletal Muscle After Ethanol

Several studies have indicated that ethanol has a wide range of effects on skeletal muscle morphology. For example, in the adult, alterations in the morphological characteristics of muscle have been observed after chronic ingestion of alcohol for as brief a time as 4 wk.[11,12] These investigators observed intracellular edema, dilation of sarcoplasmic reticulum, increases in cytoplasmic lipid and glycogen granules, and swollen and irregular mitochondria.[11,13] Although ethanol induced changes occur to varying degrees in all muscle types, type II muscle fibers appear to be most sensitive to the chronic effects of ethanol.[11,13,14] These fibers exhibit a decrease in fiber area and weight after chronic ethanol, whereas type I fibers are relatively unaffected. Although the specific mechanisms for the changes are unknown, type II fibers exhibit faster myosin isozyme ATPase activity and higher calcium pumping activity as compared with type I fibers.[10,15] Limited information is available to date, but it is possible that ethanol may specifically inhibit the synthesis or activity of one type of myosin ATPase or hinder calcium pumping capacity leading to a deterioration of type II fibers.

Mechanisms of Ethanol-Induced Alterations in Skeletal Muscle Function

Various investigators, including our laboratory, have identified at least four areas where acute or chronic ethanol consumption can impact skeletal muscle function. These areas include, but are not limited to:

1. Membrane fluidity;
2. Muscle contractility;
3. Protein synthesis; and
4. Hormonal influences.

Although there is evidence that suggests that ethanol influences each of these areas, there is a high degree of interaction among these processes and it is not immediately clear which effects are directly related to ethanol and which effects are secondary to changes in other systems. Further research will be needed to confirm many of these studies and identify the specific intracellular changes induced by acute and chronic ethanol. In addition, it is clear that ethanol affects neural activity, which influences both muscle activity and function. This area has recently been reviewed in detail[16] and, therefore, is not included in this chapter.

Membrane Fluidity

The cell membrane is critical to virtually all aspects of cell function. The actions of the cell membrane include maintaining active and passive transport of compounds into the cell, providing a matrix for the binding of extracellular compounds to specific receptors, transducing signals via second messenger systems, and maintaining osmotic gradients. The characteristics of the membrane together with the activity of various ion pumps result in the establishment of electrical properties that are essential to the function of these cells and regulate the response of these cells to extracellular signals.[10]

Recent studies suggest that ethanol may alter the structure and lipid composition of membranes. Analysis of the fluidity of membranes using spin labeling of 5-doxylstearic acid followed by spin resonance have indicated an increase in membrane fluidity after administration of ethanol in vitro.[17–21] However, other studies indicate that chronic ethanol administration results in the formation of a more rigid structure, which is resistant to the fluidizing effect of the drug.[18,19,21,22] These effects are correlated with decreases in the proportion of linoleic acid in the membrane, whereas oleic, stearic, and palmitic acids increase.[23] Such alterations in response to chronic ethanol treatment have led to the concept that the maintenance of membrane fluidity is an actively regulated process that compensates for increased fluidity induced by ethanol, creating a more rigid cell structure. After chronic exposure to the drug, the membrane becomes rigid in the absence of ethanol. Because of the adaptations of the membrane to the effects of ethanol, some investigators have considered these changes a manifestation of tolerance at the membrane level.[18,19,21–23]

There are several functional changes within the cell that are associated with increased rigidity induced by ethanol. Some studies have described a decrease in amino acid uptake through the cell membrane,[24] whereas other studies suggest that there is greater sensitivity to the toxic effects of various agents owing to impaired ability to regulate ion flux through a compromised cell membrane.[19] Although the disruption of specific ion fluxes is difficult to assess, ion movements have been measured indirectly by following changes in the membrane potential of muscle tissue. Acute ethanol has been shown to cause membrane depolarization[25] and influence the activity of sodium/potassium ATPase, an enzyme responsible for the regulation of the gradients for sodium and potassium ions across the cell membrane.[26–28] Recent studies using cultured skeletal myotubes from fetal rats confirmed that acute ethanol caused a dose-dependent depolarization of these cells.[27] However, after suppression of the sodium/potassium pump with ouabain, ethanol had little effect on the membrane potential. These results suggested that the effects of ethanol are mediated by a specific inhibition of the sodium/potassium pump. This conclusion was confirmed by measurement of ^{86}Rb uptake (via the sodium/potassium pump) in the presence of ethanol. Chronic treatment with ethanol in vitro over a 9-d period, however, resulted in a compensatory increase in sodium/potassium ATPase activity and a "normalization" of the membrane potential.[28] These results are consistent with the hypothesis that ethanol induces changes in membrane fluidity and suggest that alterations in fluidity can induce functional changes in membrane proteins responsible for the maintenance of the internal milieu of the cell.

Muscle Contractility

Early studies on the actions of acute ethanol administration indicated that 200 m*M* ethyl alcohol inhibited contractility of both diaphragm and sartorius muscle.[29–35] Although acute studies have produced consistent results, chronic studies have been more controversial. At least one investigator has reported that administration of 20% ethanol in drinking water for 27 wk had no effect on contractility of the rectus abdominis muscle in mice.[36] However, this study used a tissue with a high proportion of Type I fibers and control animals were both malnourished and dehydrated. It is possible that alterations in nutrition may have masked the effects of ethanol in this study. More recent investigations, in which nutrition was more carefully controlled, have observed reduced twitch and tetanic tension in gastrocnemius muscle of rats after chronic ethanol.[33]

Studies of the in vitro actions of ethanol on the activity of actin and myosin in muscle have been complex and, in some instances, misleading. In one study, it was reported that ethanol diminished actinomycin precipitation (used as an index of association of these proteins) and delayed the increased precipitation in response to Mg-ATP or ADP.[3,37] Similar results were found with acetaldehyde suggesting that ethanol and its metabolites interfered with the native contractile response of these proteins. However, later studies suggested that ethanol can directly inhibit the ATP-induced nucleation that is necessary for the in vitro precipitation of the actinomycin complex.[38] Since nucleation of actin and myosin appears to be the response specifically inhibited by ethanol in vitro, but is not required for normal muscle function in vivo, the results of this study raised concerns about the adequacy of the in vitro model for the actions of ethanol on muscle contraction.

In skeletal muscle, it is well-known that the crucial events in contraction and relaxation of muscle are coupled to the release and reuptake of calcium by the sarcoplasmic reticulum.[10] Earlier studies had confirmed that ethanol had little or no effect on the ability of troponin to bind calcium. However, concentrations of 0.1–1% ethanol appeared to enhance calcium release from sarcoplasmic reticulum.[39] This effect did not appear to be mediated by alterations in calcium pump activity since independent experiments confirmed that ethanol in this dose range had little effect on the activity of the pump. However, at low concentrations of ethanol, it was observed that the sarcoplasmic reticulum was more permeable to calcium — this was especially true of the heavy sarcoplasmic reticulum, which included the terminal cisternae and transverse tubules. The authors suggested that ethanol may interact with a subunit of the gated calcium channel either by increasing the size of the channel or by altering conformation (possibly via changes in membrane fluidity). Therefore, the result of ethanol exposure may be a loss of calcium storage in the sarcoplasmic reticulum, a decrease in calcium release after depolarization, and reduced muscle contractility. This hypothesis is consistent with experiments demonstrating that calcium partially reverses the ethanol-induced decrease in contraction of the longitudinal muscle.

Protein Synthesis

Many recent studies have indicated that relative rates of protein synthesis are decreased in skeletal muscle of ethanol as compared to pair-fed control animals. In response to acute alcohol administration, protein synthesis in the gastrocnemius muscle was reduced by approx 30% after correction for the specific activity of the amino acid in the intracellular pool.[40,41] In another study, fractional rates of protein synthesis were reduced by 15–35% in soleus, plantaris, gastrocnemius, diaphragm, and stomach.[42] Within the gastrocnemius muscle, separation of proteins into sarcoplasmic, stromal, and myofibrillar components revealed equivalent reductions in all protein types.[43,44] These studies also revealed that protein synthesis in type II (anaerobic, fast twitch) muscle fibers was inhibited more than type I fibers by ethanol suggesting that the increased damage in these muscle fibers was closely correlated with the reduced protein synthesis induced by ethanol.

Longer feeding regimens of ethanol to rats using the pair-feeding model (Fig. 2) demonstrated similar effects of ethanol on protein synthetic mechanisms.[45–49] In immature rats, ethanol decreased bone, liver, skin, and skeletal mass by 7–21% compared to pair-fed animals.[44] Fractional and absolute rates of protein synthesis were similarly reduced (13–30%) in both immature and mature animals. Similar to the results of the acute studies, analysis of stromal, soluble, and myofibrillar protein fractions of gastrocnemius muscle indicated an equivalent decrease in each area in response to chronic ethanol feeding. Analysis also revealed that the changes in protein synthesis were not a result of diminished insulin levels[45] or increased protein

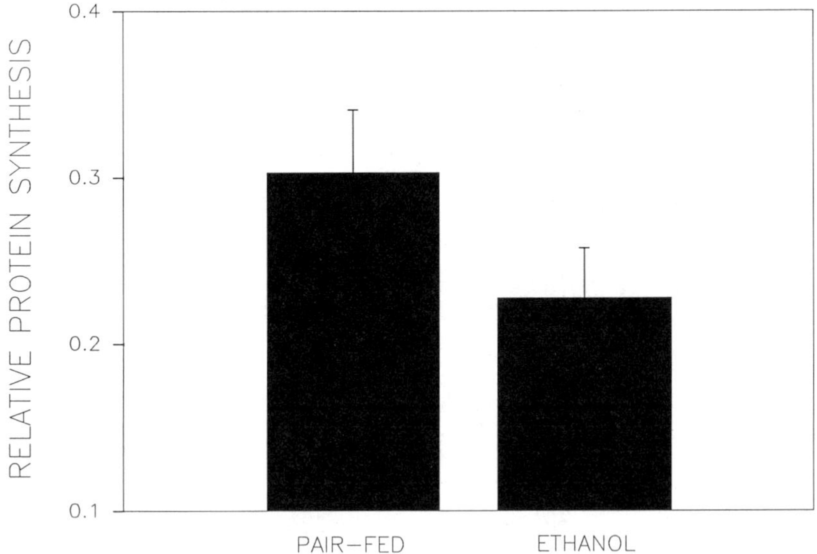

Fig. 2. Relative protein in diaphragm muscle from ethanol and pair-fed control rats. Diaphragms were removed and incubated in medium with ³H-phenylalanine. Protein synthesis was calculated as a ratio of phenylalanine specific activity in protein to phenylalanine specific activity in the free amino acid pool. Data are expressed as mean ± SEM and indicate a 27% reduction in relative protein synthesis after ethanol (Sonntag, unpublished observations).

catabolism (catabolism decreased by 13 and 19% in immature and mature rats, respectively).[50] Therefore, the results of these studies provide convincing evidence that ethanol inhibits protein synthesis in skeletal muscle and that the decline is not reversed with continued ethanol treatment as was observed for other effects of ethanol (i.e., sodium potassium ATPase activity).

The mechanisms responsible for the inhibition of protein synthesis are unclear. Ethanol may have direct effects on gene transcription, RNA processing and transport, or on translational processes. Alternatively, the effects of ethanol on gene expression may be secondary to perturbations in cellular processes, such as mitochondrial or membrane activity. Recent studies using high concentrations of ethanol (0.21–0.84M) in cell free systems have suggested additional actions of ethanol on the regulation of protein synthesis.[51] Ethanol was shown to inhibit ternary complex formation between initiation factor (eIF-2), GTP, and initiator methionine t-RNA. The authors also found evidence that ethanol may activate a specific translational inhibitor to suppress protein synthesis. This conclusion was reached since

1. Ethanol inhibited protein synthesis after a 60-min incubation period;
2. A peak that suppressed protein synthesis was resolved by chromatography; and
3. The inhibitor eluted in the same position as heme-controlled repressor.

These results indicated that ethanol may inhibit polypeptide synthesis by both activation of an inhibitory compound within the cell and by suppression of ternary complex formation.

Hormonal Regulation

Insulin-like Growth Factors

Somatomedins or insulin-like growth factors (IGFs) are a family of peptides structurally related to insulin that induce mitogenic activity in cultured fibroblasts, anabolic activity in cartilage, and DNA and protein synthesis in many other tissues.[52] IGFs are produced by a number of tissues (90% of which is produced by the liver) and circulate in high concentrations in blood. Recent studies have indicated that these hormones have an autocrine/paracrine role in tissue growth and hypertrophy. For example, IGF-1 has been shown to have a role in the differentiation of muscle in the newborn mouse,[53] the regeneration of muscle after damage induced by hypoxia or the snake venom, taipoxin,[54] and renal hypertrophy after unilateral nephrectomy.[55] IGF-II concentrations are elevated in many tissues of fetal animals, but in adults are usually found in high concentrations only in the brain and anterior pituitary. The IGFs generally circulate in plasma bound to specific carrier proteins that have been hypothesized to regulate IGF activity and recent studies have demonstrated that IGF-1 activity is enhanced when the protein is bound to specific carrier proteins.[56] Because of their important anabolic effects on tissue, we and others have proposed that a decline in plasma levels of these hormones may contribute to the reduction in muscle protein synthesis in response to ethanol.

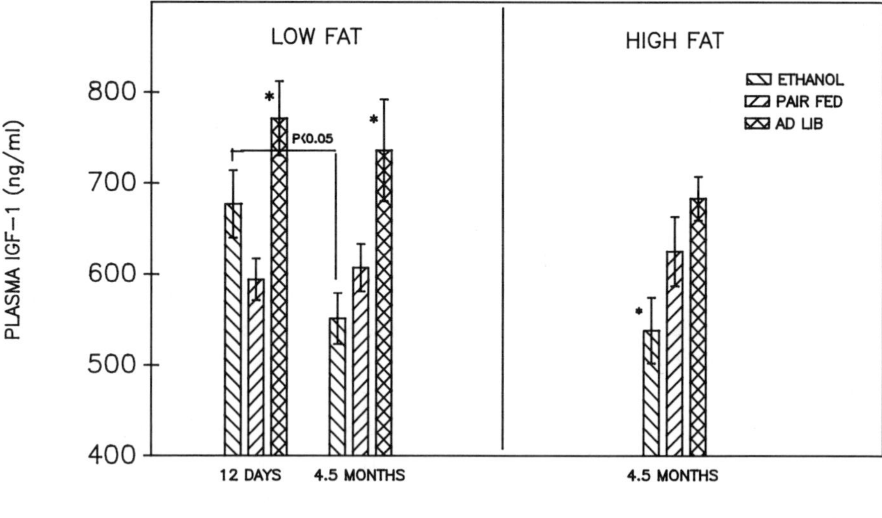

Fig. 3. Effects of ethanol on plasma levels of IGF-1 in male rats. *Left:* Effects of a low fat (12%) Lieber-DiCarli diet for either 12 d or 4.5 mo on IGF-1 levels. Animals were pair-fed a 5% ethanol diet or an isocaloric maltose-dextrin (control) diet. Additional animals received the control diet *ad libitum. Right:* Effects of a high fat (35%) Lieber-DiCarli diet for 4.5 mo on IGF-1 levels. Groups were the same as previously described. Values represent mean ± SEM. ⊠ = ethanol; ⊘ = pair-fed; ⊠ = *ad libitum.* (Data summarized from Sonntag et al., ref. 57.)

Although there are few studies on the effects of ethanol on IGF-1 activity, recent experiments have suggested that plasma levels of IGF-1 may decrease in both animals and humans in response to chronic ethanol. In our own laboratory (Fig. 3), for example, short-term ethanol feeding has little or no effect on plasma IGF-1 concentrations. However, continued ethanol feeding for 4.5 mo resulted in a decline in plasma IGF-1 concentrations compared to either *ad libitum* or pair-fed animals.[54] These changes occurred despite relatively low levels of alcohol over the course of the experiment. Several earlier investigations have also reported a decline in plasma levels of IGF-1 in patients diagnosed with alcohol-induced liver cirrhosis.[58] However, because of the nutritional alterations that normally accompany alcoholism, these reports were unable to conclude that alcohol specifically influenced the secretion of this hormone. In our studies, moderate dietary restriction, which is characteristic of chronic alcoholics, was shown to inhibit plasma levels of IGF-1. However, we found that the effects of dietary restriction were clearly separable from the effects of ethanol since the dietary effects on IGF-1 had a rapid onset (12 d) and remained relatively constant thereafter. The effects of ethanol on IGF-1 were observed after chronic feeding and the magnitude of inhibition was greater than that observed with dietary restriction alone. Therefore, the data indicate that ethanol has a direct effect on plasma levels of IGF-1.

More recent data from our laboratory indicate that the effects of chronic ethanol treatment on plasma IGF-1 are mediated by alterations in IGF-1 gene expression.[59] Comparison of male rats fed alcohol for 12 d or 4.5 mo revealed a significant reduction in IGF-1 mRNA at 4.5 mo compared to pair-fed animals. No significant differences between the ethanol and pair-fed animals were observed at 12 d. These results are in close agreement with IGF-1 concentrations in plasma and suggest that ethanol suppresses hepatic IGF-1 gene expression. Studies currently in progress should reveal whether the effects of ethanol are mediated by alterations in the number of IGF-1 secretory cells or are related to an inhibition of IGF-1 gene transcription.

Growth Hormone

The secretion of IGF-1 is regulated by the release of growth hormone from the anterior pituitary gland. Growth hormone secretion occurs in high amplitude secretory bursts at 3–4 h intervals in male rats, but is limited to a single episode occurring approx 2 h after the onset of sleep in humans.[60] The pulses are regulated by two hypothalamic hormones: somatostatin (which inhibits growth hormone release)[61] and growth hormone releasing hormone (GRF, which stimulates growth hormone release).[62] Somatostatin is a tetradecapeptide, but has a higher mol wt form (somatostatin-28), which is more potent in inhibiting growth hormone release than somatostatin-14. The interactions between these neuropeptides are responsible for the normal high amplitude secretion of growth hormone.[63]

Several previous studies have reported that ethanol administration reduces plasma growth hormone levels. Redmond, for example, reported that 3 or 4 g/kg intravenous ethanol significantly diminished the amplitude of growth hormone pulses when administered acutely to male rats.[64,65] Similar findings have been reported after intragastric infusion of 4 g/kg ethanol into prepubertal and adult female rats.[66] However, no differences were observed in response to hypothalamic growth hormone releasing hormone indicating that these decreases were not a result of ethanol-induced alterations in pituitary sensitivity. Therefore, the authors concluded that the actions of ethanol on growth hormone pulse amplitude are mediated by a hypothalamic mechanism (i.e., release of GRF or somatostatin).

In humans, ethanol administration reduces growth hormone pulse amplitude and inhibits the response to insulin-induced hypoglycemia or propranolol glucagon.[68–71] The changes in growth hormone are assumed to be responsible for the decrease in IGF-1 levels that has been observed in these subjects. However, the doses of ethanol used in the acute animal studies are high and there appear to be few long-term studies of the effects of ethanol administration on plasma growth hormone secretory dynamics. Recent results from our own laboratory[72] demonstrate that when ethanol is fed chronically (5% of liquid diet for 4.5 mo), blood concentrations are not sufficiently elevated in animals to influence the hypothalamic neurons responsible for regulating growth hormone secretion and, therefore, no major alterations in growth hormone secretory dynamics are observed. Rather, the effects of chronic ethanol exposure appear to be manifest on IGF-1 secretion by hepatic tissue owing to locally high ethanol levels before metabolism by hepatic enzymes. Alternatively, IGF-1 secretory cells may be more sensitive to the damaging effects of ethanol resulting in a reduction in this cell type. During chronic alcoholism in humans, high blood ethanol concentrations most likely affect both growth hormone secretory bursts and hepatic IGF-1 gene expression.

Testosterone

It is well known that testosterone stimulates the formation of muscle mass in skeletal muscle and is responsible for the maintenance of many secondary sexual characteristics of the male. Products of testosterone metabolism, such as dihydrotestosterone are also important for maintaining secondary sexual characteristics and organs. Because of the close interrelationship between steroid hormones, interference in the synthesis of either androgens or estrogens has a wide range of effects on the synthesis, blood concentrations, and metabolism of a multitude of other steroid hormones as well as the function of many organs.

There is a substantial volume of literature that indicates that plasma levels of testosterone decline in response to acute or chronic ethanol administration in both animal and human subjects.[73–76] Many of the effects of testosterone appear to be related to the direct effects of ethanol on steroid biosynthesis. Alcohol, for example, has been shown to inhibit the conversion of pregnenolone to progesterone in vivo and other investigators have reported that ethanol and acetaldehyde inhibit the conversion of androstenedione to testosterone in vitro.[81,82] In addition, hCG stimulation of testosterone release from the testis is reduced after alcohol administration.[77–79] Levels of luteinizing hormone release from the pituitary gland also decrease after acute or chronic ethanol and these changes appear to be associated with decreased gonadotropin hormone releasing hormone (GnRH) release from hypothalamic neurons.[83] Therefore, the decrease in testosterone is the result of a direct action on the testis as well as indirect effects via the hypothalamus.

In addition to changes in testosterone steroidogenesis, there appear to be marked changes in the metabolism of the steroid. In hepatic tissue, 5-reductase activity is enhanced after alcohol administration, which results in a decrease in serum testosterone levels. However, in response to alcohol administration over long periods of time, 5-reductase activity decreased — resulting in lower dihydrotestosterone levels in secondary organs.[84–88] Concomitant with these changes in testosterone is an increase in circulating levels of estrogens owing to an increase in hepatic aromatase activity.[88,89] To our knowledge, there have been no studies of the effects of alcohol on testosterone binding protein or studies of the effects of ethanol on androgen receptors in target tissues — specifically skeletal muscle.

Summary

Several studies have clearly suggested that ethanol has profound effects on skeletal muscle function although the specific mechanisms for the effects of ethanol remain unclear. At least part of the difficulty in assessing the actions of alcohol results from variations between studies in the time, method, and dose of ethanol administration, the types of diets utilized, and the adequacy of control groups. These differences result in a wide range of blood alcohol levels, different stages of liver disease, and variations in nutritional status both within and between studies. The resulting data create difficulties in interpretation of results and comparison of results between laboratories.

Despite the limitations of the animal model, several changes consistently occur in skeletal muscle in response to ethanol. These alterations include, but are not limited to, a decrease in membrane fluidity, muscle contractility, and protein synthesis. In addition to the direct effects, several hormones that regulate skeletal muscle metabolic activity, such as insulin-like growth factor-1 and testosterone, decline after ethanol administration and may contribute to the decline in protein synthesis. Alterations in mitochondrial function are also possible although to our knowledge this has not been studied specifically in skeletal muscle. A decrease in mitochondrial function (as has been observed in hepatic tissue) would contribute to the decline in skeletal muscle function. Therefore, alcohol abuse appears to influence skeletal muscle function at many levels. Further research will be necessary to elucidate which processes are most sensitive to alcohol and lead to a decline in skeletal muscle function.

Acknowledgment

This work was supported in part by grant AA 08536 to WES.

References

[1] E. Rubin (1979) Alcohol myopathy in heart and skeletal muscle. *N. Engl. J. Med.* **301,** 28–33.

[2] S. K. Song and E. Rubin (1972) Ethanol produced muscle damage in human volunteers. *Science* **175,** 327,328.

[3] E. Rubin, A. M. Katz, C. S. Lieber, E. P. Stein, and S. Puszkin (1976) Muscle damage produced by chronic alcohol consumption. *Am. J. Pathol.* **83,** 499–516.

[4] F. Martin, K. Ward, G. Slavin, J. Levi, and T. J. Peters (1985) Alcoholic skeletal myopathy, a clinical and pathological study. *Q. J. Med.* **55,** 233–251.

[5] P. D. Saville and C. S. Lieber (1965) Increases in skeletal calcium and femur cortex thickness produced by undernutrition. *J. Nutr.* **99,** 141–144.

[6] C. Hed, C. Lunkmark, and H. Fahlgren (1962) Acute muscular syndrome in chronic alcoholism. *Acta Med. Scand.* **171,** 585–599.

[7] G. T. Perkoff, P. Hardy, and E. Velez-Garcia (1966) Reversible acute muscular syndrome in chronic alcoholism. *N. Engl. J. Med.* **274,** 1277–1285.

[8] G. T. Perkoff, M. M. Dioso, V. Bleisch, and G. Klinkerfuss (1967) A spectrum of myopathy associated with alcoholism. I. Clinical and laboratory features. *Ann. Intern. Med.* **67,** 481–492.

[9] R. E. Worden (1976) Pattern of muscle and nerve pathology in alcoholism. *Ann. NY Acad. Sci.* **273,** 351–359.

[10] W. F. Ganong (1989) *Review of Medical Physiology*, 14th Ed. Appleton & Lange, Norwalk, CT.

[11] A. Hanid, G. Slavin, W. Mair, C. Sowter, P. Ward, J. Webb, and J. Levi (1981) Fiber type changes in striated muscle of alcoholics. *J. Clin. Pathol.* **34,** 991–995.

[12] K. H. Kiessling, L. Pilström, A. C. Bylund, K. Piehl, and B. Saltin (1975) Effects of chronic ethanol abuse on structure and enzyme activities of skeletal muscle in man. *Scand. J. Clin. Lab. Invest.* **35,** 601–607.

[13] G. Slavin, F. Martin, P. Ward, J. Levi, and T. Peters (1983) Chronic alcohol excess is associated with selective but reversible injury to type 2B muscle fibers. *J. Clin. Pathol.* **36,** 772–777.

[14] F. C. Martin, K. Ward, G. Slavin, A. J. Levi, and T. J. Peters (1985) Alcohol skeletal myopathy, a clinical and pathological study. *Q. J. Med.* **55,** 233–251.

[15] A. G. Guyton (1986) *Textbook of Medical Physiology.* W.B. Saunders, Philadelphia.

[16] L. A. Pohorecky (1982) Influence of alcohol on peripheral neurotransmitter function. *Fed. Proc.* **41,** 2452–2455.

[17] P. Seeman (1972) The membrane actions of anesthetics and tranquilizers. *Pharmacol. Rev.* **24,** 583–655.

[18] J. H. Chin and D. B. Goldstein (1977) Drug tolerance in biomembranes: A spin label study of the effects of ethanol. *Science* **196,** 684,685.

[19] E. Rubin and H. Rottenberg (1982) Ethanol-induced injury and adaptation in biological membranes. *Fed. Proc.* **41,** 2465–2471.

[20] J. M. Vanderkooi (1979) Effects of ethanol on membranes: A fluorescent probe study. *Alcohol. Clin. Exp. Res.* **3,** 60–63.

[21] J. H. Chin and D. P. Goldstein (1977) Effects of low concentrations of ethanol on the fluidity of spin-labelled erythrocyte and brain membranes. *Mol. Pharmacol.* **13,** 435–441.

[22] A. Waring, H. Rottenberg, T. Ohnishi, and E. Rubin (1981) Membranes and phospholipids of liver mitochondria from chronic alcoholic rats are resistant to membrane disordering by alcohol. *Proc. Natl. Acad. Sci. USA* **78,** 2582–2586.

[23] J. M. Littleton, S. J. Grieve, P. J. Griffiths, and G. R. John (1980) Ethanol-induced alteration in membrane phospholipid composition: Possible relationship to development of cellular tolerance to ethanol. *Adv. Exp. Med. Biol.* **126,** 7–19.

[24] J. Rosa and E. Rubin (1980) Effects of ethanol on amino acid uptake by rat liver cells. *Lab. Invest.* **43,** 366–372.

[25] E. Knutsson (1961) Effects of ethanol on the membrane potential and membrane resistance of frog muscle fibre. *Acta Physiol. Scand.* **52,** 242–253.

[26] K. Hara and M. Kasai (1977) The mechanism of increase in the ATPase activity of sarcoplasmic reticulum vesicles treated with *n*-alcohols. *J. Biochem.* (Tokyo) **82,** 1005–1017.

[27] C. Brodie and S. R. Sampson (1987) Effects of ethanol on electrophysiological

properties of rat skeletal myotubes in culture. *J. Pharmacol. Exp. Ther.* **242**, 1098–1103.

[28] C. Brodie and S. R. Sampson (1987) Effects of chronic ethanol treatment on membrane potential, its electrogenic pump component and Na-K pump activity of cultured rat skeletal myotubes. *J. Pharmacol. Exp. Ther.* **242**, 1104–1108.

[29] P. W. Gage (1965) The effects of *n*-ethyl, ethyl, and *n*-propyl alcohol on neuromuscular transmission in the rat. *J. Pharmacol. Exp. Ther.* **150**, 236–243.

[30] A. R. Khan (1981) Influence of ethanol and acetaldehyde on electro-mechanical coupling of skeletal muscle fibres. *Acta Physiol. Scand.* **III**, 425–430.

[31] S. A. Cooper and K. L. Dretchen (1975) Biphasic action of ethanol on contraction of skeletal muscle. *Eur. J. Pharmacol.* **31**, 232–236.

[32] F. Inour and G. B. Frank (1967) Effects of ethyl alcohol on excitability and on neuromuscular transmission in frog skeletal muscle. *Br. J. Pharmacol.* **30**, 186–189.

[33] D. A. Martyn and T. L. Munsat (1980) The effects of acute and chronic ethanol administration on twitch and tetanic force production by rat gastrocnemius muscle *in situ*. *Neurology* **30**, 139–143.

[34] L. C. Mendoza, K. Hellberg, A. Rickart, G. Tillich, and R. J. Bing (1971) Alcohol influences muscle contractility in vitro. *J. Clin. Pharmacol.* **11**, 165–176.

[35] T. J. Regan, G. Koroxenidis, C. B. Moscos, H. A. Oldewartel, P. H. Lehan, and H. K. Hellems (1966) Effects of acute ethanol on skeletal muscle ion transport and contractility. *J. Clin. Invest.* **45**, 270–280.

[36] S. L. Berk, P. J. Block, P. A. Toselli, and W. C. Ullrick (1975) The effects of chronic alcohol ingestion in mice on contractile properties of cardiac and skeletal muscle: A comparison with normal and dehydrated-malnourished controls. *Experientia* **31**, 1302,1303.

[37] S. Puszkin and E. Rubin (1975) Adenosine diphosphate effect on contractility of human muscle actomyosin: Inhibition by ethanol and acetaldehyde. *Science* **188**, 1319,1320.

[38] Y. Ishii, S. T. Ohnishi, and E. Rubin (1985) Action of ADP and ethanol on muscle proteins *in vitro. Biochem. Pharmacol.* **34**, 203–210.

[39] S. T. Ohnishi, J. L. Flick, and E. Rubin (1984) Ethanol increases calcium permeability of heavy sarcoplasmic reticulum in skeletal muscle. *Arch. Biochem. Biophys.* **233**, 588–594.

[40] J. M. Tiernan and L. C. Ward (1986) Acute effects of ethanol on protein synthesis in the rat. *Alcohol Alcohol.* **21**, 171–178.

[41] V. R. Preedy, P. Duane, and T. J. Peters (1988) Comparison of the acute effects of ethanol on liver and skeletal muscle protein synthesis in the rat. *Alcohol Alcohol.* **23**, 155–161.

[42] V. R. Preedy and T. J. Peters (1988) Acute effects of ethanol on protein synthesis in different muscles and muscle protein fractions of the rat. *Clin. Sci.* **74**, 461–466.

[43] V. R. Preedy, C. J. Bateman, A. B. Price, and T. J. Peters (1987) Changes in Type I and Type II fibre-rich muscles following chronic ethanol ingestion in the young rat. *Clin. Sci.* **74 (Suppl. 18),** 19P.

[44] V. R. Preedy and T. J. Peters (1989) The effect of chronic ethanol ingestion on synthesis and degradation of soluble, contractile and stromal protein fractions of skeletal muscles from immature and mature rats. *Biochem. J.* **259,** 261–266.

[45] V. R. Preedy and T. J. Peters (1988) The effect of chronic ethanol feeding on body and plasma composition and rates of skeletal muscle protein turnover in the rat. *Alcohol Alcohol.* **23,** 217–226.

[46] V. R. Preedy, S. Venkatesan, T. J. Peters, D. M. Nott, J. Yates, and S. A. Jenkins (1989) Effect of chronic ethanol ingestion on tissue RNA and blood flow in skeletal muscle with comparative reference to bone and tissues of the gastrointestinal tract of the rat. *Clin. Sci.* **76,** 243–247.

[47] V. R. Preedy, P. Duane, and T. J. Peters (1988) Biological effects of chronic ethanol consumption. A reappraisal of the Lieber-De Carli liquid-diet model with reference to skeletal muscle. *Alcohol Alcohol.* **23,** 151–160.

[48] V. R. Preedy and T. J. Peters (1987) The young rat as a model for alcohol-induced skeletal muscle myopathy. *Biochem. Soc. Trans.* **15,** 1166,1167.

[49] P. Duane and T. J. Peters (1988) Nutritional status in alcoholics with and without muscle myopathy. *Alcohol Alcohol.* **23,** 271–276.

[50] F. C. Martin and T. J. Peters (1985) Assessment *in vitro* and *in vivo* of muscle degradation in chronic skeletal muscle myopathy of alcoholism. *Clin. Sci.* **68,** 693–700.

[51] J. M. Wu (1981) Control of protein synthesis in rabbit reticulocytes: Inhibition of polypeptide synthesis by ethanol. *J. Biol. Chem.* **256,** 4164–4167.

[52] W. H. Daughaday and P. Rotwein (1989) Insulin like growth factors I and II. Peptide, messenger ribonucleic acid and gene structures, serum and tissue concentrations. *Endocr. Rev.* **10,** 68–81.

[53] E. Jennische and H. A. Hanssen (1987) Transient expression of insulin-like growth factor-1 immunoreactivity in skeletal muscle cells during post-natal development in the rat. *Acta Physiol. Scand.* **131,** 619–622.

[54] E. Jennische, A. Skottner, and H. A. Hansson (1987) Satellite cells express the trophic factor IGF-1 in regenerating skeletal muscle. *Acta Physiol. Scand.* **129,** 9–16.

[55] A. D. Stiles, I. R. S. Sosenko, A. J. O'Ercole, and B. T. Smith (1985) Relation of kidney tissue somatomedin C/insulin-like growth factor-1 to post-nephrectomy renal growth in the rat. *Endocrinology* **117,** 2397–2401.

[56] R. G. Elgin, W. H. Busby, and D. R. Clemmons (1987) An insulin-like growth factor binding protein enhances the biological response to IGF-1. *Proc. Nat. Acad. Sci. USA* **84,** 3254–3258.

[57] W. E. Sonntag and Boyd R.L (1988) Chronic ethanol inhibits plasma levels of insulin-like growth factor-1. *Life Sci.* **43,** 1325–1330.

[58] F. Salerno, V. Locatelli, and E. E. Müller (1987) Growth hormone hyper-responsiveness to growth hormone releasing hormone in patients with severe liver cirrhosis. *Clin. Endocrinol.* **27,** 183–190.

[59] W. E. Sonntag and R. L. Boyd Reduced insulin-like growth factor-1 gene expression in liver of chronically alcohol fed rats (submitted for publication).

[60] R. N. Prinz, E. D. Weitzmann, G. R. Cunningham, and I. Karacan (1983) Plasma growth hormone during sleep in young and aged men. *J. Gerontol.* **38,** 519–524.

[61] Y. C. Patel and C. B. Srikant (1986) Somatostatin mediation of adenohypophysial secretion. *Ann. Rev. Physiol.* **48,** 551–567.

[62] M. C. Gelato and G. R. Merriam (1986) Growth hormone releasing hormone. *Ann. Rev. Physiol.* **48,** 569–591.

[63] G. S. Tannenbaum, N. Ling, and P. Brazeau (1976) Somatostatin-28 is longer acting and more selective than somatostatin-14 on pituitary and pancreatic hormone release. *Endocrinology* **98,** 562–570.

[64] G. P. Redmond (1980) Effect of ethanol on endogenous rhythms of growth hormone secretion. *Alcohol. Clin. Exper. Res.* **4,** 50–58.

[65] G. P. Redmond (1981) Effect of ethanol on spontaneous and stimulated growth hormone secretion. *Prog. Biochem. Pharmacol.* **18,** 58–74.

[66] W. L. Dees, C. W. Skelley, V. Rettori, M. S. Kentroti, and S. M. McCann (1988) Influence of ethanol on growth hormone secretion in adult and prepubertal female rats. *Neuroendocrinology* **48,** 495–499.

[67] P. N. Prinz, T. A. Roehrs, P. P. Vitaliano, M. Linnoila, and E. D. Weitzman (1980) Effect of alcohol on sleep and nighttime plasma growth hormone and cortisol concentrations. *J. Clin. Endocrinol. Metab.* **51,** 759–764.

[68] D. Andreani, G. Tamburrano, and M. Javicoli (1976) Alcohol hypoglycemia: Hormonal changes. *Horm. Metab. Res.* **6 (Suppl),** 99–102.

[69] H. A. Priem, B. C. Shanley, and C. Malan (1976) Effect of alcohol administration on plasma growth hormone response to insulin-induced hypoglycemia. *Metabolism* **25,** 397–403.

[70] R. J. Chalmers, E. H. Bennie, R. H. Johnson, and H. B. Kinnell (1977) The growth hormone response to insulin induced hypoglycemia in alcoholics. *Psychol. Med.* **7,** 607–611.

[71] R. J. Chalmers, E. H. Bennie, R. H. Johnson, and G. Masterton (1978) Growth hormone, prolactin, and corticosteroid responses to insulin hypoglycemia in alcoholics. *Br. Med. J.* **1,** 745–748.

[72] W. E. Sonntag and R. L. Boyd (1989) Diminished insulin-like growth factor-1 levels after chronic ethanol: Relationship to pulsatile growth hormone release. *Alcohol. Clin. Exp. Res.,* **13,** 3–11.

[73] T. J. Cicero (1980) Common mechanisms underlying the effects of ethanol and narcotics on neuroendocrine function, in *Advances in Substance Abuse*. N. K. Mello, ed. JAI, Greenwich, CT, p. 201.

[74] T. J. Cicero, D. Bernstein, and T. M. Badger (1978) Effects of acute alcohol administration on reproductive endocrinology in the male rat. *Alcohol. Clin. Exp. Res.* **2,** 249–257.

[75] G. G. Gordon, A. L. Southern, and C. S. Lieber (1979) Hypogonadism and feminization in the male: A triple effect of alcohol. *Alcohol. Clin. Exp. Res.* **3,** 210.

[76] T. J. Cicero (1981) Neuroendocrinological effects of alcohol. *Ann. Rev. Med.* **32,** 123–142.

[77] J. Ellingboe and C. C. Varanelli (1979) Ethanol inhibits testosterone biosynthesis by direct action on leydig cells. *Res. Commun. Chem. Pathol. Pharmacol.* **24,** 87–102.

[78] T. J. Cicero, E. R. Meyer, and R. D. Bell (1978) Effects of ethanol on the hypothalamic-pituitary-luteinizing hormone axis and testicular steroidogenesis. *J. Pharmacol. Exp. Ther.* **208,** 210–215.

[79] E. P. Murono, T. Lin, J. Osterman, and H. R. Nankin (1980) Direct inhibition of testosterone synthesis in rat testis interstitial cells by ethanol: Possible sites of action. *Steroids* **36,** 619–631.

[80] F. M. Badr, A. Bartke, S. Dalterio, and W. Bulger (1977) Suppression of testosterone production by ethyl alcohol. Possible mode of action. *Steroids* **30,** 647–655.

[81] J. Ellingboe and C. C. Varanelli (1979) Ethanol inhibits testosterone biosynthesis by direct action on Leydig cells. *Res. Commun. Chem. Pathol. Pharmacol.* **24,** 87–102.

[82] T. J. Cicero, E. R. Meyer, and R. D. Bell (1979) Effects of ethanol on the hypothalamic-pituitary-luteinizing hormone axis and testicular steroidogenesis. *J. Pharmacol. Exp. Ther.* **208,** 210–215.

[83] T. J. Cicero and T. M. Badger (1977) Effects of alcohol on the hypothalamic-pituitary-gonadal axis in the male rat. *J. Pharmacol. Exp. Ther.* **201,** 427–433.

[84] C. Bode, G. A. Martini, and J. C. Bode (1978) Effect of alcohol on microsomal cortisol 4 en-5-α-reductase in the liver of rats fed on a standard or low protein diet. *Horm. Metab. Res.* **10,** 62–64.

[85] G. G. Gordon, A. L. Southern, and C. S. Lieber (1978) The effects of alcoholic liver disease and alcohol ingestion on sex hormone levels. *Alcohol. Clin. Exp. Res.* **2,** 259–266.

[86] A. L. Southern and G. G. Gordon (1976) Effects of alcohol and alcoholic cirrhosis on sex hormone metabolism. *Fertil. Steril.* **27,** 202–205.

[87] E. Rubin, C. S. Lieber, K. Altman, G. G. Gordon, and A. L. Southern (1976) Prolonged ethanol consumption increases testosterone metabolism in the liver. *Science* 191, 563,564.

[88] G. G. Gordon, J. Olivo, F. Rafii, and A. L. Southern (1975) Conversion of androgens to estrogens in cirrhosis of the liver. *J. Clin. Endocrinol. Metab.* **40,** 1018–1026.

[89] G. G. Gordon, A. L. Southern, J. Vittek, and C. S. Lieber (1979) The effect of alcohol ingestion on hepatic aromatase activity and plasma steroid hormone in the rat. *Metabolism* **28,** 20–24.

Alcohol and Liver Damage

Xanthine Oxidase

Thomas M. Soranno and Lester G. Sultatos

Introduction

Damage to cellular constituents by oxygen-derived free radicals has been implicated in many human disease states.[1,2] Among the various cells, organelles, and enzymes capable of generating biologically reactive oxygen metabolites is the enzyme xanthine oxidase (XO) (EC 1.1.3.22), which oxidizes hypoxanthine and xanthine.[3,4] This enzyme has received considerable attention regarding ischemia-reperfusion injury of heart, intestine, kidney, and liver.[4,5] In healthy tissue, oxidation of hypoxanthine and xanthine is thought to occur primarily (80–90%) through a xanthine dehydrogenase (XD) (EC 1.1.1.204) form,[5,6] which unlike XO does not produce free radicals. Numerous animal studies have suggested that during an ischemic event XD is converted to XO.[5,7–10] Therefore, subsequent reperfusion of the ischemic tissue can result in the generation of superoxide radicals ($O_2^{\cdot-}$) and/or hydrogen peroxide (H_2O_2) by XO. In turn, through transition metal-

From: *Drug and Alcohol Abuse Reviews, Vol. 2: Liver Pathology and Alcohol*
Ed: R. R. Watson ©1991 The Humana Press Inc.

catalyzed reactions, these fairly reactive oxygen metabolites can give rise to the highly reactive hydroxyl radical (OH•). The favored hypothesis surrounding the toxic effects of oxygen-derived free radicals is that they initiate cell injury through mechanisms, such as lipid peroxidation and/or protein and nucleic acid damage.[11]

In 1975, Israel et al.[12] proposed that ethanol-induced liver necrosis may result from hypoxia caused by an increase in hepatic oxygen consumption. Several studies have supported this hypoxia-theory as playing a role in the hepatotoxic effects of ethanol.[13,14] Based on these observations, Thurman and coworkers suggested that "alcoholic liver injury needs to be considered in the same light as ischemic heart disease."[14] In view of the potential involvement of the XD/XO enzyme system in ischemia-reperfusion injury, XD to XO conversion and the consequential XO-induced oxidative stress are currently being investigated as a possible mechanism in the pathogenesis of alcohol-induced liver disease (ALD).

In the US there are an estimated 18 million adults, 18 years or older, experiencing problems related to alcohol consumption.[15] ALD is perhaps the most prevalent medical disorder associated with alcohol abuse.[16] Hepatotoxic effects of alcohol range from reversible fatty liver to end stage alcoholic cirrhosis[17,18] which is the eighth leading cause of death in the US.[19]

Despite years of considerable progress toward understanding the molecular mechanism(s) involved in the hepatotoxic effects of alcohol, the pathogenesis of ALD has remained relatively elusive. Identification of the direct pathway(s) leading to cell injury after alcohol consumption has been hampered by the enormous range and extreme complexity by which ethanol and its metabolites interact with hepatocellular components. These complex interactions have been well documented in several recent reviews.[20–22] Moreover, the initiating event(s) of ALD is (are) difficult to distinguish from subsequent or coincidental changes that may occur within hepatocytes. The vast amount of information available concerning the cellular effects of ethanol seems to have culminated in the rationalization that multiple mechanisms are most likely involved in the genesis of ethanol-induced hepatocellular injury.[23]

The purpose of this chapter is to summarize evidence regarding the possible involvement of XO in the development of ALD. In this effort, biochemical and physiological features of XO and its precursor XD are also reviewed.

Biochemical Properties and Physiological Functions of Xanthine Dehydrogenase and Xanthine Oxidase

Biochemical Properties

The end product of purine nucleotide degradation in humans is the urinary metabolite uric acid. In this pathway under normal conditions the XD/XO enzyme system, with XD most likely accounting for the majority of total activity[5,6] catalyzes the sequential oxidations of hypoxanthine to xanthine and then to uric acid. This activity occurs in most tissues with the highest levels found in liver and intestine.

One of the most perplexing characteristic features of this enzyme system is its seeming ability to exist in several interconvertible forms, the aforementioned XD and XO (reversible and irreversible) as well as a transient intermediate dehydrogenase/oxidase (D/O).[6,7] The functional difference between XO and its native XD form is its specificity for an electron acceptor. XD preferentially reduces nicotinamide adenine dinucleotide (oxidized form) (NAD$^+$) to NADH (reduced form), whereas, XO transfers electrons to molecular oxygen (O$_2$) forming the potentially toxic O$_2^{-\bullet}$ and/or H$_2$O$_2$, as shown in the following.

$$\text{Hypoxanthine} + \text{H}_2\text{O} + \text{NAD}^+ \xrightarrow{\text{XD form}} \text{Xanthine} + \text{NADH} + \text{H}^+ \qquad (1)$$

$$\text{Hypoxanthine} + \text{H}_2\text{O} + 2\text{O}_2 \xrightarrow{\text{XO form}} \text{Xanthine} + \text{O}_2^{-\bullet} + \text{H}_2\text{O}_2 \qquad (2)$$

Similarly, both forms of the enzyme oxidize xanthine to uric acid.

These molybdenum flavoproteins consist of two dissociable subunits. A molybdenum atom, one flavin adenine dinucleotide (FAD) molecule, and two iron–sulfur (Fe$_2$/S$_2$) complexes are integral parts of each subunit.[4] Conversion of the NAD$^+$-utilizing dehydrogenase to the O$_2$-dependent oxidase has been well established in vitro to occur reversibly by sulfhydryl oxidation or irreversibly by proteolytic action.[7,24,25] As free sulfhydryl groups are oxidized to disulfides, enzyme conformation is altered and the electron acceptor binding site, FAD, acquires an increased affinity for O_2, whereas the attraction for NAD^+ decreases. Hence, reactive oxygen intermediates can be produced. Before the transformation to reversible XO is complete, a transient intermediate D/O may exist that can use either NAD^+ or O_2 as a cosubstrate. Conversion through sulfhydryl oxidation can be reversed by thiol reagents, such as dithiotreitol, which reduce the disulfide bonds and restore XD conformation and NAD^+ utilization. Proteolytic or irreversible conversion to XO occurs through cleavage of a polypeptide fragment from a subunit of either XD or reversible XO. Loss of this fragment results in an irreversible conformational change to the free radical producer XO. Calcium-dependent proteases, most notably calpain thiol-proteases,[26] have been postulated to facilitate this irreversibility.[5] On the contrary, Stack et al.[26] have reported that calpains are most likely not involved and suggested a calcium-dependent metalloprotease to be responsible for the irrevocable conversion.

Physiological Functions

Xanthinuria is a rare genetic disorder resulting from a deficiency of XD/XO activity. Besides having hypouricemia and an increased urinary excretion of hypoxanthine and xanthine, these patients are otherwise asymptomatic and lead normal lives. This suggests that XD/XO activity is not physiologically vital. Nevertheless, many interesting and potentially important biological functions have been proposed for this enzyme system.[4] Of course, XD/XO has long been recognized as the terminal oxidase in purine degradation. Several proposed functions potentially relevant to XO's suspected role in the development of ALD include:

1. Regulation of purine metabolism by directing purine flux between catabolic and salvage pathways;
2. Involvement in iron homeostasis by contributing to the intestinal mucosal processing of absorbed iron and catalyzing the release of iron from ferritin; and
3. Production of uric acid, which may act as an antioxidant.

Although a true role of XD/XO activity in humans and other species remains to be clarified, this enzyme most likely has varied functions.

Regulation of Purine Metabolism

In 1981, Kaminski and Jezewska[27] proposed that XD and its conversion to XO play a regulatory role in purine intermediary metabolism. They proposed that XD activity determines whether hypoxanthine is oxidized to xanthine through the XD catabolic route (*see* Reaction 1) or recycled through the purine salvage pathway. Purine salvage is simpler and much less costly than purine *de novo* biosynthesis. In a study by Della Corte and Stripe[28] they found that NADH inhibits XD but not XO. This led Kaminski and Jezewska to speculate that the overall controlling factor in their proposed XD regulatory function was cellular $NADH/NAD^+$ ratios. As a result, conditions, such as hypoxia, that increase this ratio may inhibit the XD catabolic route and therefore increase the availability of hypoxanthine to enter the salvage pathway. Furthermore, since XO is not inhibited by NADH, XD to XO conversion in vivo could eliminate the $NADH/NAD^+$ controlling factor and therefore decrease the availability of hypoxanthine for use in the salvage pathway by oxidizing it through the XO catabolic route (*see* Reaction 2).

Hepatic biotransformations of ethanol and its metabolite acetaldehyde by alcohol dehydrogenase (ADH) (EC 1.1.1.1) and aldehyde dehydrogenase (ALDH) (EC 1.2.1.3), respectively, have clearly been shown to generate an excess of NADH.[20–22] Interestingly, and detailed further in the section on "Ethanol-Induced Lipid Peroxidation," Kato et al.[29] recently suggested that an ethanol-induced increase of NADH may inhibit XD activity and shift the metabolism of hypoxanthine and xanthine to constituent XO. This increased flow through XO may subsequently produce free radicals contributing to ethanol-induced hepatotoxicity.

Iron Homeostasis Involvement

Dietary iron is absorbed through the small intestine and incorporated into transferrin. The uptake of iron by transferrin, for transport to various tissues, has been shown to be mediated by XO.[30] Bolann and Ulvik[31] and Biemond et al.[32] have shown in vitro that XO, largely through $O_2^{-\bullet}$ generation, can function as a catalyst in the release of ferrous ion (Fe^{2+}) from the principal iron-storage protein ferritin. Regardless of the exact physiological purpose for XO to interact with iron, mobilization of Fe^{2+} from ferritin can, however, have serious consequences regarding cellular injury caused by reactive oxygen molecules. In vitro and in vivo, an excess of unbound iron has clearly been associated with lipid peroxidative damage.[33] This nonprotein-bound iron can complex directly with oxygen to yield reactive perferryl ($Fe^{2+}O_2$) and ferryl ($Fe^{4+}O$) ions or reduce H_2O_2 through a Fenton-type reaction to form the highly toxic OH• as shown in the following:

$$H_2O_2 + Fe^{2+} \longrightarrow OH^- + OH\bullet + Fe^{3+} \tag{3}$$

Furthermore, the ferric ion (Fe^{3+}) produced can be reduced back to Fe^{2+} by $O_2^{-}\bullet$:

$$Fe^{3+} + O_2^{-}\bullet \longrightarrow Fe^{2+} + O_2 \tag{4}$$

As outlined by Nordman et al.,[34] these two reactions can be added to obtain the Haber-Weiss reaction:

$$H_2O_2 + O_2^{-}\bullet \xrightarrow{\text{Iron catalysis}} OH^- + OH\bullet + O_2 \tag{5}$$

Taken together, iron mobilization and $O_2^{-}\bullet/H_2O_2$ generation by XO could significantly enhance tissue damage through production of OH• and/or other reactive species.

Uric Acid Production

There are many intracellular defense mechanisms available to protect cells against oxidative stress. Major enzymatic defense systems include superoxide dismutase (SOD) (EC 1.15.1.1), catalase (CAT) (EC 1.11.1.6), and glutathione peroxidase (GSH-Px) (EC 1.11.1.9). For the most part, SOD and CAT activity can "clean up" $O_2^{-}\bullet$ and H_2O_2, respectively, and decrease their availability to enter the Haber-Weiss reaction. GSH-Px utilizes reduced glutathione (GSH) to detoxify peroxides through reduction mechanisms. Nonenzymatic defense mechanisms include ascorbic acid, reduced GSH, selenium, and vitamin E. Ames et al.[35] have provided evidence that uric acid in vitro can function to scavenge reactive oxygen metabolites. Using perfused rat liver to study reperfusion injury, Zhong et al.[36] recently reported that infusion of uric acid, in a dose-dependent manner, protected against ischemic-reperfusion damage. These studies suggest that XD/XO generated uric acid may function to protect cells against oxidative stress.

The antioxidant forces function to eliminate or at least minimize oxidative cell injury from toxic foreign chemicals and normal oxidants formed during regular aerobic metabolic events. However, compromise/loss of these antioxidant resources and/or an increase in oxidative stress beyond the protective threshold of these antioxidants may result in cellular oxidative damage.

Ethanol-Induced Lipid Peroxidation: Does Xanthine Oxidase Play a Role?

Lipid Peroxidation and Oxidative Stress

Cellular oxidative stress commonly refers to the presence of strong oxidizing agents that may cause cell injury or undergo detoxification by antioxidant defenses. In the liver, these oxidants can be O_2-derived free radicals[37] or metabolically activated products of exogenous chemicals, such as carbon tetrachloride.[38] The cellular damage most commonly associated with oxidative stress is the lipid peroxidation of polyunsaturated fatty acids, which are major structural components of biological membranes. However, proteins, nucleic acids, and carbohydrates can be damaged through oxidative stress,[11] but the contribution of such processes to tissue injury is relatively unexplored.

The lipid peroxidative process is initiated when fatty acids undergo attack by reactive electrophilic molecules abstracting hydrogen atoms from methylene carbons of the long hydrocarbon chains. Addition of O_2 to these sites form lipid peroxy radicals, which are also capable of removing hydrogen atoms from adjacent fatty acids. This leads to autooxidation reactions termed chain propagation. One initiation event has been estimated to convert, through propagation, hundreds of fatty acid side chains into lipid hydroperoxides.[39] Lipid peroxy radicals and hydroperoxides can degenerate, upsetting membrane integrity, into a variety of products, such as ketones, esters, aldehydes, and alkanes. Propagation is terminated when the free radicals involved are depleted.

The numerous functions carried out by structurally sound membranes are essential for tissue viability. This vital role of membranes, in conjunction with the peroxidative loss of membrane integrity as described earlier led to the development of widespread hypotheses suggesting lipid peroxidation as the basis of tissue injury resulting from ischemia-reperfusion or chemically induced oxidative stress.[33,37–39] Caution must be taken, however, when interpreting data in support of these hypotheses since lipid peroxidation could be an effect rather than a cause of tissue injury.[33] Tribble et al.[33] point out that a causal role for lipid peroxidation in pathological processes has not been firmly established. Reviews that describe lipid peroxidation and its biological consequences in detail are available.[37–39]

Despite a few conflicting reports,[40,41] many investigators, utilizing a wide variety of techniques, have detected enhanced hepatic lipid peroxidation in animals following acute[29,42–45] or chronic[46–49] ethanol intake. Moreover, lipid peroxidation has been demonstrated in the serum and livers of alcoholics.[50–52] Although far from being conclusive, these studies support the theory that lipid peroxidation resulting from ethanol-induced oxidative stress may be an important pathogenic mechanism of ALD in humans.[53,54]

Proposed Mechanisms for the Promotion of Oxidative Stress by Ethanol

Cederbaum[23] has compiled a list of possible mechanisms by which ethanol exposure may induce hepatic oxidative stress and lipid peroxidation. Ethanol can:

1. Decrease the levels of antioxidants, such as GSH, vitamin E, and selenium;
2. Directly disturb membrane fluidity thereby increasing membrane susceptibility to peroxidative damage;
3. Generate oxidants through the metabolism of acetaldehyde;
4. Cause mitochondrial damage thereby disrupting respiratory chain function, which can result in oxyradical formation;
5. Increase hepatic levels of iron;
6. Promote hepatic infiltration and activation of polymorphonuclear leukocytes;
7. Increase the activities of cytochromes P450, aldehyde oxidase (EC 1.2.3.1), and XO yielding an excess of $O_2^{-\bullet}$ and H_2O_2.

Despite such a list, the mechanism(s) responsible, either alone or in combination with other factors, for ethanol-induced oxidative stress and lipid peroxidation remains unclear. Furthermore, this list, which is not fully comprehensive, signifies what has plagued ALD research for years, that is, the multitude of hepatic effects caused by ethanol.

Proposed Mechanisms for the Increase of Hepatic Xanthine Oxidase Activity by Ethanol

The proposed involvement of XO in ethanol-induced oxidative stress leading to lipid peroxidation and the development of ALD seems to have grown out of studies[4–6] originally implicating this enzyme in ischemia-reperfusion injury of the intestine and heart. Since a few reports[55–57] suggest that there is no contribution of XO activity to ischemia-reperfusion injury, it is fitting that any potential involvement of XO in ethanol hepatotoxicity be viewed with caution.

Within liver lobules, blood enters the periportal region (zone 1) and flows through sinusoids to the perivenular region (zone 3) draining into the central vein. Since O_2 diffuses from blood into hepatocytes lining the sinusoids, a normal decreasing O_2 gradient exists between periportal cells and cells of the perivenular region.[14,58]

With the support of several studies,[12–14,58] ethanol has been proposed to steepen this O_2 gradient through a mechanism(s) involving an increased rate of O_2 uptake by the liver. Israel et al.[12] proposed that ethanol steepens the normal O_2 gradient to such a degree that the perivenular region lacks an adequate supply of O_2. These investigators observed that brief exposure to hypoxia produced greater perivenular necrosis in ethanol-treated than in control rats. In the same study the antithyroid drug propylthiouracil, which decreases tissue metabolic rates, decreased the perivenular damage. Moreover, using propylthiouracil, Ji et al.[58] prevented this ethanol-enhanced O_2 gradient in perfused rat liver. Based on the foregoing considerations, ethanol-induced perivenular hypoxia has therefore been implicated in the pathogenesis of ethanol hepatotoxicity. In support of this implication, a distinct histological feature of ALD is a predominance of perivenular damage.[22] Interestingly, zonal distribution of XO in rat liver has been reported to prevail in the perivenular region.[29,53] This distribution of XO, however, needs further conformation.

A model proposed by McCord[5] has suggested that since ATP levels in hypoxic tissues are rapidly depleted, proper cation gradients across cellular membranes cannot be maintained and cytosolic calcium concentrations may rise. In turn, calcium-dependent proteases could become activated and convert XD to XO. Moreover, ATP catabolism in hypoxic tissue results in the accumulation of the XO substrate hypoxanthine and other corresponding metabolites. Under these conditions, XO activity could be elevated producing an excess of $O_2^{\bullet-}$ and H_2O_2.

Six and twelve hours after a single dose of ethanol (5 g/kg) in rats, Oei et al.[59] and Sultatos,[60] respectively, have demonstrated a significant conversion of hepatic XD to XO. In agreement with Sultatos,[60] but in contrast with Oei et al.,[59] Kato et al.[29] did not detect conversion in rat liver 6 h after ethanol treatment. Although Abbandanza et al.[61] did not find conversion 4 h after ethanol treatment (5 g/kg), they did observe XD to XO conversion in rat liver following daily doses of ethanol (6 g/kg) over 9 d. Similarly, proteolytic XD to XO conversion in the ischemic liver seems to occur at slow rates.[10,29] Such low rates suggest that XD to XO conversion may not play a role in the early stages of ischemia and/or ethanol-induced liver damage. However, as discussed later, Kato et al.[29] speculate that XD to XO conversion may not be necessary for the XD/XO system to be involved in ethanol hepatotoxicity. Although the ethanol-dependent conversions reported earlier could have occurred through a mechanism similar to McCord's hypoxia model, acetaldehyde was also implicated as a potential causative agent through interaction with a sulfhydryl group(s) on XD.[59,60]

Frequently, an XD/XO inhibitor, allopurinol, is utilized to discriminate between XO-dependent tissue injury and injury resulting from other potential sources of oxidative stress. Kera et al.[62] reported that rats pretreated with allopurinol (100 mg/kg) were not protected from ethanol-induced lipid peroxidation. In another study, similar results were obtained with perfused livers and isolated hepatocytes.[54] Conversely, Kato et al.[29] demonstrated that allopurinol pretreatment (40 mg/kg) significantly decreased ethanol-induced hepatic lipid peroxidative damage in rat as measured by malondialdehyde levels. Similarly, other groups[13,59] observed allopurinol to be protective against ethanol hepatotoxicity. In addition to differences in methodology, two factors that may be contributing to these apparent discrepancies are: (a) since allopurinol and its metabolite oxypurinol have an intrinsic ability to act as powerful scavengers of free radicals from any source,[63] these agents may not discriminate XO-induced injury from other free radical sources of injury and (b) since uric acid has been proposed to function as an antioxidant[35,36] and protect tissues from oxidative damage, the extent to which XO is inhibited by allopurinol may be critical to whether or not XO activity causes tissue injury. These factors have questioned the dependability of allopurinol in XO research.[63]

As previously mentioned, recent evidence suggests that the conversion of hepatic XD to XO may not be required for the XD/XO system to be involved in ethanol toxicity.[29] Kato and coworkers[29] treated rats with a single dose of ethanol (5 g/kg) and 6 h later did not detect conversion of hepatic XD to XO. Despite this lack of conversion, hepatic lipid peroxidation was observed and was significantly decreased following pretreatment with allopurinol. In addition, the levels of hepatic NADH, AMP, hypoxanthine, and xanthine were significantly increased over control values. Recall that hypoxic conditions also result in the hepatic accumulation of ATP metabolites, such as AMP and hypoxanthine.[5] The concentration of hepatic NADH corresponding to that measured in vivo after ethanol treatment inhibited 60–70% of XD activity in vitro. Based on these findings and, as discussed earlier, the proposed regulatory role of XD/XO in purine metabolism,[27] Kato et al.[29] speculated that after ethanol intake, the observed increase in hepatic NADH inhibits XD and results in a shift of substrate flux through constituent XO. This shift in activity to XO may contribute, without actual XD to XO conversion, to ethanol-induced lipid peroxidative damage in the liver.

Regardless of the mechanism, excess XO activity resulting from ethanol exposure could lead to production of O_2^- and H_2O_2, which in turn could form OH• through the iron-catalyzed Haber-Weiss reaction.[34] This XO-induced oxidative stress may contribute to the enhancement of hepatic lipid peroxidation observed after ethanol exposure[53] and hence the development of ALD.

Conclusions and Summary

Since the molecular events responsible for the cellular damage to ALD are not known with certainty, specific therapeutic intervention remains a problem. There are many promising hypotheses regarding the development of liver injury following excess ethanol intake. This indicates that multiple mechanisms are most likely responsible for the pathogenesis of ALD. The present chapter has summarized one theory that an ethanol-induced increase in the activity of XO may contribute, through cellular oxidative damage, to the hepatotoxicity of ethanol. Although far from being conclusive, lipid peroxidation is the oxidative damage that has been associated with an excess of XO activity and ethanol-induced liver damage. It must be emphasized that before XO can be regarded as a significant factor in ALD, the role of lipid peroxidation in cell injury and death must be more completely understood. Lipid peroxidation could be a consequence rather than a cause of cell death. Until a direct molecular pathway(s) leading to ethanol hepatotoxicity can be identified, the best prevention and treatment of ALD is perhaps alcohol abstinence.

References

[1] C. Cross (1987) Oxygen radicals and human disease. *Ann. Intern. Med.* **107**, 526–545.

[2] B. Halliwell (1987) Oxidants and human disease: Some new concepts. *FASEB J.* **1**, 358–364.

[3] R. C. Bray (1975) Molybdenum iron-sulfur flavin hydroxylases and related enzymes, in *The Enzymes*, vol. 12. P. D. Boyer, ed. Academic, New York, pp. 299–417.

[4] D. A. Parks and D. N. Granger (1986) Xanthine oxidase: Biochemistry, distribution and physiology. *Acta Physiol. Scand.* **548 (Suppl.)**, 87–99.

[5] J. M. McCord (1985) Oxygen derived free radicals in postischemic tissue injury. *N. Engl. J. Med.* **312**, 159–163.

[6] D. A. Parks, T. K. Williams, and J. S. Beckman (1988) Conversion of xanthine dehydrogenase to oxidase in ischemic rat intestine: A reevaluation. *Am. J. Physiol.* **254**, G768–G774.

[7] E. Della Corte and F. Stirpe (1972) The regulation of rat liver xanthine oxidase. Involvement of thiol groups in the conversion of the enzyme activity from dehydrogenase (type D) into oxidase (type O) and purification of the enzyme. *Biochem. J.* **126**, 739–745.

[8] N. R. Waud and K. V. Rajagopalan (1976) Purification and properties of the NAD^+-dependent (type D) and O_2-dependent (type O) form of rat liver xanthine dehydrogenase. *Arch. Biochem. Biophys.* **172**, 354–364.

[9] D. N. Granger, G. Rutili, and J. M. McCord (1981) Role of superoxide radicals in intestinal ischemia. *Gastroenterology* **811**, 22–29.

[10] T. D. Engerson, T. G. McKelvey, D. B. Phyme, E. B. Boggio, S. J. Snyder, and H. P. Jones (1987) Conversion of xanthine dehydrogenase to oxidase in ischemic rat tissues. *J. Clin. Invest.* **79**, 1564–1570.

[11] S. J. Weiss (1986) Oxygen, ischemia and inflammation. *Acta Physiol. Scand.* **548 (Suppl.)**, 9–37.

[12] Y. Israel, H. Kalant, H. Orrego, J. M. Khanna, L. Videla, and J. M. Phillips (1975) Experimental alcohol-induced hepatic necrosis: Suppression by propyl-thiouracil. *Proc. Natl. Acad. Sci. USA* **72**, 1137–1141.

[13] M. Younes and O. Strubelt (1987) Enhancement of hypoxic liver damage by ethanol. *Biochem. Pharmacol.* **36**, 2973–2977.

[14] R. G. Thurman, S. Ji, and J. J. Lemasters (1986) Lobular oxygen gradients: Possible role in alcohol-induced hepatotoxicity, in *Regulation of Hepatic Metabolism*. R. G. Thurman, F. C. Kauffman, and K. Jungermann, eds. Plenum, New York, pp. 293–316.

[15] US Department of Health and Human Services (1987) Alcohol and Health, Rockville, MD [DHHS publication (ADM) 87–1519]. pp. 1–23.

[16] R. L. Berkelman, M. Ralston, J. Herndon, M. Gwinn, D. Bertolucci, and M. Dufar (1986) Patterns of alcohol consumption and alcohol-related morbidity and mortality. *Morbidity and Mortality Weekly Rep.* **35,** 1ss-5ss.

[17] A. Baptista, L. Bianchi, J. deGroote, V. J. Desmet, P. Gedigk, G. Korb, R. N. M. MacSween, H. Popper, H. Poulsen, P. J. Schever, M. Schmid, H. Thaler, and W. Wepler (1981) Alcoholic liver disease: Morphological manifestations. *Lancet* **1,** 707–711.

[18] C. S. Lieber and K. S. Guadagnini (1990) The spectrum of alcoholic liver disease. *Hospital Practice* **29–2A,** 51–69.

[19] J. Galambus (1985) Epidemiology of cirrhosis in the United States of America, in *Alcoholic Liver Disease.* P. Hall, ed. Wiley, New York, p. 230.

[20] L. G. Sultatos and T. M. Soranno (1991) Alcohol-induced liver disease, in *Biochemistry and Physiology of Substance Abuse,* vol. 3. R. R. Watson, ed. CRC, Boca Raton, FL, pp. 71–92.

[21] C. S. Lieber (1988) Metabolic effects of ethanol and its interaction with other drugs, hepatotoxic agents, vitamins, and carcinogens: A 1988 update. *Sem. Liver Dis.* **8,** 47–68.

[22] C. S. Lieber (1988) Biochemical and molecular basis of alcohol-induced injury to liver and other tissues. *N. Engl. J. Med.* **319,** 1639–1650.

[23] A. I. Cederbaum (1989) Introduction: Role of lipid peroxidation and oxidative stress in alcohol toxicity. *Free Rad. Biol. Med.* **7,** 537–539.

[24] F. Stirpe and E. Della Corte (1969) The regulation of rat liver xanthine oxidase. Conversion *in vitro* of the enzyme activity from dehydrogenase (type D) to oxidase (type O). *J. Biol. Chem.* **244,** 3855–3863.

[25] W. R. Waud and K. V. Rajagopalan (1976) The mechanism of conversion of rat liver xanthine dehydrogenase from an NAD^+-dependent form (type D) to an O_2-dependent form (type O). *Arch. Biochem. Biophys.* **172,** 365–379.

[26] K. Stark, P. Seubert, G. Lynch, and M. Baudry (1989) Proteolytic conversion of xanthine dehydrogenase to xanthine oxidase: Evidence against a role for calcium-activated protease (calpain). *Biochem. Biophys. Res. Comm.* **165,** 858–864.

[27] Z. W. Kaminski and M. M. Jezewska (1981) Effect of NADH on hypoxanthine hydroxylation by native NAD^+-dependent xanthine oxidoreductase of rat liver, and possible biological role of this effect. *Biochem. J.* **200,** 597–603.

[28] E. Della Corte and F. Stirpe (1970) The regulation of xanthine oxidase inhibition by reduced nicotinamide-adenine dinucleotide of rat liver xanthine oxidase type D and of chick xanthine dehydrogenase. *Biochem. J.* **117,** 97–100.

[29] S. Kato, T. Kawase, J. Alderman, N. Inatomi, and C. S. Lieber (1990) Role of xanthine oxidase in ethanol-induced lipid peroxidation in rats. *Gastroenterology* **98,** 203–210.

[30] R. W. Topham, M. C. Walker, M. P. Calisch, and R. W. Williams (1982)

Evidence for the participation of intestinal xanthine oxidase in the mucosal processing of iron. *Biochemistry.* **21,** 4529–4535.

[31] B. J. Bolann and R. J. Ulvik (1987) Release of iron from ferritin by xanthine oxidase. *Biochem. J.* **243,** 55–59.

[32] P. Biemond, A. J. G. Swaak, C. M. Beindorff, and J. F. Koster (1986) Superoxide-dependent and -independent mechanisms of iron mobilization from ferritin by xanthine oxidase. *Biochem. J.* **239,** 169–173.

[33] D. L. Tribble, T. Y. Aw, and D. P. Jones (1987) The pathophysiological significance of lipid peroxidation in oxidative cell injury. *Hepatology* **7,** 377–387.

[34] R. Nordmann, C. Ribiere, and H. Rouach (1987) Involvement of iron and iron-catalyzed free radical production in ethanol metabolism and toxicity. *Enzyme* **37,** 57–69.

[35] B. N. Ames, R. Cathcart, E. Schwiers, and P. Huschstein (1981) Uric acid provides an antioxidant defense in human against oxidants and radicals causing aging and cancer: A hypothesis. *Proc. Natl. Acad. Sci. USA* **78,** 6859–6862.

[36] Z. Zhong, J. J. Lemasters, and R. G. Thurman (1989) Role of purines and xanthine oxidase in reperfusion injury in perfused rat liver. *J. Pharmacol. Exp. Ther.* **250,** 470–475.

[37] G. L. Plaa and H. Witschi (1976) Chemicals, drugs, and lipid peroxidation. *Ann. Rev. Pharmacol. Toxicol.* **16,** 125–141.

[38] H. Kappus and H. Sies (1981) Toxic drug effects associated with oxygen metabolism: Redox cycling and lipid peroxidation. *Experentia* **37,** 1233–1358.

[39] J. M. C. Gutteridge and B. Halliwell (1990) The measurement and mechanism of lipid peroxidation in biological systems. *TIBS* **15,** 129–135.

[40] S. Hashimoto and P. O. Recknagel (1968) No chemical evidence of hepatic lipid peroxidation in acute ethanol toxicity. *Exp. Mol. Pathol.* **8,** 225–242.

[41] H. Speisky, D. Bunout, H. Orrego, H. G. Giles, A. Gunasekara, and Y. Israel (1985) Lack of changes in diene conjugate levels following ethanol induced glutathione depletion or necrosis. *Res. Commun. Chem. Pathol. Pharmacol.* **48,** 77–90.

[42] N. R. DiLuzio (1966) A mechanism of the acute ethanol-induced fatty liver and the modification of liver injury by antioxidants. *Lab. Invest.* **15,** 50–63.

[43] L. A. Videla, V. Fernandez, G. Ugarte, A. Valenzuela, and A. Villanueva (1980) Effect of acute ethanol intoxication on the content of reduced glutathione of the liver in relation to its lipoperoxidative capacity in the rat. *FEBS Lett.* **111,** 6–10.

[44] U. Koster, D. Albrecht, and H. Kappus (1977) Evidence for carbon tetrachloride- and ethanol-induced lipid peroxidation *in vivo* demonstrated by ethane production in mice and rats. *Toxicol. Appl. Pharmacol.* **41,** 639–648.

[45] A. Valenzuela, N. Fernandez, V. Fernandez, G. Urgarte, L. A. Videla, R. Guerra, and A. Villanueva (1980) Effect of acute ethanol ingestion on lipoperoxidation and on the activity of the enzymes related to peroxide metabolism in rat liver. *FEBS Lett.* **111,** 11–13.

[46] S. Shaw, E. Jayatilleke, W. A. Ross, E. R. Gordon, and C. S. Lieber (1981) Ethanol-induced lipid peroxidation: Potentiation by long-term feeding and attenuation by methionine. *J. Lab. Clin. Med.* **98,** 417–424.

[47] R. C. Reitz (1975) A possible mechanism for the peroxidation of lipids due to chronic ethanol ingestion. *Biochem. Biophys. Acta* **380,** 145–154.

[48] M. Koes, T. Ward, and S. Pennington (1974) Lipid peroxidation in chronic ethanol treated rats: *In vitro* uncoupling of peroxidation from reduced nicotine adenosine dinucleotide phosphate oxidation. *Lipids* **9,** 899–904.

[49] H. Remmer, D. Albrecht, and H. Kappus (1977) Lipid peroxidation in isolated hepatocytes from rats ingesting ethanol chronically. *Naunyn-Schmiedeber's Arch. Pharmacol.* **298,** 107–113.

[50] S. Shaw, K. P. Rubin, and C. S. Lieber (1983) Depressed hepatic glutathione and increased diene conjugates in alcoholic liver disease: Evidence of lipid peroxidation. *Dig. Dis. Sci.* **28,** 585–589.

[51] T. Suematsu, T. Matsumura, N. Sato, T. Miyamoto, T. Ooka, T. Kamada, and H. Abe (1981) Lipid peroxidation in alcoholic liver disease in humans. *Alcohol. Clin. Exp. Res.* **5,** 427–430.

[52] A. R. Tanner, I. Bantock, L. Hinks, B. Lloyd, N. R. Turner, and R. Wright (1986) Depressed selenium and vitamin E levels in an alcoholic population. Possible relationship to hepatic injury through increased lipid peroxidation. *Dig. Dis. Sci.* **31,** 1307–1312.

[53] L. A. Videla and A. Valenzuela (1982) Alcohol ingestion, liver glutathione, and lipoperoxidation: Metabolic interrelation and pathological implications. *Life Sci.* **31,** 2395–2407.

[54] A. Muller and H. Sies (1987) Alcohol, aldehydes and lipid peroxidation: Current notions. *Alcohol Alcohol.* **1 (Suppl.),** 67–74.

[55] D. A. Parks and D. N. Granger (1988) Ischemia-reperfusion injury: A radical view. *Hepatology* **8,** 680–682.

[56] J. Metzger, S. P. Dore, and B. H. Lauterburg (1988) Oxidant stress during reperfusion of ischemic liver: No evidence for a role of xanthine oxidase. *Hepatology* **8,** 580–584.

[57] S. W. Werns and B. R. Lucchesi (1990) Free radicals and ischemic tissue injury. *TIPS* **11,** 161–166.

[58] S. Ji, J. J. Lemasters, V. Christenson, and R. G. Thurman (1982) Periportal and pericentral pyridine nucleotide fluorescence from the surface of the perfused liver: Evaluation of the hypothesis that chronic treatment with ethanol produces pericentral hypoxia. *Proc. Natl. Acad. Sci. USA* **79,** 5415–5419.

[59] H. H. H. Oei, H. C. Zoganas, J. M. McCord, and S. W. Schafer, (1986) Role of acetaldehyde and xanthine oxidase in ethanol-induced oxidative stress. *Res. Com. Chem. Path. Pharmacol.* **51,** 195–203.

[60] L. G. Sultatos (1988) Effects of acute ethanol administration on the hepatic

xanthine dehydrogenase/oxidase system in the rat. *J. Pharmacol. Exp. Ther.* **246,** 946–949.

[61] A. Abbondanza, M. G. Battelli, M. Soffritti, and C. Cessi (1989) Xanthine oxidase status in ethanol-intoxicated rat liver. *Alcohol. Clin. Exp. Res.* **13,** 841–844.

[62] Y. Kera, Y. Ohbora, and S. Komura (1988) The metabolism of acetaldehyde and not acetaldehyde itself is responsible for *in vivo* ethanol-inducible lipid peroxidation in rats. *Biochem. Pharmacol.* **37,** 3633–3638.

[63] P. C. Moorhouse, M. Grootveld, B. Halliwell, J. G. Quinlan, and J. M. C. Gutteridge (1987) Allopurinol and oxypurinol are hydroxyl radical scavengers. *FEBS Lett.* **213,** 23–28.

Polymorphisms of Alcohol and Aldehyde Dehydrogenases and Their Significance for Alcohol Liver Diseases

Akira Yoshida and Akitaka Shibuya

Introduction

Family pedigree studies and adoption studies have now demonstrated significant hereditary contributions in alcoholism.[1,2] Genetic differences in alcohol-seeking behavior, sensitivity of the central nervous system, and tissue susceptibility to alcohol and its metabolites, would affect the development of alcoholism and other alcohol-related problems. These multiple genetic factors and their interactions with environmental, social, and psychological factors have not yet been well understood.

More than 80% of ethanol ingested at a moderate level is oxidized by alcohol dehydrogenase, and acetaldehyde thus produced is further oxidized to nontoxic acetate by aldehyde dehydrogenase. Differences in the alcohol-metabolizing system would affect alcohol sensitivity and indirectly influence the development of alcohol-related diseases. Large numbers of alcohol dehydrogenase isozymes and aldehyde dehydrogenase isozymes have been

From: *Drug and Alcohol Abuse Reviews, Vol. 2: Liver Pathology and Alcohol*
Ed: R. R. Watson ©1991 The Humana Press Inc.

found in humans and other mammals. In recent several years, genetic variations and polymorphisms of some of these enzymes have been elucidated at the gene level. In this chapter, we will summarize characteristics of alcohol dehydrogenase and aldehyde dehydrogenase isozymes and discuss possible relationships between the genetic variations of these enzymes, alcohol sensitivity, and alcoholic liver diseases.

Alcohol Dehydrogenase

Isozymes and Their Physiological Roles

Alcohol dehydrogenase (alcohol: NAD^+ oxidoreductase, EC 1.1.1.1, abbreviation ADH) is a group of enzymes catalyzing the oxidation of varieties of alcohols to the corresponding aldehydes. ADH isozymes of humans and other mammals are grouped in three distinctive "classes" based on their enzymatic characteristics. The isozymes that exhibit high catalytic activity for oxidation of shortchain aliphatic alcohol, such as ethanol, and are strongly inactivated by pyrazole, are grouped as class I ADH.[3] Another type (class II) of ADH isozymes, exhibits a high activity for oxidation of longchain aliphatic alcohols and aromatic alcohols, and is less sensitive to pyrazole.[4] Other ADH isozymes, which have virtually no activity for ethanol oxidation, but exhibit high activity for oxidation of longchain alcohols, and are completely insensitive to pyrazole, are classified as class III ADH.[5]

The human class I ADH isozymes include homo- and heterodimers consisting of three types of subunit (α, β, and γ), which are controlled by three nonallelic structural loci, ADH_1, ADH_2, and ADH_3 (Table 1). The human class II ADH is a homodimer of π subunit which is controlled by ADH_4 gene, and the class III ADH is a homodimer of χ subunit controlled by ADH_5 gene. The three class I ADH genes are clustered on chromosome 4q21–23 within about 80 kilo base pairs.[6,7] Other ADH genes are also on chromosome 4q21-25.[8,9]

The class I ADHs are most abundant in the liver, and exist also in other tissues including the intestine, lung, and kidney, but are not detectable in the brain, skin fibroblasts, and red blood cells.[10] The class II ADH ($\pi\pi$) is primarily found in the liver.[11] Similar isozyme(s) is also detected in the gastrointestinal tract.[12] However, it remains to be elucidated whether the stomach isozyme is identical to the liver $\pi\pi$ ADH or stomach contains other ADH isozyme(s) (*see* later discussion). The class III ADH is found in all tissues examined, including the brain, testis, and red blood cells.[13,14]

Table 1
ADH Genes and Polymorphisms

ADH class	Alleles		Subunit	Mutation site	Gene frequencies
	Locus	Common			
I	ADH_1	ADH_1	α		~100%
	ADH_2	ADH_2^1	β_1		Wild type, >90% in Caucasians
		ADH_2^2	β_2	Arg→His at position 47	Common in Orientals (~70%)
		ADH_2^3	β_3	Arg→Cys at position 369	Common in Blacks (~16%)
	ADH_3	ADH_3^1	γ_1		Wild type, >90% in Orientals
		ADH_3^2	γ_2	Arg→Glu at position 271	Common in Caucasians (~40%)
				Ile→Val at position 349	
II	ADH_4	ADH_4^1	π_1		
		ADH_4^2	π_2	Arg→Lys at position 302	
				Val→Ile at position 312	
III	ADH_5	ADH_5	χ		
	ADH_6	ADH_6		(new gene and locus, *see text*)	

The value of ADH_2^2 frequency was obtained from references;[27,44,84,85] that of ADH_2^3 from reference;[28] and that of ADH_3^1 and ADH_3^2 from references.[12,29] The possible existence of at least two common alleles for the ADH_4 locus was suggested in reference.[39]

Ethanol ingested is mainly oxidized by the class I isozymes in the liver, particularly by that consisting of β subunit, which is predominant in the adult liver. The class II ADH ($\pi\pi$ enzyme), which has a higher K_m for ethanol than the class I ADHs, may also participate in ethanol oxidation, when tissue ethanol level exceeds 20 mM.[4] There are two other systems for ethanol metabolism, i.e., catalase located in the peroxisomes and the NADPH⁺-dependent microsomal ethanol oxidizing systems (MEOS) located in the endoplasmic reticulum.[15–17] The MEOS system may play a significant role in alcoholics and habitual heavy drinkers with high blood alcohol levels. However, in general, it is considered that ethanol is mainly oxidized by the ADH system.[18]

It has been known that females are more susceptible to developing alcoholic liver injury than males. Recently it was reported that a significant portion of orally administered ethanol was metabolized in the stomach of males, but not in females, and that ADH activity of stomach mucous membrane is substantially higher in males than females.[19] We recently cloned a new human ADH gene (designated as *ADH₆*), which does not belong to any known ADH class.[20] The *ADH₆* gene is far more strongly expressed in the stomach than in the liver (unpublished observation). Whether or not the *ADH₆* encodes sex-dependent ADH in the stomach mucous membrane remains to be elucidated.

The class I ADHs metabolize dopamine and serotonin,[11,21] and the class II ADH also oxidize serotonin and norepinephrine,[13,21] suggesting relationships between alcoholism and metabolism of neurotransmitters. The class I ADH isozymes containing γ-subunit exhibit 3β-hydroxy-5β-steroid dehydrogenase activity, and testosterone was found to be an allosteric regulator.[22] The class I ADHs can efficiently oxidize 16-hydroxyhexa-decanoic acid, hence the enzymes may take part in fatty acid metabolism.[23] The rat liver class I ADH, and presumably also human ADHs, can convert the endogenously generated toxic aldehyde, 4-hydroxynonenal, to the less toxic alcohol form.[24] Exogenously ingested ethanol would compete with the endogenous substrates and disturb the physiological detoxification, resulting in tissue damage.

The molecular identity of rat class III ADH and glutathione-dependent formaldehyde dehydrogenase (EC 1.2.1.1) was recently demonstrated.[25] The human class III ADH may also exhibit similar aldehyde dehydrogenase activity (i.e., oxidation of *S*-hydroxymethyl-glutathione to *S*-formyl-glutathione in the presence of NAD⁺). Rat retina and hamster testis contain

ADH, which converts transretinol to retinaldehyde.[26,27] This ADH isozyme may play a role in activation of vitamin A in respective organs. Analogous ADH isozyme may also exist in humans. Genetic abnormalities, and consequent alterations of activity and kinetic properties of any one of these ADH isozymes, would affect ethanol oxidation, and/or metabolism of neurotransmitters, fatty acids, and biogenic toxic metabolites, and could change one's vulnerability in developing alcohol-related diseases.

Genetic Variants and Polymorphisms

Three common alleles, i.e., ADH_2^1 for β1, ADH_2^2 for β2, and ADH_2^3 for β3, have been recognized in the ADH_2 locus. The wild type ADH_2^1 is predominant in Caucasians (gene frequency >90%), whereas the atypical ADH_2^2 is prevalent (~70%) among Orientals,[27] and the ADH_2^3 is fairly common (~16%) in American Blacks.[28] Two common alleles, i.e., ADH_3^1 for γ_1 and ADH_2^2 for γ_2, are found in Caucasians, but not in Orientals.[12,29]

The molecular differences, at both the protein level and the gene level, of these variant genes and gene products (i.e., variant enzymes) have been elucidated.

The difference between the wild type β_1 and the Oriental atypical β_2 subunit is a single amino acid substitution Arg→His at the 47th position generated by the G/C→A/T base transition on exon 3 (Fig. 1).[30–33] The isozyme consisting of atypical β_2 subunit exhibits about 100 times higher catalytic activity for ethanol oxidation than the usual $\beta_1\beta_1$ isozyme at the physiological pH.[30]

The amino acid substitution between the wild type β_1 and the variant β_3 (β Indianapolis) was reported to be Arg→Cys at the 369th position.[34] Deducing from the nucleotide sequence of the ADH_2^1 gene, this substitution was generated by the C/G→T/A base transition in exon 9. The catalytic activity of isozyme consisting of variant β_3 subunit is two orders of magnitude higher than that of the usual $\beta_1\beta_1$ isozyme.[35]

From the nucleotide sequences of cDNAs for γ_1 and γ_2 subunits, two amino acid differences, i.e., Arg→Glu at the 271st position, and Ile→Val at the 349th position, were detected.[36] The 276th position of γ subunit as originally reported as Val based on protein sequencing.[37] From the cDNA sequence, this position should be Met.[38] The difference is apparently an error in protein sequencing and is not due to genetic polymorphism.

Discrepancies were found between the amino acid sequences of the π subunit and the nucleotide sequence of πcDNA, i.e., the position 303 is

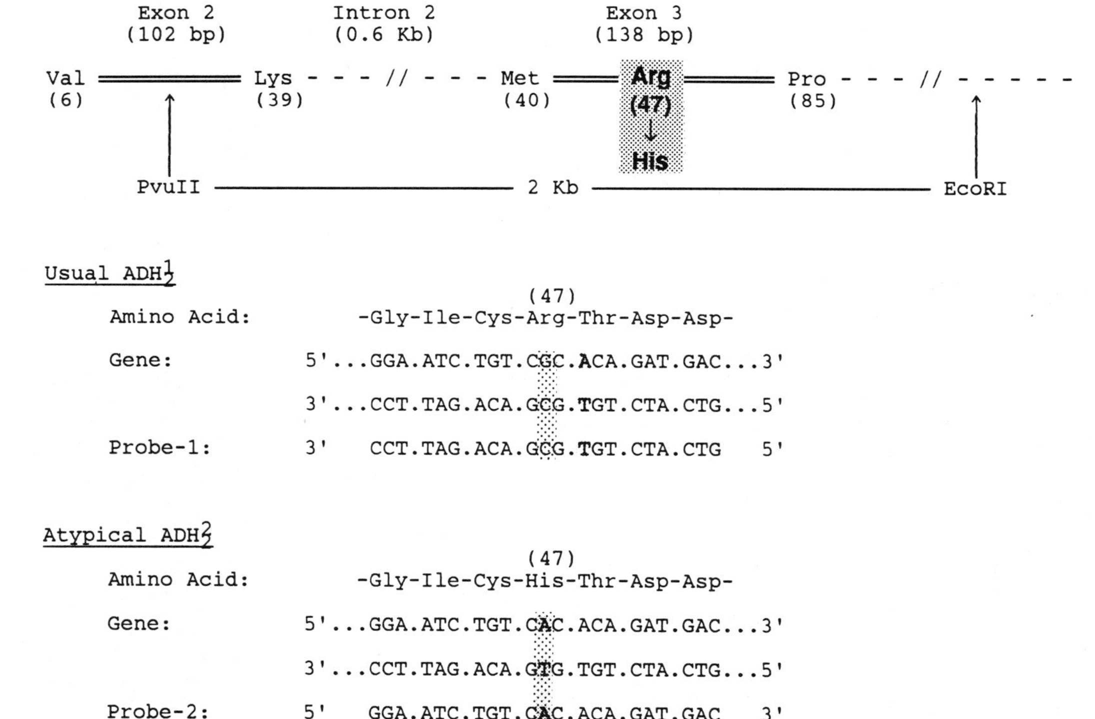

Fig. 1. Mutation site of the *ADH₂* locus. Nucleotide sequences and amino acid sequences of the mutation region are shown. The sequences of allele specific probes for genotype determination are also shown. Data were obtained from reference.[44] The mutation position is shown in shadowed boxes. Detailed genomic structure and restriction sites were described in references.[32,101]

Arg in cDNA but Lys in protein, and the position 312 is Val in cDNA but Ile in protein.[39] Two or more common alleles might exist in the ADH_4 locus. cDNA for the π subunit can encode 391 amino acid residues, instead of 379 residues determined by protein sequencing.[39] The size difference could be owing to posttranslational cleavage of the COOH-terminal region, not to genetic polymorphism.

A cDNA clone for the χ subunit can encode 373 amino acid residues matched with the amino acid sequence data,[40] whereas another cDNA differed by one residue (Tyr→Asp at 166) and could encode additional 19 amino acid residues starting from an upstream initiation codon.[41] It remains to be further examined whether or not polymorphisms exist in the ADH_5 locus, and posttranslational cleavage of the NH_2-terminal occurred in the χ subunit.

Restriction fragment length polymorphisms (RFLP) have been observed in the ADH loci. Because of the high degree of similarity (~95% identity in coding exons) in the three class I ADH loci, restriction fragment patterns are very complex, when Southern blot hybridization is carried out using cDNA or exon probes. Using a βcDNA as a probe, PvuII polymorphism was found in the ADH cluster locus.[42] Using less homologous intron sequences, one from the ADH_2 (β) gene, and two from the ADH_3 (γ) gene as probes, RsaI polymorphism was found in the ADH_2 locus, and XbaI, MspI, and StuI polymorphisms were found in the ADH_3 locus.[43] Frequencies of these RFLP differ widely between Caucasians and Orientals. The mutation, G/C→A/T on exon 3 of the ADH_2 locus, occurring in the Oriental atypical ADH_2^2 allele, generates a MaeIII cleavage site in the atypical allele, creating RFLP in Orientals.[44] SacI haplotype was found to be polymorphic in the ADH_5 locus.[45] RFLP of the ADH_4 locus has not yet been reported.

Aldehyde Dehydrogenase

Isozymes and Their Physiological Roles

Aldehyde dehydrogenases (Aldehyde: NAD^+ oxidoreductase, EC 1.2.1.3, ALDH) are a group of enzymes catalyzing the conversion of aldehydes to corresponding acids via a NAD^+-dependent irreversible reaction. Many human ALDH isozymes are distinguished based on the separation by physicochemical methods, tissue and subcellular distributions, and enzymatic properties (Table 2). The cytosolic liver $ALDH_1$ and the mitochon-

Table 2

Biochemical Properties of Purified Human ALDH Isozymes[a]

Isozymes	Major tissues	Subcellular[b] localization	pI[c]	K_m (μM) Acetaldehyde, pH	Preferred[d] aldehyde, pH	Disulfiram sensitivity, 20 μM	Subunit mol. wt	Subunit/ native molecule
ALDH$_1$	Liver	C	5.1	22 (7.5)		+	54,000	4
ALDH$_2$	Liver	M	4.9	3.5 (7.5)		±	54,000	4
γ-ABDH	Liver	N	5.3 (major)	50.4 (7.4)	13.8 (7.4)	−	54,000	4
			5.45 (minor)	40.3 (7.4)	8.0 (7.4)	−	54,000	4
ALDH$_3$	Liver Stomach	C	5.9–6.4	83000 (8.5)	11 (8.5)	−	54,000	2
ALDH$_4$	Liver	M	6.77 6.89	5000 (7.0)	100 (7.0)	−	70,600	2
ALDH$_x$	Liver Testis	M	N	N	N	N	54,000	N
ALDH$_{2a}$	Brain	M	4.9	1 (9.0)	1 (9.0)	+	54,000	4
ALDH$_{2b}$ Saliva	Brain	M	5.0	1 (9.0)	0.5 (9.0)	−	54,000	4
ALDH	Saliva	C	6.5–7.0	106 (8.0)	N	N	48,000	N

[a]Data for ALDH$_1$ and ALDH$_2$ were obtained from reference,[46] for γ-ABDH from reference,[49] for ALDH$_{2a}$ and ALDH$_{2b}$ from references,[50,51] and for saliva ALDH from reference.[53]

[b]c = cytosol; M = mitochondrial.

[c]pI (isoelectric point) determined by different laboratories showed ±0.2 differences.

[d]Preferred aldehydes are: γ-aminobutyraldehyde for γ-ABDH; heptaldehyde for ALDH$_3$; glutamic-γ-semialdehyde for ALDH$_4$; and dopaldehyde for ALDH$_{2a}$ and ALDH$_{2b}$.

N = Not known.

drial $ALDH_2$, which exhibit high catalytic activity for oxidation of acetaldehyde, are considered to play a major role in acetaldehyde detoxification in the liver. The cytosolic $ALDH_1$ has a higher K_m for acetaldehyde (apparent $K_m = 22\mu M$ at pH 7.5) and a lower K_m for NAD ($5\mu M$) than the mitochondrial $ALDH_2$ ($3.5\mu M$ for acetaldehyde and $16\mu M$ for NAD).[46] Although the mitochondrial $ALDH_2$ is generally considered to play a major role, the relative importance of these two isozymes in aldehyde detoxification in vivo is controversial. The $ALDH_3$ exhibits optimal activity for oxidation of benzaldehyde.[47] $ALDH_4$ is most active for glutamic-γ–semialdehyde as substrate, and thus the enzyme is classified as glutamic-γ–semialdehyde dehydrogenase.[48] A unique ALDH (γ–ABDH) has low K_m for acetaldehyde, but it is most active for oxidation of γ–aminobutyraldehyde (γ–AB) at the physiological pH, and thus is classified as γ–ABDH.[49]

Human brain ALDH isozymes have attracted attention because of their role in metabolism of neurotransmitters, besides the acetaldehyde oxidation. The brain cytosolic $ALDH_1$ corresponds to, and most likely is identical to, the liver $ALDH_1$. The brain contains two mitochondrial ALDH isozymes, $ALDH_{2a}$ and $ALDH_{2b}$, which are active for acetaldehyde oxidation.[50,51] These two isozymes may be different from the liver $ALDH_2$ and can oxidize DOPAL (3,4-dihydroxyphenyl-acetaldehyde).[51] Cerebellum, corpus striatum, and pons show a high activity for DOPAL oxidation.[52] Brain ALDH isozymes with activity for DOPAL oxidation remain to be further characterized. Human saliva contains ALDH isozyme which can oxidize acetaldehyde (K_m 100μM for acetaldehyde).[53] The biochemical and immunological data suggest that the saliva ALDH is different from liver $ALDH_1$ and $ALDH_2$, not a product of secondary modification.

Genomic and cDNA clones for a new ALDH (tentatively designated as $ALDH_x$) were recently obtained.[20] Judging from the deduced amino acid sequence, the gene is for a unique ALDH isozyme.[20] The enzyme produced by *ALDH*$_x$ gene oxidizes propionaldehyde but not benzaldehyde (unpublished observation).

The characteristics of the nine known human ALDH isozymes discussed previously are summarized in Table 2. The oligomeric forms of saliva ALDH and $ALDH_x$ isozyme are unknown. $ALDH_3$ and $ALDH_4$ are dimeric and the rest of the isozymes are tetrameric. The subunit mol wt of $ALDH_4$ is 70,600, that of saliva ALDH is 48,000, and the rest of the isozymes are approx 54,000.

Activities of $ALDH_2$, $ALDH_3$, and $ALDH_4$ isozymes were reported to be very low or absent in various fetal tissues, whereas $ALDH_1$ was found to be expressed in early developmental stages.[54,55] However, a recent study indicated that $ALDH_1$, $ALDH_2$, and $ALDH_4$ all existed in fetal livers that were obtained quickly after abortion or death and carefully preserved.[56] Thus, the fetus is capable of detoxifying acetaldehyde transferred from the mother.

Genetic Variants and Polymorphisms

Approximately 50% of Orientals lack $ALDH_2$ activity in their livers, but virtually none of the Caucasians exhibits $ALDH_2$ deficiency.[57] An enzymatically inactive but immunologically crossreactive material (CRM) corresponding to $ALDH_2$ was found in ALDH-deficient Japanese livers.[58] Thus, the $ALDH_2$ deficiency in Orientals is a result of a structural mutation in the *ALDH_2* gene, and not deletion of the gene. The molecular difference between the active $ALDH_2{}^1$ enzyme and the catalytically inactive $ALDH_2{}^2$ enzyme is a single amino acid substitution Glu→Lys at the 14th position from the COOH-terminal (or at the 487th position from the NH$_2$-terminal), originated by G/C→A/T base transition in exon 12 of the *ALDH_2* locus (Fig. 2).[59–61]

In contrast to the high frequency of *ALDH_2*^{2} variant observed in the Orientals, $ALDH_1$ variants were found to be less common. A variant, with severely diminished catalytic activity but strong immunological crossreactivity, was found in one out of ten Japanese livers.[62] Apparently, the same variant was also found in two out of 60 Japanese livers.[63] Another $ALDH_1$ variant associated with different electrophoretic mobility was found in two Oriental subjects.[64]

Recently, two $ALDH_1$ kinetic variants, $ALDH_1$-Columbo and $ALDH_1$-Harrow, were found in Caucasian alcohol flushers[65] (*see next section*).

Polymorphism at the *ALDH_3* locus was proposed based on the observed multiplicity of $ALDH_3$ bands in stomach samples.[66] It was argued that the variation could be due to secondary modification, and not due to genetic polymorphism.[67] However, later studies supported the existence of genetic polymorphism.[68,69] It was proposed that the two common alleles, i.e., *ALDH_{3b}*^{1} and *ALDH_{3b}*^{2}, exist in the *ALDH_{3b}* locus, based on the variations in isoelectric focusing patterns of $ALDH_3$ isozymes in Chinese stomach samples.[70] In the model proposed, *ALDH_{3a}* locus is expressed in the liver as well as in the stomach and lung, whereas *ALDH_{3b}* locus is not expressed

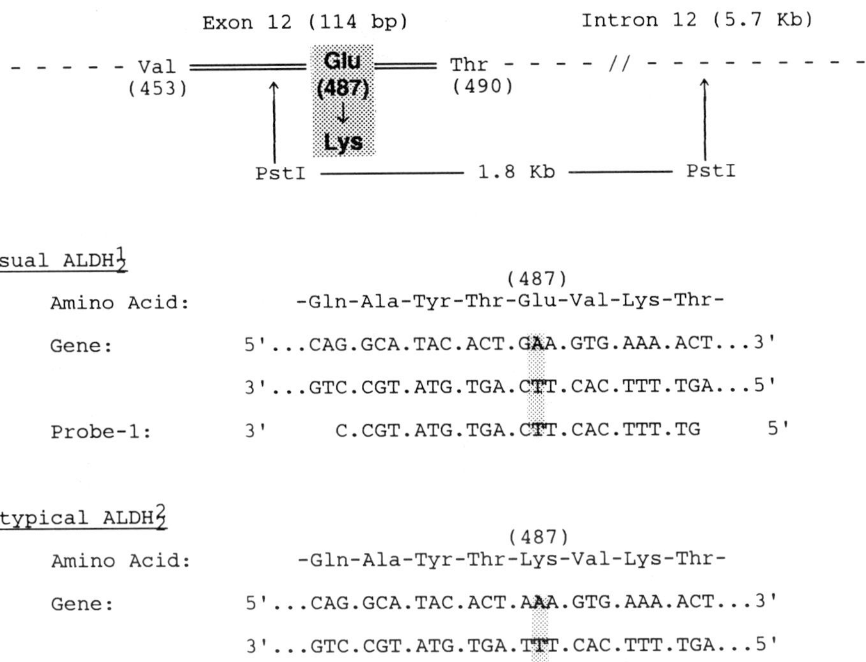

Fig. 2. Mutation site of the *ALDH₂* locus. Nucleotide sequences and amino acid sequences of the mutation region are shown. The sequences of allele specific probes are also shown. Data were obtained from references.[81,86] The mutation position is shown in shadowed boxes. Detailed genomic structure and restriction sites were described in references.[60,61]

in the liver.[70] The frequencies of $ALDH_{3b}{}^1$ and $ALDH_{3b}{}^2$ are estimated to be 0.14 and 0.86, respectively, in Chinese.

The nucleotide sequences determined from the genomic DNA clone (G) and testis cDNA clone (C) of $ALDH_x$ revealed discrepancies at three positions resulting in two amino acid exchanges, Val→Ala at position 69 and Arg→Leu at position 90.[20] When the genomic DNA samples from unrelated individuals were subjected to polymerase chain reaction of the targeted region followed by nucleotide sequence analysis, seven were found to be (C) type, only one was (G) type, and two were the recombinant type with other nucleotide changes. Therefore, the $ALDH_x$ locus is polymorphic. Difference in enzyme activity and electrophoretic mobility was observed when (G) and (C) types of DNA were expressed in the CHO-20 cells (unpublished observation).

Saliva ALDH deficiency was found in about 30% of Japanese.[53] It remains to be clarified whether or not the deficiency is really due to genetic polymorphism in the saliva ALDH locus. Polymorphisms of known ALDH loci are summarized in Table 3.

In the study of restriction fragment length polymorphisms, TaqI haplotype of the $ALDH_1$ locus was found to be polymorphic in Orientals but not in Caucasians.[71] MspI haplotype of the $ALDH_1$ locus is polymorphic in both populations, but the frequencies are different. In the $ALDH_2$ locus, MspI haplotype is polymorphic in both populations, and the frequencies are the same.[71] Thus far, no polymorphism was found in EcoRI and PstI haplotypes.

Genetic Polymorphisms of ADH and ALDH, and Alcohol-Related Problems

Individual and racial differences in alcohol sensitivity have been recognized for a long time. "Alcohol sensitive" persons ("alcohol flusher") exhibit rapid facial flushing, elevation of skin temperature, increase in pulse rate, and hypertension, when they drink a moderate amount (0.3–0.5 mL ethanol per 1 kg body wt) of alcohol. The first systematic study on racial differences of alcohol sensitivity was reported by Wolff, who observed alcohol flushing in about 80% of Mongoloids but only in about 5% of Caucasoids.[72] The difference could not be due to acquired habit, since the racial differences were clearly observed also in young infants. Several other investigators confirmed Wolff's observation, although figures differ among the reports, i.e., the frequency of alcohol flusher in Orientals is 71% in the study of Ewing et al.,[73] 50–60% in the studies by Wilson et al.,[74] and Zeiner et al.[75] Only about 5–8% of Caucasians were found to be alcohol sensitive in these studies.

Stamatoyannopoulos et al. observed that nearly 90% of Orientals exhibit much higher ADH activity in their livers than Caucasians, and suggested that a high incidence of alcohol sensitivity in Orientals could be caused by the rapid acetaldehyde formation by the more active ADH_2 variant.[76] On the other hand, Goedde et al. found that approximately 50%

Table 3
ALDH Genes and Polymorphisms

Isozyme	Locus	Common alleles	Mutation site	Gene frequency	Chromosome assignment
ALDH$_1$	ALDH$_1$	ALDH$_1$	—	~100%	9q21
ALDH$_2$	ALDH$_2$	ALDH$_2^1$		Wild type, ~100% in Caucasians	12q24
		ALDH$_2^2$	Glu→Lys at position 487	Common in Orientals (~30%)	12q24
ALDH$_3$	ALDH$_{3a}$				17
	ALDH$_{3b}^1$	ALDH$_{3b}^1$		Wild type	[a]
		ALDH$_{3b}^2$		Common in Chinese (86%)	[a]
ALDH$_4$	ALDH$_4$				
ALDH$_x$	ALDH$_x$	ALDH$_x^1$			9
		ALDH$_x^2$	Val→Ala at position 69		[b]
			Arg→Leu at position 90		[b]

[a]From isoelectric focusing patterns of Chinese stomach samples.[70]

[b]From nucleotide sequences of genomic DNA samples from ten unrelated individuals.[20] Data of ALDH$_1$ and ALDH$_2$ were obtained from references;[59–61,87,90,100] that of ALDH$_3$ from references;[47,70] that of ALDH$_x$ from an unpublished observation.

453

of Orientals lack mitochondrial $ALDH_2$ activity in their livers, and proposed that the alcohol sensitivity is a consequence of an accumulation of acetaldehyde due to $ALDH_2$ deficiency.[57,77] The high incidence of alcohol sensitivity could result from a combination of these two polymorphisms in Orientals. The alcohol sensitivity might discourage individuals from drinking, thus decreasing the risk of alcohol-related problems in the subjects with the abnormalities.

In order to verify these possibilities, genotypes of ADH_2 locus and $ALDH_2$ locus of control subjects, alcohol-sensitive and nonsensitive subjects, and patients with alcoholic diseases have to be determined.

It was reported that most of Japanese alcoholics and those with alcoholic liver disease had the active $ALDH_2$ isozyme in their livers.[63,78,79] However, neither the phenotypes and genotypes of the ADH_2 locus, nor the genotypes of the $ALDH_2$ locus were examined in these studies. It was suggested that Japanese alcohol flushers might be homozygous atypical $ALDH_2^2/ALDH_2^2$, but not heterozygous $ALDH_2^1/ALDH_2^2$, at the $ALDH_2$ locus.[80] The findings are questionable since the genotyping method used does not seem to be reliable.

Genotypes of the ADH_2 locus and the $ALDH_2$ locus can be determined by the hybridization of endonuclease-digested genomic DNA samples;[44,81] or polymerase chain reaction (PCR) amplified DNA,[82–84] with allele specific oligonucleotide probes (Figs. 1 and 2). The ADH_3^1 and ADH_3^2 alleles can also be distinguished by the same procedure.[84]

In 49 unrelated control Japanese individuals examined, the frequency of atypical ADH_2^2 allele is 0.71 and that of usual ADH_2^1 is 0.29, and the frequencies of genotypes determined were compatible to the Hardy-Weinberg expectation.[44] The frequencies of ADH_2^1 and ADH_2^2 alleles were previously estimated from the isozyme patterns of liver samples observed in electrophoresis or isoelectric focusing. Since the atypical β_2 subunit, which is a product of the atypical ADH_2^2 allele, is overwhelmed in the isozyme activity stain, the distinction of heterozygous atypical ADH_2^1/ADH_2^2 and homozygous atypical ADH_2^2/ADH_2^2 is ambiguous in electrophoretic examination. The distinction of the homozygous atypical and heterozygous atypical is more clear in the isoelectric focusing. The frequency of the atypical ADH_2^2 allele estimated from isoelectric focusing patterns ranged from 0.62 to 0.74 in Japanese.[85,86]

In the same 49 control subjects, the frequency of atypical $ALDH_2^2$ allele is 0.35 and that of the usual $ALDH_2^1$ is 0.65.[87] None of the Caucasians examined had the atypical $ALDH_2^2$ gene. The frequencies of genotypes determined were compatible to the Hardy–Weinberg expectation, indicating the reliability of the genotyping method.

Since about 50% of Japanese lack $ALDH_2$ activity, the data imply that the heterozygous atypical $ALDH_2^1/ALDH_2^2$ subjects as well as the homozygous atypical $ALDH_2^2/ALDH_2^2$ subjects lack liver $ALDH_2$ activity, i.e., the atypical $ALDH_2^2$ gene is dominant in expression of enzyme activity.[87] The notion was supported by other investigators.[83]

The severe $ALDH_2$ deficiency in heterozygous $ALDH_2^1/ALDH_2^2$ status (i.e., dominant expression of the variant $ALDH_2^2$) is not readily compatible to the commonly accepted assumption (and observation on other loci) that both usual and variant genes would be expressed in heterozygous status and hybrid oligomeric enzymes would exhibit catalytic activity. In conjunction with this problem, the following points should be considered. The direct genotyping method only examines the targeted nucleotide region, which includes the $ALDH_2^2$ mutation site (Fig. 2). Therefore, the possibility of the existence of other variant allele(s) is not excluded. Another common variant allele, $ALDH_2^3$, which produces a defective subunit could exist in Japanese. Assuming that

1. The frequencies of $ALDH_2^1 = 0.3$, $ALDH_2^2 = 0.35$, and $ALDH_2^3 = 0.35$;
2. Subjects with $ALDH_2^1/ALDH_2^1$, $ALDH_2^1/ALDH_2^2$, and $ALDH_2^1$ exhibit the enzyme activity; and
3. Subjects with $ALDH_2^2/ALDH_2^2$, $ALDH_2^2/ALDH_2^3$, and $ALDH_2^3/ALDH_2^3$ lack the activity, the observed frequency of $ALDH_2$ deficiency (about 50%) can be explained by the three allele model.

The model predicts that approx 40% of Japanese with the enzyme activity are heterozygous $ALDH_2^1/ALDH_2^2$. However, none of the Japanese livers with $ALDH_2$ activity thus far examined had the atypical $ALDH_2^2$ gene;[56,82,86] thus the three allele model is rejected. Formation of catalytically inactive and/or very labile heterotetramers may account for the dominant expression of the defective $ALDH_2$ gene at the heterozygous status.[87]

Genotypes of Japanese alcohol flushers, nonflushers, and patients with alcoholic liver diseases are summarized in Table 4. All patients (23 unrelated subjects) were habitual heavy drinkers over a period of more than 5 yrs, and, based on histological criteria, were diagnosed as alcoholic fatty liver (2 subjects), alcoholic fibrosis (5 subjects), alcoholic liver cirrhosis

Table 4
Genotypes of *ADH₂* and *ALDH₂* Loci in Japanese

ADH_2 locus	Genotypes			Gene frequency	
	1-1	1-2	2-2	ADH_2^1	ADH_2^2
Control ($n = 49$)	4	20	25	0.29	0.71
Patients with alcoholic liver disease ($n = 23$)	3	6	14	0.26	0.74
Alcohol flusher ($n = 8$)	0	1	7	0.06	0.94
Nonflusher ($n = 6$)	0	3	3	0.25	0.75

$ALDH_2$ locus	Genotypes			Gene frequency	
	1-1	1-2	2-2	$ALDH_2^1$	$ALDH_2^2$
Control ($n = 49$)	21	22	6	0.65	0.35
Patients with alcoholic liver disease ($n = 23$)	20	3	0	0.93	0.07
Alcohol flusher ($n = 9$)	0	7	2	0.39	0.61
Nonflusher ($n = 6$)	5	1	0	0.92	0.08

Data were obtained from references.[44,87,89] Difference in frequencies of the $ALDH_2^1$ and $ALDH_2^2$ between the controls and alcoholic liver patients is statistically significant ($p < 0.005$). Difference in frequencies of the $ALDH/_2^2$ and $ALDH/_2^2$ between the alcohol flushers and nonflushers is statistically different ($p < 0.01$).

(15 subjects), and alcoholic liver cirrhosis accompanied by hepatocellular carcinoma (1 subject).[88]

No difference was found between the subjects with alcoholic liver diseases and controls in the frequency of the atypical ADH_2^2.[88] The frequency of the ADH_2^2 was found to be higher in alcohol flushers than in nonflushers, but the statistical significance was not established in the sample size analyzed.[88] More cases have to be examined to settle the correlation between ADH₂ genotypes and alcohol flushing.

The genotype analysis indicates that all Japanese alcohol flushers are either heterozygous $ALDH_2^1/ALDH_2^2$ or homozygous atypical $ALDH_2^2/ALDH_2^2$, and conversely, most of Japanese with alcoholic liver diseases are homozygous usual $ALDH_2^1/ALDH_2^1$.[88,89] One can conclude that Japanese with genotypes $ALDH_2^1/ALDH_2^2$ or $ALDH_2^2/ALDH_2^2$ are alcohol sensitive, and thus they are at low risk in developing alcoholic liver diseases and presumably other alcohol-related diseases.

The frequency of the atypical $ALDH_2^2$ allele is high also in other Orientals, i.e., 0.15 in South Koreans and 0.20 in Chinese.[90] Atypical subjects, either homozygous or heterozygous at the $ALDH_2^2$ loci in these populations are likely to be alcohol sensitive and less vulnerable in developing alcohol-related diseases.

The fetal alcohol syndrome is characterized by physical and mental anomalies that occur in children whose mothers drank alcohol during pregnancy. As described earlier, $ALDH_2$ is expressed in early embryos,[56] hence, the Oriental atypical $ALDH_2^2$ gene, which is a preventive factor against alcohol-related diseases in adult life, could be a risk factor in developing the fetal alcohol syndrome. The possibility can be tested by genotyping affected Oriental families.

The ALDH genotyping of American Indians has been a subject of interest. Both American Indians and Orientals are of Mongoloid origin. A high frequency (50–70%) of alcohol flushing was observed in a North American Indian tribe.[91] However, unlike Orientals, American Indians have higher frequencies of the alcohol-related problems. North American Indians (Sioux, Navajo, Pueblo, Oklahoma) showed a low (or no) frequency of $ALDH_2$ deficiency, whereas approx 40% of South American Indians (Atacameños, Mapuche, Shuara) lack $ALDH_2$ activity.[92–95] Recently, $ALDH_2$ genotypes of 28 South American (Mapuche) Indians were determined and it was found that none of them has the atypical $ALDH_2^2$ gene (i.e., frequency of $ALDH_2^2$ is less than 2%).[96]

Should about 40% of the Mapuche Indians lack $ALDH_2$ activity, another defective mutant $ALDH_2$ gene, which is different from the atypical Oriental type $ALDH_2^2$ gene, might exist at a high frequency in this population. Further confirmation on the $ALDH_2$ deficiency in South American Indians is necessary, since the previous phenotyping of South American Indians was performed using hair root extracts, but not using the more reliable liver samples. Systematic studies of the reliable $ALDH_2$ phenotyping and genotyping, together with characterization of their alcohol-flushing characters and other alcohol-related problems may elucidate the relationship between the $ALDH_2$ types and physiological manifestations found in American Indians.

Approximately 5–8% of Caucasians exhibit alcohol-flushing character.[72–74] In addition, about 6–10% of Caucasians are reported to be chlorpropamide-induced alcohol flushers and exhibit alcohol flushing when they take chlorpropamide, a commonly used drug for diabetics.[97] The character seems to be a dominantly inherited trait. By contrast to Oriental alcohol flushers, no significant elevation in blood acetaldehyde levels nor hypertension were observed in these Caucasian alcohol flushers (personal communication from R. J. Ward and T. J. Peters). However, a significant elevation of blood acetaldehyde level and slower rate of acetaldehyde oxidation were observed in chlorpropamide-induced alcohol flushers.[98] Thus, physiological background differs between alcohol flushers and chlorpropamide-induced alcohol flushers in Orientals and Caucasians.

By examining properties of $ALDH_1$ existing in blood samples from nine unrelated Caucasian alcohol flushers, two types of $ALDH_1$ variants were found.[65] One variant (Harrow variant) exhibited very low activity (10–20% of control) and altered electrophoretic mobility. The enzyme deficiency and alcohol-flushing character are inherited in relatives of the propositus. From the pedigree data, it is evident that the $ALDH_1$ deficiency and alcohol-flushing character are expressed in heterozygous variant status,[65] (also, unpublished observation). Another $ALDH_1$ variant (Columbo variant) found in a Caucasian alcohol flusher exhibited moderately reduced activity and altered kinetic properties.[65] The frequencies of these two variants among Caucasians have not yet been determined.

Relationships between the RFLPs of these *ADH* and *ALDH* loci and alcohol-related problems have not been systematically examined.

In the recent study, no association was found between the MspI RFLP at the ADH_3 locus and alcoholism.[99]

Concluding Remarks

The intimate positive correlation between the Oriental atypical $ALDH_2^2$ gene with alcohol sensitivity and the negative correlation with development of alcoholic liver diseases have been proven. Caucasians with the variant $ALDH_1$ genes, even at heterozygous status, are also alcohol sensitive; hence, they are at low risk of developing alcoholic diseases.

Similar genetic studies have not yet been carried out in the ADH_2^3 gene (for β_3 subunit), which is common in Blacks, ADH_3^2 (for γ_2 subunit) which is common in Caucasians, the locus, which may be polymorphic, the $ALDH_{3b}$ locus, which may be polymorphic in Chinese and other populations, and the polymorphic $ALDH_x$ locus. As reviewed earlier, alcohol dehydrogenases and aldehyde dehydrogenases not only participate in ethanol detoxification, but also play roles in metabolism of neurotransmitters, fatty acid oxidation, and detoxification of biogenic metabolites. Recent technological development of molecular genetics allows us to determine these mutation sites and determine genotypes using readily available genomic DNA samples. Possible significance of genetic variations of these loci in alcohol-related problems may be elucidated through this approach.

A strong association of RFLP at the dopamine D_2 receptor locus with alcoholism was recently reported.[98] Genetic abnormalities and polymorphisms of ADHs and ALDHs involved in neurotransmitters may affect alcohol-seeking behavior and in developing alcohol-related diseases. Our knowledge on brain ADH and ALDH isozymes with such activity is very limited, at both the enzyme and the gene levels, and needs to be extended.

Acknowledgment

This study was supported by the US Public Health Service Grant AA05763.

References

[1] M. A. Schuckit, D. W. Goodwin, and G. Winokur (1972) A study of alcoholism in half-siblings. *Am. J. Psychiat.* **128,** 1132–1136.

[2] D. W. Goodwin, F. Schulsinger, L. Hermansen, and G. Winokur (1973) Alcohol problems in adoptees raised apart from alcoholic biological parents. *Arch. Gen. Psychiat.* **28,** 238–243.

[3] D. J. Strydom and B. L. Vallee (1982) Characterization of human alcohol dehydrogenase isozymes by high-performance liquid chromatographic peptide mapping. *Anal. Biochem..* **123,** 422–429.

[4] T. K. Li, W. F. Bosron, W. P. Defeldecker, L. G. Lange, and B. L. Vallee (1977) Isolation of π-alcohol dehydrogenase of human liver: Is it a determinant of alcoholism? *Proc. Natl. Acad. Sci. USA* **74,** 4378–4381.

[5] A. Adinoffi, M. Adinoffi, and D. A. Hopkinson (1984) Immunological and biochemical characterization of the human alcohol dehydrogenase chi-ADH isozyme. *Ann. Hum. Genet.* **48,** 1–10.

[6] M. Tsukahara and A. Yoshida (1989) Chromosomal assignment of alcohol dehydrogenase cluster locus to human chromosome 4q21–23 by in situ hybridization. *Genomics* **4,** 218–220.

[7] M. Yasunami, I. Kikuchi, D. Sarapata, and A. Yoshida (1990) The human class I alcohol dehydrogenase gene cluster: Three genes are tandemly organized in an 80 kb long segment of the genome. *Genomics* **7,** 152–158

[8] J. D. McPherson, M. Smith, C. Wagner, J. Wasmuth, and J.-O. Höög (1989) Mapping of the class II alcohol dehydrogenase gene locus to 4q22. *Cytogenet. Cell. Genet.* (abstract) **51,** 1043.

[9] L. Carlock, S. Hiroshige, J. Wasmuth, and M. Smith (1985) Assignment of the gene coding for class III ADH to human chromosome 4: 4q21–25. *Cytogenet. Cell. Genet.* (abstract) **40,** 598.

[10] M. Smith, D. A. Hopkinson, and H. Harris (1971) Developmental changes and polymorphism in human alcohol dehydrogenase. *Ann. Hum. Genet.* **34,** 251–272.

[11] G. Mårdh and B. L. Vallee (1986) Human class I alcohol dehydrogenase catalyze the interconversion of alcohols and aldehydes in the metabolism of dopamine. *Biochemistry* **25,** 7279–7282.

[12] M. Smith, D. A. Hopkinson, and H. Harris (1972) Alcohol dehydrogenase isozymes in adult human stomach and liver: Evidence for activity of the ADH(3) locus. *Ann. Hum. Genet.* **35,** 243–253.

[13] V. Consalvi, G. Mårdh, and B. L. Vallee (1986) Human alcohol dehydrogenases and serotonin metabolism. *Biochem. Biophys. Res. Comm.* **139,** 1009–1016.

[14] A. J. McEvily, B. Holmquist, S. Auld, and B. L. Vallee (1988) 3β-Hydroxy-5β-steroid dehydrogenase activity of human liver alcohol dehydrogenase is specific to γ-subunit. *Biochem.* **27,** 4284–4288.

[15] C. S. Lieber and L. M. DeCarli (1968) Ethanol oxidation by hepatic microsomes: Adaptive increase after ethanol feeding. *Science* **162,** 690–691.

[16] C. S. Lieber and L. M. DeCarli (1970) Hepatic microsomal ethanol oxidizing system: In vitro characteristics and adaptive properties in vivo. *J. Biol. Chem.* **245,** 2505–2512.

[17] H. Ishii, J.-G. Joly, and C. S. Lieber (1973) Effect of ethanol on the amount and enzyme activities of hepatic rough and smooth microsomal membranes. *Biochem. Biophys. Acta* **291,** 411–420.

[18] K. J. Isselbacher and E. A. Carter (1970) Ethanol oxidation by liver microsomes: Evidence against a separate and distinct enzyme system. *Biochem. Biophys. Res. Comm.* **39,** 530–537.

[19] M. Frezza, C. di Padova, G. Possato, M. Terpin, E. Baraona, and C. S. Lieber (1990) High blood alcohol levels in women: The role of decreased gastric alcohol dehydrogenase activity and first-pass metabolism. *N. Eng. J. Med.* **322,** 95–99.

[20] A. Yoshida, L. C. Hsu, and M. Yasunami (1991) Genetics of human alcohol-metabolizing enzymes. *Prog. Nucleic Acid Res. and Mol. Biol.* **40,** 255–287.

[21] G. Mårdh, A. L. Dingley, D. S. Auld, and B. L. Vallee (1986) Human class II (π) alcohol dehydrogenase has a redox-specific function in norepinephrine metabolism. *Proc. Natl. Acad. Sci. USA* **83,** 8908–8912.

[22] G. Mårdh, K. H. Falchuck, D. S. Auld, and B. L. Vallee (1986) Testosterone allosterically regulates ethanol oxidation by homo- and heterodimeric γ-subunit-

containing isozymes of human alcohol dehydrogenase. *Proc. Natl. Acad. Sci. USA* **83,** 2836–2840.

[23] F. W. Wagner, A. R. Burger, and B. L. Vallee (1983) Kinetic properties of human liver alcohol dehydrogenase: Oxidation of alcohols by class I isoenzymes. *Biochemistry* **22,** 1857–1863.

[24] H. Esterbauer, H. Zollner, and J. Lang (1985) Metabolism of the lipid peroxidation product 4-hydroxynonenal by isolated hepatocytes and liver cytosolic fractions. *Biochem. J.* **228,** 363–373.

[25] M. Koivusalo, M. Baumann, and L. Votila (1989) Evidence for the identity of glutathione-dependent formaldehyde dehydrogenase and class III alcohol dehydrogenase. *FEBS Lett.* **257,** 105–109.

[26] P. Julià, J. Farrés, and X. Parés (1987) Characterization of three isozymes of rat alcohol dehydrogenase: Tissue distribution and physical and enzymatic properties. *Eur. J. Biochem.* **162,** 179–189.

[27] W.-M. Keung (1988) A genuine organ specific alcohol dehydrogenase from hamster testes: Isolation, characterization and developmental changes. *Biochem. Biophys. Res. Commun.* **156,** 38–45.

[28] W. F. Bosron, T.-K. Li, and B. L. Vallee (1980) New molecular forms of human liver alcohol dehydrogenase: Isolation and characterization of ADH (Indianapolis). *Proc. Natl. Acad. Sci. USA* **77,** 5784–5788.

[29] Y.-S. Teng, S. Jehan, and L. E. Lie-Injo (1979) Human alcohol dehydroenase ADH_2 and ADH_3 polymorphisms in ethnic Chinese and Indians of West Malaysia. *Hum. Genet.* **53,** 87–90.

[30] A. Yoshida, C. C. Impraim, and I.-Y. Huang (1981) Enzymatic and structural differences between usual and atypical human liver alcohol dehydrogenases. *J. Biol. Chem.* **256,** 12430–12436.

[31] H. Jörnvall, J. Hempel, B. T. Vallee, W. F. Bosron, and T.-K. Li (1984) Human liver alcohol dehydrogenase: Amino acid substitution of the $\beta_2\beta_2$ Oriental isozyme explains functional properties, establishes an active site structure, and parallels mutational exchanges in the yeast enzyme. *Proc. Natl. Acad. Sci. USA* **81,** 3024–3028.

[32] T. Ikuta, T. Fujiyoshi, K. Kurachi, and A. Yoshida (1985) Molecular cloning of a full-length cDNA for human alcohol dehydrogenase. *Proc. Natl. Acad. Sci. USA* **82,** 2703–2707.

[33] T. Ehring, J. P. von Wartburg, and B. Wermuth (1988) cDNA sequence of the β_2-subunit of human liver alcohol dehydrogenase. *FEBS Lett.* **234,** 53–55.

[34] J. C. Burnell, L. G. Carr, F. E. Dwulet, H. J. Edenberg, T.-K. Li, and W. F. Bosron (1987) The human β_3 alcohol dehydrogenase subunit differs from β_1 by a Cys for Arg-369 substitution which decreases NAD(H) binding. *Biochem. Biophys. Res. Commun.* **146,** 1227–1233.

[35] C. L. Stone, J. C. Burnell, T.-K. Li, and W. F. Bosron (1989) Relationships

between the kinetics of alcohol or coenzyme oxidoreduction and amino acid sequence of human liver alcohol dehydrogenase isozymes, in *Enzymology and Molecular Biology of Carbonyl Metabolism,* vol. 2. H. Weiner and T. G. Flynn, eds. Liss, New York, pp. 155–165.

[36] J.-O. Höög, L.-O. Hedén, K. Larsson, H. Jörnvall, and H. von Bahr-Lindström (1986) The γ_1 and γ_2 subunits of human alcohol dehydrogenase: cDNA structures two amino acid replacements, and compatibility with changes in the enzymatic properties. *Eur. J. Biochem.* **159,** 215–218.

[37] J. Hempel, R. Bühler, R. Kaiser, B. Holmquist, C. de Zalenski, J. P. von Wartburg, et al. (1984) Human liver alcohol dehydrogenase 2: The primary structure of the γ_1 protein chain. *Eur. J. Biochem.* **145,** 447–453.

[38] T. Ikuta, S. Szeto, and A. Yoshida (1986) Three human alcohol dehydrogenase subunits: cDNA structure and molecular and evolutionary divergence. *Proc. Natl. Acad. Sci. USA* **83,** 634–638.

[39] J.-O. Höög, H. von Bahr-Lindström, L.-O. Hedén, B. Holmquist, K. Larsson, J. Hempel, B. L. Vallee, and H. Jörnvall (1987) Structure of the class II enzyme of human liver alcohol dehydrogenase: Combined cDNA and protein sequence determined of the π subunit. *Biochemistry* **26,** 1926–1932.

[40] C. P. Sharma, E. A. Fox, B. Holmquist, H. Jörnvall and B. L. Vallee (1989) cDNA sequence of human class III alcohol dehydrogenase. *Biochem. Biophys. Res. Commun.* **164,** 631–637.

[41] P. R. Giri, J. F. Krug, C. Kozak, et al. (1989) Cloning and comparative mapping of a human class III (χ) alcohol dehydrogenase cDNA. *Biochem. Biophys. Res. Commun.* **164,** 453–460.

[42] T. Shah, A. J. S. MacPherson, R. J. Ward, T. J. Peters, and A. Yoshida (1989) A PvuII RFLP in the human ADH_2 gene. *Nuc. Acid Res.* **17,** 7549.

[43] M. Smith (1988) Molecular genetic studies on alcohol and aldehyde dehydrogenase: Individual variation, gene mapping and analysis of regulation. *Biochem. Soc. Trans.* **16,** 227–230.

[44] T. Ikuta, A. Shibuya, A. Yoshida (1988) Direct determination of usual (Caucasian type) and atypical (Oriental type) alleles of class I human alcohol dehydrogenase-2 locus. *Biochem. Genet.* **26,** 519–525.

[45] M. Dean, C. Stewart, P. R. Giri, J. Krug, T. Moretti, H. Seuanez, et al. (1989) Identification of an RFLP in the ADH_3 gene. *Cytogenet. Cell. Genet.* (abstract) **51,** 985.

[46] M. Ikawa, C. C. Impraim, G. Wang, and A. Yoshida (1983) Isolation and characterization of aldehyde dehydrogenase isozymes from usual and atypical human livers. *J. Biol. Chem.* **258,** 6282–6287.

[47] I. Santisteban, S. Povey, L. F. West, J. M. Parrington, and D. A. Hopkinson (1985) Chromosome assignment, biochemical and immunological studies on a human aldehyde dehydrogenase, ALDH3. *Ann. Hum. Genet.* **49,** 87–100.

48 C. Forte-McRobbie and R. Pietruszko (1986) Purification and characterization of human liver "high Km" aldehyde dehydrogenase and its identification as glutamic γ-semialdehyde dehydrogenase. *J. Biol. Chem.* **261**, 2154–2163.

49 G. Kurys, W. Ambroziak, R. Pietruszko (1989) Human aldehyde dehydrogenases: Purification and characterization of a third isozyme with low Km for γ-aminobutyraldehyde. *J. Biol. Chem.* **264**, 4715–4721.

50 M. T. Ryzlak and R. Pietruszko (1987) Purification and characterization of aldehyde dehydrogenase from human brain. *Arch. Biochem. Biophys.* **255**, 409–418.

51 M. T. Ryzlak and R. Pietruszko (1989) Human brain glyceraldehyde-3-phosphate dehydrogenase, succinic semialdehyde dehydrogenase and aldehyde dehydrogenase isozymes: Substrate specificity and sensitivity to disulfiram. *Alcohol. Clin. Exp. Res* **13**, 755–761.

52 G. Hafer, D. P. Agarwal, H. W. Goedde (1987) Human brain aldehyde dehydrogenase: Activity with DOPAL and isozyme distribution. *Alcohol* **4**, 413–418.

53 S. Harada, T. Muramatsu, D. P. Agarwal, and H. W. Goedde (1989) Polymorphism of aldehyde dehydrogenase in human saliva. *Prog. Clin. Biol. Res.* **290**, 133–139.

54 D. A. Hopkinson, I. Santisteban, S. Povey, and M. Smith (1985) Biochemical genetic analysis of human and rodent aldehyde dehydrogenase (ALDH). *Alcohol* **2**, 73–78.

55 T. Braun, E. Bober, J. Schaper, et al. (1987) Human mitochondrial aldehyde dehydrogenase: mRNA expression in different tissues using specific probe isolated from a cDNA expression library. *Alcohol Alcohol.* Suppl. 1, 161–165.

56 A. Yoshida, A. Shibuya, V. Davé, M. Nakayama, and A. Hayashi (1990) Developmental changes of aldehyde dehydrogenase isozymes in human livers: Mitochondrial $ALDH_2$ isozyme is expressed in fetal livers. *Experientia* **46**, 747–750.

57 H. W. Goedde, S. Harada, and D. P. Agarwal (1979) Racial differences in alcohol sensitivity: A new hypothesis. *Hum. Genet.* **51**, 331–334.

58 C. Impraim, G. Wang, and A. Yoshida (1982) Structural mutation in a major human aldehyde dehydrogenase gene results in loss of enzyme activity. *Am. J. Hum. Genet.* **34**, 837–841.

59 A. Yoshida, I.-Y. Huang, and M. Ikawa (1984) Molecular abnormality of an inactive aldehyde dehydrogenase variant commonly found in Orientals. *Proc. Natl. Acad. Sci. USA* **81**, 258–261.

60 L. C. Hsu, K. Tani, K. Fujioyoshi, K. Kurachi, and A. Yoshida (1985) Cloning of cDNA for human aldehyde dehydrogenase 1 and 2. *Proc. Natl. Acad. Sci. USA* **82**, 3771–3775.

61 L. C. Hsu, R. E. Bendel, and A. Yoshida (1988) Genomic structure of the human mitochondrial aldehyde dehydrogenase gene. *Genomics* **2**, 57–65.

62 A. Yoshida (1983) A possible structural variant of human cytosolic aldehyde dehydrogenase with diminished enzyme activity. *Am. J. Hum. Genet.* **35**, 1115,1116.

[63] R. Kanayama, Y. Matsuda, S. Takase, and A. Takada (1984) Human liver aldehyde dehydrogenase isozymes. *Alcohol Metab. Liv.* (Japanese) **2**, 223–234.

[64] R. Eckey, D. P. Agarwal, N. Saha, and H. W. Goedde (1986) Detection and partial characterization of a variant form of cytosolic aldehyde dehydrogenase isozyme. *Hum. Genet.* **72**, 95–97.

[65] A. Yoshida, R. J. Ward, and T. J. Peters (1989) Cytosolic aldehyde dehydrogenase (ALDH1) variants found in alcohol flushers. *Ann. Hum. Genet.* **53**, 1–7.

[66] Y.-S. Teng (1981) Stomach aldehyde dehydrogenase: Report of a new locus. *Hum. Genet.* **31**, 74–77.

[67] D. Mainer-Tackmann, D. P. Agarwal, N. Saha, and H. W. Goedde (1984) Aldehyde dehydrogenase isozymes in stomach autopsy specimens from Germans and Chinese. *Enzyme* **32**, 170–177.

[68] D. A. Hopkinson, I. Santisteban, S. Povey, and M. Smith (1985) Biochemical genetic analysis of human and rodent aldehyde dehydrogenase (ALDH). *Alcohol* **2**, 73–78.

[69] J. A. Duley, O. Harris, and R. S. Holmes (1985) Analysis of human alcohol- and aldehyde-metabolizing isozymes by electrophoresis and isoelectric focussing. *Alcohol. Clin. Exp. Res.* **9**, 263–271.

[70] S.-J. Yin, T.-C. Cheng, C.-P. Chang, Y.-J. Chen, Y.-C. Chao. H.-S. Tang, T.-M. Chang, and C.-W. Wu (1988) Human stomach alcohol and aldehyde dehydrogenase (ALDH): A genetic model proposed for ALDH III isozymes. *Biochem. Genet.* **26**, 345–360.

[71] A. Yoshida and S.-H. Chen (1989) Restriction fragment-length polymorphism of human aldehyde dehydrogenase-1 and aldehyde dehydrogenase 2 loci. *Hum. Genet.* **83**, 204.

[72] P. H. Wolff (1972) Ethnic differences in alcohol sensitivity. *Science* **175**, 449,450.

[73] J. A. Ewing, B. A. Rouse, and E. D. Pellizzari (1974) Alcohol sensitivity and ethnic background. *Am. J. Psychiat.* **131**, 206–210.

[74] J. R. Wilson, G. E. McClearn, and R. C. Johnson (1978) Ethnic variation in the use and effects of alcohol. *Drug Alcohol Depend.* **3**, 147–151.

[75] A. R. Zeiner, A. Paredes, and H. Dix Christensen (1979) The role of acetaldehyde in mediating reactivity to an acute dose of ethanol among different racial groups. *Alcohol. Clin. Exp. Res.* **3**, 11–18.

[76] G. Stamatoyannopoulos, S.-H. Chen, and M. Fukui (1975) Liver alcohol dehydrogenase in Japanese: High population frequency of atypical form and its possible role in alcohol sensitivity. *Am. J. Hum. Genet.* **27**, 789–796.

[77] Y. Mizoi, I. Ijiri, Y. Tatsuno, T. Kijima, S. Fujiwara, and J. Adachi (1979) Relationship between facial flushing and blood acetaldehyde levels after alcohol intake. *Pharmacol. Biochem. Behav.* **10**, 301–311.

[78] S. Harada, D. P. Agarwal, and H. W. Goedde (1985) Aldehyde dehydrogenase polymorphism and alcohol metabolism in alcoholics. *Alcohol* **2,** 391–392.

[79] H. Yoshihara, N. Sato, T. Kamada, and H. Abe (1983) Low Km ALDH isozyme and alcoholic liver injury. *Pharmacol. Biochem. Behav.* **18,** 425–428.

[80] H. W. Goedde and D. P. Agarwal (1987) Polymorphism of aldehyde dehydrogenase and alcohol sensitivity. *Enzyme* **37,** 29–44.

[81] L. C. Hsu, R. E. Bendel, and A. Yoshida (1987) Direct detection of usual and atypical alleles on human aldehyde dehydrogenase-2 ($ALDH_2$) locus. *Am. J. Hum. Genet.* **41,** 996–1001.

[82] K. Gennari, B. Wermuth, D. Muellener, T. Ehring, and J.-P. von Wartburg (1988) Genotyping of human class 1 alcohol dehydrogenase: Analysis of enzymatically amplified DNA with allele-specific oligonucleotides. *FEBS Lett.* **228,** 305–309.

[83] D. W. Crabb, H. J. Edenberg, W. F. Bosron, and T.-K. Li (1989) Genotypes of aldehyde dehydrogenase deficiency and alcohol sensitivity: The inactive $ALDH_2$ allele is dominant. *J. Clin. Inv.* **83,** 314–316.

[84] Y. Xu, L. Carr, W. F. Bosron, T. K. Li, and H. J. Edenberg (1988) Genotyping of human alcohol dehydrogenases at the ADH_2 and ADH_3 loci following DNA sequence amplification. *Genomics* **2,** 209–214.

[85] S.-J. Yin, W. F. Bosron, T.-K. Li, K. Ohnishi, K. Okada, H. Ishii, et al. (1984) Polymorphism of human liver alcohol dehydrogenase: Identification of ADH_2 2-1 and ADH_2 2-2 phenotypes in the Japanese by isoelectric focussing. *Biochem. Genet.* **22,** 169–180.

[86] M. Kogame and Y. Mizoi (1985) The polymorphism of alcohol and aldehyde dehydrogenase in Japanese and the significance in ethanol metabolism. *Jpn. J. Alcohol Drug Depend.* **20,** 122–124.

[87] A. Shibuya and A. Yoshida (1988) Frequency of the atypical aldehyde dehydrogenase-2 gene ($ALDH_2{}^2$) in Japanese and Caucasians. *Am. J. Hum. Genet.* **43,** 741–743.

[88] A. Shibuya and A. Yoshida (1988) Genotypes of alcohol-metabolizing enzymes in Japanese with alcohol liver diseases: A strong association of the usual Caucasian type aldehyde dehydrogenase gene (*$ALDH_2{}^1$*) with the disease. *Am. J. Hum. Genet.* **43,** 744–748.

[89] A. Shibuya, M. Yasunami, and A. Yoshida (1989) Genotypes of alcohol dehydrogenase and aldehyde dehydrogenase loci in Japanese alcohol flushers and nonflushers. *Hum. Genet.* **82,** 14–16.

[90] S. Singh, G. Fritz, B. Fang, S. Harada, Y. K. Paik, R. Eckey, D. P. Agarwal, and H. W. Goedde (1989) Inheritance of mitochondrial aldehyde dehydrogenase: Genotyping in Chinese, Japanese and South Korean families reveals dominance of the mutant allele. *Hum. Genet.* **83,** 119–121.

[91] P. H. Wolff (1973) Vasomotor sensitivity to alcohol in diverse Mongoloid

populations. *Am. J. Hum. Genet.* **25,** 193–199.

[92] H. W. Goedde, D. P. Agarwal, S. Harada, F. Rothhammer, J. O. Wittaker, and R. Liskar (1986) Aldehyde dehydrogenase polymorphism in North American South American, and Mexican Indian populations. *Am. J. Hum. Genet.* **38,** 395–399.

[93] A. R. Zeiner, J. M. Girardot, N. Nichols, and D. Jones-Saumty (1984) ALDH I isozyme deficiency among North American Indians. *2nd Cong. Int. Soc. Biomed. Res. Alcohol.* (abstract) p. 129.

[94] D. Rex, W. F. Bosron, J. E. Smialek, and T.-K. Li (1985) Alcohol and aldehyde dehydrogenase isozymes in a North American Indian population. *Alcohol. Clin. Exp. Res.* **9,** 147–152.

[95] W. F. Bosron, D. K. Rex, C. A. Harden, and T. K. Li (1988) Alcohol and aldehyde dehydrogenase isozymes in Sioux North American Indians. *Alcohol. Clin. Exp. Res.* **12,** 454–455.

[96] B. F. O'Dowd, F. Rothhammer, and Y. Israel (1990) Genotyping of mitochondrial aldehyde dehydrogenase locus of native South American Indians. *Alcohol. Clin. Exp. Res.*

[97] J. N. Baramuk, R. B. Murray, and W. G. Mabbee (1987) Naloxone, ethanol, and the chlorpropamide alcohol flush. *Alcohol. Clin. Exp. Res.* **11,** 518–520.

[98] A. H. Barnett, C. Gonzales-Auvert, D. A. Pyke, J. B. Saunders, R. Williams, C. J. Dickenson, and M. D. Rawlins (1981) Blood concentrations of acetaldehyde during chlorpropamide alcohol flush. *Br. Med. J.* **283,** 939–941.

[99] K. Blum, E. P. Noble, P. J. Sheridan, A. Montgomery, T. Ritche, P. Jagadeeswaran, et al. (1990) Allelic association of human dopamine D_2 receptor gene in alcoholism. *JAMA* **263,** 2055–2060.

[100] L. Ragunthan, L. C. Hsu, I. Klisak, et al. (1988) Regional localization of human genes for aldehyde dehydrogenase-1 ($ALDH_1$) and aldehyde dehydrogenase-2 ($ALDH_2$). *Genomics* **2,** 267–269.

[101] G. Duester, M. Smith, V. Bilanchone, R. S. Sparks, A. Yoshida, and T. Mohaudas (1986) Molecular analysis of human class I alcohol dehydrogenase gene family and nucleotide sequence of the gene encoding the subunit. *J. Biol. Chem.* **261,** 2027–2033.

Effects of Alcohol and Cocaine Abuse on the Antioxidant Systems, Nutritional Status, and Liver Damage

*Olalekan E. Odeleye
and Ronald R. Watson*

Introduction

It has been known for several years that the abuse of drugs such as alcohol (ethanol) and cocaine disrupt hepatic structure and functions. The mechanisms of these drug-induced hepatotoxicities are now thought to be intricately related to changes in the functional activities of inherent enzyme antioxidant systems (e.g., superoxide dismutase, catalase, glutathione peroxidases, and the selenoenzymes). These systems and the dietary antioxidant status[1–4] of tocopherols, ascorbate, and beta-carotene protect the biological system against oxidative damage.[5–8] The ability of the hepatic cells to maintain their viability and integrity against insults from xenobiotics, including commonly used drugs of abuse, is in part dependent on these antioxidant defense mechanisms. The role of xenobiotics generating free radi-

From: *Drug and Alcohol Abuse Reviews, Vol. 2: Liver Pathology and Alcohol*
Ed: R. R. Watson ©1991 The Humana Press Inc.

cals and their conversion to reactive electrophiles generating species during their intracellular metabolic and detoxification process and their role in cellular damage is fully elucidated.[9,10] The generation and role of free radicals in liver damage is reviewed in another chapter of this volume.

Alcohol and cocaine are commonly abused drugs.[11] This review will discuss the metabolism and hepatotoxicity of these two drugs. Another recently recognized aspect of liver damage reviewed in this section is the liver antioxidant system, including dietary nutrients that confer some protection against the drug-induced hepatotoxicity. In addition, since nutritional status of the drug abuser affects the extent of damages commonly observed, this review, therefore, will discuss some of the nutritional deficiencies associated with cocaine and alcohol abuse.

Metabolism and Related Hepatotoxicity of Alcohol Abuse

Metabolism of Alcohol

Alcohol is oxidized almost exclusively in the liver by three main pathways, each located in a different subcellular compartment of the hepatocyte: the alcohol dehydrogenase pathway of the cytosol; the microsomal ethanol-oxidizing system (MEOS) in the endoplasmic reticulum; and catalase of the peroxisomes.[12] The activation of each of these pathways may be associated with the generation of reactive electrophiles, resulting in hepatic damage.

Alcohol Dehydrogenase Pathway

Alcohol dehydrogenase (ADH) catalyzes the conversion of ethanol to acetaldehyde in a series of reactions that requires nicotinamide adenine dinucleotide (NAD) as a cofactor. The overall result of ethanol oxidation is the generation of excess reducing equivalents as free NADH in hepatic cytosol, mainly because the metabolic systems involved in NADH removal are not able to fully affect the accumulation of NADH. The acetaldehyde produced in the reaction is further converted to acetate ADH in the mitochondria.[13,14] Also in the oxidation step, NAD functions as a coenzyme and NADH is formed. The increased NADH/NAD ratio results in a major change in liver metabolism of lipids[15] and protein,[16] and consequent liver damages associated with alcohol abuse. The net result of ethanol oxidation by the hepatic ADH is acetate, which is released into the bloodstream to be further oxidized to carbon dioxide and water in the peripheral tissues.[17,18]

It is commonly accepted that hepatic ADH activity is the only rate-limiting step of ethanol metabolism, although numerous studies have reported the lack of correlation between the rates of ethanol oxidation and ADH activity.[19–21] Although chronic ethanol administration to rats decreases ADH activity in perivenous and periportal hepatocytes, the rate of ethanol elimination nevertheless increases.[22,23] Even in human subjects who have the atypical ADH with a higher activity than normal, the rate of alcohol metabolism is not higher than observed in normal subjects.[24] Theorell and coworkers calculated that when the amount of NADH produced in the ADH reaction goes beyond the immediate metabolic needs, its concentration increases with subsequent inhibition of the ADH reaction.[25] Other factors may also affect the rate of alcohol oxidation by ADH: the intracellular acetaldehyde concentrations, the activity of the shuttle mechanisms transporting reducing equivalents into the mitochondria, and the activity of the mitochondrial respiratory chain.[26]

Microsomal Ethanol Oxidizing System and Catalase

The cytochrome P-450 microsomal ethanol oxidizing system (MEOS) and the catalase system in various cell fractions, including peroxisomes and microsomes, provide alternate pathways for ethanol oxidation.[27,28] The quantitative roles of these alternate pathways for ethanol metabolism is less than 20% in normal conditions.[29] However, the contribution of the MEOS to metabolic oxidation of ethanol increases during chronic alcohol consumption. The MEOS is localized in the endoplasmic reticulum using reduced nicotinamide adenine dinucleotide phosphate (NADPH) and oxygen. It increases in activity after chronic ethanol consumption, which is associated with rapid growth of the smooth endothelial reticulum.[30] Compared to ADH, the MEOS requires higher ethanol levels for full saturation and maximal velocity. Therefore, at high blood ethanol concentrations, the contribution of this non-ADH pathway is markedly increased.[31]

Catalase

Catalase is also capable of oxidizing ethanol in vivo in the presence of H_2O_2-generating system. The H_2O_2-mediated ethanol peroxidation by catalase is limited by the rate of H_2O_2 generated. Since the physiological rate of H_2O_2 production is low, the contribution of catalase to in vivo ethanol elimination is not of great importance.[32]

Hepatotoxicity Associated with Alcohol Abuse

The mechanisms whereby alcohol produce hepatic injury remain a central concern in the toxicology of ethanol. This problem has been pursued largely by following the intracellular fate of alcohol. The results have led to two major conclusions: First, some of the effects are caused by a direct action of ethanol or its reactive metabolites, acetaldehyde and acetate; and part of its effects are mediated by hormonal changes that accompany alcohol abuse.[33] Other changes are dependent on the nutritional status of the abuser,[34] the level of ethanol administered,[35] and the duration of ethanol intake.[36] Changes in immune functions may also play a role in the ultimate liver pathology.

The pathogenic mechanisms of alcohol hepatotoxicity resulting in alcoholic liver disease (ALD) is accompanied by a multitude of biological factors, including reduced nutritional intake, improper digestion and absorption, and increased requirement for some nutrients. The complex interrelated cascade of changes result in vicious cycles leading to increasing severity of alcoholic hepatotoxicity. Alcohol abuse causes a broad spectrum of pathologic, morphologic, histologic, and biochemical changes in the liver. Some of these changes are the subjects of recent reviews,[37–41] and other sections of this volume. Although alcohol has many effects on the liver, all of these effects, except cirrhosis, are partially reversible on cessation of alcohol ingestion. Cirrhosis is irreversible and ultimately fatal. The pathological features of ALD can be divided into three broad categories — fatty liver changes, alcoholic hepatitis with or without fibrosis, and cirrhosis. This division is artificial for three major reasons. First, the categories represent a continuum of disease; second, at any given time, one or more combinations may be present in the liver; and third, if a liver biopsy is performed after a period of abstinence from alcohol, the alcohol-related changes may not be seen.

The role of alcohol in the pathogenesis of fatty liver is well documented[40–44] and the consensus of available evidence is that fatty changes alone probably have no role in the development of cirrhosis, outside of other nutritional factors.[45] The hepatic fatty changes induced by alcohol include fat cysts, lipogranuloma, megamitochondria, hepatocyte swelling, and Mallory bodies that appear after excessive alcohol ingestion, usually visible within 3–7 d.[46] On cessation of drinking, the changes may disappear within a few days but in severe cases, it takes 4–6 wks for these changes to clear.[47] Some of these changes are not specific to ALD and are seen in many other conditions including alimentary disorders, abetalipoprotenemia, and in prolonged steroid use.[48] Although it may appear that these nonspecific changes are unimportant, their presence in association with other more specific changes often lead to a correct diagnosis of ALD.

Alcoholic hepatitis is characterized by the presence of Mallory bodies in hepatocyte, with a surrounding neutrophil and mononuclear cellular infiltrate. Mallory bodies are discrete collections of eosinophilic hyaline intracytoplasmic materials commonly situated around the nucleus causing the hepatocyte to be swollen.

In cirrhotic livers, hepatocytes containing Mallory bodies are most frequently found at the interphase between regenerating nodules and fibrous septa. Alcoholic hepatitis is often accompanied by or results in fibrosis. The fibrosis typically occurs as fine strands surrounding individual hepatocytes seen in pericellular fibrosis. Individual hepatocytes gradually disappear and larger foci of fibrosis are formed, eventually resulting in solid, often stellate, septa of fibrosis, radiating from the central vein. A late complication of cirrhosis, immunosuppression, and dietary deficiencies is hepatocellular cancer.[49] Although it is clear that ethanol consumption is hepatotoxic, some of the other mechanisms of damage include alterations in hepatic plasma membrane fluidity[50,51] and increased lipid peroxidation[52,53] are yet to be fully elaborated.

Another hepatotoxic effect of alcohol is the increased susceptibility of the alcoholic to the adverse effects of various drugs. Ethanol is an inducer not only of its own metabolism but also those of a number of other drugs. The administration of ethanol results in inhibition or acceleration of drug detoxification depending on the dosage and the time interval between the administration of ethanol and the drug. Ethanol, in vitro, is a competitive inhibitor of anilase, pentobarbital hydroxylases, and a mixed inhibitor of the demethylation of aminopyrine and ethylmorphine.[54] It also alters the metabolism of drugs such as 4-hydroxyphenazon and 4-aminoantipyrine from the major oxidative to the minor conjugative pathways[55] and inhibits the rates of disappearance of phenobarbital and meprobamate from the blood of humans[54] and animals.[55] The concomitant administration of ethanol and drugs such as barbiturates and chloral hydrate result in the enhanced depressant effect of these drugs on the central nervous system. The effect of ethanol and chloral hydrate given in combination is greater than the simple summation of the effects obtained when either drug is given alone. This potentiation of effect appears to be owing to the mutual inhibition of the metabolism of drugs.[56] Commonly used H_2-receptor antagonists, such as cimetidine, decrease ADH activity and enhance periportal blood levels of ethanol, precipitating liver damage.[57,58] Ethanol also interacts with narcotics to potentiate hepatotoxicity. In humans, the combined use of morphine and alcohol potentiates the effects of both drugs and increases chronic hepatic damages and the probability of death.[59] Similarly, the combined treatment of ethanol and cocaine to adult male mice potentiated cocaine-induced toxicity characterized by elevated serum transaminase activity and frank intralobular necrosis,[60a,60b] reduced hepatic glutathione,[61] and increased hepatic lipoperoxidation.[60b,62] Chronic ethanol consumption also increased chemically induced tumors[63,64] by inhibiting repair of alkylated DNA,[65] and served as a promoter of hepatocellular carcinoma.[66]

The mechanisms of increased susceptibility of alcohol abusers to the adverse effects of various drugs has been recently reviewed.[67] These include the effect of ethanol on rate of drug uptake, increasing drug-plasma protein binding thus increasing toxicity of the drug, increasing hepatic blood flow and hepatic uptake of drug and alcohol, the binding of ethanol to the cytochrome P-450 system and the subsequent spectrum modification, and the alteration of the ADH system by ethanol.[66]

Metabolism and Related
Hepatotoxicity of Cocaine Abuse

Cocaine is an alkaloid that causes powerful and rapid stimulation of the central nervous and cardiovascular systems. The abuse of this drug has increased greatly over the last several years, and has spread to all ages and socioeconomic groups, and has nearly doubled in the adolescent population.[68] This widespread use has resulted in the increased incidence of acute cocaine poisoning cases seen in emergency clinics and sudden death of chronic abusers.[69]

Metabolism of Cocaine

The metabolism of cocaine occurs by two separate pathways: The major pathway involves the hydrolysis of cocaine to ecogonine methyl esters and benzoic acid by serum cholinesterase and esterases.[70,71] Other hydrolytic metabolite of cocaine, benzoyl ecogonine, is produced by hydrolysis of the methyl ester group formed by spontaneous hydrolysis of cocaine. More recent studies have confirmed this enzymatic reaction and have shown that liver esterases also catalyze this biotransformation.[70] The second route of cocaine metabolism involves a hepatic cytochrome P-450 and FAD-containing monooxygenase pathway.[72,73] Although the FAD-containing monooxygenase pathway is of minor importance in humans under very light usage, it is responsible for the production of the hepatotoxic metabolites of cocaine metabolism in heavy users.[74]

Hepatotoxicity of Cocaine Abuse

The first evidence of hepatic damage following cocaine use was demonstrated in a group of human cocaine and heroin users that exhibited elevated serum transaminase levels.[75] Animal models have also shown that acute or chronic cocaine use precipitated severe liver damage in the form of fatty infiltration, mitozonal and periportal necrosis, and elevated serum transaminases.[60b,76] This cocaine-mediated hepatic injury has been demonstrated in both induced[61] and noninduced[77] mice. Studies by Thompson et al.[74] showed that the cytochrome P-450 system is responsible for all the detoxification of the metabolites of cocaine, norcocaine, *N*-hydroxycocaine, and norcocaine nitroxide, and the liver damage associated with cocaine abuse. However, recent studies also ascribe cocaine-induced liver damage to the observed depletion of hepatic glutathione[61] and to increased hepatic lipid peroxidation.[78]

Enzymes and Nonenzyme System Involved in Alcohol and Cocaine Hepatotoxicity

The morbidity and mortality associated with alcohol and cocaine abuse relates to its pervasive effects on all major organ systems and particularly so in the liver. Because the liver is the major site of the metabolism of cocaine and alcohol, the increased oxidative stress and increased formation of free radicals and enhanced lipid peroxidation occurring in this organ profoundly affect hepatic antioxidants defense systems, which are designed to protect against this oxidative injury.

The antioxidant system may be divided into two major groups: the endogenous enzymic antioxidants, which include superoxide dismutase

(SOD), glutathione peroxidase (GSH-peroxidase), catalase, uric acid, and others; and the dietary supplied antioxidants, such as vitamins E and C, the carotenoids and some vitamin A related compounds, and selenium. These antioxidant systems detoxify the hepatotoxic free radicals, reactive electrophiles and lipid peroxides formed by the interaction of O_2 species with unsaturated lipids of the cell.

Endogenous Antioxidant Enzyme System

Glutathione Peroxidase

Glutathione peroxidase (GSH) is made up of four protein subunits, each of which contain one atom of the element selenium at its active site.[79] Deficiency of this element causes a fall in the activity of this enzyme to very low levels, often to less than 5% of control activity.[80] The enzyme is found at high activity in the livers of those who do not abuse drugs.[81]

The role of GSH-enzymes against lipid peroxidation is controversial. An early report by McCay et al.[82] suggested that GSH-peroxidase prevented lipid peroxidation. Later reports proposed that the lipoperoxidative actions of GSH-peroxidase was due to other proteins and not selenium-dependent.[83] However, recent studies by Mercurio et al.[84] and Takahashi et al.[85] support an antioxidant defense role for selenium-dependent GSH.

The depletion of GSH, one of the major defenses against oxidative stress, renders the cell more susceptible to the development of peroxidation, cell damage, and lysis.[86] Ethanol enhances GSH depletion and potentiates acute hepatotoxicity.[87] Videla and coworkers demonstrated that the administration of a single dose of 5.8 of ethanol/kg body wt to rats fasted overnight induced a drastic decrease in liver GSH after 6 h of intoxication.[88,89] In humans[90] and rats,[91] acute ethanol consumption leads to an increase in plasma malondialdehyde and plasma GSH, reflecting increased utilization and loss of the enzyme from the liver. The mechanism by which ethanol exerts this effect include

1. An inhibition of hepatic GSH synthesis;[92]
2. Binding of GSH to acetaldehyde produced in the degradation of ethanol;[93]
3. Oxidation of GSH by lipid peroxides produced by ethanol;[94] and
4. Binding of acetaldehyde to cystine, a precursor of GSH[95] to form the 2-mTCA derivative.[96]

Similarly, the in vivo depletion of hepatic GSH after cocaine administration,[97] and the importance of GSH in protecting against cocaine-mediated cellular injury[98,99] have been demonstrated.

Catalase

In animals, catalase is present in all major organs, being especially concentrated in liver and erythrocytes.[100] Purified catalases consist of four protein subunits, each unit containing a heme (Fe [III]-protoporphyrin) group bound to its active site. Each subunit also usually contains one molecule of NADPH bound to it, which helps to stabilize the enzyme.[1]

The catalase reaction may be written as follows:

$$\text{catalase} - \text{Fe (III)} + H_2O_2 \rightleftharpoons \text{Compound I}$$
$$\text{Compound I} + H_2O_2 \rightleftharpoons \text{Catalase} - \text{Fe (III)} + H_2O_2$$
$$+ O_2$$

The presence of peroxidatic substrates for catalase in vivo decreases the concentration of compound I, causing more free catalase to be formed.[101]

The catalase activity of animals is largely located in subcellular organelles bound by a single membrane called peroxisomes. The peroxisomes also contain some of the cellular H_2O_2-generating enzymes, such as glycollate oxidase, urate oxidase, and the flavoprotein dehydrogenases involved in the beta-oxidation of fatty acids. Ethanol's oxidation by catalase in vivo occurs in the peroxisomes and because ethanol is a substrate for the peroxidative actions of catalase, it reduces the concentration of Compound I and also reduces pyridine nucleotide, which is a substrate for the alcohol dehydrogenase that converts NAD^+ to NADH.[102,103]

Superoxide Dismutases (SODs)

The SOD are metalloenzymes that catalyze the conversion of O_2^- to H_2O_2 and thus prevent accumulation of the oxygen radicals generated during alcohol and drug metabolism from accumulating.

Antioxidant Nutrients and Liver Damage

Chronic alcohol and/or cocaine abuse have profound effects in depleting hepatic levels of the antioxidant nutrients, thus increasing liver damage common among such individuals. This section focuses on the mechanism of protection conferred by these nutrients against alcohol-induced hepatotoxicity.

Nutrients act at different levels in the oxidative sequence by:

1. Decreasing localized oxygen radical concentration;
2. Preventing first-chain initiation by scavenging chain-initiating radicals such as OH°;
3. Binding metal ions in forms that will not generate such chain-initiating species as OH°, ferryl, or $Fe^{2+}/Fe^{3+}/O_2$ and/or will not decompose lipid peroxides to peroxy or alkoxy radicals;
4. Decompose peroxides by converting them to nonradical products such as alcohol; and
5. Chain-breaking or scavenging intermediate radicals such as peroxy and alkoxy radicals to prevent continuing hydrogen abstraction.[104]

Many antioxidants have multiple mechanisms of action. Some are preventive antioxidants, some are chain-breaking antioxidants, and others are repairing antioxidants, which diminish the rate of lipid peroxidation.

Vitamin E (Tocopherol)

Vitamin E is a group of closely related family of compounds called the tocopherols. There are four major tocopherols with antioxidant activity. Alpha-tocopherol is the most biologically important of the group,[105] and the terms alpha-tocopherol and vitamin E are now used interchangeably. Although vitamin E, compared to a number of synthetic phenol (butylated hydroxytoluene) used industrially, is a relatively poor antioxidant, it is the most important antioxidant in humans.[106]

Vitamin E is a fat-soluble molecule and, being hydrophobic, it tends to concentrate in the interior of membranes susceptible to oxidative damage. For example, the mitochondrial membranes contain about one molecule of alpha-tocopherol per 2,100 molecules of phospholipid of blood lipoproteins and in the adrenal glands. Both the cortex and the medulla contain high levels of vitamin E because of their high content of oxygenase enzymes, which increases their susceptibility to oxidative damage.[107,108]

Vitamin E functions in vivo as a protector of lipid peroxidation as indicated by decreased ethane exhalation and hepatic malondialdehyde formation.[109,110] It prevents lipid peroxidation by both quenching and reacting with singlet oxygen radicals. It is oxidized by the superoxide generating system and, like most molecules, it also reacts with OH• at an almost diffusion-controlled rate in this reaction.[111] During its action as a chain-breaking antioxidant in membranes, alpha-tocopherol is consumed and converted to the radical form.[112] However, mechanisms exist in vivo for reducing the radical back to alpha-tocopherol. A synergism between vitamins E and C in trapping free radical is suggested.[113] Recent studies[114,115] have confirmed that ascorbic acid reduces the alpha-tocopheryl radical back to alpha-tocopherol in intact membranes. Thus, the addition of ascorbate to membranes containing vitamin E can have antioxidant as well as pro-oxidant effects.[116] Furthermore, recent findings showed that vitamin E may also protect against peroxidation by modifying hepatic lipid components,[117] thus maintaining membrane structure. In that experiment, rats fed alcoholic diets supplemented with vitamin E showed hepatic lipid composition and fatty acid profiles similar to the control rats.

Vitamin A Related Compounds

Vitamin A consists of a large group of related substances with various structural characteristics and biological activity of which the most important are the carotenoids.[118] Excluding the *cis-trans* isomers of a given carotenoids, the number of carotenoids is estimated at 563.[119] However, using singlet oxygen quenching as the biological action for classification purposes, these carotenoids may be divided into four major categories. These categories together with examples may be defined as:[216]

1. Biologically active and nutritionally active (beta-carotene);
2. Biologically active but nutritionally inactive (canthaxanthin);
3. Biologically inactive but nutritionally active (beta-apo-14-carotenal); and
4. Biologically and nutritionally inactive (phytoene).

The mechanism(s) via which beta-carotene (BC) exert a protective effect in biological systems have generated considerable interest. It has been proposed that BC deactivates reactive chemical species such as singlet oxygen and free radicals,[120] which would otherwise initiate harmful reactions such as lipid peroxidation. The effectiveness of BC as a quencher of both singlet oxygen and reactive triplets sensitizers has been clearly demonstrated.[121,122]

Although BC does not have the structural features commonly associated with chain-breaking antioxidants,[122] its carbon-centered radical, beta-car°, reacts rapidly and reversibly with oxygen to form a new chain-carrying peroxyl radical, B-car-00.[104] The role of BC as an antioxidant can be summarized as shown:

$$B\text{-carotene} + R00^{\circ} \longrightarrow B\text{-car}^{\circ}$$
$$B\text{-car}^{\circ} + O_2 \rightleftharpoons B\text{-Car-00}^{\circ}$$

Dietary canthaxanthin is also shown to increase resistance to lipid peroxidation by enhancing membrane alpha-tocopherol and by providing antioxidant activities.[123]

Vitamin C (Ascorbic Acid)

Ascorbic acid is required in vivo as a cofactor for several enzymes including proline hydroxylase and lysine hydroxylase, which are involved in the biosynthesis of collagen. Analysis of rat tissues show that next to the adrenala cortex and the kidney, the liver has the highest levels of semihydroascorbate reductase activity.[124]

Ascorbate acts as a reducing agent (electron donor), thus it reduces Fe (III) to Fe (II).[125] This property is important in promoting iron uptake from the gut. The observations that dietary ascorbate inhibit the carcinogenic actions of several nitroso-compounds fed to animals can be attributed to its ability to reduce them to inactive forms.[126] Ascorbate may detoxify various organic radicals in vivo by a similar process. Donation of one electron by ascorbate gives the semidehydroascorbate radical, which can be further oxidized to give dehydroascorbase. The semidehydroascorbate radical is not particularly reactive and mainly undergoes a disproportionate reaction:

$$2 \text{ semidehydroascorbate} \rightleftharpoons \text{ascorbate} + \text{dehydroascorbate}$$

Dehydroascorbate is unstable and breaks down rapidly, producing oxalic acid and threonic acids.[127] Measurement of the quantitative yield of four isomeric conjugated diene hydroperoxides using methyl linoleate as a substrate by Nikki et al.[128] showed that vitamin C scavenges the chain-carrying peroxy radicals and suppresses the oxidation of the substrate.

Ascorbate is also shown to scavenge OH^- and singlet oxygen and react with O_2^-,[129] and inhibit ethane and pentane (indices of peroxidation) in guinea pigs.[130] In addition, ascorbate regenerates the chain-breaking antioxidant alpha-tocopherol in biological membranes. It is yet to be seen if similar observations are made with the reactive electrophiles generated from ethanol's oxidation and cocaine metabolism.

Effects of Alcohol and Cocaine Abuse on Nutritional Status

Nutrient Deficiencies in Alcoholism

Alcoholism has profound deteriorating effects on nutritional status.[131] The several alcohol-induced nutrient deficiencies in turn affect the metabolism of alcohol thus aggravating alcohol's hepatotoxicity and further worsening the nutritional status of the alcoholic. For example, alcohol depresses appetite, displaces other foods and nutrients from the diet, and decreases the value of food by interfering with digestion and absorption. Even when nutrients are absorbed, alcohol prevents them from being fully utilized by altering their transportation, storage, and excretion. Patients hospitalized for medical complications associated with alcoholism may be severely malnourished in several nutrients, including protein and energy deficiencies. Such medical complications are known to be due to the direct and indirect effect of alcoholism on nutrient availability and utilization.[132]

Interactions of Ethanol with Specific Nutrients

Macronutrients

Protein. When ethanol is consumed as additional calories, it may spare nitrogen utilization, thus preventing muscles and other organs from breaking down their proteins for use as energy sources. When ethanol replaces carbohydrate calories, there is an increase in nitrogen losses as urea.[133] Also, the ingestion of ethanol depresses whole body protein synthesis and inhibits hepatic and muscular mitochondrial protein synthesis,[134] depresses serum albumin fraction and total protein,[135] impairs absorption and secretion of amino acids by liver and increased serum concentration of branched-chain amino acids,[136] and inhibits the secretion of albumin and plasma lycoprotein by the liver.[137,138a,138b]

Carbohydrate and Energy Balance. The effects of alcohol on carbohydrate and energy balance in epidemiological and clinical studies in human and experimental animals is recently reviewed.[139] This section, therefore, will focus on the mechanism of changes elicited by alcohol.

The calories in ethanol are inefficiently utilized by the body, especially when the dose is high or when the drinker is an alcoholic. Even when ethanol is ingested as extra calories, it causes less weight gain than did calorically equivalent amount of carbohydrate or fat,[140] and no weight gain in lean individuals.[141] The lack of energy gained from alcohol is a direct toxic effect of ethanol metabolism in the liver. The MEOS induced or activated by chronic consumption of high alcohol levels consumes NADPH-related compounds without creating new ones.[142] Consequently, the energy released from the system is dissipated as heat. Chronic ethanol consumption results in a generalized depression in hepatic mitochondria energy metabolism. It decreases both the rate and efficiency of ATP synthesis via the oxidative phosphorylation system.[138a] Also, hormonal imbalances leading to reduced hepatic ATP content[143] and increased ATPase activity,[144] decreased oxygen utilization,[145] and the inhibition of glucose metabolism under oxygen-poor conditions may explain the lack of weight gain commonly observed in alcohol abusers. Furthermore, ethanol, unlike carbohydrates, induces lipogenic enzymes by reducing the activity of lactate dehydrogenase and malic enzymes, increases ATP citrate lyase,[146] increases blood acetaldehyde,[147] and depresses cardiac microsomal protein synthesis.[148] Finally, high ethanol consumption may affect absorption of nutrients and hence weight gain.

Alcohol also affects carbohydrate metabolism via its regulation of pancreatic enzymes. SanKaran et al. showed that the acinar content of amylase and the acinar response to cholecystokinin-octapeptide is significantly lower in rats fed diets containing 26% ethanol-derived calories.[149] Human alcohol abusers with liver cirrhosis have decreased insulin sensitivity and glucose-6-phosphatase, increased hexokinase activity, low or absent glucokinase activity, and a reduced glucokinase/hexokinase ratio.[150] The resultant changes in these pancreatic enzymes lead to the glucose intolerance and insulin resistance observed in chronic alcohol abusers.

Lipids. Many biochemical abnormalities in lipid metabolism result from intoxication or chronic alcohol usage. When alcohol is present in the system, it displaces fat as the primary fuel in the liver, resulting in hepatic accumulation of fat. The lipids that accumulate in the liver originate from three main sources: dietary lipids, which reach the blood stream and the liver as chylomicrons; adipose tissue lipids, which are transported to the liver as free fatty acids; and lipids synthesized in the liver. Metabolic disturbances in the equilibrium resulting from ethanol ingestion affect hepatic lipid accumulation by:

1. Increasing the amounts of precursors for hepatic lipid synthesis;
2. Increasing hepatic lipogenesis via the stimulation of lipogenic enzymes;
3. Decreasing lipid breakdown;
4. Decreasing hepatic secretion of lipids; and
5. Enhancing hepatic uptake of circulating lipids.

Increased Availability of Substrates for Hepatic Lipid Biosynthesis. Ethanol interferes with the supply of precursors of lipogenesis from extrahepatic sources by providing reducing equivalents and carbon units for lipid biosynthesis.[151] The altered redox state inhibits the oxidation of fatty acids and diverts them into esterification, which is further enhanced by the increased concentration of glycerol-3-phosphate.[152–154] Ethanol also increases the amount of fatty acid transported from the adipose tissue and the small intestine into the liver where they are then deposited.[155]

Increased Activity of the Lipid Synthetic Enzymes. In addition to ethanol having the effect of increasing the supply of precursors, it may also increase the rate of triglyceride synthesis by stimulating the enzymes catalyzing triglyceride synthesis. Both acute and chronic ethanol consumption stimulate phosphatidate phosphohydrolase in the microsomal and soluble fractions of the mitochondria,[156] and the increase in the enzyme activity leads to the accumulation of hepatic triglycerides.[157]

Similarly, the increased phospholipid content of the liver after chronic ethanol administration[158] is accounted for by the increased activity of two enzymes involved in the synthesis of phosphatidyl choline: choline phosphotransferase and phosphatidyl ethanol amine methyltransferase.[159]

Decreased Lipid Breakdown and Secretion from the Liver. The accumulation of esterified lipids in the alcoholic fatty liver result from an impaired capacity of lysosomal lipase and esterase to hydrolyze the glycerol esters. Chronic ethanol administration decreased or did not alter the activity of lysosomal enzymes,[160,161] but it did decrease the activity of microsomal and cytosolic phospholipase A[162] required for the hydrolysis of hepatic cholesterol. Furthermore, ingestion of ethanol increases bile acids in the liver[163] while it depresses its glandular secretion.[164] This reduction in biliary secretion of bile acids is secondary to the diminution in cholesterol-7-alpha-hydroxylase activity and the accumulation of cholesteryl esters in the liver.[165]

Effects of Chronic Alcoholism on Lipid Composition. Chronic alcohol exposure is reported to increase,[166,167] decrease,[168] or have no effect[169,170] on tissue cholesterol levels. Some authors have observed little changes in hepatic phospholipids,[158,171,172] whereas others have reported only minor changes in the brain phospholipid composition.[173,174] The variations of these results may be owing to differences in the species studied, the route of administration, the dose and duration of alcohol delivered, and the constituents of the administered diet.

More significant effects of alcohol are noted in the fatty acid distribution. Reduction of arachidonic acid, a polyunsaturated fatty acid, have been observed in rat liver,[173,175,176] red blood cells,[177–179] platelets,[180,181] and the heart.[182]

The lipid composition of the brain is considered resistant to dietary influences; however, several studies have reported alcohol-induced alterations in brain fatty acid composition. Littleton et al.[183] reported a significant decline in docosanhexaenoic acid (22:6 or 3) in mouse brain after a 2-h ethanol exposure. Similar changes in mouse brain synaptic membrane content of 22:6 or 3 in the phosphatidyl serine were observed following 7 d of dietary ethanol.[174] It is, therefore, evident that ethanol metabolism exerts a degree of plasticity of the hepatic and brain polyunsaturated fatty acids composition in animals.

Minerals

Calcium. Alcohol abuse directly or indirectly affects calcium balance. It may affect calcium balance directly by affecting water balance through its diuretic effects.[184] Negative calcium balance may also occur secondarily to fat malabsorption in human alcoholic patients[185] and in rodents.[186] However, because abnormalities of bone metabolism are prominent in alcohol abusers, some other factors distinct from reduced absorption may be involved in the negative calcium balance accompanying alcoholism.

Magnesium. Severe depletion of magnesium and its associated enzymatic activities is a frequent occurrence in alcohol abusers.[187] This depletion is attributed to decreased magnesium intake, malabsorption, and alcohol-induced magnesium losses in the urine, vomiting, and diarrhea.[187] However, a positive balance occurs on withdrawal from alcohol, and magnesium therapy can be used to revert the low levels of the mineral in magnesium-deficient alcohol abusers.[188]

Iron. Iron is a constituent of hemoglobin and certain enzymes involved in energy production. Alcohol abusers frequently are iron deficient, which is a complicated physiological occurrence. For example, elevated serum iron is often seen in active alcohol abusers, but this high level drops quickly with abstinence.[189] Patients with alcoholic liver disease show a sevenfold increase in erythrocyte ferritin content.[190] This increase occurs from the high iron content of the alcoholic beverages consumed, increased secretion of hydrochloric acid produced in the stomach by alcohol, and the alcoholic inhibition of a coenzyme, pyridoxal kinase, which interrupts utilization resulting in increased serum iron levels.[189] In some cases, iron deficiency may occur from increased gastrointestinal blood loss secondary to gastritis or cirrhosis.[191] Other reports[192] found increased rather than decreased iron absorption in chronic alcoholism. This increased hepatic iron content, resulting in siderosis, may be damaging to the liver.

Zinc. A depleted zinc status is a common finding in chronic and acute alcohol abusers.[193,194] Depletion can be as low as 60% of normal levels in chronic alcohol abusers with cirrhotic livers.[196,197] It is argued that reduced food intake during alcohol consumption may play a significant role in the maintenance of serum zinc levels. Richard et al.[198] reported that acute intake of ethanol in humans did not affect plasma zinc concentration anymore than that seen by the low intake of food alone. Similarly, in rats, moderate doses of alcohol as part of an adequate diet resulted in decreases of both serum and hepatic zinc levels similar to those caused by dietary zinc deficiency alone.[199]

Zinc is a component of various enzyme systems, and it is required for the maintenance of healthy skin, bones, and hair, and in the storage and mobilization of vitamin A. The impaired night vision commonly seen in alcohol abusers is a result of the derangement of vitamin A metabolism secondary to zinc deficiency.[194,200] Zinc is associated with insulin in the beta-cells of the pancreas and for optimum humoral immune defense.[201,202] Several of the biochemical and physiological functions of zinc are affected by alcohol intake.[199]

Alcohol and zinc interact to impair each others metabolism.[199,203] For example, administration of a high zinc diet (10 ppm) containing 30% of ethanol as calories to pregnant and lactating rats and their offsprings lowered maternal zinc status to values similar to those fed low zinc diets (2 ppm) without alcohol. Furthermore, the levels of serum zinc and alkaline phosphatase were depressed in the offsprings in the alcohol fed rats.[203]

Selenium. In trace quantities, selenium is an essential nutrient and an antioxidant. Low blood selenium levels is associated with abnormal liver structure and functions.[195,204] Alcohol abusers tend to be deficient in selenium in the absence of severe liver disease or inadequate intake.[205] This low serum level may contribute to hepatic injuries via increased lipid peroxidation and the associated damage of liver-cell membranes.[206] Again, selenium depletion in alcohol abusers has been attributed to poor dietary intake.[204] Plasma selenium also decreases in patients with nonalcoholic liver injury.[207,208] Therefore, although selenium deficiency may contribute to alcoholic liver injury, low selenium levels may be, in part, a consequence of liver injury.

Water-Soluble Vitamins

Thiamine. Although severe thiamine deficiency is uncommon in the industrialized countries, an appreciable number of alcohol abusers are mildly deficient. This deficiency status results in disastrous neurological and cardiac disorders.[209]

Deficient thiamine status has been found in many alcohol abusers. In a study of a drinking population, Leevy et al.[210] found that 30% of malnourished alcohol abusers had blood thiamine level 20% less than the lower limit range of healthy volunteers. A low or deficient excretion of thiamine in the urine was found in 272 of alcohol abusers admitted to a hospital.[211] Similarly, between 20–73% of an alcoholic population were found to have a high risk of a thiamine deficiency, as estimated by erythrocyte transketolase activity.[212] Alcoholism is a major cause of thiamine deficiency seen in hospitals with 43% low in B_1 status, and 65% of those found to be deficient in B_1 were alcohol abusers.[213]

This poor thiamine status in alcohol abusers is partly owing to impaired intestinal absorption.[214] In animal experiments, ethanol disturbs both in vitro and in vivo the active transport of thiamine across the intestinal wall.[215] It is postulated that in addition to alcohol, the associated malnutrition contributes significantly to the high increase of thiamine deficiency.[210,216] Over 70% of alcohol abusers were found to have a deficient intake of thiamine estimated by the 7-d dietary recall.[217,218] The amount of alcohol ingested is also shown to affect the thiamine status of alcohol abusers.[211] However, the ease and safety of the administration of thiamine during treatment of alcoholism revealed that it reverses some of the clinical deficiency symptoms and the neurological disorders of alcohol-induced thiamine deficiency.[219,220]

Riboflavin (B₂). Riboflavin deficiency is seen in many alcohol abusers.[221,222] This deficiency seems to be mainly from the poor dietary intake, as no effect of ethanol on the absorption of the vitamin[223] or a correlation between ethanol intake and riboflavin status has been noted.[224] However, riboflavin deficiency can complicate chronic alcoholism,[225] and chronic alcohol feeding can induce riboflavin deficiency when intake of the vitamin is marginal.[226,227]

Pyridoxine (B₆). Pyridoxine (vitamin B_2) is required for normal cellular metabolism, growth, and development, particularly of the brain and central nervous system. In surveys of the B_6 status of alcohol abusers, lower than normal mean circulating levels have been noted.[228–231] About 50% of alcohol abusers studied have deficient levels of the vitamin and its cofactor, 5-pyridoxal phosphate. Also, 65 of 113 alcohol abusers showed an abnormal handling of tryptophan,[232] indicative of a B_6 deficiency.

The main reason for the low circulating levels seen in alcohol abusers seems to be an abnormal handling of vitamin B_6 by alcohol abusers. Ethanol does not interfere with the passive diffusion of B_6, but it does inhibit enzymes in the intestinal lining that remove the phosphate groups of phosphorylated B_6.[192] Alcohol and acetaldehyde accelerate intracellular degradation of 5-pyridoxal phosphate,[233,234] decrease its activation by inhibiting pyridoxine kinase,[235] and reduce the availability of dietary pyridoxine.[236]

Alcohol-induced vitamin B6 deficiencies also cause depression[237] via decreased neurotransmitter synthesis and reduced brain neurotransmitter synthesis. Vitamin B_6 deficiency also reduces cellular transfer of amino acids via deficient pituitary growth hormone secretion.[236]

Folic Acid. Folate deficiency is predominantly associated with alcoholism, poverty, and old age.[238] In the US folate deficiency is found in about 20–50% of alcohol abusers[231,238,239] and the anemia seen in alcohol abusers is frequently associated with impaired folate status and activity.[240,241]

Several factors contribute to these low folate levels in alcohol abusers. These include decreased food intake,[241] the type and amount of alcoholic beverage consumed,[242] decreased folate absorption,[243] interference with folate storage and release, and the interference of folate utilization in the functional tissue pool by alcohol.[244]

Alcohol ingestion accelerates the rate of decrease in circulating folate levels[245,246] and reduces the absorption[247] and tissue uptake[248] of folic acid, thus causing a further decrease in circulating folate levels. The reduced folate status in turn provides a malabsorption of folic acid.[243,249] This leads eventually to depletion of the body folate stores and overt signs of folate deficiency.

Cobalamin (Vitamin B$_{12}$). Vitamin B$_{12}$ functions mainly as a coenzyme involved in carbohydrate and fat metabolism. The effect of chronic and acute alcoholism on B$_{12}$ status has been recently reviewed.[250] In a study of alcohol abusers, no abnormal B$_{12}$ levels were found,[251] but impaired absorption of labeled vitamin B$_{12}$, as measured by the percentage of the oral dose excreted in the feces, was observed in alcoholic cirrhotic patients.[252] As most alcoholic drinks contain considerable amounts of folate, which masks the gross deficiency symptoms of B$_{12}$, the deficiency of this vitamin is not seen frequently in alcohol abusers. However, absorption is impaired in chronic alcohol abusers,[253,254] probably through interference at the site of active transport in the terminal portion of the small intestine.

Niacin. There are conflicting reports on alcohol effects on niacin levels in alcohol abusers. Some studies reported low circulating levels,[255,256] whereas others found no differences in circulating niacin levels[223,257] or in urinary excretion of *n*-methyl nicotinamide[211] between alcohol abusers and controls. Niacin intake did not differ greatly between alcohol abusers and abstainers,[253,259] especially when the intake of tryptophan, which can be partially converted into niacin, is also considered.

Pantothenic Acid. The few studies investigating pantothenic acid status in alcohol abusers found reduced urinary excretion[260] and mean circulating levels[254,256] in alcoholic patients than those found in nondrinking subjects. However, the mechanisms leading to these reduced levels in alcohol abusers have not been elucidated. Human alcohol abusers with liver diseases have been shown to have depleted pantothenic acid levels related to the extent of liver damage.[259] These findings could also be interpreted in terms of duration of alcoholism and thus of duration of reduced pantothenic acid intake. Alcohol does not affect the pantothenic status of humans[261] and rats[262] fed a nutritionally adequate diet. Nevertheless, the decrease in pantothenic acid secretion found in rehabilitated alcohol abusers[260] may indicate a problem in utilization of this vitamin.

Biotin. The role of biotin in human and animal nutrition is not yet completely elucidated.[263] In alcohol abusers, both circulating levels and liver contents of biotin are reduced.[264] This low level is generally associated with the development of fatty liver. As no effect of ethanol *per se* has been noted on circulating and hepatic biotin levels, the low levels found in alcohol abusers are probably of nutritional origin.[264]

Ascorbic Acid (Vitamin C). Surprisingly, very few studies on the vitamin C status in alcohol abusers have been published. These investigations found not only reduced mean circulating levels but also a high frequency of deficient levels.[228,265,266] Vitamin C deficiency in chronically alcohol-fed guinea pigs reduced the efficiency of the microsomal ethanol oxidizing system,[265] and produced a lower rate of decline of infused ethanol.[267] Ascorbic acid protects against the harmful effect of acetaldehyde on the heart,[268,269] causes weight gain,[267] and protects against toxicity[270] in alcohol-fed animals.

Fat-Soluble Vitamins

Vitamin A. Although dietary vitamin A deficiency is not a serious health problem in the general population, its level is adversely affected in chronic alcohol abusers.[271,272] Change in vitamin A levels may be owing in part to inadequate intake. People who derive less than 20% of their daily dietary calories from alcohol ingest a normal amount of vitamin A,[273] whereas heavier drinkers consume 75% or less of the recommended daily allowance of vitamin A.[274] Low vitamin A status has also been observed in Norwegians who consume large amounts of alcohol.[275] Ethanol and vitamin A consumption synergistically increase tracheal cancers in alcohol abusers,[276] and deficiency of vitamin A increases the susceptibility to neoplasia and carcinogenesis.[277] However, decreased nutritional intake alone does not fully explain why patients with alcoholic liver disease have very low hepatic vitamin A at all stages in the development of the disease. Experimental administration of ethanol in normal nutritionally adequate diets, and even with vitamin A supplemented diets, resulted in a depression of liver vitamin A stores.[278] Thus, the low vitamin A stores of alcohol abusers may not be attributed to insufficient vitamin A consumption or to impaired absorption by the digestive system alone.[279]

Other mechanisms proposed to explain the interaction of ethanol's depletion of vitamin A status include the increased mobilization of vitamin A from the liver to other organs. This view is consistent with the observation that after chronic ethanol consumption, vitamin A in peripheral tissue increased, even when hepatic vitamin A was depleted.[279–281] An acute, nonlethal dose of ethanol significantly increased retinyl esters in serum lipoprotein and decreased hepatic vitamin A stores.[282] These findings suggest that a shift of vitamin A from the liver to other organs through lipoprotein-bound retinyl esters occurs as a result of ethanol administration.

The second mechanism for hepatic depletion of vitamin A following ethanol consumption involves increased catabolism. Retinol is mobilized from the liver on a retinol binding protein, which can be metabolized to retinal and retinoic acid via the cytosolic and retinol and retinal dehydrogenase.[283] Retinoic acid, in turn, can be degraded through a microsomal cytochrome P-450-mediated enzyme activity. Therefore, ethanol consumption could decrease hepatic vitamin A, in part through increased metabolism in the liver. Indeed, we recently showed that rats fed ethanol exhibited increased lipid peroxidation and reduced vitamin A levels, whereas rats fed diets supplemented with vitamin E showed reduced lipid peroxidation and increased hepatic vitamin A levels.[284] We hypothesized that this result can be explained by the sparring action of vitamin E on vitamin A stores in alcoholism.

Vitamin D. Vitamin D metabolism is adversely affected by chronic alcohol abuse. In alcohol abusers with or without liver disease, significantly lower plasma levels of vitamin D have been reported in about 45% of the population studied.[285,286] The reasons for these low levels have not yet been fully elucidated. However, the reasons for this depletion are multifactorial and include poor diet, reduced exposure to sunshine, malabsorption — especially in cases of fat malabsorption[286,287] — and increased rate of vitamin D degradation.[288]

The reduction in circulating vitamin D levels in alcohol abusers results in reduced bone mass and low calcium levels, arising from reduced absorption and mobilization.[184,289] Also, since vitamin D plays a vital role in glucose metabolism via a direct regulatory role in maintaining insulin levels,[290,291] alcohol-induced vitamin D deficiencies result in impairment of insulin response by a reduced secretion and a delayed response to glucose.[292,293]

Vitamin E. Vitamin E, because of its antioxidant properties, has received tremendous attention in human nutrition. As the major antioxidant in the membrane, vitamin E is often referred to as the backbone of defense against alcohol and drug-induced lipid peroxidation.[294,295] Studies indicate that ethanol consumption reduced the mean circulating and hepatic stores of vitamin E in rats[284,296,297] and in human alcohol abusers.[298–300]

Mechanism(s) leading to reduced circulating levels of vitamin E in alcohol abusers have not yet been fully explained. However, dietary intake, malabsorption, and B-lipoprotein deficiency in liver disease may all contribute.[301] Ethanol feeding to rats was shown to result in increased hepatic alpha-tocopheryl quinone, a metabolite of alpha-tocopherol by free radical reaction,[302] thus indicating that ethanol enhances the degradation of vitamin E by free radicals. The supplementation of a low vitamin E ethanolic diet with the vitamin decreases the susceptibility of living systems to free radical attack and the consequent cell damage.[62,109]

Vitamin K. Vitamin K is present in a variety of foods. It is required only in relatively small amounts by humans, and since part of the vitamin K requirement may be covered by intestinal synthesis, a significant deficiency status would be very rarely encountered and very difficult to produce in humans. However, a combination of sterilization of the large intestine, pancreatic insufficiency, cholestasis, or an abnormality secondary to folate deficiency may lead to vitamin K deficiency. Nevertheless, lengthening of prothrombin time has been observed only in patients with severe liver disease such as alcoholic and nonalcoholic cirrhosis, and chronic active hepatic disease.[303] Although the prevalence of this reduced prothrombin tissue has not been compared in alcohol-induced liver disease and nonalcoholic liver disease, this reduced prothrombin time in alcoholics shows that alcohol-induced liver injury interferes with vitamin K utilization.

Nutritional Deficiencies Associated with Cocaine Abuse

Despite the prevalence of cocaine abuse in our population, its effects on the nutritional status on humans has not been intensively studied as that that accompany alcohol abuse. Comprehensive studies of the nutritional status of cocaine abusers would provide valuable information on the depletion of specific nutrients in such individuals, and this information may be incorporated into the treatment programs of chronic cocaine users.

The nutritional effects caused by use of drugs of abuse has been recently reviewed.[304] Habitual cocaine use suppresses the appetite[305,306] and decreases the motivation for food,[307] which in turn reinforces the need for the drug.[308] This cascade effect worsens the nutritional status of the abuser, a phenomenon observed in humans.[309] Cocaine use alters food selection and increases the tendencies for eating disorders. Epidemiological surveys by Castro et al.[310] comparing the dietary habits of adult cocaine users and their nonusing peers found that cocaine users ate significantly fewer complete or balanced meals, drank more alcoholic beverages, consumed more cups of coffee, and had lower fat food intake compared to the nonusers. Cocaine users also have higher rates of eating disorders such as anorexia nervosa and bulimia.[311] Furthermore, coca-leaf chewers have increased frequency of hookworm anemia, inferior personal hygiene and increased bouts of illness,[309] factors that increase the nutritional requirements for protein, energy, and vitamins. Intravenous cocaine users usually exhibit hepatotoxicity with damaged liver tissues, which may regenerate following the cessation of cocaine use and return of adequate food and nutrients intake.[312] Cocaine use increases utilization of dietary proteins[313] and promotes weight losses.[314,315] The increased utilization of dietary protein is the result of the noninductive increases in the cocaine-*n*-demethylase enzyme activities,[316,317] which retard the incorporation of dietary protein into body tissues. Although available evidence suggests that cocaine abuse leads to deterioration of the nutritional status of the abuser, studies where sensitive markers of nutritional deficiency of essential nutrients is correlated to the duration of abuse is much needed.

Summary and Conclusions

Alcohol and cocaine abuse are leading causes of hepatic damage, as well as the various physiological and biochemical abnormalities that accompany liver damage. From the variety of abnormalities observed, it is most likely that the etiology of alcohol and cocaine-induced hepatotoxicity is multifactorial.

Chronic alcohol and cocaine abusers show evidence of nutritional deficiencies owing to decreased intake, poor absorption, and impaired storage, utilization, and metabolism of essential nutrients. In addition, drug abuse depletes tissue levels and/or activities of the inherent antioxidant enzymes and dietary antioxidants, which protect the biological system against reactive electrophiles generated from the oxidative degradation or metabolism of these drugs. Thus the multifactorial effect of drug abuse on nutritional status is an undisputed factor in the pathogenesis of liver damage.

Many nutrients, including protein and amino acid, fatty acids, carbohydrates, folic acids, thiamine, ascorbic acid, riboflavin, zinc, selenium, and iron, have been examined in humans and animals abusing cocaine and alcohol. Of these, protein-, vitamin E-, and vitamin A-related substances and selenium are the most studied. Data so far accumulated consistently indicate that nutritional deficiencies in the abusers clearly potentiate ethanol and cocaine hepatotoxicity. However, results from some recent studies suggest that when the abuser is in an adequate nutritional state, the effect of ethanol and other drug abuse on liver damage may not be as severe. Nutrient supplementation and alteration of the dietary constituents used in alcohol studies have been investigated, but results from these investigations are not consistent.

Clearly, more extensive investigations are needed, including studies of a dose–response relationship, and effect of cocaine abuse on the nutritional status, in order to establish the beneficial effects of supplementation on improving not only the nutritional status but also the antioxidant defense systems. Results from such studies may provide necessary information in nutritional programs designed to "treat" alcohol- and drug-related hepatotoxicity.

Acknowledgments

This review and our studies cited here is supported by NIAAA Grant 08037 and NIDA grant 04827. We acknowledge and appreciate our collaborations with Professor Cleamond D. Eskelson, Department of Surgery, The University of Arizona, Tuscon, Arizona.

References

[1] G. W. Burton (1989) Antioxidant actions of carotenoids. *J. Nutr.* **119,** 109–111.

[2] C. Kim, M. A. Leo, N. Lowe, and C. S. Lieber (1988) Differential effects of retinoids and chronic ethanol consumption on membranes in rats. *J. Nutr.* **118,** 1097–1103.

[3] E. Nikki, T. Saito, and Y. Kamiya (1983) The role of vitamin C as an antioxidant. *Chem. Lett.* (Japan) **14,** 631–632.

[4] G. W. Burton and K. U. Ingold (1985) Vitamin E as an in vitro and in vivo antioxidant. *Ann. NY Acad. Sci.* **570,** 7–22.

[5] H. N. Kirkman, S. Galiano, and G. F. Gaetani (1987) The function of catalase bound NADPH. *J. Biol. Chem.* **262,** 660–666.

[6] I. A. Watkins, S. Kawanishi, and W. S. Caughey (1985) Autoxidation reactions of hemoglobin A free from other red cell components: A minimal mechanism. *Biochem. Biophys. Res. Commun.* **132,** 742–748.

[7] I. Fridovich (1986) Superoxide dismutases. *Adv. Enzymol.* **58,** 61–97.

[8] R. F. Burk (1990) Protection against free radical injury by selenoenzymes. *Pharmacol. Ther.* **45,** 383–385.

[9] A. B. Freeman and J. D. Crapo (1982) Biology of disease: Free radicals and tissue injury. *Lab. Invest.* **47,** 412–416.

[10] M. Comporti (1985) Biology of disease: Lipid peroxidation and cellular damage in toxic liver injury. *Lab. Invest.* **53,** 599–622.

[11] H. D. Kleber (1988) Cocaine abuse: Historical, epidemiological and psychological perspectives. *J. Clin. Psychiat.* **49,** 3–6.

[12] C. S. Lieber and M. Savolainen (1983) Ethanol and lipids. *Alcohol. Clin. Exp. Res.* **8,** 409–423.

[13] M. E. Lebsak, E. R. Gordon, and C. S. Lieber (1981) The effect of chronic ethanol consumption on aldehyde dehydrogenase activity. *Biochem. Pharmacol.* **30,** 2273–2277.

[14] S. Tottman, H. Petterson, and K. H. Kiessling (1973) The subcellular distribution and properties of aldehyde dehydrogenase in rat liver. *Biochem. J.* **135,** 577–586.

[15] C. S. Lieber (1984) Metabolism and metabolic effects of alcohol. *Med. Clin. North Am.* **68,** 3–31.

[16] D. S. Tuma, R. K. Zetterman, and M. F. Sorrell (1980) Inhibition of glycoprotein secretion by ethanol and acetaldehyde in rat liver slices. *Biochem. Pharmacol.* **29,** 35–38.

[17] R. R. Watson, M. E. Mohs, C. D. Eskelson, R. E. Sampliner, and B. Hartman (1986) Identification of alcohol abuse and alcoholism with biological parameters. *Alcohol. Clin. Exp. Res.* **10,** 364–385.

[18] S. C. Cunnane, K. R. McAdoo, and D. F. Horrobin (1987) Long-term ethanol consumption in the hamster: Effects of tissue lipids, fatty acids and erythrocyte hemolysis. *Ann. Nutr. Metab.* **31,** 265–271.

[19] C. S. Lieber and L. M. DeCarli (1970) Hepatic microsomal ethanol oxidized system: In vitro characteristics and adaptive properties in vivo. *J. Biol. Chem.* **245,** 2505–2512.

[20] G. Ugarte, H. Ituoriaga, and T. Pereda (1977) Possible relationship between the role of ethanol metabolism and the severity of hepatic damage in chronic alcoholic. *Dig. Dis.* **22,** 406–410.

[21] L. Videla and Y. Israel (1970) Factors that modify the metabolism of ethanol in rat liver and adaptive changes produced by its chronic administration. *Biochem. J.* **118,** 225–281.

[22] H. Vaananen, K. O. Lindros, and M. Salaspuro (1984) Distribution of ethanol metabolism in periportal and perivenous rat hepatocytes after chronic ethanol treatment. *Liver* **4,** 72.

[23] H. Vaananen, M. Salaspuro, and K. O. Lindros (1984) Ethanol metabolizing

enzymes in isolated periportal and perivenous rat hepatocytes: Changes after chronic ethanol injection. *Hepatology* **4,** 862–866.

[24] J. A. Edward and D. A. Price-Evans (1967) Ethanol metabolism in subjects possessing typical and atypical liver dehydrogenase. *Clin. Pharmacol. Ther.* **8,** 824–829.

[25] H. Theorell and R. Bonnichsen (1951) Studies in liver dehydrogenase. Equilibra and initial reaction velocities. *Acta Chem. Scand.* **5,** 1105–1126.

[26] A. I. Cederbaum (1980) Regulation of pathways of alcohol metabolism in the liver. *Mount Sinai Med.* **47,** 317–328.

[27] D. R. Koop, E. T. Morgan, G. E. Taff, and M. J. Coon (1982) Purification and characterization of a unique isozopure of cytochrome P-450 from liver microsomes of ethanol-treated rabbits. *J. Biol. Chem.* **257,** 8472–8480.

[28] R. G. Thurman and H. J. Brentzel (1977) The role of alcohol dehydrogenase in microsomal ethanol oxidation and the adaptive increase in ethanol metabolism due to chronic treatment with ethanol. *Alcohol. Clin. Exp. Res.* **1,** 33–38.

[29] R. G. Thurman, W. R. McKenna, J. H. Brentzel, and A. Hesse (1975) A Significant pathway of ethanol metabolism. *Fed. Proc.* **34,** 2075–2084.

[30] H. Ishii, J. G. Joly, and C. S. Lieber (1973) Effect of ethanol on the amount and enzyme activities of hepatic rough and smooth microsomal membranes. *Biochim. Biophys. Acta* **291,** 411–420.

[31] T. Takagi, I. Alderman, and C. S. Lieber (1985) In vivo roles of alcohol dehydrogenetics (ADH), catalase and the microsomal ethanol oxidized system (MEOS) in deer mice. *Alcohol* **2,** 9–12.

[32] E. Baroana, S. Shaw, and C. S. Lieber (1982) Alcohol induced changes in amino acids and protein metabolism, in *Medical Disorders of Alcoholism: Pathogenesis and Treatment.* C. S. Lieber, ed. W. B. Saunders, Philadelphia, pp. 178–206.

[33] C. S. Lieber and M. Savolainen (1984) Ethanol and lipids. *Alcohol. Clin. Exp. Res.* **8,** 409–423.

[34] D. Bunout, V. Gattas, H. Ituoriaga, C. Perez, T. Pereda, and G. Ugarte (1983) Nutritional studies of alcoholic patients: Its possible relationship to alcoholic liver damages. *Am. J. Clin. Nutr.* **38,** 469–473.

[35] G. A. Rao, D. E. Riley, and E. C. Larkin (1987) Dietary carbohydrate stimulates alcohol ingestion, promotes growth and prevents fatty liver in rats. *Nutr. Res.* **7,** 81–87.

[36] G. A. Martini and R. Teschke (1988) Alcohol abstinence in alcoholic liver disease. *Acta Med. Scand.* **703 (Suppl.),** 185–194.

[37] P. J. Scheuer (1982) The morphology of alcoholic liver disease. *Br. Med. Bull.* **38,** 63–65.

[38] V. J. Desmet (1988) Alcohol liver disease. Histoloical features and evolution. *Acta Med. Scand.* **703,** 111–126.

[39] R. N. MacSween (1983) Alcoholic liver disease, in *Recent Advances in Hepatology.* A. C. Thomas and R. N. MacSween, eds. Churchill Livingstone, Edinburh, pp. 71–88.

[40] H. Popper, S. N. Thung, and M. A. Gerber (1981) Pathology of alcoholic liver disease. *Semin. Liver Dis.* **1,** 203–216.

[41] S. Sherlock (1988) Alcoholic liver disease: Clinical patterns and dianosis. *Acta Med. Scand.* **703,** 103–110.

[42] J. Szebeni, C. D. Eskelson, R. Sampliner, B. Hartman, J. Griffin, T. Dormandy, and R. R. Watson (1988) Plasma fatty acid pattern including diene conjugates linoleic acid in ethanol users and in patients with ethanol related liver disease. *Alcohol. Clin. Exp. Res.* **18,** 647–652.

[43] E. Mezey (1976) Ethanol metabolism and ethanol–drug interaction. *Biochem. Pharmacol.* **25,** 869–875.

[44] M. J. World, P. R. Ryle, and A. D. Thomson (1985) Alcoholic malnutrition and the small intestine. *Alcohol Alcohol.* **20,** 89–124.

[45] H. Orrego, Y. Israel, and L. M. Blendis (1981) Alcoholic liver disease: Information in search of knowledge. *Hepatology* **1,** 267–283.

[46] E. Rubin and C. S. Lieber (1967) Early five structural changes in the human liver induced by alcohol. *Gastroenterology* **52,** 1–13.

[47] C. S. Lieber and E. Rubin (1968) Ethanol— an hepatotoxic drug. *Gastroenterology* **54,** 557–565.

[48] R. S. Patrick and J. D. McGee (1980) Inhibition of drug metabolism by acute ethanol intoxication: A hepatic microsomal mechanism, in *Biopsy Pathology of Liver.* F. Walker and A. M. Neville, eds. Chapman T. Hall, London, pp. 189–191.

[49] C. S. Lieber, A. Garro, M. A. Leo, K. M. Mak, and T. Warner (1986) Alcohol and cancer. *Hepatology* **6,** 1005–1019.

[50] M. A. Polokoff, T. J. Simon, R. A. Harris, F. R. Simon, and M. Iwahashy (1985) Chronic ethanol increases liver plasma membrane fluidity. *Biochemistry* **24,** 3114–3120.

[51] A. Schuller, J. Moscat, E. Diez, C. Checa-Fernandez, F. E. Gavilanes, and A. Municio (1984) The fluidity of plasma membrane from ethanol-treated rat liver. *Mol. Cell Biochem.* **64,** 89–95.

[52] M. U. Dianzani (1985) Lipid peroxidation in ethanol poisoning: A critical reconsideration. *Alcohol Alcohol.* **20,** 161–173.

[53] S. Worrall, J. De-Jersey, B. C. Shanley, and P. A. Wilce (1989) Ethanol induces the production of antibodies to acetaldehyde-modified epitopes in rats. *Alcohol Alcohol.* **24,** 217–223.

[54] E. Rubin, H. Gang, P. S. Misra, and C. S. Lieber (1970) Inhibition of drug metabolism by acute ethanol intoxication: A hepatic microsomal mechanism. *Am. J. Med.* **49,** 801–806.

[55] R. Schuppel (1969) The influence of acute ethanol administration on drug conjugation in the rat. *Nauyn-Schmiedeberg Arch. Exp. Path. Pharmacol.* **265,** 233–243.

[56] H. L. Kaplan, N. C. Jain, R. B. Forney, and A. B. Richards, (1969) Chloral hydrate-ethanol interactions in the mouse and dog. *Toxicol. Appl. Pharmacol.* **14,** 127–137.

[57] J. Caballeria, E. Baroana, M. Rodamilans, and C. S. Lieber (1989) Effect of cimetidine on gastric alcohol dehydrogenase activity and blood ethanol level. *Gastroenterology* **97,** 388–392.

[58] J. Caballeria, E. Baroana, M. Rodamilans, and C. S. Lieber (1989) Cimetidine and alcohol absorption. *Gastroenterology* **97,** 1067–1068.

[59] B. Kissing (1974) Interactions of ethyl alcohol and other drugs, in *The Biology of Alcoholism, Clinical Pathology,* vol. 3. B. Kissing and H. Begleiter, eds. Plenum, New York, pp. 109–161.

[60a] A. Smith, R. N. Freeman, and R. D. Harbison (1981) Ethanol enhancement of cocaine-induced hepatotoxicity. *Biochem. Pharmacol.* **30,** 453–458.

[60b] O. E. Odeleye, R. R. Watson, C. D. Eskelson, and A. A. Odeleye (1991) Synergistic hepatotoxic effects of ethanol on cocaine metabolism and lipid peroxidation. *Fed. Am. Soc. Exp. Biol. J.* **5,** 4135.

[61] C. S. Boyer and D. R. Petersen (1990) Potentiation of cocaine-mediated hepatotoxicity for acute and chronic ethanol. *Alcohol. Clin. Exp. Res.* **14,** 28–31.

[62] O. E. Odeleye and R. R. Watson (1990) Is the Lieber-DeCarli diet adequate in vitamin E? *Alcohol Alcohol.* **25,** 433–434.

[63] R. Teschke, M. Minzlaff, H. Oldiges, and H. Frenzel (1983) Alcohol consumption and tumor incidence due to diamethylnitrosamine administration. *Alcohol Alcohol.* **18,** 129–133.

[64] S. I. Mufti, G. Becker, and I. G. Sipes (1989) Effect of chronic dietary ethanol consumption on the initiation and promotion of chemically-induced esophageal carcinogenesis in experimental rats. *Carcinogenesis* **10,** 303–309.

[65] S. I. Mufti, M. Salvagnini, C. S. Lieber, and A. T. Garro (1988) Chronic ethanol consumption inhibit repair of dimethylnitrosamine-induced DNA alkylation. *Biochem. Biophys. Res. Commun.* **152,** 423–431.

[66] K. Ohnishi, H. Terabayashi, T. Unuma, A. Takahashi, and K. Okuda (1987) Effect of habitual alcohol intake and cigarette smoking on the development of hepatocellular carcinoma. *Alcohol. Clin. Exp. Res.* **11,** 45–48.

[67] C. S. Lieber (1990) Interaction of ethanol with drugs, hepatotoxic agents, carcinogens and vitamins. *Alcohol Alcohol.* **25,** 157–176.

[68] M. S. Gold, L. Semlitz, C. A. Dackis, and T. Extein (1985) The adolescent cocaine epidemic. *Semin. Adolesc. Med.* **1,** 303–309.

[69] R. K. Mittleman and C. U. Wethi (1984) Death caused by recreational cocaine use. An update. *J. Am. Med. Assoc.* **252,** 1889–1893.

[70] D. J. Stewart, T. Inaba, M. Larcassen, and W. Kalow (1979) Cocaine metabolism: Cocaine and norcocaine hydrolysis by liver and serum esterases. *Clin. Pharmacol. Ther.* **25,** 464–468.

[71] D. J. Stewart, T. Inaba, B. K. Tan, and W. Kalow (1977) Hydrolysis of cocaine in human plasma by cholinesterase. *Life Sci.* **20,** 1557–1564.

[72] M. W. Kloss, G. M. Rosen, and E. J. Rauckman (1984) Cocaine mediated hepatotoxicity, a critical review. *Biochem. Pharmacol.* **33,** 169–173.

[73] M. W. Kloss, J. Cavagnaro, C. M. Rosen, and E. J. Rauckman (1982) Involvement of FAD-containing monooxygenase in cocaine induced hepatotoxicity. *Toxicol. Appl. Pharmacol.* **64,** 88–93.

[74] M. L. Thompson, L. Shuster, and K. Shaw (1979) Cocaine induced hepatic necrosis in mice—the role of cocaine metabolism. *Biochem. Pharmacol.* **28,** 2389–2395.

[75] V. Marks and P. A. Chapple (1967) Hepatic dysfunction in heroin and cocaine users. *Br. J. Addict.* **62,** 189–195.

[76] C. D. Klaasen and G. L. Plaa (1969) Comparison of the biochemical alterations elicited in livers from rats treated with carbon tetrachloride, chlorform, 1,1,2-trichloroethane and 1,1,1-trichloroethane. *Biochem. Pharmacol.* **18,** 2019–2027.

[77] M. W. Kloss, G. M. Rosen, and E. J. Rauckman (1982) Acute cocaine-induced hepatotoxicity in DBA/2Ha male mice. *Toxicol. Appl. Pharmacol.* **65,** 75–83.

[78] M. W. Kloss, G. M. Rosen, and E. J. Rauckman (1983) Evidence of enhanced in vivo lipid peroxidation after acute cocaine administration. *Toxic. Lett.* **15,** 65–70.

[79] B. Chance, H. Sies, and A. Boveris (1979) Hydroperoxide metabolism in mammalian organ. *Physiol. Rev.* **59,** 527–605.

[80] R. F. Burk (1990) Protection against free radical injury by seleno enzymes. *Pharmacol. Ther.* **45,** 383–385.

[81] S. L. Marklund (1987) Caeruloplasm extracellular superoxide dismutase and scavenging, superoxide anion radicals. *J. Free Rad. Biol. Med.* **2,** 255–260.

[82] P. B. McCay, D. D. Gibson, K. L. Fong, and K. R.Hornbrook (1976) Effect of glutathione peroxidase activity on lipid peroxidation in biological membranes. *Biochim. Biophys. Acta* **431,** 459–465.

[83] R. F. Burk, R. A. Lawrence, and J. M. Lane (1980) Liver necrosis and lipid peroxidation in the rat as the result of paraquat and diquat administration. *J. Clin. Invest.* **65,** 1024–1031.

[84] S. D. Mercurio and G. F. Combs (1986) Selenium-dependent glutathione peroxidase inhibitors increase toxicity of pro-oxidant compounds. *J. Nutr.* **116,** 1726–1734.

[85] K. Takahashi, P. E. Newberger, and H. J. Cohen (1986) Glutathione peroxidase protein. Absence of selenium deficiency states and correlation of enzymatic activity. *J. Clin. Invest.* **77,** 1402–1404.

[86] R. Nordmann, C. Ribiere, and H. Rovach (1990) Ethanol-induced peroxidation and oxidative stress in extrahepatic tissues. *Alcohol Alcohol.* **25,** 231–237.

[87] O. Strubelt, M. Yones, and R. Pentz (1987) Enhancement by glutathione depletion of ethanol-induced acute hepatotoxicity in vitro and in vivo. *Toxicology* **45,** 213–223.

[88] L. A. Videla, F. G. Ugarte, and A. Valenzuela (1980) Effect of acute ethanol intoxication on the content of glutathione of the liver in relation to its lipoperoxidative capacity in the rat. *FEBS Lett.* **111,** 6–10.

[89] V. Fernandez and L. A. Videla (1981) Effect of acute and chronic ethanol ingestion on the content of reduced lutathione of various tissues of the rat. *Experimentia* **37,** 392–394.

[90] G. Vendemials, E. Altomase, I. Grattagliano, and O. Albano (1989) Increased plasma levels of glutathione and malondialdehyde after acute ethanol ingestion in humans. *J. Hepatol.* **9,** 359–365.

[91] J. L. Pierson and M. C. Mitchell (1986) Increased hepatic efflux of glutathione after chronic ethanol feeding. *Biochem. Pharmacol.* **35,** 1533–1537.

[92] H. Spiesky, A. McDonald, G. Giles, H. Orrego, and Y. Israel (1985) Increased loss and decreased synthesis of hepatic lutathione after acute ethanol administration. *Biochem. J.* **225,** 565–572.

[93] J. Vina, J. N. Estrella, D. Guerri, and F. J. Romero (1980) Effect of ethanol on glutathione concentration in isolated hepatocyte. *Biochem. J.* **188,** 549–552.

[94] L. A. Videla and A. Valenzuela (1982) Alcohol ingestion, liver glutathione and lipoperoxidation. Metabolic interrelationship and patholoical implication. *Life Sci.* **31,** 2395–2407.

[95] C. S. Lieber (1988) Metabolic effects of ethanol and its interaction with other drugs, hepatotoxic agents, vitamins and carcinogens: A 1988 update. *Semin. Liver Dis.* **8,** 47–68.

[96] H. T. Nagasawa, J. A. Elberling, and E. G. DeMaster (1980) Structural requirements for the sequestration of metabolically enerated acetaldehyde. *J. Med. Chem.* **23,** 140–143.

[97] E. J. Rauckman, J. Cavagnaro, and G. M. Rosen (1982) Norcocaine nitroxide. A potential hepatotoxic metabolite of cocaine. *Mol. Pharmacol.* **21,** 458–463.

[98] M. A. Evans (1983) Role of protein building in cocaine-induced hepatic necrosis. *J. Pharmacol. Exp. Ther.* **224,** 73–79.

[99] K. A. Suarez, P. Bhonste, and D. L. Richardson (1986) Protective effect of N-acetylcysteine treatment against cocaine induced hepatotoxicity and lipid peroxidation in the mouse. *Res. Comm. Subst. Abuse* **7,** 7–18.

[100] S. F. Marklund, N. G. Westman, E. Lundgren, G. Roos (1982) Copper and zinc containing superoxide dismutase, manganese-containing superoxide dismutase, catalase, and glutathione peroxidase in normal and neoplastic human cell lines and normal human tissues. *Cancer Res.* **42,** 1955–1961.

[101] P. Nicholls and G. R. Schonbaum (1963) Catalases, in *The Enzymes*, vol. 8. P. D. Boyer, H. Hardy, and H. Myrback, eds. Academic, New York, pp. 147–225.

[102] A. I. Cedarbaum and E. Dicker (1983) Inhibition of microsomal oxidation of alcohol's and of hydroxyl radical scavenging agents by the iron-chelating agent desferrioxamine. *Biochem. J.* **210**, 107–113.

[103] R. Nordman, C. Ribiere, and H. Rovach (1987) Involvement of iron and iron catalysed free radical production in ethanol metabolism and toxicity. *Enzyme* **37**, 57–69.

[104] B. Halliwell and J. M. Gutteridge (1989) *Free Radical in Biology and Medicine.* Clarendon, Oxford, pp. 189–276.

[105] J. T. Brown and B. V. Charlwood (1986) The accumulation of essential oils, tissue cultures of *Pelargonium frarans* (wild). *FEBS Lett.* **205**, 117–120.

[106] I. C. U. Ingold, A. C. Webb, D. Willer, G. W. Burton, T. A. Metcalfe, and D. P. Muller (1987) Vitamin E remains the major lipid soluble, chain breaking antioxidant in human plasma even in individuals suffering severe vitamin E deficiency. *Arch. Biochem. Biophys.* **259**, 224–225.

[107] E. H. Gruger and A. L. Tappel (1971) Reactions of biological antioxidants. Composition of biological membranes. *Lipids* **6**, 147–148.

[108] A. Benedetti and M. Comporti (1987) Formation, reactions and toxicity of aldehydes produced in the course of lipid peroxidation in cellular membranes. *Bioelectrochem. Bioenerg.* **18**, 187–196.

[109] O. E. Odeleye, C. D. Eskelson, C. O. Watson, R. R. Watson, S. I. Mufti, and M. Chvapil (1991) Vitamin E reduction of lipid peroxidation products in rats fed cod liver oil and ethanol. *Alcohol* (in press).

[110] C. J. Dillard and A. L. Tappel (1980) Lipid peroxidation products in biological tissues. *Free Radical Biol. Med.* **7**, 193-196.

[111] L. J. Machlin (1984) Anti-oxidant nutrients, in *Handbook of Vitamins*. L. J. Machlin, ed. Marcel Dekker, New York, pp. 96–146.

[112] E. Niki, T. Saito, A. Kawakani, and Y. Kamiya (1984) Inhibition of oxidation of methyl linoleate in solution by vitamin E and vitamin C. *J. Biol. Chem.* **259**, 4177–4182.

[113] H. W. Leung, M. J. Vang, and R. D. Mavis (1981) The cooperative interraction between vitamin E and vitamin C in suppression of peroxidation of membrane phospholipids. *Biochim. Biophys. Acta.* **664**, 266–272.

[114] J. E. Packer, T. F. Slater, and R. L. Willson (1979) Direct observation of a free radical interraction between vitamin A and vitamin C. *Nature* **278**, 737–738.

[115] E. Niki, J. Tsuchiya, and Y. Tanimura (1982) ESR study of radicals reactions with vitamin C, glutathione and thiophenol. *Chem. Lett.* 789–792.

[116] H. Wafers and H. Sies (1988) The protection by ascorbate and glutathione against lipid peroxidation is dependent on vitamin E. *Eur. J. Biochem.* **174**, 353–357.

[117] O. E. Odeleye, C. D. Eskelson, R. R. Watson, S. I. Mufti, and D. Earnest (1991) The effects of chronic ethanol and cod liver oil consumption on rat liver lipid composition: Modulatory role of vitamin E. Submitted to *Alcohol Alcohol.*

[118] A. Bendich and J. A. Olson (1988) Biological actions of the carotenoids. *FASEB J.* **48,** 292–383.

[119] O. Straub (1987) *Key to Carotenoids,* 2nd Ed. H. Pfander, ed. Biekhausen Vexlag, Basel, pp. 1–296.

[120] G. W. Burton (1989) Antioxidant actions of carotenoids. *J. Nutr.* **119,** 109–111.

[121] C. S. Foote (1976) Photosensitized oxidation and singler oxygen: Consequences in biological membranes, in *Free Radical in Biology,* vol. 2. W. A. Pryor, ed. Academic, New York, p. 85–124.

[122] G. W. Burton and K. U. Ingold (1984) B-carotene: An unusual type of lipid antioxidant. *Science* **224,** 569–573.

[123] S. T. Mayne and R. E. Parker (1989) Antioxidant activity of dietary canthaxanthin. *Nutr. Cancer* **12,** 225–236.

[124] E. J. Diliberto, G. Dean, C. Carter, and P. L. Allen (1982) Tissue, subcellular and submitochondral, distribution of semidehydroascorbate reductase. Possible role of semidehydroascorbate reductase in cofactor regeneration. *J. Neurochem.* **39,** 563–568.

[125] L. G. Forni and R. L. Willson (1983) Vitamin C and consecutive hydrogen atom and electron transfer reaction in free radical protection: A novel catalytic role for glutathione, in *Protective Agents in Cancer.* D. C. McBrien and T. F. Slatter, eds. Academic, London, pp. 159–173.

[126] G. Kallitratos, E. Fasske, A. Donos, A. Vadalouka-Kalfaka, and V. Kou (1983) The prophylactic and therapeutic effect of vitamin C on experiential malignant tumors, in *Protective Agents in Cancer.* D. C. McBrien and T. F. Slatter, eds. Academic, London, pp. 221–242.

[127] A. Bendich (1986) The antioxidant role of vitamin C. *Adv. Free Rad. Biol. Med.* **2,** 419–425.

[128] E. Nikki, T. Saito, and Y. Kamiya (1983) The role of vitamin C as an antioxidant. *Chem. Lett.* (Japan), 631–632.

[129] B. Halliwell, M. Wasil, and M. Grootveld (1987) Biologically-significant scavenging of the myeloperoxidase-derived oxidant hypochlorous acid by ascorbic acid. *FEBS Lett.* **213,** 15–18.

[130] K. J. Kunert and A. L. Tappel (1983) The effect of vitamin C on in vivo lipid peroxidation in guinea pigs as measured by pentane and ethane exhalation. *Lipids* **18,** 271–274.

[131] R. C. Denney and R. Johnson (1984) Nutrition, alcohol, and drug abuse. *Proc. Nutr. Soc.* **43,** 265–279.

[132] C. S. Lieber (1988) The influence of alcohol on nutritional status. *Nutr. Rev.* **46,** 241–254.

[133] D. Brenout, M. Peterman, G. Ugarte, G. Barrera, and H. Ituoriaga (1987) Nitrogen economy in alcoholic patients without liver disease. *Metabolism* **36,** 651–653.

[134] S. S. Schreiber, M. Dratz, M. A. Rothschild, F. Reff, and C. Evans (1974) Alcoholic carcinopathy. II. Inhibition of cardiac microsomal protein synthesis by acetaldehyde. *J. Mol. Cell. Cardiol.* **6,** 207–214.

[135] D. Stamm, E. Hansert, and W. Feurlein (1984) Excessive consumption of alcohol in men as biological influence factor in clinical laboratory investigations. *J. Clin. Chem. Clin. Biochem.* **22,** 65–77.

[136] C. S. Lieber (1989) Alcohol and nutrition: An overview. *Alcohol Health Res. World* **13,** 197–205.

[137] D. J. Tuma, C. A. Casey, and M. F. Sorrell (1990) Effects of ethanol on hepatic protein trafficking. Impairment of receptor-mediated endocytosis. *Alcohol Alcohol.* **25,** 117–125.

[138a] C. C. Cunningham, W. B. Coleman, and P. Spach (1990) The effect of chronic ethanol consumption hepatic mitochondrial energy metabolism. *Alcohol Alcohol.* **25,** 127–136.

[138b] D. J. Tuma and M. F. Sorrell (1988) Effects of ethanol on protein trafficking in the liver. *Semin. Liver Dis.* **8,** 69–80.

[139] M. E. Mohs and R. R. Watson (1989) Changes in nutrient status and balance associated with alcohol abuse, in *Diagnosis of Alcohol Abuse.* R. R. Watson, ed. CRC, Boca Raton, FL, pp. 125–146.

[140] R. C. Pirola and C. S. Lieber (1972) The energy cost of the metabolism of drugs including ethanol. *Pharmacology* **7,** 185–196.

[141] J. R. Crouse and S. M. Grundy (1984) Effect of alcohol on plasma lipoproteins, cholesterol and triglyceride metabolism in man. *J. Lipid Res.* **25,** 486–496.

[142] M. Tsutsumi, J. M. Laskez, M. Shiniqu, A. S. Rosman, and C. S. Lieber (1989) The intralobular distribution of ethanol-inducible P450IIE1 in rat and human liver. *Hepatology* **10,** 437–446.

[143] P. I. Spait, R. E. Bottenus, and C. C. Cunningham (1982) Control of adenine mitochondria from rats with ethanol-induced fatty liver. *Biochem. J.* **202,** 445–452.

[144] M. Arai, E. R. Gordon, and C. S. Lieber (1984) Decreased cytochrome oxidase activity in hepatic mitochondria after chronic ethanol consumption and the possible role of decreased cytochrome aa3 content and changes in phospholipid. *Biochim. Biophys. Acta* **797,** 327.

[145] C. S. Lieber, E. Baroana, Hernandez-Munoz, S. Kubota, N. Sato, S. Kawano, T. Natsumura, and N. Inatomi (1989) Impaired oxygen utilization: A new mechanism for the hepatotoxicity of ethanol in sub-human primates. *J. Clin. Invest.* **83,** 1682–1690.

[146] G. D. Guthrie, K. J. Myers, E. J. Gesser, G. W. White, and J. R. Koehl (1990) Alcohol as a nutrient: Interactive between ethanol and carbohydrate. *Alcohol. Clin. Exp. Res.* **14,** 17–22.

[147] S. Takase, M. Yasuhura, A. Takada, and Y. Ueshima (1990) Changes in blood acetaldehyde levels after ethanol administration in alcoholics. *Alcohol* **7**, 37–41.

[148] E. Rubin, D. S. Beattie, and C. S. Lieber (1970) Effect of ethanol on the biogenesis of mitohondrial functions. *Lab. Invest.* **23**, 620–627.

[149] H. SanKaran, C. Y. Nishimura, J. C. Lin, E. C. Larkin, and G. A. Rao (1989) Regulation of pancreatic amylase by dietary carbohydrase in chronic alcoholic rats. *Pancreas* **4**, 733–738.

[150] E. A. Sotaniemi, K. Keinamen, J. T. Lahtela, R. D. Costas, M. Cruz-Vidal, R. D. Abbott, and R. J. Havik (1985) Carbohydrate intolerance associated with reduced hepatic lucose phosphorylating and releasing enzymes activities and peripheral insulin resistance in alcoholics with liver cirrhosis. *J. Hepatology* **1**, 277–290.

[151] M. Arakawa, S. Taketomi, K. Furuno, T. Matsuo, H. Iwatsuka, and S. Suzuoki (1975) Metabolic studies on the development of ethanol-induced fatty liver in KK-AY mice. *J. Nutr.* **105**, 1500–1508.

[152] M. P. Salaspuro, W. A. Ross, E. Jayatilleke, S. Shaw, and C. S. Lieber (1981) Attenuation of the ethanol induced hepatic redox change after chronic alcohol consumption in baboons: Metabolic consequences in vivo and in vivo. *Hepatology* **1**, 33–38.

[153] R. Blomstrand, L. Kager, and O. Lantto (1973) Status on studies on the ethanol-induced decrease of fatty acid oxidation in rats and human liver slices. *Life Sci.* **13**, 1131–1141.

[154] E. A. Nikkila and K. Ojala (1963) Role of hepatic L-alpha-glycero phosphate and triglyceride synthesis in production of fatty acid liver by ethanol. *Proc. Soc. Exp. Biol. Med.* **113**, 814–817.

[155] H. Brunengraber, M. Boutry, L. Lowenstein, and J. M. Lowenstein (1974) The effect of ethanol on lipogenesis by the perfused liver, in *Alcohol and Aldehyde Metabolizing Systems.* R. G. Wurman, T. Yonetani, J. R. Williamson, and B. Chance, eds. Academic, New York, pp. 329–337.

[156] M. J. Savolainen and T. E. Hassinen (1980) Effect of ethanol on hepatic phosphotidate phosphohydroxylase. Dose-dependent enzyme induction and its abolition by adrenalectomy and pyrazole treatment. *Arch. Biochem. Biophys.* **201**, 640–645.

[157] M. J. Savolainen (1977) Stimulation of hepatic phosphotidate phosphohydrolase activity by a single dose of ethanol. *Biochem. Biophys. Res. Commun.* **75**, 511–518.

[158] O. E. Odeleye, C. D. Eskelson, R. R. Watson, and S. I. Mufti (1991) Composition of hepatic lipids after ethanol, cod liver oil and vitamin E feeding in rats. *Adv. Exp. Med. Biol.* **283**, 785–788.

[159] E. O. Uthus, D. N. Skurdal, and W. E. Cornatzer (1976) Effect of ethanol ingestion on choline phosphotransferase and phosphatidyl ethanol amine methyltransferase activities in liver microsomes. *Lipids* **11**, 641–644.

[160] E. Nezey, J. J. Potter, R. T. Slusser, D. Brandes, J. Romero, T. Tanura, and C. H. Halsted (1980) Effect of ethanol feeding on hepatic lysosomes in the monkey. *Lab. Invest.* **43**, 83–93.

[161] E. Nezey, J. J. Potter, and R. A. Ammon (1976) Effect of ethanol administration on the activity of hepatic lysosomal enzymes. *Biochem. Pharmacol.* **25**, 2663–2667.

[162] N. Takeuchi, N. Ito, and Y. Yamamura (1974) Esterification of cholesterol and hydrolysis of cholesteryl ester in alcohol induced fatty liver of rats. *Lipids* **9**, 353–357.

[163] J. L. Boyer (1972) Effect of chronic ethanol feeding on bile formation and secretion of lipids in the rat. *Gastroenterology* **62**, 294–301.

[164] A. F. Lefevre, L. N. DeCarli, and C. S. Lieber (1972) Effect of ethanol on cholesterol and bile acid metabolism. *J. Lipid Res.* **13**, 48–55.

[165] S. C. Cunnane, K. R. McAdoo, and D. F. Horrobin (1987) Long-term ethanol consumption in the hamster: Effects on tissue lipids, fatty acids and erythrocyte hemolysis. *Ann. Nutr. Metab.* **31**, 265–271.

[166] M. R. Lakshmanan and R. L. Veech (1977) Short- and long-term effect of ethanol administration in vivo on rat liver HMG-CoA reductase and cholesterol 7-hydroxylase activities. *J. Lipid Res.* **18**, 325–330.

[167] H. Rottenberg (1986) Membrane solubility of ethanol in chronic alcoholism: The effect of ethanol feeding and its withdrawal on the protection by alcohol of rat red blood cells from hypotonic hemolysis. *Biochem. Biophys. Acta* **855**, 211–212.

[168] A. Benedetti, A. M. Birabell, E. Brunell, G. Curatola, G. Feretti, U. Del-Prete, A. M. Jezequel, and F. Orlandi (1987) Modification of lipid composition of erythrocyte membranes in chronic alcoholism. *Pharm. Res. Commun.* **19**, 657–662.

[169] R. A. Harris, D. M. Baxter, M. A. Mitchell, and R. J. Hitzemann (1984) Physical properties and lipid composition of brain membranes from ethanol tolerant dependent mice. *Mol. Pharm.* **25**, 401–409.

[170] T. F. Taraschi, J. S. Ellingson, A. G. Wu, R. Zimmerman, and E. Rubin (1986) Membrane tolerance to ethanol is rapidly lost after withdrawal: A model for studies of membrane adaptation. *Proc. Natl. Acad. Sci. USA* **83**, 3669–3673.

[171] R. C. Aloia, J. Paxton, J. S. Daviau, O. Van Gelb, W. Mlekusch, W. Truppe, J. A. Meyer, and E. S. Bralles (1985) Effect of chronic ethanol consumption on brain microsome lipid composition, membrane fluidity and Na+-K+-ATPase activity. *Life Sci.* **36**, 1003–1017.

[172] C. Alling, L. Gustavsson, A. A. S. Kristensson, and S. Wallersteid (1984) Changes in fatty acid composition of major glycerophospholipids in erythrocyte membranes from chronic alcoholics during withdrawal. *Scand. J. Clin. Lab. Invest.* **44**, 283–289.

[173] S. C. Cunnane, Y. S. Huang, and D. F. Horrobin (1986) Dietary manipulation of ethanol preference in the Syrian Golden Hamster. *Pharm. Biochem. Behav.* **25**, 1285–1292.

[174] R. A. Harris, D. M. Baxter, M. A. Mitchell, and R. J. Hitzemann (1984) Physical properties and lipid composition of brain membranes from ethanol tolerant-dependent mice. *Mol. Pharm.* **25**, 401–409.

[175] J. Neiman, T. Cursted, and T. Cronholm (1987) Composition of platelets phosphatidylinositol and phosphatidycholine after ethanol withdrawal. *Thrombosis Res.* **46**, 295–301.

[176] N. Salem, Jr. and J. W. Karanian (1988) Polyunsaturated fatty acids and ethanol. *Adv. Alcohol Subst. Abuse* **7**, 183–197.

[177] P. La-Droitte, Y. Lamboeuf, G. DeSaint-Blanquat, and J. P. Bezaury (1985) Sensitivity of individual erythrocyte membrane phospholipid to changes in fatty acid composition in chronic alcoholic patients. *Alcohol. Clin. Exp. Res.* **9**, 135–137.

[178] D. F. Horrobin and M. S. Manku (1980) Possible role of prostaglandin E1 in affective disorders and in alcoholism. *Br. Med. J.* **280**, 1363–1366.

[179] E. Glen, L. MacDonnell, I. Glen, and J. Mackenzie (1984) Possible pharmacological approaches to the prevention and treatment of alcohol related CNS impairment: Results of a double blind trial of essential fatty acid, in *Pharmacological Treatments for Alcoholism*. G. Edward and J. Littleton, eds. Methuen, New York, pp. 331–350.

[180] J. Nieman, M. Hillbom, G. Benthin, and E. E. Anggard (1987) Urinary excretion of 2,3-dinor-6-keto prostaglandin F1 alpha and platelets thromboxane formation during ethanol withdrawal in alcoholics. *J. Clin. Pathol.* **5**, 512–515.

[181] M. M. Engler, J. W. Karanian, and N. Salem, Jr. (1987) The effect of gamma-linoleic acid (18, 3 w-6) on alcohol-induced changes in fatty acid composition, blood pressure and its reactivity. *Fed. Proc.* **46**, 1467.

[182] R. C. Reitz, E. Helsabeck, and D. P. Mason (1973) Effect of chronic alcohol ingestion on the fatty acid composition of the heart. *Lipids* **8**, 80–84.

[183] J. H. Littleton, G. R. John, and S. J. Grieve (1979) Alterations in phospholipid composition in ethanol tolerance and dependence. *Alcohol. Clin. Exp. Res.* **3**, 50–56.

[184] N. McIntyre (1984) The effects of alcohol on water, electrolyte and minerals, in *Clinical Biochemistry of Alcoholism*. S. E. Rosalski, ed. Churchill Livingstone, New York, pp. 117.

[185] M. Y. Morgan (1982) Alcohol and the endocrine system. *Med. Bull.* **38**, 35–42.

[186] E. L. Krawitt (1973) Ethanol inhibits intestinal calcium transport in rats. *Nature* **243**, 88–89.

[187] E. B. Flink (1986) Magnesium deficiency in alcoholism. *Alcohol. Clin. Exp. Res.* **10**, 590–594.

[188] L. T. Iseri, J. Freed, and A. R. Bures (1975) Magnesium deficiency and cardiac disorders. *Am. J. Med.* **58**, 837–846.

[189] W. N. Burton and L. Gladstone (1982) M.I.L.T. Laboratory clues to the diagnosis of alcoholism. *Med. J.* **161**, 265–268.

[190] M. B. Van der Weyden, H. Fong, H. H. Salem, R. G. Batey, and F. J. Dudley (1983) Erythrocyte ferritin content in idiopathic haemochromatosis and alcoholic liver disease with iron overload. *Br. Med. J. (Clin. Res.)* **286,** 752–754.

[191] D. Savage and J. Lindenbaum (1986) Anemia in alcoholics. *Medicine* (Baltimore) **65,** 322–327.

[192] L. Feinman (1989) Absorption and utilization of nutrients in alcoholism. *Alcohol Health Res. World* **13,** 207–210.

[193] C. T. Wu, J. N. Lee, and W. W. Shen (1984) Serum zinc, copper, and ceruloplasmin levels in male alcoholics. *Biol. Psychiatry* **19,** 1333–1338.

[194] C. J. McClain and L. C. Su (1983) Zinc deficiency in the alcoholics: A review. *Alcohol. Clin. Exp. Res.* **7,** 510.

[195] A. R. Tanner, I. Bantock, L. Hinks, B. Lloyd, N. R. Turner, and R. Wright (1986) Depressed selenium and vitamin E levels in an alcoholic population: Possible relationship to hepatic injury through lipid peroxidation. *Dig. Dis. Sci.* **31,** 1307–1312.

[196] J. Canalese, R. B. Sewell, L. Poston, and R. Williams (1985) Zinc abnormalities in fulminant hepatic failure. *Aust. NZ J. Med.* **15,** 7–9.

[197] C. J. McClain, D. R. Antonow, D. A. Cohen, and S. I. Shedlofsky (1986) Zinc metabolism in alcoholic liver disease. *Alcohol. Clin. Exp. Res.* **10,** 582–589.

[198] B. Richard, D. M. Flint, and M. L. Wahlquist (1981) Acute effects of food and ethanol on plasma zinc concentration. *Nutr. Rep. Int.* **23,** 939–943.

[199] Review (1985) Zinc deficiency impairs ethanol metabolism. *Nutr. Rev.* **43,** 158–159.

[200] R. M. Aturokala and C. A. Herath (1985) Zinc and vitamin A status of alcoholics in Sri Lanka, *13th Int. Cong. Nutr.* Brighton, UK, Aug. 18, pp. 136 (Abstract).

[201] T. R. Hartoma, E. A. Sotaniemi, and J. Maathanen (1979) Effects of zinc on some biochemical indices of metabolism. *Nutr. Metab.* **23,** 203–294.

[202] R. R. Chandra and B. Au (1980) Single nutrient deficiency and cell mediated immune responses. 1. Zinc. *Am. J. Clin. Nutr.* **33,** 736–738.

[203] L. C. Yeh and F. L. Cerklewski (1985) Interaction between ethanol and low dietary zinc during gestation and lactation in the rat. *J. Nutr.* **114,** 2027–2033.

[204] S. K. Dutta, P. A. Miller, L. B. Greenberg, and O. A. Levander (1983) Selenium and acute alcoholism. *Am. J. Clin. Nutr.* **38,** 713–718.

[205] B. Dworkin, W. S. Rosenthal, R. H. Jankowski, and D. Haldea (1985) Low blood selenium levels in alcoholics with and without advanced liver disease: Correlation with clinical and nutritional status. *Dig. Dis. Sci.* **30,** 838–844.

[206] H. Rorpela, J. Kampulainen, and P. V. Luoma (1985) Decreased serum selenium in alcoholics as related to liver structure and function. *Am. J. Clin. Nutr.* **42,** 147–151.

[207] M. J. Valimaki, K. J. Harju, and R. H. Ylikahri (1983) Decreased serum

selenium in alcoholics: A consequence of liver dysfunctions. *Clin. Chem. Acta* **130,** 291–296.

[208] H. Shah, A. Smith, and M. F. Picciano (1985) Plasma selenium levels in alcoholic liver disease and primary biliary cirrhosis. *Nutr. Res.* **5 (Suppl. 1),** S-385–S-387.

[209] B. Wood and K. J. Breen (1979) Vitamin deficiency in alcoholism with particular reference to thiamine deficiency. *Clin. Exp. Pharm. Physiol.* **6,** 457–458.

[210] C. M. Leevy, H. Baker, W. Tenhove, O. Frank, and G. R. Cherrick (1965) B-complex vitamins in liver disease of the alcoholic. *Am. J. Clin. Nutr.* **16,** 339–346.

[211] J. N. Neville, J. A. Eagles, G. Samson, and R. E. Olson (1968) Nutritional status of alcoholics. *Am. J. Clin. Nutr.* **21,** 1329–1340.

[212] M. Baines (1978) Detection and incidence of B and C vitamin deficiency in alcohol-related illnesses. *Ann. Clin. Biochem.* **15,** 307–312.

[213] A. S. Truswell, T. Konno, and J. D. Hansen (1972) Thiamine deficiency in adult hospital patients. *S. Afr. Med. J.* **46,** 2079–2082.

[214] H. Baker and O. Frank (1978) Absorption, utilization and clinical effectiveness of allithiamines compared to water-soluble thiamines. *J. Nutr. Sci. Vitaminol.* **22 (Suppl.),** 63–68.

[215] A. M. Hoyumpa, K. J. Breen, S. Schenker, and F. A. Wilson (1975) Thiamine transport across the rat intestine. II. Effect of ethanol. *Lab. Clin. Med.* **86,** 803–816.

[216] J. Fennelly, O. Frank, H. Baker, and C. M. Leevy (1964) Peripheral neuropathy of the alcoholic: I, Aetiological role of aneurin and other B-complex vitamins. *Br. Med. J.* **2,** 1290–1292.

[217] P. W. Kershaw (1967) Blood thiamine and nicotine acid levels in alcoholism and confusional states. *Br. J. Psychiat.* **113,** 387–393.

[218] D. S. McLaren, M. A. Docherty, and D. H. Boyd (1980) *Proc. Nutr. Soc.* **39,** 24A.

[219] V. G. Periera, Z. Masuda, A. Katz, and V. Tronchini (1984) Shonstin beri-beri report of two successfully treated patients with hemodynamic documentation. *Am. J. Cardiol.* **53,** 1467.

[220] K. F. Whyte, M. G. Dunnigan, and W. B. McIntosh (1982) Excessive beer consumption and beri-beri. *Scott. Med. J.* **27,** 288–291.

[221] M. Baines (1978) Detection and incidence of B and C vitamin deficiency in alcohol-related illnesses. *Anal. Clin. Biochem.* **15,** 307–318.

[222] M. Shehata and S. Saad (1978) The effect of aliphatic alcohol on certain vitamins of the B-complex group in the liver of the rat. *Pol. J. Pharmacol. Pharm.* **30,** 35–39.

[223] A. D. Thomson, H. Baker, and C. M. Leevy (1970) Patterns of [13]S-thiamine hydrochloride absorption in the malnourished alcoholic patient. *J. Lab. Clin. Med.* **76,** 34–45.

[224] A. Lemoine, A. Monges, J. L. Codaccioni, P. Bermond, and W. F. Korner (1972) Effect of alcohol intake and riboflavin status of human. *Alcoholism* **18,** 199–217.

[225] L. Pekkanen and M. Rusi (1979) The effects of dietary niacin and riboflavin on voluntary intake and metabolism in rats. *Pharmacol. Biochem. Behav.* **11,** 575–579.

[226] W. S. Rosenthal, N. F. Adham, R. Lopez, and J. M. Cooperman (1973) Riboflavin deficiency in complicated chronic alcoholism. *Am. J. Clin. Nutr.* **26,** 858–860.

[227] C. I. Kim and D. A. Roe (1985) Development of riboflavin deficiency in alcohol fed hamsters. *Drug Nutr. Inter.* **3,** 99–107.

[228] M. Baries (1978) Detection and incidence of B and C vitamins deficiency in alcohol related illness. *Ann. Clin. Biochem.* **15,** 307–312.

[229] M. P. Walsh, P. Howorth, and V. Marks (1966) Pyroxidine deficiency and tryptophan metabolism in chronic alcoholics. *Am. J. Clin. Nutr.* **19,** 379–383.

[230] L. Lumeng and T. K. Li (1974) Vitamin B_6 metabolism in chronic alcohol abuse. *J. Clin. Invest.* **53,** 693–704.

[231] R. E. Davis and R. K. Smith (1974) Pyroxidal and folate deficiency in alcoholics. *Med. J. Austr.* **2,** 357–360.

[232] R. Pluvinage (1975) Alcohol intake and vitamin deficiencies. *C. M. de France* **82,** 3915–3920.

[233] M. S. Devgun, A. Fiabane, C. R. Paterson, and P. Zarembski (1981) Vitamin and mineral nutrition in chronic alcoholics including patients with Korsakoff's psychosis. *Br. J. Nutr.* **45,** 469–473.

[234] R. E. Vanderlinde (1986) Review of pyridoxal phosphate and the transaminase in liver disease. *Ann. Clin. Lab. Sci.* **16,** 79–93.

[235] R. L. Veitch, L. Lumeng, and T. K. Li (1974) The effect of ethanol and acetaldehyde on vitamin B_6 metabolism in liver. *Gastroenterology* **66,** 868.

[236] P. R. Ryle and A. D. Thomson (1984) Nutrition and vitamins in alcoholism, in *Clinical Biochemistry of Alcoholism.* S. B. Rosalski, ed. Churchill Livingstone, New York, pp. 188.

[237] F. Fatteb (1985) Alcohol is dangerous to your health. *J. Am. Med. Assoc.* **20,** 2959–2960.

[238] D. G. Weir, P. G. McGing, and J. M. Scott (1985) Folate metabolism, the enterohepatic circulation and alcohol. *Biochem. Pharmacol.* **34,** 1–7.

[239] V. Herbert, R. Zalusky, and C. S. Davison (1968) Correlation of folate deficiency with alcoholism and associated macrocytosis, anemia and liver disease. *Ann. Intern. Med.* **58,** 977–988.

[240] R. E. Davis (1986) Clinical chemistry of folic acid. *Adv. Clin. Chem.* **25,** 233–294.

[241] C. H. Halsted (1980) Folate deficiency in alcoholism. *Am. J. Clin. Nutr.* **33,** 2736–2741.

[242] A. Wu, I. Chanarin, G. Slavin, and A. J. Levi (1975) Folate deficiency in the alcoholic—its relationship to clinical and haematological abnormalities, liver disease and folate stress. *Br. J. Hematol.* **29,** 469–478.

[243] C. H. Halsted, E. A. Robles, and E. Mezey (1973) Intestinal malabsorption in folate-deficient alcoholics. *Gastroenterology* **64,** 526–532.

[244] R. M. Russell, I. H. Rosenberg, P. D. Wilson, F. L. Iber, E. B. Daks, A. C. Biovetti, C. L. Otradovac, P. A. Karowski, and W. A. Press (1983) Increased urinary excretion and prolonged turnover time of folic acid during ethanol ingestion. *Am. J. Clin. Nutr.* **38,** 64–70.

[245] E. R. Eichner and R. S. Hillman (1973) Effect of alcohol on serum folate level. *J. Clin. Invest.* **52,** 584–591.

[246] C. Paine, E. R. Eichner, and V. Dickson (1973) Concordance of radio-immunoassay and microbiological assay in the study of the ethanol-induced fall in serum folate level. *Am. J. Med. Sci.* **266,** 135–138.

[247] C. H. Halsted, R. C. Griggs, and J. W. Harris (1967) The effect of alcoholism on the absorption of folic acid (H^3-PGA) evaluated by plasma levels and urine excretion. *J. Lab. Clin. Chem.* **69,** 116–131.

[248] F. Lane, P. Goff, R. McGuffin, E. R. Eichner, and R. S. Hillman (1976) Folic acid metabolism in normal, folate deficient and alcoholic man. *Br. J. Hematol.* **34,** 489–500.

[249] C. H. Halsted, E. A. Robles, and E. Mezey (1971) Decreased jejunal uptake of labeled folic acid (3H-PGA) in alcoholic patients: Roles of alcohol and nutrition. *N. Engl. J. Med.* **285,** 701–706.

[250] J. P. Bonjour (1980) Vitamins and alcoholism. II. Folate and B12. *Int. J. Vit. Nutr. Res.* **50,** 96–121.

[251] E. R. Eichner, B. Buchanan, J. W. Smith, and R. S. Hillman (1972) Variation in the hematologic and medical status of alcoholics. *Am. J. Med. Sci.* **263,** 35–42.

[252] C. Kimber, D. J. Deller, R. N. Ibbotson, and H. Lander (1965) The mechanism of anemia in chronic liver disease. *Q. J. Med.* **34,** 33–64.

[253] J. Lindenbaum and C. S. Lieber (1969) Alcohol induced malabsorption of vitamin B_{12} in man. *Nature* **224,** 806.

[254] J. Lindenbaum and C. S. Lieber (1975) Effects of chronic ethanol administration on intestinal absorption in man in the absence of nutritional deficiency. *Ann. NY Acad. Sci.* **252,** 228–234.

[255] D. K. Dastur, Q. Santhadevi, E. V. Quadros, F. C. Avari, N. H. Wadia, M. M. Desai, and E. P. Bharucha (1976) The B-vitamins in malnutrition with alcoholism. *Br. J. Nutr.* **36,** 143–159.

[256] J. Fennelly, O. Frank, H. Baker, and C. M. Leevy (1964) Effect of alcohol on excretion of some water soluble vitamins. *Br. Med. J.* **2,** 1290–1292.

[257] J. E. Rossouw, D. Labadarios, M. Davis, and R. Williams (1978) The degradation of tryptophan in severe liver disease. *Int. J. Vitam. Nutr. Res.* **48,** 281–289.

[258] J. J. Barboriak, C. B. Rooney, T. H. Leitshuh, and A. J. Anderson (1978) Alcohol and nutrient intake of elderly men. *J. Am. Diet. Assoc.* **72**, 493–495.

[259] I. R. Payne, G. H. Lu, and K. Meyer (1974) Relationship of dietary tryptophan and niacin to tryptophan metabolism in alcoholics and non-alcoholics. *Am. J. Clin. Nutr.* **27**, 572–579.

[260] H. G. Tao and H. M. Fox (1976) Measurements of urinary pantothenic acid excretions of alcoholic patients. *J. Nutr. Sci. Vitaminol.* **23**, 333–337.

[261] H. Baker, O. Frank, R. K. Zetterman, K. S. Rajan, W. Tenhove, and C. M. Leevy (1975) Inability of chronic alcoholics with liver disease to use food as a source of folates thiamin and vitamin B_6. *Am. J. Clin. Nutr.* **28**, 1377–1380.

[262] M. Lhuissier and M. Suschetet (1979) Concentrations du foie en quelques vitamins hydrosolubles chez la rat recevant, isolement ou en association, de metabasulfite de potassium, de l'acide tannique et de l'ethanol. *Int. J. Vitam. Nutr. Res.* **49**, 312–316.

[263] National Academy of Science Recommended Dietary Allowance. Biotin. Washington, DC, pp. 120–122.

[264] J. P. Bonjour (1977) Biotin in man's nutrition and therapy — a review. *Int. J. Vitam. Nutr. Res.* **47**, 107–118.

[265] J. Dow and A. Goldberg (1975) Ethanol metabolism in the vitamin C deficient guinea pig. *Biochem. Pharmacol.* **24**, 863–866.

[266] I. U. Shugalei (1987) Features of vitamin C metabolism and the functional status of the liver in alcoholism and alcoholic delirium in the stage of detoxification therapy. *Zh. Neuropathol. Psychiatry* **87**, 240–257.

[267] A. A. Yunice, J. M. Hsu, A. Fahmy, and S. Henry (1984) Ethanol-ascorbate interrelationship in acute and chronic alcoholism in the guinea pig. *Proc. Soc. Exp. Biol. Med.* **177**, 262–280.

[268] H. Sprince, C. M. Parker, G. G. Smith, and L. J. Gonzalez (1975) Protection against acetaldehyde toxicity by ascorbic acid plus reserpine or atropine. *Fed. Proc.* **2**, 34.

[269] H. Sprince, C. M. Parker, G. G. Smith, and L. J. Gonzalez (1975) Protection action of ascorbic acid and sulfur compounds aainst acetaldehyde toxicity: Implications in alcoholism and smoking. *Agents Actions* **5**, 164–172.

[270] R. L. Susick, Jr. and V. G. Zannoni (1984) Ascorbic acid and alcohol oxidation. *Biochem. Pharmacol.* **33**, 3963–3969.

[271] R. M. Russell (1980) Vitamin A and zinc metabolism in alcoholism. *Am. J. Clin. Nutr.* **33**, 2741–2746.

[272] S. K. Majundar, G. K. Shaw, and A. D. Thomson (1983) Blood B-carotene status in chronic alcoholics — a good biochemical marker for malnutrition. *Drug Alcohol Depend.* **12**, 113.

[273] H. W. Gruchow, K. A. Sobocinski, J. J. Barboriak, and J. G. Scheller (1985)

Alcohol consumption, nutrient intake and relative body weight among US adults. *Am. J. Clin. Nutr.* **422,** 289–297.

[274] V. N. Hillers and L. K. Massey (1985) Interrelationship of moderate and high alcohol consumption with diet and health status. *Am. J. Clin. Nutr.* **41,** 356–362.

[275] G. Kvale, E. Bjelke, and J. J. Gart (1983) Dietary habits and lung cancer risk. *Int. J. Cancer* **31,** 397–405.

[276] K. M. Mak, M. A. Leo, and C. S. Lieber (1984) Ethanol potentiates squamous metaplasia of the rat trachea caused by vitamin A deficiency. *Trans. Assoc. Am. Physicians* **98,** 210–221.

[277] P. Nettesheim and M. L. Williams (1976) The influence of vitamin A on the susceptibility of the rat lung by 3-methylcholanthrease. *Br. J. Cancer* **17,** 351–357.

[278] M. A. Leo and C. S. Lieber (1982) Hepatic vitamin A depletion in alcoholic liver injury. *N. Engl. J. Med.* **307,** 597–601.

[279] M. Sato and C. S. Lieber (1981) Hepatic vitamin A depletion after chronic ethanol consumption in the baboons and rats. *J. Nutr.* **111,** 2015–2023.

[280] M. A. Leo, C. Kim, and C. S. Lieber (1986) Increased vitamin A in esophagus and other extrahepatic tissues after chronic ethanol consumption in the rat. *Alcohol. Clin. Exp. Res.* **10,** 487–492.

[281] M. A. Leo and C. S. Lieber (1988) Hypervitaminoses A: A livers lovers lament. *Hepatology* **8,** 412–417.

[282] M. Sato and C. S. Lieber (1982) Changes in vitamin A status after acute ethanol administration in the rat. *J. Nutr.* **112,** 1188–1196.

[283] D. S. Goodman and W. S. Blaner (1984) Biosynthesis, absorption, and hepatic metabolism of retinol, in *The Retinoids.* H. B. Sporn, A. B. Roberts, and D. S. Goodman, eds. Academic, New York, pp. 2–34.

[284] O. E. Odeleye, C. D. Eskelson, J. I. Alak, R. R. Watson, M. Chvapil, and S. I. Mufti (1991) The effects of vitamin E supplementation on hepatic levels of vitamin A and E in ethanol and cod liver oil fed rats. *Int. J. Vitam. Nutr. Res.* (in press)

[285] R. K. Long, R. K. Skinner, M. R. Willis, and S. Sherlock (1978) Formation of vit. D metabolites from 3A & 14C-radiolabelled vit D-3 in chronic liver disease. *Lancet* **2,** 650–652.

[286] D. B. Posner, R. M. Russell, S. Absood, T. B. Connor, C. Davis, L. Martin, J. B. Williams, A. H. Norris, and C. Merchant (1978) Effective 25-hydroxylation of vitamin D_2 in alcoholic cirrhosis. *Gastroenterology* **74,** 866–870.

[287] S. K. Dutta, B. S. Costa, R. M. Russell, and T. B. Connor (1979) Fat soluble vitamin deficiency in treated patients with pancreatic insufficiency. *Gastroenterology* **76,** 1126.

[288] R. T. Jun, M. Davis, J. O. Hunter, T. M. Chalmer, and D. E. Lawson (1978) Abnormal vitamin D metabolism in cirrhosis. *Gut* **19,** 290–293.

[289] E. Mezey (1985) Metabolic effects of alcohol. *Fed. Proc.* **44**, 134–138.

[290] O. Gedik and S. Akaline (1986) Effects of vitamin D deficiency and repletion on insulin and glucagon secretion in man. *Diabetologia* **29**, 142–145.

[291] B. L. Nyomba, R. Bouillon, and P. DeMoor (1984) Influence of vitamin D status on insulin secretion and glucose tolerance in the rabbit. *Endocrinology* **115**, 191–197.

[292] S. A. Clark, W. E. Stumpf, and M. Sar (1981) Effect of 1,25-dihydroxyvitamin D_3 on insulin secretion. *Diabetes* **30**, 382–386.

[293] S. Kadawaki and A. W. Norman (1984) Demonstration that the vitamin D metabolite $1,25(OH)_2$–vitamin D_3 and not $24,25(OH)_2$-vitamin D_3 is essential for normal insulin secretion in the perfused rat pancreas. *Diabetes* **34**, 315–320.

[294] P. B. McCay (1985) Vitamin E. Interaction with free radicals and ascorbate. *Annu. Rev. Nutr.* **5**, 323–340.

[295] E. Nikki (1987) Interaction of ascorbate and alpha-tocopherol. *Ann. NY Acad. Sci.* **498**, 186–199.

[296] G. E. Bjorneboe, A. Bjorneboe, B. F. Hagen, J. Morland, and C. A. Drevon (1987) Reduced hepatic alpha-tocopherol content after long-term administration of ethanol to rats. *Biochim. Biophys. Acta* **918**, 236–241.

[297] A. Bjorneboe, G.A. Bjorneboe, E. Bodd, B. F. Hagen, N. Kveseth, and C. A. Drevon (1986) Transport and distribution of alpha-tocopherol in lymph, serum and liver cells in rats. *Biochim. Biophys. Acta* **889**, 310–315.

[298] G. E. Bjorneboe, J. Johnsen, A. Bjorneboe, J.-E. Bache-Wigg, J. Morland, and G. A. Drevon (1988) Diminished serum concentrations of vitamin E and selenium in alcoholics. *Ann. Nutr. Metab.* **32**, 56–61.

[299] G. E. Bjorneboe, J. Johnsen, A. Bjorneboe, S. L. Marklund, N. Skylv, A. Hoiseth, J.-E. Bache-Wigg, J. Morland, and C. A. Drevon (1988) Some aspects of antioxidant status in blood from alcoholics. *Alcohol. Clin. Exp. Res.* **12**, 806–810.

[300] E. M. Dworkin, W. S. Rosenthal, G. G. Gordon, and R. H. Jankowski (1984) Diminished serum concentration of selenium and vitamin E in alcoholics. *Alcohol. Clin. Exp. Res.* **8**, 535–538.

[301] J. P. Bonjour (1981) Vitamins and alcoholism. X. Vitamin D, XI. Vitamin E, XII. Vitamin K. *Int. J. Vitam. Nutr. Res.* **51**, 307–318.

[302] T. Kawase, S. Kato, and C. S. Lieber (1989) Lipid peroxidation and antioxidant defense system in rats liver after chronic ethanol feedin. *Hepatology* **10**, 815–821.

[303] A. G. Moran, J. Kelleher, B. E. Walker, M. S. Losowsky, H. Droller, and R. S. Middleton (1972) Increased prothrombin time in chronic liver disease. *Int. J. Vitam. Nutr. Res.* **45**, 448–462.

[304] M. E. Mohs and R. R. Watson (1989) Nutritional effects of selected drugs of abuse, in *Biochemistry and Physiology of Substance Abuse*, vol. 1. CRC, Boca Raton, FL, pp. 59-76.

[305] G. R. Gay (1981) You've come a long way, baby! Coke time for the new

American lady of the eighties. *J. Psychoactive Drugs* **13**, 297–318.

[306] F. J. Burczynski, R. L. Boni, J. Erickson and J. Vitti (1987) The effect of erythroxylum coca, cocaine and ecogonine methyl ester as dietary supplement on energy metabolism in the rat. *Enthnopharmacology* **16**, 153–166.

[307] Anonymous (1979) Coca-leaf chewing and public health. *Lancet* **i**, 963.

[308] T. P. Oei (1983) Effect of body weight reduction and food deprivation on cocaine self-administration. *Pharmacol. Biochem. Behav.* **19**, 453–455.

[309] A. A. Buck, T. T. Sasaki, J. J. Hewitt, and A. A. Macrae (1968) Coca chewing and health. An epidemioloic study among residents of a Peruvian village. *Am. J. Epidemiol.* **88**, 159–177.

[310] F. G. Castro, M. D. Newcomb, and K. Cadish (1987) Lifestyle differences between young adult cocaine users and their non-user peers. *J. Drug Ed.* **17**, 89–111.

[311] R. R. Watson and M. E. Mohs (1990) Effects of morphine, cocaine and heroin on nutrition. *Prog. Clin. Biol. Res.* **325**, 413–418.

[312] V. Marks and P. A. Chapple (1967) Hepatic dysfunction in heroin and co-caine users. *Br. J. Addict.* **62**, 189–195.

[313] R. Ramos-Aliaga (1970) Effect of cocaine on the intermediate metabolism of test animals in different nutritional states. *Bol. Soc. Quim. Peru* **36**, 70–98.

[314] R. C. Denney and R. Johnson (1984) Nutrition, alcohol, and drug abuse. *Proc. Nutr. Soc.* **43**, 265–279.

[315] H. F. Havas, G. Dellaria, G. Schiffman, E. Gellez, and M. Adler (1987) Effect of cocaine on the immune response and host resistance in BALB/c mice. *Int. Arch. Allergy Appl. Immunol.* **83**, 377–383.

[316] R. Ramos-Aliaga and J. Cheriboga (1970) Enzymatic n-demethylation of cocaine and nutritional status. *Arch. Latinoam. Nutr.* **20**, 415–428.

[317] R. Ramos-Aliaga and G. Puma (1981) Adaptive increases in liver cocaine N-demethylation induced by the drug in rats receiving different levels of utilization protein: I. Its relationship with protein efficiency. *Comm. Subst. Abuse* **2**, 27–46.

Caffeine Metabolism

Disposition in Liver Disease
and Hepatic-Function Testing

Charles P. Denaro
and Neal L. Benowitz

Introduction

Caffeine is probably the most commonly consumed drug in the world. Caffeine is 1,3,7-trimethylxanthine (137X) and is metabolized by N-demethylation to dimethylxanthines (Fig. 1). All these compounds are pharmacologically active.[1,2] This chapter will describe the metabolism of caffeine and the changes in caffeine metabolism that occur in people with liver disease. We will also examine the use of caffeine to assess cytochrome P-450 function, acetylator status, and liver function in general.

Metabolism

Oral absorption of caffeine is rapid and complete.[3,4] Only a small fraction (1–4%) of caffeine is excreted unchanged in the urine.[4–10] Caffeine is extensively metabolized by the liver. Evidence to support hepatic metabolism includes in vitro studies demonstrating biotransformation of caffeine by human liver microsomes,[11,12] observations of impaired clearance of caffeine in people with liver disease,[13–16] and the well-known effects of induc-

From: *Drug and Alcohol Abuse Reviews, Vol. 2: Liver Pathology and Alcohol*
Ed: R. R. Watson ©1991 The Humana Press Inc.

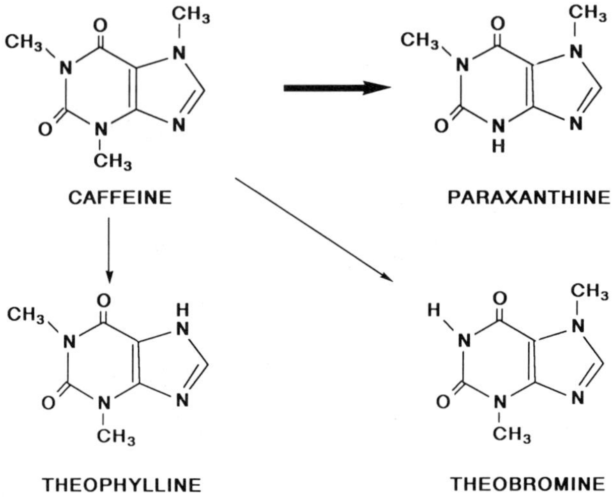

Fig. 1. Chemical structures of caffeine, paraxanthine, theobromine, and theophylline.

ers and inhibitors of hepatic microsomal enzymes on caffeine metabolism.[17–19] Since caffeine is completely bioavailable, the extent of extraction from the blood in each pass through the liver must be low (i.e., a low-extraction drug). Caffeine is bound to plasma proteins (presumably albumin) with binding reported to range from 10 to 35%.[1,20,21]

Table 1 lists the pharmacokinetic parameters of caffeine from nine studies in healthy subjects given single doses of caffeine.[6,10,13,15,22–26] There is a wide interindividual variation in clearance with values ranging almost ninefold. Although some of this variation is attributable to the influence of cigaret smoking on caffeine metabolism, studies in nonsmokers showed a three- or fourfold difference.

The known metabolic pathways of caffeine in humans are illustrated in Fig. 2. The major routes of metabolism are indicated by the heavy arrows. Details of the discovery of these metabolic pathways have been reviewed by Arnaud.[27] The primary and major pathway for the metabolism of caffeine is *N*3-demethylation to paraxanthine (17X).[5] About 80% of caffeine is metabolized via 17X. Approximately 10% of caffeine is *N*1-demethylated to theobromine (37X) and 4% is *N*7-demethylated to theophylline.[28] These dimethylxanthines undergo further *N*-demethylation to

Table 1
Pharmacokinetic Parameters of Caffeine
from Single-Dose Studies[a]

Reference	Volume of distribution, L/kg	Clearance, L/h/kg	Half-life, h
Tang-Liu, 1983[6]	0.52[b]	0.096	5.4
	(0.46–0.58)	(0.038–0.203)	(2.8–9.9)
Denaro, 1990[10]	0.57[c]	0.118	4.0
	(0.41–0.69)	(0.072–0.203)	(2.6–6.1)
Desmond, 1980[13]	0.54[d]	0.084	5.2
	(±0.17)	(±0.03)	(±2.4)
Scott, 1989[15]	0.41[e]	0.088	4.0
	(0.23–0.63)	(0.052–0.146)	(2.1–8.1)
George, 1986[22]	0.84[d]	0.177	3.6
	(0.52–1.14)	(0.077–0.331)	(2.3–5.1)
Lelo, 1986[23]	0.71[c]	0.124	4.1
	NA	(±0.058)	(±1.3)
May, 1982[24]	0.65[d]	0.149	3.2
	(0.56–0.80)	(0.100–0.230)	(2.2–4.0)
Campbell, 1987[f,25]	0.63[d]	0.069	7.3
	(0.50–0.80)	(0.041–0.155)	(2.2–12.1)
Carbo, 1989[26]	0.73[d]	0.153	4.7
	(0.43–1.29)	(0.067–0.293)	(1.0–13.5)
Mean	0.62	0.118	4.6
Range	0.23–1.29	0.038–0.331	1.0–13.5

[a]Results are individual mean values from each study; range or standard deviation given in parentheses. NA = not available.

[b]Extrapolated volume of distribution.

[c]Steady-state volume of distribution.

[d]Volume of distribution calculated from clearance and terminal rate constant — V area.

[e]Volume of distribution calculated from fitted polyexponential curves — presumably steady-state volume of distribution.

[f]Pharmacokinetic values based on salivary concentrations.

monomethylxanthines, in particular 1-methylxanthine (1MX), and all methylxanthines may undergo ring oxidation (hydroxylation) to methyluric acids. Cornish and Christman in 1957 showed that demethylation of caffeine and its metabolites does not go beyond the monomethylated state.[29] Another important pathway is the acetylation of a 17X metabolite

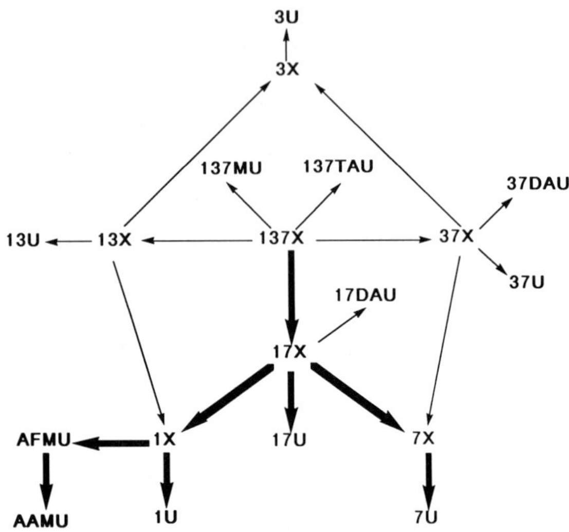

Fig. 2. Metabolic pathways of caffeine. 137X: 1,3,7 dimethylxanthine (caffeine); 17X: 1,7-dimethylxanthine (paraxanthine); 37X: 3,7-dimethylxanthine (theobromine); 13X: 1,3-dimethylxanthine (theophylline); 17U: 1,7-dimethyluric acid; 13U: 1,3-dimethyluric acid; 1X: 1-methylxanthine; 3X: 3-methylxanthine; 7X: 7-methylxanthine; 1U: 1-methyluric acid; 3U: 3-methyluric acid; 7U: 7-methyluric acid; 137MU: 1,3,7-trimethyluric acid; AFMU: 5-acetylamino-6-formylamino-3-methyluracil; AAMU: 5-acetylamino-6-amino-3-methyluracil; 137TAU: 6-amino-5[*N*-formylmethylamino]-1,3-dimethyluracil; 17DAU: 6-amino-5[*N*-formylmethyl-amino]-3-methyluracil; 37DAU: 6-amino-5[*N*-formylmethylamino]-1-methyluracil.

to 5-acetylamino-6-formylamino-3-methyluracil (AFMU).[30,31] AFMU is unstable in vitro and spontaneously transforms to 5-acetylamino-6-amino-3-methyluracil (AAMU).[31]

Table 2 summarizes the urinary recoveries of the various metabolites from seven studies.[4–10] A wide range of recoveries is reported by different investigators. The tabulated coefficient of variation is derived from the mean values in Table 2. The true coefficient of variation for individual values would be larger. This variability probably represents both individual variation in metabolism and methodological problems with various assays. Our experience suggests that the latter may be an important source of variability. The assay for measuring all of these metabolites is technically difficult, and good quality control data for various assays are rarely published. Ratios of the

Table 2
Mean Urinary Recoveries of Caffeine Metabolites, from Literature[a]

Reference	137X	17X	37X	13X	1X	1U	AFMU AAMU	17U	13U	137U	7X	7U	3X	3U	37U
Bonati, 1982[4]	1.2	4.4	2.4	—	12.8	43.6	—	7.4	2.9	—	6.9	—	2.5	—	—
Arnaud, 1981[5]	1.0	6.0	3.0	0.7	11.7	11.7	5.4	9.0	2.6	2.0	6.4	1.4	2.6	.0.1	0.8
Tang-Liu, 1983[6]	3.7	7.1	1.2	0.8	10.0	21.0	—	7.3	2.9	2.5	4.0	4.7	2.3	—	—
Callahan, 1983[7,b]	1.8	4.8	1.1	—	12.2	15.7	14.4	7.1	2.7	0.9	1.9	1.0	2.1	0.6	—
Grant, 1983[8]	—	4.8	1.1	—	10.1	11.8	4.3	6.0	1.2	—	2.5	—	1.5	—	—
Blanchard, 1985[9,c]	2.2	3.5	1.6	0.7	9.2	30.1	—	10.2	3.1	2.8	2.4	7.7	1.2	—	—
Denaro, 1990[10,d]	1.3	4.2	1.3	0.4	8.2	12.5	12.2	4.1	1.3	0.2	3.3	1.5	1.9	—	—
Mean	1.9	5.0	1.7	0.6	10.6	20.9	9.1	7.3	2.4	1.7	3.9	3.3	2.0	—	—
CV[e]	54	24	41	33	16	57	55	27	34	65	51	89	26	—	—

[a]Expressed as mean molar percentage of dose administered. For abbreviations, *see* Fig. 2.
[b]Average of three different populations studied.
[c]Average of two different populations studied.
[d]Average of two different dosing regimens given to same population.
[e]Coefficient of variation expressed as a percentage.

metabolites and their subsequent products in the urine can be used to characterize acetylator phenotype and to indicate the activity of *N*-demethylation, hydroxylation and xanthine oxidase drug-metabolizing enzymes.[8,32,33] This will be discussed in more detail later.

N-Demethylation of caffeine is carried out by the P-450IA subfamily of P-450 enzymes.[11,12,17,34] The nomenclature used comes from the recently proposed classification based on amino acid homology.[35] (This enzyme was previously known as aryl hydrocarbon hydroxylase [AHH] or polycyclic aromatic hydrocarbon inducible P-450, P-448, P_1-450, P-450c.) Ring oxidation (or hydroxylation) to methyluric acids is carried out in part by P-450IA, but a large and variable part is mediated by other enzymes that are not influenced by polycyclic aromatic hydrocarbons.[11]

A clinical implication of the role of P-450IA in metabolizing caffeine is that many drugs that induce or inhibit the metabolism of caffeine interact with theophylline in the same manner. Cigaret smoke and such drugs as phenytoin accelerate caffeine metabolism,[18,36] whereas phenobarbital has little effect.[17,34] Numerous compounds have been shown to inhibit the metabolism of caffeine. These include cimetidine,[19,24] oral contraceptives,[7,21] some quinolone antibiotics,[26,37] mexiletine,[38] methoxsalen,[39] disulfiram,[40] and alcohol (acute ingestion).[22,41] Longer half-lives of caffeine are seen in pregnant women.[42] Erythromycin is expected to interfere with caffeine metabolism, based on its inhibitory effects on the clearance of theophylline.

Neonates lack the capacity to *N*-demethylate caffeine, and they eliminate caffeine primarily by renal excretion, which is very slow.[43] The average half-life of caffeine ranges from 65–103 h at birth[44,45] compared to the average half-life of 4.6 h in adults (Table 1). Carrier et al. showed that total, *N*3-, and *N*7-demethylation rates increase exponentially with postnatal age, with a plateau reached by 120 d of age.[46]

There is considerable evidence that the elimination of caffeine is a nonlinear process. Because the major pathway of metabolism of caffeine, as well that of its primary metabolites, is *N*-demethylation, end-product inhibition of *N*-demethylation is a good possibility. Support for this idea comes from studies showing that both theobromine and caffeine inhibit theophylline metabolism in rat liver slices,[47] that the coadministration of caffeine prolongs the elimination half-life of theophylline in humans,[48] that the clearance of theobromine falls with exposure to other methylxanthines or with chronic dosing of theobromine,[49] and that paraxanthine infusion reduces the clearance of caffeine in rabbits.[50] There is also evidence to suggest that paraxanthine clearance falls as caffeine concentrations increase.[6]

If end-product inhibition occurs in vivo, one would expect to find dose-dependent changes in caffeine clearance. The higher the dose, the more competition between caffeine and dimethylxanthines is expected. Dose-dependency of methylxanthine metabolism is supported by several observations. Dose-related saturable metabolism of theophylline has been demonstrated.[51,52] With a breath test used to measure N-demethylation of labeled caffeine, the excretion rate of labeled CO_2 plateaued as the dose of labeled caffeine increased from 3 to 5 mg/kg.[53] Tang-Liu et al.[6] showed that plasma concentrations of caffeine decayed in a nonlinear fashion. In an overdose of an estimated 6–8 g of caffeine, the calculated elimination half-life was approx 16 h,[54] much longer than the half-life of caffeine in healthy subjects after lower doses of caffeine. Dose-dependent metabolism of caffeine has also been observed in some animal species.[55]

Recently, the dose-dependency of the metabolism of caffeine in humans was established directly.[10] Prior studies of the issue of dose-dependency of caffeine employed single doses of caffeine that would not be expected to generate levels of metabolites adequate to produce end-product inhibition.[4,56] In contrast, we examined the metabolism of caffeine while caffeine was given repeatedly, as it is consumed by most people.[10] Our experiment was conducted when concentrations of caffeine and its dimethylxanthine metabolites were at steady state, so that the possibility of competition among caffeine and its metabolites for N-demethylation would be maximized. Intravenous doses of stable isotope-labeled caffeine were administered to characterize the disposition kinetics of caffeine in the face of ongoing consumption of caffeine.

Three treatments were compared in a crossover experiment in seven healthy nonsmokers. Isotope-labeled caffeine (25 mg) was given after 3 d of placebo, 4.2 mg/kg/d of caffeine in six divided doses (low), and 12 mg/kg/d of caffeine in six divided doses (high). The average concentrations of isotope-labeled caffeine for each treatment are shown in Fig. 3. This figure demonstrates a progressive reduction in elimination rate and a higher AUC of isotope-labeled caffeine as the dose of oral caffeine increased. The average clearance of caffeine fell significantly, from 0.118 L/h/kg in the placebo to 0.069 L/h/kg in the low-dose to 0.054 L/h/kg in the high-dose periods. The average half-lives were 4.0, 6.1, and 8.7 h for the placebo, low-, and

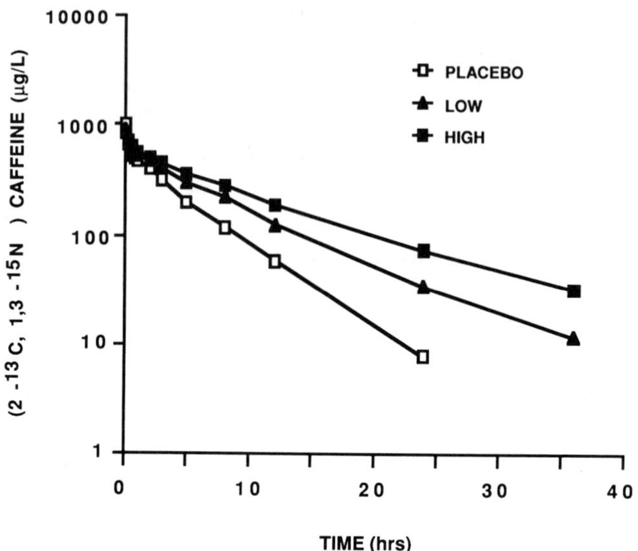

Fig. 3. Mean plasma concentrations of $(2\text{-}^{13}C, 1,3\text{-}^{15}N_2)$caffeine; 25 mg given intravenously to subjects during differing caffeine-consumption conditions: –□–, placebo; –▲–, low-dose (4.2 mg/kg/d); –■–, high-dose (12 mg/kg/d). From C. P. Denaro, C. R. Brown, M. Wilson, P. Jacob, and N. L. Benowitz (1990) Dose-dependency of caffeine metabolism with repeated dosing. *Clin. Pharmacol. Ther.* **48**, 277–285.

high-dose periods, respectively. The formation and metabolic clearance of paraxanthine fell, consistent with what is expected if there is competition for *N*-demethylation.

Whether caffeine can induce its own metabolism has not been thoroughly studied. Demonstration of induction would be complicated by end-product inhibition. In one study, following 1 wk of methylxanthine abstinence, 480 mg/d of caffeine was administered to healthy subjects for 1 wk, followed by a 48-h washout period.[22] Caffeine pharmacokinetics were no different on the first day of caffeine and after the washout, but the duration of abstinence or the duration of the consumption of caffeine may have been inadequate to show induction of metabolism.

Caffeine Metabolism
in Liver Disease

Numerous studies have shown that the metabolism of caffeine is impaired in liver disease. Plasma clearance and half-life are prolonged, and there is wide interpatient variation. Some of this variation is related to the severity of liver dysfunction. Statland and Demas[57] studied two patients with severe liver dysfunction and three healthy controls. Half-lives in the controls ranged from 5 to 6.25 h; in patients with liver disease, the half-lives were 60 and 168 h. A formal study of the pharmacokinetics of caffeine in liver disease was carried out by Desmond et al.[13] They compared 10 patients with cirrhosis and 15 healthy volunteers. Unfortunately, they sampled plasma for only 48 h after caffeine dosing and, in the two patients with the most severe liver disease, there was minimal decline in caffeine concentrations over that interval of time. Half-life and clearance could not be estimated for these two subjects. When the remaining cirrhotic patients were compared with controls, clearance was reduced by an average of 35%. Half-life was prolonged only slightly, because there was a trend for the volume of distribution (V) to be smaller in the cirrhotic group. Plasma binding of caffeine was 30% in control and 25% in cirrhotic individuals. This correlated to the differences in serum albumin. The time to maximum concentration and the concentration at that time was similar in cirrhotic compared to control individuals, suggesting that the absorption kinetics of caffeine are similar in both groups.

In another study,[14] eight cirrhotic patients, seven patients with stage IV primary biliary cirrhosis (PBC), 11 patients with noncirrhotic liver disease, and 10 healthy controls were compared. The cirrhotic patients were not classified as to the severity of their disease, and plasma sampling of caffeine concentrations was carried out for only 8 h after the caffeine dose. Thus, estimates of pharmacokinetic parameters of caffeine in the patients with severe liver dysfunction would be approximate at best. The average plasma clearance of caffeine was reduced in all three liver-disease groups compared to controls. In the cirrhotic and PBC groups, clearance was reduced by more than 50%. In these two groups there was an approximate tenfold range in values for clearance and half-life, whereas only a threefold range was seen in the control group. This could be explained, in part, by failure to characterize the disposition curve of caffeine adequately, but more likely this variation is attributable to differences in the severity of liver disease in patients within these two groups. Concentrations of caffeine taken in the morning after an overnight fast were four- to eightfold higher in the cirrhotic and PBC groups than in the control group. The clearance of caffeine was slightly reduced in the noncirrhotic liver-disease group, compared with controls, and seven of the 11 patients had clearances within the range of the normal controls. Using a 48-h sampling paradigm, other investigators have also shown that there were only minor differences between caffeine clearance in controls and that in noncirrhotic liver-disease patients.[16]

Two research groups have assessed the metabolism of caffeine with respect to the severity of hepatic dysfunction in cirrhotic patients. Scott et al.[15] classified 19 cirrhotic individuals as "compensated" and "decompensated" using the Child-Turcotte-Pugh scoring system.[58] In the decompensated group, clearance was reduced by 85% compared to controls, and half-life was always >10 h in this group. There was only a 20% decrease in clearance in compensated cirrhosis compared to controls. However, all controls were nonsmokers and 50% of the compensated group were smokers. Thus, the clearance values for the compensated cirrhotic individuals may have shown an upward bias. In the other study, involving 26 cirrhotic patients, the percentage of smokers was the same in both the control and the cirrhotic group.[16] The patients were classified in three groups with respect to severity of hepatic dysfunction. In the compensated cirrhotic group, which was analogous to the group in Scott's study, there was a 50% decrease in clearance. Both studies demonstrated a significant correlation between the Child-Turcotte-Pugh scoring system and the clearance of caffeine. This clinical scoring system accounted for approx 50% of the variance in the clearance of caffeine. Unfortunately, there was still wide variability in clearance even within subgroups. Of note, the clearance of caffeine correlated significantly to prothrombin time and serum concentrations of albumin and bilirubin.[16]

The urinary metabolite profile of caffeine in patients with liver disease has also been studied by Scott et al.[59] However, caffeine excretion was assessed for only 48 h, which would only be approximately one half-life in decompensated cirrhosis, and AFMU/AAMU were not measured. Without measuring these major metabolites (AFMU/AAMU), the extent of demethylation, hydroxylation, and acetylation, as estimated by using various ratios of metabolites of caffeine (*see below*), could not be compared between groups. In the decompensated cirrhotic group there was, as expected, a delay in the excretion of the metabolites of caffeine and an increased elimination of unchanged caffeine. After 48 h there were trends for a reduced recovery of 1X and1U, but this could have reflected inadequate time of collection.

The Use of Caffeine to Assess Hepatic Enzyme Activity

P-450IA Activity

Measurement of the activity of this enzyme system is important, since the level of its activity has been correlated to carcinogenesis and teratogenesis in animal studies.[60,61] These enzymes are induced by various xenobiotics and may transform these compounds into toxic intermediates.[62,63] Since caffeine is primarily metabolized by P-450IA, measures of caffeine metabolism have been employed as tests to assess the activity of this enzyme. Such tests could be useful in large-scale epidemiological studies.

Direct measurement of the clearance of caffeine would reflect P-450IA activity, but formal measurement is too cumbersome for large numbers of subjects. A simpler way to estimate the clearance of caffeine is to collect two caffeine samples of either plasma or saliva after a dose of caffeine.[64] Although this test may be useful in the assessment of liver function in hepatic disease (*see below*), it may still be impractical for screening of large populations.

A noninvasive method to measure the rate of *N*-demethylation of caffeine is the caffeine breath test (CBT).[17,53] Caffeine is labeled with ^{13}C or ^{14}C at all three (1,3, and 7) methyl groups, or singularly at the 3 or 7 methyl group. Labeled CO_2 is measured in expired-air collections. The rate of CO_2 excretion from trilabeled caffeine is proportional to the dose for up to 3 mg/kg, and the 2-h cumulative CO_2 excretion of both tri- and monolabeled caffeine is correlated to caffeine clearance.[14,53] At doses above 3 mg/kg of labeled caffeine, the excretion rate of CO_2 plateaus, suggesting that the P-450IA enzyme(s) involved with caffeine demethylation are saturable (*see above*).[53] The CBT has been shown to be sensitive to known inducers of P-450IA, and the rate of CO_2 excretion was reduced in liver disease. However, this test, although noninvasive, is still too technical and too costly to be useful in screening large numbers of subjects for epidemiological studies.

An alternative technique for assessing P-450IA activity, which might be amenable for screening large numbers of subjects, is the use of ratios of metabolites of caffeine recovered in the urine. An advantage of metabolite ratios is that they relate concentrations of metabolites to each other and are essentially independent of total recovery from the urine.[8] A number of possible ratios could be used to assess the demethylation of caffeine. The ratio of (AFMU + 1U + 1X) / 17U—or AUX/17U, where AUX = (AFMU + 1U + 1X)—has been proposed as an in vivo index of P-450IA activity.[25] In theory, this is a ratio of products catalyzed by two different enzymes. The numerator represents the sum of the 7-*N*-demethylation products of paraxanthine (P-450IA-mediated), and the denominator is the 8-hydroxylation product of paraxanthine (mediated by another P-450 enzyme). The ratio assumes that all 1X formation comes from 17X, and ignores the small contribution from 13X. The AUX/17U ratio reflects P-450IA activity in vitro,[11] and in single-dose studies this ratio was shown to be correlated to the clearance of caffeine.[25] Figure 4 shows how the ratio distinguishes children, smokers, and users of oral contraceptives from the general adult population. Inhibition of P-450IA activity by cimetidine was demonstrated by a 38% decrease in the pretreatment value of AUX/17U.[65] In the two subjects investigated, this ratio was stable with multiple dosing, and in eight individuals a single urine sample provided information similar to that of a 24-h urine collection.[25] More subjects under different dosing conditions will have to be investigated to confirm those conclusions.

In vitro studies, however, have shown that 8-hydroxylation of paraxanthine is mediated both by P-450IA and by another P-450 enzyme.[11] In microsomal preparations with high activity of P-450IA, hydroxylation is carried out mainly by P-450IA. In preparations with low P-450IA activity, another P-450 enzyme is the dominant enzyme involved with paraxanthine hydroxylation. Thus, there might be a loss of sensitivity in this ratio in individuals with high P-450IA activity, since the ratio then has largely P-450IA-mediated products in both numerator and denominator. The study of cimetidine's effect on the ratio (quoted above)[65] used nonsmokers. Possibly, the result would be less clear in smokers, in whom P-450IA activity is higher.

The use of this ratio assumes that the relative excretion rate of various metabolites will not change with changes in urine flow. Although the excretion of caffeine and dimethylxanthines has been shown to be dependent on urine flow,[8,66] it is assumed that the monomethylated xanthines and

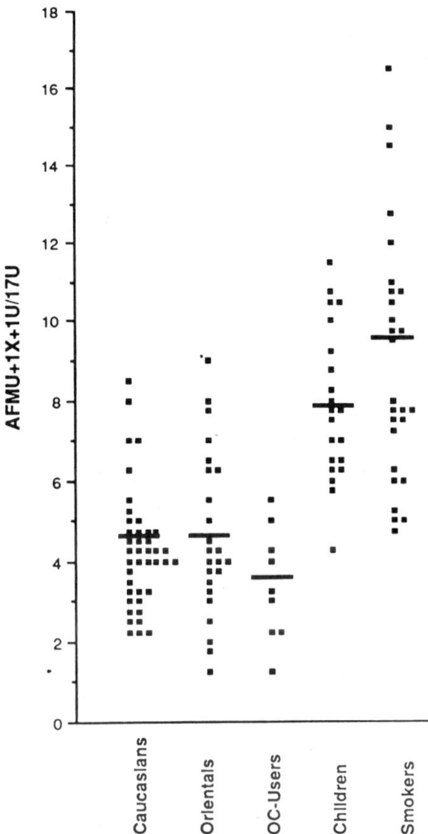

Fig. 4. Comparison of AFMU + 1U + 1X/17U ratios in five different populations. Horizontal bars mark population means (OC, oral contraceptive). From M. E. Campbell, S. P. Spielberg, and W. A. Kalow (1987) A urinary metabolite ratio that reflects systemic caffeine clearance. *Clin. Pharmacol. Ther.* **42,** 157–165. Reprinted with permission.

uric acids are so polar that reabsorption in the renal tube does not occur. However, this has not been actively investigated. As seen in Fig. 4, there is a large degree of variability remaining with AUX/17U, even when it is stratified for children, adults, and environmental factors. Part of this variability could be caused by differences in urine flow and timing of urine collections.

Another possible metabolite ratio that could assess P-450IA activity is (AFMU + 1X + 1U)/17X. This ratio of the sum of the *N*-demethylation products of paraxanthine to paraxanthine reflects *N*3-demethylation activity. However, this ratio varies 30-fold in the adult population,[8] and, although some of this variability may be caused by induction and inhibition of P-450IA activity, the influence of urine flow on 17X excretion may also be an important factor.

Obviously, genetic and environmental factors will contribute to the variability in urine metabolite ratios, but the influences of increasing age, caffeine dose, and renal and hepatic disease also require further investigation. The clearance of caffeine is 35% lower in subjects over 70 years old.[67] As described previously, caffeine demonstrates nonlinear metabolism when studied under multiple dosing conditions, and the ratio could change with different doses. What happens to these ratios in the presence of renal disease is unknown, and since AUX/17U is a ratio of products from two or more separate enzymes, the ratio may not reflect caffeine clearance in liver disease, since both numerator and denominator may be affected. Whether the ratio remains a good discriminator of P-450IA induction in liver disease remains to be investigated. A technical concern in the measurement of the ratios is that AFMU is unstable. The use of AAMU, to which AFMU degrades and can be wholly chemically converted, would improve the precision of this ratio.

We correlated several urine metabolite ratios with the clearance of caffeine under steady-state conditions during two different multiple-dose regimens of oral caffeine (4.2 and 12 mg/kg/d) in seven subjects.[68] The experimental design was described in the metabolism section of this chapter. The clearance of caffeine was measured using intravenous doses of stable isotope-labeled caffeine, and the ratios were measured from 24-h urine collections. In addition to the two ratios described above (but using AAMU instead of AFMU), we also investigated ratios suggested by Carrier et al. to assess *N*-demethylation of caffeine,[46] and ratios that would assess hydroxylation and acetylation of caffeine and xanthine oxidase activity.[8] The ratios proposed by Carrier et al. are based on the number of methyl groups removed by the enzyme(s) divided by the total number of methyl groups that one would recover from the urine had there been no demethylation. Correlations between different urine-metabolite ratios and the clearance of caffeine are listed in Table 3.

Table 3
Caffeine-Metabolite Ratios and Correlation to Caffeine Clearance
During Different Caffeine-Dosing Conditions

Ratio[a]	Low[b]	High	Regression[c] Low	Regression[c] High
AUX/17X	8.60	8.22	0.139	0.196
			26%	17%
AUX/17U	8.84	8.18	0.009	0.139
			73%	26%
Total demethylation	0.58	0.57	0.043	0.048
			51%	49%
N3-demethylation	0.90	0.86[d]	0.623	0.063
			0%	44%
N7-demethylation	0.73	0.67[d]	0.560	0.123
			0%	29%
N1-demethylation	0.13	0.18[d]	0.182	0.288
			19%	7%
17U/17X	1.00	1.05	0.858	0.703
			0%	0%
17U/(17X + AUX)	0.11	0.12	0.011	0.154
			71%	23%
AAMU/AUX	0.35	0.36	0.599	0.759
			0%	0%
1U/1X	1.66	1.46	0.637	0.311
			0%	4%

[a]AUX = AAMU + 1U + 1X; total demethylation = (DX + DU) + [(MX + MU + AAMU) · 2]/total · 3 where total = DX + DU + MX + MU + AAMU + TX + TU and DX = all dimethylxanthines, DU = all dimethyluric acids, MX = all monomethylxanthines, MU = all monomethyluric acids, TX = caffeine, and TU = 1,3,7 trimethyluric acid; N3-demethylation = (17X + 17U + 1X + 1U + 7X + 7U + AAMU)/total; N7-demethylation = (13X + 13U + 1X + 1U + 3X + 3U + AAMU)/total; and N1-demethylation = (37X + 37U + 3X + 3U + 7X + 7U)/total.

[b]Low = 4.2 and High = 12 mg/kg/d of caffeine; results expressed as means.

[c]Regression of caffeine clearance on each ratio; results are the p value for the regression and, immediately below, the r^2 value.

[d]Significantly different from Low ($p < 0.05$).

The mean values of some of the ratios change with the change in dose, although only slightly. Since we have observed that most of the fall in the clearance of caffeine occurs between a single 25-mg dose and 4.2 mg/kg/d of caffeine at steady state, we would expect that the ratios would also change in value at lower steady-state doses. AUX/17U is highly correlated to caffeine clearance at the low, but not at the high, dose. The total demethylation ratio looks equally useful under both dosing conditions, despite the use in the ratio of some compounds with excretion rates known to be influenced somewhat by urine flow. These conclusions were confirmed by analyzing the data using stepwise multiple regression.

Acetylator Phenotype

The formation of AFMU, an acetylated metabolite, is a unique characteristic of caffeine metabolism in humans.[1] As seen in Fig. 2, AFMU is formed from 1X. However, this is probably an oversimplification, in that AFMU is not recovered when 1X is ingested.[8] It has been proposed that AFMU is formed from an unstable open-ringed intermediate arising after *N*7-demethylation of 17X, which is quickly acetylated in fast acetylators, whereas in slow acetylators the open ring closes and more 1X is formed instead. Grant et al. demonstrated that slow acetylators excrete more 1X + 1U than fast acetylators, but the overall excretion of AFMU + 1X + 1U did not differ between the groups.[8] Various ratios, such as AFMU/(AFMU + 1U + 1X + 17U + 17X); AFMU/1X; AAMU/(1X + 1U); and AAMU/(AAMU + 1U + 1X) (or AAMU/AUX), were shown to classify the subjects studied into two groups, with a classification in complete concordance with other methods of acetylator phenotyping.[8,32,69,70]

AAMU/(1X + 1U) and AAMU/AUX seem to be the best ratios to use to assess acetylation phenotype. The use of AAMU rather than AFMU improved precision in defining acetylator phenotype and the addition of 1U to the denominator reduced intrasubject variability, since xanthine oxidase activity (measured by the 1X/1U ratio) is quite variable in individual subjects.[70] Using the ratio AAMU/AUX, a value of 0.36 was proposed as the cutoff value between fast and slow acetylators. Although spot urine samples after a single dose of caffeine can be employed to characterize acetylation phenotype,[69] a reduction in the intrasubject variability occurred when subjects consumed their normal multiple-dose intake of caffeine and a first morning urine sample was collected.[70]

The influences of dose, and of inducers and inhibitors of P-450IA activity, on caffeine acetylation ratios have not been fully investigated. In our study (*see* Table 3), the mean AAMU/AUX ratio did not change for the two doses examined. However, we did not have equal numbers of fast and slow acetylators. If 0.36 is used as the cutoff value to distinguish between slow and fast acetylators, then one individual would have changed classification as his or her dose of caffeine was increased. Assessment at lower doses than we used would be important. The influence of such factors as smoking or the use of cimetidine and the oral contraceptive pill on the caffeine acetylation ratio should be evaluated, since calculation of the ratio involves the use of metabolites derived from demethylation pathways.

Assessment of Hepatic Function in Liver Disease

Routine liver-function tests measure hepatocellular injury, bilirubin excretion, and synthesis capacity of the liver. In chronic liver disease, serum transaminase levels are poorly correlated to prognosis, and bilirubin and albumin plasma concentrations and prothrombin time are relatively inaccurate measures, as well as being influenced by many extrahepatic factors. Drug metabolism is an important function of the liver, and tests that assess drug-metabolizing capacity might characterize hepatic function with greater accuracy than currently available clinical tests. Quantification of hepatic metabolism is potentially useful in a number of clinical areas. In decompensated liver disease, such assessment could help determine the optimal time for transplantation and could be useful in appraising donor liver function. They could be also employed to modify the dosage of drugs that are metabolized by the liver, in the way that serum creatinine is used to adjust the doses of renally excreted drugs. Finally, accurate measures of hepatic function would be invaluable in clinical trials of treatments of liver disease.

In the research setting, a variety of tests to measure metabolism, such as galactose elimination capacity, antipyrine clearance, aminopyrine breath test, indocyanine green clearance, and lidocaine elimination, have been employed. They are not employed in routine clinical practice, since the tests require the administration of exogenous (and, in the case of aminopyrine, radioactive) agents that have potentially adverse effects; they are cumbersome, time-consuming, expensive, often require multiple sampling, and require patient cooperation. Although these tests have been shown to be useful in predicting outcome in liver disease,[71–73] it is unclear whether they have any superiority over the Child-Turcotte classification (with or without modifications) in prognosis assessment.[74–76] The lack of a clear advantage in the use of these tests probably results from the great degree of interindividual variation; since these tests are difficult to perform, they are often used only once in the course of a patient's disease. This is not how other tests of liver function are used, and, if a simple test of hepatic metabolism could be designed, then multiple assessments in one individual could be carried out to determine the stability of an individual's liver function over time. Prognosis of chronic liver disease is determined not only by the remaining hepatic function, but also by the rate of progression of the disease.[77]

Measures of caffeine metabolism fit a number of criteria that are desirable in a test of hepatic function, and it is possible that a simple, reliable, and inexpensive test utilizing caffeine could be designed. Caffeine is a ubiquitously consumed drug that is thought to have no serious adverse effects in normal dosages; it is easily measured, completely absorbed, and virtually totally metabolized by the liver. Caffeine has a low extraction ratio; its metabolism depends on hepatocellular function and is not influenced by changes in hepatic blood flow. This last feature may or may not be an advantage, since liver blood-flow perturbations occur in cirrhosis.

The measurement of the clearance of caffeine could be a useful measure of hepatic metabolism as it is correlated to the severity of cirrhosis (using the Child-Turcotte-Pugh severity score)[15,16] and is also correlated to other tests of drug metabolism, such as the aminopyrine breath test and, to a lesser extent, to indocyanine green clearance and galactose-elimination capacity.[14,16,64] However, formal measurement of caffeine clearance requires multiple sampling. Jost et al. suggested the use of a dose of caffeine followed by two salivary concentrations 8 h apart to estimate caffeine clearance.[64] There is a close relationship between plasma and salivary concentrations.[56,64,78] Clearance was calculated by multiplying an averaged population value for volume of distribution with the slope of caffeine disposition that was estimated from the two sampled concentrations. They measured caffeine clearance in cirrhotic and noncirrhotic liver-disease patients and in healthy controls, and demonstrated significant differences between all three groups. As expected, there was an overlap in values between liver-disease subjects and controls, especially between those with noncirrhotic liver disease and controls. Reproducibility was assessed in a subgroup of subjects by measuring clearance again at 2 wk or at 6 mo, and the coefficient of variation was <20%.

Whether this test accurately assesses hepatic metabolism depends on how closely it reflects true caffeine clearance. However, this validation was not performed. The use of two concentrations only 8 h apart would not adequately define the slope of the elimination curve for caffeine disposition in patients with prolonged caffeine half-lives. An average population volume of distribution may be inappropriate for patients with liver dysfunction, particularly in the presence of edema and ascites. Even though the average volume of distribution has been reported to be similar in patients with liver disease and in healthy controls in some studies,[13,14] other studies have reported differences.[15,16] The use of pharmacokinetic techniques, such as Bayesian forecasting and optimal sampling theory, might improve the precision in the measurement of caffeine clearance when only two concentrations are available.

The other major drawback of this proposed test is a practical one. One must ensure that an adequate caffeine dose has been given recently, two samples have to be collected over a relatively long period of time, and no further caffeine can be consumed between the samples.

A caffeine breath test has been shown to correlate well to caffeine clearance, and the CO_2 excretion rate is reduced in patients with cirrhosis.[14] However, this test does not seem to offer any advantages over the aminopyrine breath test.

Renner et al. proposed that a single fasting caffeine concentration might be used to assess hepatic metabolism. They showed, in a group of patients with liver disease, a hyperbolic correlation between fasting caffeine concentrations and caffeine clearance, aminopyrine breath test, and indocyanine green clearance.[14,79] The average fasting caffeine concentration was significantly higher in cirrhotic patients than in controls, but substantial overlap was seen. Other investigators, however, have found little correlation between fasting levels and the clearance of caffeine.[80–82] This disparity occurs because clearance is the ratio of dosing rate and the average plasma concentration at steady state. To see a high degree of correlation between caffeine clearance and fasting concentrations of caffeine, the daily dose of caffeine in the whole population (healthy subjects as well as liver-disease patients) should be uniform. Furthermore, the amount of caffeine consumed by an individual over time should not vary if repeated measurements to assess the progression of disease in that patient are performed. Also, fasting concentrations are not the same as daily average concentrations and are influenced by the time at which caffeine was last ingested. Caffeine concentrations in the afternoon or night after multiple caffeine doses during the day have been shown to correlate better than trough concentrations to the average caffeine concentration.[80]

To circumvent the problem of nonuniformity in dosage, other groups have proposed the use of standardized doses of caffeine, with measurement of caffeine concentrations 12 h or more later.[64,82,83] Marchesini et al. showed that, after 2 d of controlled caffeine consumption, the next morning caffeine concentration was closely correlated to clearances of caffeine and antipyrine.[82] Wang et al. studied cirrhotic and noncirrhotic liver-disease patients and healthy controls after 4 d of abstinence from caffeine.[83] They then gave a standardized dose of caffeine and found that the 12-h caffeine concentration completely distinguished the three groups of subjects from one another. This separation was superior to that observed when measuring fasting caffeine concentrations. However, all of these tests are still somewhat cumbersome for routine clinical use, and direct measurement of caffeine clearance would probably be just as easy to perform.

An alternative method for assessing caffeine metabolism is the use of urine metabolite ratios. Some of these ratios are correlated to caffeine clearance (*see* Table 3), and standardization of caffeine intake is not required. The ratio AUX/17U may not be useful, since the amount of metabolites in both numerator and denominator would be expected to diminish in hepatic dysfunction, but this would not be the case with the total-demethylation ratio. If a single urine sample conveys the same information about caffeine clearance as a 24-h urine collection, then a simple test of hepatic metabolism that could be repeated over time in an individual patient is feasible. Metabolite ratios can also assess hydroxylation, acetylation, and xanthine oxidase activity. Estimations of the activity of multiple enzyme systems might prove superior to measuring caffeine clearance alone in the characterization of hepatic function. However, assaying all these metabolites is technically difficult, which could discourage widespread application of this test.

Whichever test is utilized, it will have to deal with the high degree of individual variation in hepatic drug metabolism. As discussed previously, caffeine disposition is influenced by environmental factors, other drugs, and the dose of caffeine itself. Smoking and mexiletine administration have been shown to influence caffeine metabolism in patients with liver disease,[84] and other drugs that inhibit caffeine metabolism are likely to do the same. However, if repeated testing of an individual is carried out and known factors that influence caffeine metabolism are kept constant, the course of liver disease in that individual might be accurately assessed by quantitating the metabolism of caffeine.

Although not yet practical for routine clinical use, the measurement of caffeine clearance has been successfully applied in the research setting. It has been used to characterize hepatic function in patients with cystic fibrosis,[85] it has demonstrated that microsomal function is maintained in the presence of jaundice associated with severe extrahepatic infection,[86] and it has shown that microsomal drug-metabolizing activity is reduced in the elderly.[67]

Summary

Caffeine is one of the most widely consumed psychoactive drugs in the world. Absorption of caffeine is rapid and complete. It is extensively metabolized by *N*-demethylation, hydroxylation, and acetylation to at least 17 metabolites, which are renally excreted. The major pathway of metabolism is sequential *N*-demethylation, which is carried out by cytochrome P-450IA. The primary dimethylxanthine metabolites—paraxanthine, theobromine, and theophylline — are pharmacologically active. The demethylation of caffeine appears to be inhibited by competition from dimethylxanthine *N*-demethylation. As a result, caffeine disposition is dose-dependent during multiple dosing conditions.

Caffeine does not cause liver disease, but its metabolism is highly affected by the presence of hepatic dysfunction. In decompensated cirrhosis, the clearance of caffeine can be markedly decreased, resulting in half-lives of as long as 100 h or more. The severity of liver dysfunction as assessed by the Child-Turcotte-Pugh score is correlated to the reduction in caffeine clearance.

Measures of caffeine *N*-demethylation have been used to assess hepatic cytochrome P-450IA activity. Certain ratios of concentrations of caffeine metabolites found in the urine are correlated to caffeine clearance. These ratios are potentially useful in the assessment of P-450IA activity in studies requiring the screening of large numbers of people. Acetylator status can also be characterized by ratios of particular caffeine metabolites.

Hepatic reserve in liver disease may be characterized with greater accuracy with the assessment of rates of drug metabolism than with the usual tests of liver function. Caffeine meets many of the criteria of an ideal test agent. Simple measures of caffeine clearance have been employed in research studies of liver function, and there is potential for developing a practical test for routine clinical monitoring of hepatic function using measures of caffeine metabolism.

Acknowledgments

Preparation of this chapter was supported by US Public Health Service grant DA01696 from The National Institute on Drug Abuse. Charles P. Denaro is a Merck International Fellow in Clinical Pharmacology. We thank Peyton Jacob, III, and Margaret Wilson for reviewing this manuscript.

References

[1] M. J. Arnaud (1987) The pharmacology of caffeine. *Prog. Drug Res.* **31,** 273–313.

[2] C. G. A. Persson, J. A. Karlsson, and I. Erjefalt (1982) Differentiation between bronchodilation and universal adenosine antagonism among xanthine derivatives. *Life Sci.* **30,** 2181–2189.

[3] J. Blanchard and S. J. A. Sawers (1983) The absolute bioavailability of caffeine in man. *Eur. J. Clin. Pharmacol.* **24,** 93–98.

[4] M. Bonati, R. Latini, F. Galletti, J. F. Young, G. Tognoni, and S. Garatini (1982) Caffeine disposition after oral doses. *Clin. Pharmacol. Ther.* **32,** 98–106.

[5] M. J. Arnaud and C. Welsch (1981) Theophylline and caffeine metabolism in man, in *Methods in Clinical Pharmacology,* vol. 3. N. Reitbrock, G. B. Woodcook, and A. H. Staib, eds. Braunschweig/Wiesbaden, Vieweg, pp. 135–148.

[6] D. D. Tang-Liu, R. L. Williams, and S. Riegelman (1983) Disposition of caffeine and its metabolites in man. *J. Pharmacol. Exp. Ther.* **224,** 180–185.

[7] M. M. Callahan, R. S. Robertson, A. R. Branfman, M. F. McComish, and D. W. Yesair (1983) Comparison of caffeine metabolism in three nonsmoking populations after oral administration of radiolabeled caffeine. *Drug Metab. Dispos.* **11,** 211–217.

[8] D. M. Grant, B. K. Tang, and W. Kalow (1983) Variability in caffeine metabolism. *Clin. Pharmacol. Ther.* **33,** 591–602.

[9] J. Blanchard, J. A. Sawers, J. H. G. Jonkman, and D. D. Tang-Liu (1985) Comparison of the urinary metabolite profile of caffeine in young and elderly males. *Br. J. Clin. Pharmacol.* **19,** 225–232.

[10] C. P. Denaro, C. R. Brown, M. Wilson, P. Jacob, and N. L. Benowitz (1990) Dose-dependency of caffeine metabolism with repeated dosing. *Clin. Pharmacol. Ther.* **48,** 277–285.

[11] M. E. Campbell, D. M. Grant, T. Inaba, and W. Kalow (1987) Biotransformation of caffeine, paraxanthine, theophylline, and theobromine by polycyclic aromatic hydrocarbon-inducible cytochrome(s) P-450 in human liver microsomes. *Drug Metab. Dispos.* **15,** 237–249.

[12] D. M. Grant, M. E. Campbell, B. K. Tang, and W. Kalow (1987) Biotransformation of caffeine by microsomes from human liver. *Biochem. Pharmacol.* **36,** 1251–1260.

[13] P. V. Desmond, R. V. Patwardhan, R. F. Johnson, and S. Schenker (1980) Impaired elimination of caffeine in cirrhosis. *Dig. Dis. Sci.* **25,** 193–197.

[14] E. Renner, H. Wietholtz, P. Huguenin, M. J. Arnaud, and R. Preisig (1984) Caffeine: A model compound for measuring liver function. *Hepatology* **4,** 38–46.

[15] N. R. Scott, D. Stambuk, J. Chakraborty, V. Marks, and M. Y. Morgan (1989) The pharmacokinetics of caffeine and its dimethylxanthine metabolites in patients with chronic liver disease. *Br. J. Clin. Pharmacol.* **27,** 205–213.

[16] A. Holstege, M. Staiger, K. Haag, and W. Gerok (1989) Correlation of caffeine elimination and Child's classification in liver cirrhosis. *Klin. Wochenschr.* **67,** 6–15.

[17] H. Weitholtz, M. Voegelin, M. J. Arnaud, J. Bircher, and R. Preisig (1981) Assessment of the cytochrome P-448 dependent liver enzyme system by a caffeine breath test. *Eur. J. Clin. Pharmacol.* **21,** 53–59.

[18] W. D. Parsons and A. H. Neims (1978) Effect of smoking on caffeine clearance. *Clin. Pharmacol. Ther.* **24,** 40–45.

[19] L. J. Broughton and H. J. Rogers (1981) Decreased systemic clearance of caffeine due to cimetidine. *Br. J. Clin. Pharmacol.* **12,** 155–159.

[20] M. L. Eichman, D. E. Guttman, C. Van Winkle, and E. P. Guth (1962) Interactions of xanthine molecules with bovine serum albumin. *J. Pharm. Sci.* **51,** 66–71.

[21] R. V. Patwardhan, P. V. Desmond, R. F. Johnson, and S. Schenker (1980) Impaired elimination of caffeine by oral contraceptive steroids. *J. Lab. Clin. Med.* **95,** 603–608.

[22] J. George, T. Murphy, R. Roberts, W. G. E. Cooksley, J. W. Halliday, and L. W. Powell (1986) Influence of alcohol and caffeine consumption on caffeine elimination. *Clin. Exp. Pharmacol. Physiol.* **13,** 731–736.

[23] A. Lelo, D. J. Birkett, R. A. Robson, and J. O. Miners (1986) Comparative pharmacokinetics of caffeine and its primary demethylated metabolites paraxanthine, theobromine and theophylline in man. *Br. J. Clin. Pharmacol.* **22,** 177–182.

[24] D. C. May, C. H. Jarboe, A. B. Van Bakel, and W. M. Williams (1982) Effects of cimetidine on caffeine disposition in smokers and nonsmokers. *Clin. Pharmacol. Ther.* **31,** 656–661.

[25] M. E. Campbell, S. P. Spielberg, and W. Kalow (1987) A urinary metabolite ratio that reflects systemic caffeine clearance. *Clin. Pharmacol. Ther.* **42,** 157–165.

[26] M. Carbo, J. Segura, R. De la Torre, J. Badenas, and J. Cami (1989) Effect of quinolones on caffeine disposition. *Clin. Pharmacol. Ther.* **45,** 234–240.

[27] M. J. Arnaud (1984) Products of metabolism of caffeine, in *Caffeine, Perspectives from Recent Research.* P. B. Dews, ed. Springer-Verlag, Berlin, pp. 3–38.

[28] A. Lelo, J. O. Miners, R. A. Robson, and D. J. Birkett (1986) Quantitative assessment of caffeine partial clearances in man. *Br. J. Clin. Pharmacol.* **22,** 183–186.

[29] H. H. Cornish and A. A. Christman (1957) A study of the metabolism of theobromine, theophylline, and caffeine in man. *J. Biol. Chem.* **228,** 315–323.

[30] M. M. Callahan, R. S. Robertson, M. J. Arnaud, A. R. Branfman, M. F. McComish, and D. W. Yesair (1982) Human metabolism of [1-methyl-^{14}C]- and [2-^{14}C]caffeine after oral administration. *Drug Metab. Dispos.* **10,** 417–423.

[31] B. K. Tang, D. M. Grant, and W. Kalow (1983) Isolation and identification of 5-acetylamino-6-formylamino-3-methyluracil as a major metabolite of caffeine in man. *Drug Metab. Dispos.* **11,** 218–220.

[32] D. M. Grant, B. K. Tang, and W. Kalow (1983) Polymorphic *N*-acetylation of a caffeine metabolite. *Clin. Pharmacol. Ther.* **33,** 355–359.

[33] D. M. Grant, B. K. Tang, M. E. Campbell, and W. Kalow (1986) Effect of allopurinol on caffeine disposition in man. *Br. J. Clin. Pharmacol.* **21,** 454–458.

[34] R. M. Welch, S. Y. Hsu, and R. L. DeAngelis (1977) Effect of Aroclor 1254, phenobarbital, and polycyclic aromatic hydrocarbons on the plasma clearance of caffeine in the rat. *Clin. Pharmacol. Ther.* **22,** 791–798.

[35] F. J. Gonzalez (1989) The molecular biology of cytochrome P450s. *Pharmacol. Rev.* **40,** 243–288.

[36] H. Weitholtz, T. Zysset, K. Kreiten, D. Kohl, R. Buchsel, and S. Matern (1989) Effect of phenytoin, carbamazepine, and valproic acid on caffeine metabolism. *Eur. J. Clin. Pharmacol.* **36,** 401–406.

[37] W. Stille, S. Harder, S. Mieke, C. Beer, M. Pramod, M. Shah, K. Frech, and A. H. Staib (1987) Decrease of caffeine elimination in man during co-administration of 4-quinolones. *J. Antimicrob. Chemother.* **20,** 729–734.

[38] R. Joeres, H. Klinker, H. Heusler, and E. Richter (1987) Influence of mexiletine on caffeine elimination. *Pharmacol. Ther.* **33,** 163–169.

[39] D. C. Mays, C. Camisa, P. Cheney, C. M. Pacula, S. Nawoot, and N. Gerber (1987) Methoxsalen is a potent inhibitor of the metabolism of caffeine in humans. *Clin. Pharmacol. Ther.* **42,** 621–626.

[40] C. A. Beach, D. C. Mays, R. C. Guiler, C. H. Jacober, and N. Gerber (1986) Inhibition of elimination of caffeine by disulfiram in normal subjects and recovering alcoholics. *Clin. Pharmacol. Ther.* **39,** 265–270.

[41] M. C. Mitchell, A. M. Hoyumpa, S. Schenker, R. F. Johnson, S. Nichols, and R. V. Patwardhan (1983) Inhibition of caffeine elimination by short-term ethanol administration. *J. Lab. Clin. Med.* **101,** 826–834.

[42] W. D. Parsons and J. G. Pelletier (1982) Delayed elimination of caffeine by women in the last 2 weeks of pregnancy. *Can. Med. Assoc. J.* **127,** 377–380.

[43] A. Aldridge, J. V. Aranda, and A. H. Neims (1979) Caffeine metabolism in the newborn. *Clin. Pharmacol. Ther.* **25,** 447–453.

[44] J. V. Aranda, C. E. Cook, W. Gorman, J. M. Collinge, and P. M. Loughnan (1979) Pharmacokinetic profile of caffeine in the premature newborn infant with apnoea. *J. Pediatr.* **94,** 663–668.

[45] R. Corodischer and M. Karplus (1982) Pharmacokinetic aspects of caffeine in premature infants with apnoea. *Eur. J. Clin. Pharmacol.* **22,** 47–52.

[46] O. Carrier, G. Pons, E. Rey, M. Richard, C. Moran, J. Badoual, and G. Olive (1988) Maturation of caffeine metabolic pathways in infancy. *Clin. Pharmacol. Ther.* **44,** 145–151.

[47] S. M. Lohman and R. P. Meich (1976) Theophylline metabolism by the rat microsomal system. *J. Pharmacol. Exp. Ther.* **196,** 213–225.

[48] T. J. Monks, J. Caldwell, and R. L. Smith (1979) Influence of methylxanthine-containing foods on theophylline metabolism and kinetics. *Clin. Pharmacol. Ther.* **26,** 513–524.

[49] D. D. Drouillard, E. S. Vesell, and B. H. Dvorchik (1978) Studies on theobromine disposition in normal subjects. *Clin. Pharmacol. Ther.* **23,** 296–302.

[50] S. H. Dorrbecker, R. A. Ferraina, B. R. Dorrbecker, and P. A. Kramer (1987) Caffeine and paraxanthine pharmacokinetics in the rabbit: Concentration and product inhibition effects. *J. Pharmacokinet. Biopharm.* **15,** 117–132.

[51] D. D. Tang-Liu, R. L. Williams, and S. Riegelman (1982) Nonlinear theophylline elimination. *Clin. Pharmacol. Ther.* **31,** 358–369.

[52] H. Efthimion, D. J. Morgan, L. Ioannides-Demos, K. Raymond, and A. J. McLean (1984) Influence of chronic dosing on theophylline clearance. *Br. J. Clin. Pharmacol.* **17,** 525–530.

[53] A. N. Kotake, D. A. Schoeller, G. H. Lambert, A. L. Baker, D. D. Schaffer, and H. Josephs (1982) The caffeine CO_2 breath test: Dose response and route of *N*-demethylation in smokers and nonsmokers. *Clin. Pharmacol. Ther.* **32,** 261–269.

[54] C. L. Leson, M. A. McGuigan, and S. M. Bryson (1988) Caffeine overdose in an adolescent male. *J. Toxicol. Clin. Toxicol.* **26,** 407–415.

[55] M. Bonati, R. Latini, G. Tognoni, J. F. Young, and S. Garattini (1984) Interspecies comparison of *in vivo* caffeine pharmacokinetics in man, monkey, rabbit, rat and mouse. *Metab. Rev.* **15,** 1355–1383.

[56] R. Newton, L. J. Broughton, M. J. Lind, H. J. Rogers, and I. D. Bradbrook (1981) Plasma and salivary pharmacokinetics of caffeine in man. *Eur. J. Clin. Pharmacol.* **21,** 45–52.

[57] B. E. Statland and T. J. Demas (1980) Serum caffeine half-lives: Healthy subjects vs. patients having alcohol hepatic disease. *Am. J. Clin. Pathol.* **73,** 390–393.

[58] R. N. H. Pugh, I. M. Murray-Lyon, J. L. Dawson, M. C. Pietroni, and R. Williams (1973) Transection of the oesophagus for bleeding oesophageal varices. *Br. J. Surg.* **60,** 646–649.

[59] N. R. Scott, D. Stambuk, J. Chakraborty, V. Marks, and M. Morgan (1988) Caffeine clearance and biotransformation in patients with chronic liver disease. *Clin. Sci.* **74**, 377–384.

[60] R. E. Kouri (1976) Relationship between labels of aryl hydrocarbon hydroxylase activity and susceptibility to 3-methylcholanthrene and benzo[a]pyrene-induced cancers in inbred strains of mice, in *Polynuclear Aromatic Hydrocarbons: Chemistry, Metabolism and Carcinogenesis.* R. I. Freundenthal and P. W. Jones, eds. Raven, New York, pp. 139–160.

[61] G. H. Lambert and D. W. Nebert (1977) Genetically mediated induction of drug metabolizing enzymes associated with congenital defects. *Teratology* **16**, 147–153.

[62] D. W. Nebert and N. M. Jensen (1979) The Ah locus: Genetic regulation of the metabolism of carcinogens, drugs and other environmental chemicals by cytochrome P-450-mediated monooxygenases. *CRC Crit. Rev. Biochem.* **6**, 401–437.

[63] D. V. Parke and C. Ioannides (1982) Role of mixed-function oxidases in the formation of biological reactive intermediates. *Adv. Exp. Med. Biol.* **136A**, 23–38.

[64] G. Jost, A. Wahllander, U. Von Mandach, and R. Preisig (1987) Overnight salivary caffeine clearance: A liver function test suitable for routine use. *Hepatology* **7**, 338–344.

[65] T. A. Shaw-Stiffel, B. K. Tang, S. P. Spielberg, and N. H. Shear (1988) Caffeine—A novel probe to assess drug effects on hepatic cytochrome P-450 activity. *Hepatology* **8**, 1385.

[66] J. Blanchard and S. J. A. Sawers (1983) Relationship between urine flow rate and renal clearance of caffeine in man. *J. Clin. Pharmacol.* **23**, 134–138.

[67] M. Schnegg and B. H. Lauterburg (1986) Quantitative liver function in the elderly assessed by galactose elimination capacity, aminopyrine demethylation and caffeine clearance. *J. Hepatol.* **3**, 164–171.

[68] C. P. Denaro and N. L. Benowitz. Correlation of metabolite ratios of caffeine with caffeine clearance. Manuscript in preparation.

[69] D. M. Grant, B. K. Tang, and W. Kalow (1984) A simple test for acetylator phenotype using caffeine. *Br. J. Clin. Pharmacol.* **17**, 459–464.

[70] B. K. Tang, D. Kadar, and W. Kalow (1987) An alternative test for acetylator phenotyping with caffeine. *Clin. Pharmacol. Ther.* **42**, 509–513.

[71] J. B. Saunders, N. Wright, and K. O. Lewis (1980) Predicting outcome of paracetamol poisoning by using ^{14}C-aminopyrine breath test. *Br. Med. J.* **280**, 279,280.

[72] J. F. Schneider, A. L. Baker, N. W. Haines, G. Hatfield, and J. L. Boyer (1980) Aminopyrine *N*-demethylation: A prognostic test of liver function in patients with alcoholic liver disease. *Gastroenterology* **79**, 1145–1150.

[73] L. Ranek, P. B. Andreasen, and N. Tygstrup (1976) Galactose elimination capacity as a prognostic index in patients with fulminant liver failure. *Gut.* **17,** 959–964.

[74] J. Lindskov (1982) The quantitative liver function as measured by galactose elimination capacity: II. Prognostic value and changes during disease in patients with cirrhosis. *Acta. Med. Scand.* **212,** 303–308.

[75] J. P. Villeneuve, C. Infante-Rivard, M. Ampelas, G. Pomier-Layrargues, P. M. Huet, and D. Marleau (1986) Prognostic value of the aminopyrine breath test in cirrhotic patients. *Hepatology* **6,** 928–931.

[76] G. Pomier-Layrargues, P. M. Huet, C. Infante-Rivard, J. P. Villenueve, D. Marleau, L. Dugay, S. Tanguay, and P. Lavuie (1988) Prognostic value of indocyanine green and lidocaine kinetics for survival and chronic hepatic encephalopathy in cirrhotic patients following elective end-to-side portacaval shunt. *Hepatology* **8,** 1506–1510.

[77] J. Bircher (1986) Assessment of prognosis in advanced liver disease: To score or to measure, that's the question. *Hepatology* **6,** 1036,1037.

[78] E. Zylber-Katz, L. Granit, and M. Levy (1984) Relationship between caffeine concentrations in plasma and saliva. *Clin. Pharmacol. Ther.* **36,** 133–137.

[79] A. Wahllander, E. Renner, and R. Preisig (1985) Fasting plasma caffeine concentration. *Scand. J. Gastroenterol.* **20,** 1133–1141.

[80] A. Lelo, J. O. Miners, R. Robson, and D. J. Birkett (1986) Assessment of caffeine exposure: Caffeine content of beverages, caffeine intake, and plasma concentrations of methylxanthines. *Clin. Pharmacol. Ther.* **39,** 54–59.

[81] R. M. Mooney, J. W. Halliday, W. G. E. Cooksley, and L. W. Powell (1984) Fasting serum caffeine (FSC) as an index of functional liver cell mass. *Hepatology* **4(58),** 1021.

[82] G. Marchesini, G. A. Checchia, G. Grossi, R. Lolli, G. D. Bianchi, M. Zoli, and E. Pisi (1988) Caffeine intake, fasting plasma caffeine and caffeine clearance in patients with liver diseases. *Liver* **8,** 241–246.

[83] T. Wang, F. Stellaard, and G. Paumgartner (1985) Caffeine elimination: A test of liver function. *Klin. Wochenschr.* **63,** 1124–1128.

[84] R. Joeres, H. Klinker, H. Heusler, J. Epping, G. Hofstetter, D. Drost, H. Reuss, W. Zilly, E. Richter (1987) Factors influencing the caffeine test for cytochrome P 448-dependent liver function. *Arch. Toxicol.* **60,** 93,94.

[85] M. G. Bianchetti, R. Kraemer, J. Passweg, J. Jost, and R. Preisig (1988) Use of salivary levels to predict clearance of caffeine in patients with cystic fibrosis. *J. Pediatr. Gastroenterol. Nutr.* **7,** 688–693.

[86] M. Pirovino, F. Meister, E. Rubli, and G. Karlaganis (1989) Preserved cytosolic and synthetic liver function in jaundice of severe extrahepatic infection. *Gastroenterology* **96,** 1589–1595.

Marijuana, Liver Enzymes, and Toxicity

Lester M. Bornheim

Introduction

Marijuana has been used by humans for thousands of years[1] for a variety of social, religious, and medical purposes.[2–6] Although used medicinally in the United States since the middle of the 19th century,[7–12] the nonmedicinal use of marijuana was made illegal in 1937; since then, concern over its possible toxicological effects has arisen cyclically. A series of studies undertaken in the 1940s by the Mayor's Committee in New York,[13] although failing to substantiate the anticipated serious effects on the physical and mental health of marijuana users, indicated the harmful potential of marijuana in certain users. Since that time, and particularly after the marked increase in marijuana consumption during the 1960s, thousands of reports have been published on the pharmacological and toxicological effects of marijuana and its constituents. Although substantial acute toxicity of marijuana use has not been reported, concern remains over the possible long-term effects. Since the effects of chronic tobacco smoking and alcohol use became apparent only after very prolonged use, it is possible that the long-term effects of marijuana use in the populace may manifest themselves in the decades to come. This chapter will focus on the known acute and chronic

From: *Drug and Alcohol Abuse Reviews, Vol. 2: Liver Pathology and Alcohol*
Ed: R. R. Watson ©1991 The Humana Press Inc.

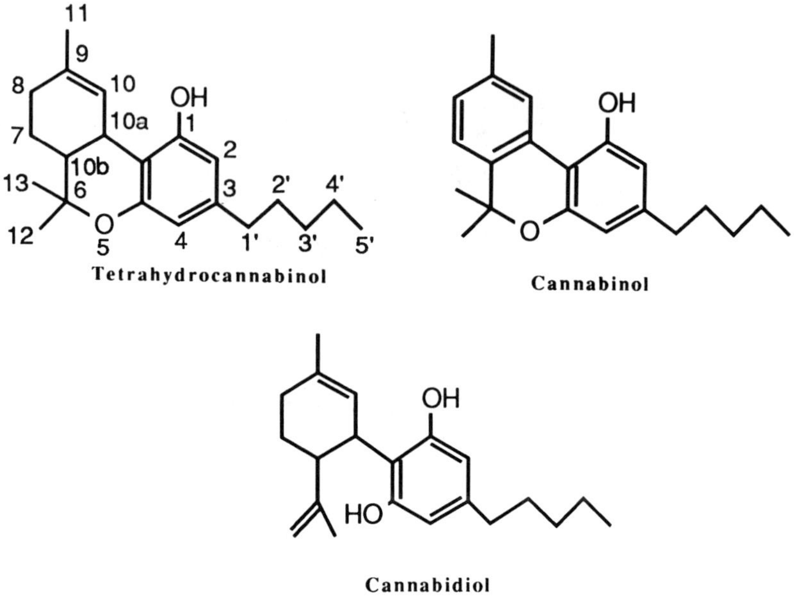

Tetrahydrocannabinol

Cannabinol

Cannabidiol

Fig. 1. Structures of major cannabinoids. Δ^9-Tetrahydrocannabinol is numbered by a benzpyrene numbering system.

effects of marijuana and its constituents on liver function and hopefully will incite an awareness of the potential toxicological effects of long-term use.

Chemistry of Marijuana

Constituents

One of the dilemmas in assessing the toxicology of marijuana use results from the extremely complicated chemical nature of marijuana. Marijuana is a complex mixture of over 400 compounds,[14] which vary in concentration according to the plant phenotype.[15] Although Δ^9-tetrahydrocannabinol (THC) is just one of more than 60 cannabinoids present,[16] it is probably responsible for most of the psychoactivity of marijuana (Fig. 1). Cannabinol (CBN), another major constituent that is only one-tenth as potent as THC,[17] probably contributes little to the overall psychoactive properties of marijuana. Cannabidiol (CBD), a third major constituent of marijuana, is devoid of psychotomimetic properties.[17,18] Several studies have characterized the anticonvulsant properties of CBD[19–21] and its potential therapeutic use as an antiepileptic agent has been proposed.[22-27] More important, because CBD can markedly affect drug metabolism (ref. 28, and refs. therein), it may alter the metabolic disposition of THC and many other drugs. These effects on drug metabolism will be discussed in greater detail later in this chapter.

Metabolism of Cannabinoids

The extensive hepatic metabolism of the cannabinoids further complicates the evaluation of the toxicity of marijuana. Over 100 hydroxylated metabolites of THC have been isolated and characterized,[16,29] and CBN and CBD yield a similar abundance of metabolites as well. Hydroxylation of THC at the carbon allylic to the double bond in the terpene ring is particularly favored (Fig. 1). The most abundant metabolite found in all species studied is 11-hydroxy-THC, although appreciable amounts of species-dependent 8α- and 8β-hydroxy-THC are also formed. In the rat and the mouse, 8α-hydroxylation predominates, but in humans and guinea pigs the reverse is true.[29] In addition to terpene-ring hydroxylation, extensive oxidation of the pentyl sidechain is also observed. Hydroxylation at the 1'-, 2'-, 3'-, and 4'-positions has been found, the relative amounts being species-dependent.[30] The hydroxylated sidechain is also known to undergo various sidechain cleavage reactions.[31] To complicate the metabolic profile even more, most of the mono-hydroxylated metabolites are susceptible to further oxidation. Oxidation can occur either at the site of the initial hydroxylation (resulting in either a carbonyl compound or a carboxylic acid) or at a different site(s), yielding di- or even tri-hydroxylated metabolites.[32] Considering the various combinations of mono-, di-, and tri-hydroxylated-metabolites and sidechain cleavage products, it is not hard to envisage the abundance of THC metabolites detected.

After primary, secondary, or tertiary oxidation, THC metabolites are usually excreted into the bile ($^2/_3$ of the dose) and urine ($^1/_3$ of the dose), either unconjugated or as glucucuronide conjugates, and are known to undergo extensive enterohepatic recirculation.[33] For this reason, and because of sequestration into various lipid compartments, elimination of THC and metabolites is quite slow. Only 50% of the dose is excreted in 4–5 d, and urinary metabolites can be detected several weeks after marijuana ingestion.[34]

CBN and CBD are found to be metabolized by pathways very similar to those of THC. However, in contrast to THC, a large amount of CBD is excreted unchanged in the feces, and CBD is also found to be excreted into the urine as the CBD–glucuronide conjugate.[35]

Metabolism of THC in the fetus has not been extensively studied. Although THC has been shown to cross the placenta, its major metabolite (11-hydroxy-THC) does not appear to cross the placenta or to be formed in the fetus.[36]

Liver Toxicity

*Short-Term Effects in Animals**

Effects on Drug Metabolism

Background. A great deal of work has been done in rodents to determine the effects of marijuana and its constituents on drug metabolism, and much of this has been recently reviewed.[28] CBD appears to affect the microsomal monooxygenase system of the liver, which metabolizes a wide variety of xenobiotics and endogenous compounds.[37–39] Cytochrome P-450 (P-450) is the terminal oxidase of this system and consists of a family of closely related hemoproteins. Because P-450s metabolize such an extensive variety of substrates, there is a very large potential for inhibitory interactions between substrates competing for the enzyme. Such interactions are minimized both by the existence of multiple P-450 isozymes with distinct but overlapping substrate specificities and by the ability of chemicals to induce these isozymes selectively. Thus, although two or more substrates may compete for a certain P-450 isozyme, other isozymes might also oxidize the substrates, albeit with different efficiencies and regioselectivities.

The P-450 superfamily of isozymes can be generally classified according to the nomenclature recently recommended by Nebert et al.[40] Table 1 summarizes the classification of these subfamilies. Many compounds are capable of selectively inducing one or more of the particular P-450 subfamilies. Barbiturates and antiepileptics induce P-450 isozymes[41–44] similar to those induced by phenobarbital (sometimes referred to as phenobarbital-inducible P-450), and are classified in the IIB subfamily. Polycyclic aromatic hydrocarbons induce P-450 isozymes sometimes referred to as P-448[41,42,44] and classified in the IA subfamily. Steroids and macrolide antibiotics induce

---

*Defined as <1 wk of exposure.

Table 1
Nomenclature for the Cytochrome P-450 Superfamily

P-450 subfamily	Trivial P-450 name	Typical inducer
IA	c,d (P-448)	3-Methylcholanthrene
IIA	a	None
IIB	b,e	Phenobarbital
IIC	g,h,i	None
	f,k	Phenobarbital (modest)
IID	db	None
IIE	j	Ethanol
IIIA	p,pcn	Dexamethasone, macrolide antibiotics

a third type of P-450 isozyme,[45,46] belonging to the IIIA subfamily. In addition, shortchain aliphatics, such as ethanol and acetone, are capable of inducing yet another subfamily (IIE) of P-450 isozymes.[47,48] Although most of the inducible P-450 isozymes purified from liver thus far can be categorized in these four classes, this classification is by no means comprehensive. In addition, many isozymes of P-450 have been found to be constitutively expressed, are not usually drug-inducible, and have been classified in the IIA, IIC, and IID subfamilies.

Inhibitory Effects. Loewe first observed prolonged barbiturate-induced sleep-time after marijuana exposure, which suggested an inhibition of hepatic drug metabolism known to be involved in barbiturate inactivation.[49] Subsequent studies found that THC was intracellularly localized in the endoplasmic reticulum and could inhibit the in vitro metabolism of aminopyrine and hexobarbital.[50]

THC was thought to inhibit P-450, since typical Type I difference spectra were demonstrated when THC was added to hepatic microsomes,[51,52] with a spectral dissociation constant (K_d) of 18.5 μM and an inhibition constant (K_i) of 15.4 μM for ethylmorphine N-demethylation. Although hexobarbital metabolism was competitively inhibited in vitro,[50] it was not comparably inhibited in vivo after THC treatment.[51] It is not likely that the hepatic concentrations of THC after a single dose are sufficiently high to cause inhibition in vivo.[49]

CBD also interacts with hepatic P-450, but, unlike THC, it was found to be an inhibitor of drug metabolism both in vivo[49, 53–58] and in vitro[53] with a potency similar to that of SKF 525-A.[54] In fact, Paton and Pertwee correlated the inhibitory actions of marijuana almost completely to that of its CBD content.[54] CBD-mediated Type I binding of microsomal cytochrome P-450 was fourfold higher than that of other cannabinoids.[59] Siemans et al.[53] determined that marijuana extracts with a proportionately higher content of CBD than THC, inhibited drug metabolism much more potently both in vivo and in vitro than when the relative ratios were reversed. CBD also significantly altered the in vivo metabolism of pentobarbital, in contrast to THC or other cannabinoids studied.[55]

In addition, acute CBD treatment of mice lowered hepatic P-450 content and significantly increased the half-time of barbiturate in the brain at a time when barbiturate-induced sleep-time was prolonged.[56] Because barbiturate metabolism is catalyzed by hepatic P-450, the persistence of barbiturate in the brain suggests a direct correlation between CBD-mediated P-450 loss and inhibition of barbiturate metabolism. Borys et al.[56] did not detect any CBD-mediated hepatic P-450 destruction in vitro, but did note the formation of carbon monoxide during in vitro CBD metabolism, which could bind up to 65% of the total P-450 present in the incubations.[57]

Hamajima et al.[58] similarly compared the effects of CBD and THC on drug metabolism in mice and found CBD to be more inhibitory than THC, with males more susceptible to inhibition than females. Because activities of hepatic δ-aminolevulinic acid synthetase or heme oxygenase (involved in heme synthesis and catabolism, respectively) were not altered after CBD treatment,[60] it is not likely that CBD affects heme turnover in the liver.

A more detailed characterization of the CBD-mediated inhibition of specific P-450 isozymes has been reported.[61,62] Administration of CBD, but not THC, to mice acutely inhibited more than 75% of the activities of hepatic microsomal erythromycin and ethylmorphine *N*-demethylases and 6β-testosterone hydroxylase.[62] These particular oxidations are effectively catalyzed by the P-450IIIA subfamily (Table 1). Since P-450 content was decreased by only 35%, whereas *p*-chloro-*N*-methylaniline *N*-demethylase activity (known to be catalyzed by P-450IA) was not significantly affected, CBD appeared to inactivate only certain P-450 isozymes selectively. Thus, the isozyme(s) inactivated by CBD possess(es) many of the same functional characteristics as the P-450IIIA subfamily,[45,46] found constitutively in male rodents and/or induced by steroids and macrolide antibiotics. However, treatment of mice with dexamethasone (a known P-450IIIA inducer) did not result in any increased inactivation of P-450 or inhibition of

P-450IIIA-dependent functional activities over that observed in nonpretreated animals.[63] The P-450IIIA subfamily is composed of several different isozymes within a given species, which are immunochemically indistinguishable by polyclonal antibodies but differ in their reactivity with monoclonal antibodies, their *N*-terminal amino acid sequences, their inducibility by drugs, and their susceptibility to chloramphenicol-mediated inactivation.[64,65] Therefore, it is plausible that the constitutive P-450IIIA isozyme is susceptible to CBD-mediated inactivation whereas the dexamethasone-inducible isozyme is resistant.

The effects of CBD on THC metabolism have also been determined. Any alteration of THC metabolism would be of great interest, since several metabolites of THC have been shown to possess pharmacological activity as well. Borys and Karler[66] found that, whereas in vitro THC metabolism with mouse hepatic microsomes was linear for 60 min, CBD metabolism was linear for only 10 min. In addition, they reported decreased in vitro THC metabolism after preincubation of microsomes with CBD, indicating that CBD could inhibit not only its own metabolism, but that of THC as well. Karler et al.[67] reported that CBD and its monohydroxylated products were metabolized and cleared from the liver very rapidly ($t_{1/2}$ = 1 h) and were virtually absent at a time when inhibition of drug metabolism still persisted. They proposed that such inhibition was most likely a result of very polar, unidentified CBD metabolites that were present in the liver at relatively high concentrations when drug metabolism was inhibited. However, it now seems likely that the inhibition is not attributable to the polar metabolites, but to inactivation of P-450 isozymes.

There has been some debate whether THC itself or its major metabolite (11-hydroxy-THC) is responsible for most of the pharmacological effects observed after marijuana consumption. Several investigators have attempted to answer this question by employing inhibitors of drug metabolism and determining their effects on the pharmacological action of THC. To assess the role of THC metabolism in its pharmacological actions, Sofia and Barry[68] examined the effect of in vivo treatment of mice with SKF 525-A, a nonspecific inhibitor of P-450. Since SKF 525-A inhibited THC metabolism in vitro in rats,[69] it should potentiate the effect of THC if the parent compound is active or decrease the effect of THC if a metabolite is active. Because SKF 525-A enhanced the action of THC, they concluded that it was the parent compound, not a metabolite, that was pharmacologically active. However, when levels of both THC and its major metabolite were measured in a subsequent study, it was found that treatment with SKF 525-A in vivo paradoxically increased THC metabolite levels in the brain threefold.[70] It was proposed that SKF 525-A might inhibit secondary metabolism of the major metabolite to a greater degree than it inhibited its formation, thus resulting in an accumulation of the major metabolite. Although in vitro SKF 525-A largely inhibits the formation of the major metabolite in hepatic microsomes,[69] it is possible that in vivo SKF 525-A inhibition may not affect its formation to the same extent as its further metabolism. Nevertheless, whatever the mechanism for the increased brain concentration of the metabolite, these data suggest that it is the metabolite, not the parent compound, that potentiates the pharmacological effect of THC, as was proposed by others.[71,72] In a similar study, CBD pretreatment also increased brain levels of the major THC metabolite,[73] as did SKF 525-A, further demonstrating that alteration of hepatic THC metabolism by inhibitors can actually stimulate production of a particular THC metabolite.

More recently, we have attempted to characterize the effects of CBD-mediated P-450 inactivation on THC metabolism in order to relate THC metabolite production to specific P-450 isozymes.[74a] After hepatic microsomal incubations with THC, monohydroxylated metabolites were extracted and separated by HPLC. Two major metabolites (identified as 11- and 8α-hydroxy-THC) accounted for >80% of the metabolites observed, and three minor metabolites were also observed. Polyclonal antibody raised against P-450IIIA, when preincubated with mouse liver microsomes, almost completely inhibited the production of the minor metabolites, but failed to affect the production of the major metabolites. In contrast, in vivo CBD treatment of mice markedly inhibited the production of the major metabolites and most of the minor metabolites. This suggests that in vivo CBD treatment resulted in the inactivation of an isozyme responsible for most of the THC metabolism, in addition to the inactivation of P-450IIIA. A P-450 isozyme (related to the IIC subfamily) that hydroxylates THC exclusively at the 11- and 8α-positions has recently been purified, and is probably inactivated in vivo by CBD.[74b] Thus, it appears that THC metabolism is specifically catalyzed by two constitutively expressed P-450 subfamilies (P-450IIC and P-450IIIA) that generate most, if not all, of the observed monohydroxylated metabolites.

Induction. Repetitive CBD treatment had been postulated to induce P-450,[54] and indirect evidence for such induction was presented in later studies.[56,57] We have described[61,62] the purification of a P-450 (related to the P-450IIB subfamily), that is absent in hepatic microsomes of untreated mice, but is readily detected immunochemically in liver microsomes from mice repetitively treated with CBD for 4 d. The induction of this P-450 is paralleled by an increase (>30-fold) in hepatic microsomal pentoxyresorufin *O*-dealkylase activity (known to be catalyzed specifically by the P-450IIB subfamily), which was also below the limits of detection in hepatic microsomes from untreated mice. This CBD-inducible isozyme possessed high hexobarbital hydroxylase activity that was resistant to CBD-mediated inactivation. It thus might explain the loss of susceptibility to CBD-mediated prolongation of barbiturate-induced sleep times previously reported after repetitive CBD treatment.[56,57]

Repeated administration to mice of Δ^8-THC or 11-hydroxy-Δ^8-THC (5 mg/kg, iv, for 3–7 d) has also been reported to increase P-450 content as well as aniline hydroxylase activity.[75] To my knowledge, this is the only report suggesting that THC and its major metabolite are capable of inducing P-450.

Teratogenesis. Limited data implicating a teratogenic potential of THC have been reported.[76] Because inducers and inhibitors of drug metabolism appear to affect THC-elicited teratogenesis, these data are discussed in this section. Low THC doses (50 mg/kg, ip to pregnant mice on gestational days 8–13) moderately increased fetal resorption rates, which were markedly potentiated by the coadministration of SKF 525-A. THC treatment by itself did not significantly increase the incidence of cleft palate, but a marked increase was observed when THC was coadministered with SKF 525-A. At higher THC doses (200 mg/kg), resorption rates were markedly increased irrespective of whether the mothers were pretreated with phenobarbital. In contrast, THC increased the incidence of cleft palate only in the animals that were exposed transplacentally to phenobarbital. The authors concluded that SKF 525-A and phenobarbital probably alter qualitatively the production of THC metabolites.

Other Effects

THC has also been found to damage the structural integrity of liver cell mitochondria in a dose-dependent manner, with internal disruption observed at 50 µg/mg protein.[77] Concentrations in this range, however, are not physiologically relevant.

In addition to its effect on hepatic P-450, CBD is also found to potentiate THC-mediated increases in hepatic tryptophan pyrrolase and tyrosine-α–ketoglutarate transaminase.[78] Since CBD itself failed to affect these enzymes, the potentiation might be attributable to a CBD-mediated decrease in THC metabolism.

Cannabinoids (marijuana extracts or THC) have been consistently reported to decrease liver glycogen,[79–81] with a concomitant increase in blood glucose. THC and 11-hydroxy-THC have been found to increase glucagon activation of liver plasma membrane adenylate cyclase.[82] Cannabinoids have also been shown to inhibit adenylate cyclase, presumably through a putative cannabinoid receptor.[83] In fact, a putative cannabinoid receptor has recently been detected in the brain,[84] and binding data closely mirrors the data for adenylate cyclase inhibition, suggesting that cannabinoids may exert their central effects through this pathway. Whether these receptors are also present in the liver remains to be determined.

Short-Term Effects in Humans

Effects on Drug Metabolism

Many conflicting reports concerning the effect of cannabinoids on clinical drug metabolism have been published. Depending on several factors, as discussed above, the cannabinoids in marijuana vary in proportion. Preparations with a high CBD content may also quantitatively and qualitatively affect THC metabolism, thereby further complicating the interpretation of the data. In addition, inhibition and/or stimulation of drug metabolism may occur, depending on the length of exposure.

CBD pretreatment influences hexobarbital metabolism, i.e., increases the area under the plasma concentration–time curve and the peak plasma concentrations of hexobarbital, and decreases its oral clearance, indicating a decrease in its systemic clearance.[85] Several other reports indicate an effect of CBD on THC metabolism. Although Agurell et al.[86] found no change in THC plasma levels on coadministration of CBD, it was suggested that CBD might affect the kinetics of metabolite formation. Hunt et al.[87] also reported no effect of CBD on the pharmacokinetics of THC, although some changes in the pattern of THC metabolites were observed after CBD pretreatment.

It is possible that a qualitative change in THC metabolism could result in an altered clinical response to THC, since several THC metabolites have been found to be pharmacologically active. The effects of CBD (when administered alone or together with THC) on the alteration of the pharmacological effects of THC were reported by Karniol et al.[88] THC was found to increase pulse rate, disturb time production tasks, and induce strong psychological reactions. Although CBD in equal or greater doses produced none of these effects, when given together with THC, CBD was able to attenuate several effects of THC. In addition, CBD also changed the type of psychological reactions induced by THC from that of general anxiety and panic to a more pleasurable experience.

Similar results have been reported by Hollister,[18] who found CBD to be devoid of the mental and physical effects of THC, and by Dalton et al.,[89] who also found CBD to be devoid of psychological effects, but capable of attenuating the maximum "high" caused by THC. CBD also significantly attenuated several of the more unpleasurable THC-influenced emotions, described by subjects as feelings of discontent, trouble, feebleness, or being withdrawn.[90]

Thus, the effects of CBD on drug metabolism in humans are still unclear. Dalton et al.[91] found no effect of CBD on the pharmacokinetics of secobarbital, in contrast to both its inhibition of hexobarbital metabolism reported by Benowitz et al.[85] and their own report on the effects of CBD treatment on the pharmacological effects of THC.[89] Although alteration of THC metabolism is suggested, competition with THC for binding at the receptor site in the brain could explain the CBD-mediated alteration of the pharmacological action of THC. However, since the binding affinity of CBD is at least two orders of magnitude lower than that of THC,[84] this competition is unlikely.

Other Effects

To my knowledge, there have not been any other clinical reports of acute effects of marijuana or cannabinoids on the liver.

Long-Term Effects in Animals

Effects on Drug Metabolism

Inhibition. In rats treated with THC (20 mg/kg by gastric gavage) daily for 90 d and then withdrawn from treatment for an additional 60 d, THC was found to decrease markedly (56% of control) the aflatoxin B_1 binding to DNA, which is catalyzed by hepatic microsomes.[92] This demonstrates the highly persistent effects of long-term THC treatment. More studies along these lines should be undertaken to distinguish between a direct hepatic effect by persistent metabolites or one that is mediated through an altered regulation of drug-metabolizing enzymes.

Induction. Marijuana extract (20 mg/kg, ip) administered to rats for 7 or 15 d significantly increased hepatic microsomal aminopyrine *N*-demethylase activity,[93] reflecting induction of drug-metabolizing enzymes. Since THC and CBD content was not quantitated, it is difficult to identify the cannabinoid reponsible for the induction, although it is clear that marijuana exposure can increase drug metabolism.

Teratogenesis. When THC and/or phenobarbital were administered to rats for the entire term of pregnancy, phenobarbital, but not THC, was found to increase the fetal resorption rate as well as to decrease litter size and pup weight.[94] When administered together, the effects observed were no greater than that found with phenobarbital alone. This is in contrast to the reported acute synergistic effects between THC and phenobarbital on resorption rate and incidence of cleft palate.[76] Differences in species used (rat vs mouse) or dose of THC (50 vs 200 mg/kg) may be the reason for the discrepancy, although altered THC metabolism after chronic THC treatment cannot be ruled out.

When the effects of marijuana extract and alcohol on pregnancy were compared,[95] Abel found that fetal resorption rate significantly increased only when the compounds were coadministered. Although ethanol may exert a direct influence, such a synergism could also result from altered THC metabolism. Since ethanol is known to induce P-450IIE,[48] it is possible that this isozyme may produce toxic THC metabolites, resulting in the increase in resorption rate. In rhesus monkeys, THC administration during early pregnancy resulted in an increased abortion rate.[96] Administration after the first third of pregnancy increased premature and stillborn births. The influence of P-450 inhibitors or inducers on these effects was not assessed.

Other Effects

Fifty THC injections to pigeons resulted in no abnormalities after gross observation of the liver.[97] Marijuana extract given to monkeys for 90 d,[98] resulted in histological liver changes, including cytoplasmic degranulation and vacuolization with a decrease in liver glycogen. Increased SGOT, SGPT, serum bilirubin, and altered lipid metabolism were also noted.

Hepatic expression of *c-k-ras* protooncogene in rats increased three-fold after 90 d exposure to THC followed by 60 d of withdrawal.[92] Although this may indicate an increased propensity for carcinogenesis, as discussed previously, this treatment also decreased the aflatoxin B_1 binding to DNA, which is catalyzed by hepatic microsomes. Thus, it can only be concluded that chronic THC treatment results in several very long-lasting effects, even after treatment is discontinued.

Long-Term Effects in Humans

Effects on Drug Metabolism

Marked inhibition of barbiturate metabolism after 5–12 d of CBD treatment was reported by Benowitz et al.[85] Inductive effects of marijuana consumption were first reported by Lemberger et al.,[99] who found that long-term marijuana users metabolized radiolabeled THC at twice the rate of nonusers. However, later studies found no evidence of increased metabolism after frequent THC administration,[100] although disappearance of antipryrine, alcohol, and pentobarbital was found to be decreased, possibly as a result of an increased volume of distribution, decreased metabolic clearance, and delayed absorption. A later study[101] confirmed the lack of change in half-life of THC after 10–12 d of THC administration. These reports, although far from conclusive, suggest that marijuana consumption, but not that of THC alone, may result in induction.

Other Effects

In a widely cited study,[102] severe necrosis was reported in an individual who used marijuana daily for three years. Study of 12 additional marijuana users showed mild liver dysfunction in eight of the 12 users. Percutaneous liver biopsy of three users revealed striking parenchymatous degeneration with swelling and vacuolization of the cytoplasm. Interpretation of these findings was difficult, since alcohol and amphetamines had also been ingested. A subsequent study[103] of 50 marijuana users found no evidence of liver dysfunction when marijuana was the sole drug abused; however, dysfunction was noted in users who also consumed large amounts of alcohol. Many other reports also cite the lack of liver toxicity in long-term marijuana users.[104–107] Concurrent marijuana and alcohol use was also studied in adolescents and found to have no effect on liver function as assessed by γ-glutamyltranspeptidase activity.[108]

Hepatotoxicity has been reported to result from THC-induced lysosomal damage,[109] and antibodies to marijuana have been found in marijuana users.[110] The significance of these findings remains to be determined.

Conclusions

From the data previously discussed in this review, it may be concluded that marijuana consumption does not result in any marked liver toxicity after either short- or long-term use. The most obvious consequence of marijuana use may be its effect on drug metabolism, although its effects in humans are far from clear. It seems likely that marijuana use may result in either induction or inhibition of drug metabolism, depending on the marijuana constituents present and whether it is used chronically or occasionally. CBD, which is likely to be ingested in pharmacologically relevant doses as a result of marijuana consumption, appears to be responsible for most of the observed inductive or inhibitory effects. Although devoid of psychotropic effects itself, CBD can alter hepatic drug metabolism and thereby affect both the psychological and physiological effects of THC and, presumably, of other drugs as well.

Other consequences of marijuana use involve its teratogenic potential. Since this appears to be influenced by drugs that affect its metabolism, it is possible that a toxic metabolite is responsible.

Overall, the toxicity of marijuana on the liver is certainly less than that of alcohol, and is probably similar to that of most lipophilic drugs consumed chronically. Cannabinoid metabolites persist in the body for weeks after discontinuance of marijuana use, and, since several physiological alterations have been detected several months after cannabinoid withdrawal, a certain amount of caution must be exercised. Research into the long-term effects of marijuana use is certainly desirable, particularly since this drug is still being used by a large fraction of the population.

Acknowledgments

I would like to acknowledge the support of NIH Grant DA-04265 and to thank Bernice Wilson for her expert typing and Almira Correia for her helpful advice and review of this manuscript.

References

[1] E. L. Abel (1980) *Marihuana, The First Twelve Thousand Years.* Plenum, New York.

[2] W. B. O'Shaugnessy (1843) On the *cannabis indica* or Indian hemp. *Pharmacol. J. Trans.* **2,** 591.

[3] A. Christison (1851) On the natural history, action, and uses of Indian hemp. *Mon. J. Med. Sci.* **13,** 26,177.

[4] I. C. Chopra and R. N. Chopra (1957) The use of cannabis drugs in India. *Bull. Narc.* **9,** 4–29.

[5] T. F. Brunner (1977) Marijuana in Ancient Greece and Rome? The literary evidence. *J. Psychedelic Drugs* **9,** 221–225.

[6] M. Touw (1981) The religious and medicinal uses of cannabis in China, India, and Tibet. *J. Psychoactive Drugs* **13,** 23–34.

[7] R. R. McMeens (1973) Report of the Ohio State Medical Committee on *Cannabis indica,* in Trans. XVth Annu. Meet., Ohio State Medical Society, 75, 1860; reprinted in *Marijuana: Medical Papers 1839–1972,* T. H. Mikuriya, Medi-Comp, Oakland, CA.

[8] H. C. Wood (1871) On the medical activity of the hemp plant as grown in North America. *Proc. Am. Philos. Soc.* **11,** 226.

[9] R. Dunglison (1856) *New Remedies.* Blanchard & Lea, Philadelphia, p. 175.

[10] J. Aulde (1890) Studies in therapeutics—*Cannabis sativa. Ther. Gaz.* **14,** 523.

[11] S. Mackenzie (1887) Indian hemp in persistent headache. *J. Am. Med. Assoc.* **9,** 732.

[12] T. L. Wright (1863) Some therapeutic effects of *Cannabis indica. Cincinnati Lancet Observer* **6,** 73.

[13] Mayor's Committee on Marihuana (1944) *The Marihuana Problems in the City of New York.* Jaques Cattell, Lancaster, PA.

[14] R. Mechoulam (1981) Chemistry of cannabis. *Handbook Exp. Pharmacol.* **55,** 119–134.

[15] P. S. Fetterman, E. S. Keith, C. W. Waller, O. Guerrero, N. Doorenbos, and M. W. Quimby (1971) Mississippi-grown *Cannabis sativa* L.: Preliminary observation on chemical definition of phenotype and variations in tetrahydrocannabinol content *versus* age, sex and plant part. *J. Pharm. Sci.* **60,** 1246–1249.

[16] C. E. Turner, M. A. Elsohly, and E. G. Boeren (1980) Constituents of *Cannabis sativa* L.: XVII. A review of the natural constituents. *J. Nat. Prod.* **43,** 169–235.

[17] M. Perez-Reyes, M. C. Timmons, K. H. Davis, and E. M. Wall (1973) A comparison of the pharmacological activity in man of intravenously administered delta-9-tetrahydrocannabinol, cannabinol, and cannabidiol. *Experientia* **29,** 1368,1369.

[18] L. E. Hollister (1973) Cannabidiol and cannabinol in man. *Experientia* **29,** 825,826.

[19] E. A. Carlini, J. R. Leite, M. Tannhauser, and A. C. Berardi (1973) Cannabidiol and *Cannabis sativa* extract protect mice and rats against convulsive agents. *J. Pharm. Pharmacol.* **25,** 664,665.

[20] I. Izquierdo and A. G. Nasello (1973) Effects of cannabidiol on maximal electroshock seizures in rats. *J. Pharm. Pharmacol.* **25,** 916,917.

[21] R. Karler, W. Cely, and S. A. Turkanis (1973) The anticonvulsant activity of cannabidiol and cannabinol. *Life Sci.* **13,** 1527–1531.

[22] P. Consroe and S. R. Snider (1986) Theraputic potential of cannabinoids in neurological disorders, in *Cannabinoids as Therapeutic Agents.* CRC, Boca Raton, FL, pp. 21–49.

[23] R. Karler and S. A. Turkanis (1981) The cannabinoids as potential antiepileptics. *J. Clin. Pharmacol.* **21,** 437S–448S.

[24] S. A. Turkanis and R. Karler (1981) Electrophysiological properties of the cannabinoids. *J. Clin. Pharmacol.* **21,** 449S–463S.

[25] R. J. Porter (1983) Efficacy of antiepileptic drugs, in *Epilepsy.* A. A. Ward, Jr., J. K. Penry, and D. Purpura, eds. Raven, New York, pp. 225–237.

[26] A. V. Delgado-Escueta, D. M. Treiman, and G. O. Walsh (1983) The treatable epilepsies. *N. Engl. J. Med.* **308,** 1576–1584.

[27] J. M. Cunha, E. A. Carlini, and A. E. Pereira (1980) Chronic administration of cannabidiol to healthy volunteers and epileptic patients. *Pharmacology* **21,** 175–185.

[28] L. M. Bornheim (1989) Effect of cannabidiol on drug metabolism, in *Biochemistry and Physiology of Substance Abuse,* vol. 1. R. R. Watson, ed. CRC, Boca Raton, FL, pp. 21–35.

[29] D. J. Harvey and W. D. M. Paton (1986) Metabolism of the cannabinoids, in *Reviews in Biochemical Toxicology.* E. Hodgson, J. R. Bend, and R. M. Philpot, eds. Elsevier, New York, pp. 221–264.

[30] D. J. Harvey, B. R. Martin, and W. D. M. Paton (1980) Identification of in vivo liver metabolites of Δ^1-tetrahydracannabinol, cannabidiol, and cannabinol produced by the guinea pig. *Pharm. Pharmacol.* **32,** 267–271.

[31] B. R. Martin, D. J. Harvey, and W. D. M. Paton (1976) Identification of new in vivo side-chain acid metabolites of Δ^1-tetrahydrocannabinol. *J. Pharm. Pharmacol.* **28,** 773,774.

[32] D. J. Harvey, B. R. Martin, and W. D. M. Paton (1977) Identification of di- and tri-substituted hydroxy and ketone metabolites of Δ^1-tetrahydrocannabinol in mouse liver. *J. Pharm. Pharmacol.* **29,** 482–486.

[33] H. A. Klausner, and J. V. Dingel (1971) The metabolism and excretion of Δ^9-tetrahydrocannabinol in the rat. *Life Sci.* Part 1 **10,** 49–59.

[34] C. A. Dackis, A. L. C. Pottash, W. Annitto, and M. S. Gold (1982) Persistence of urinary marijuana levels after supervised abstinence. *Am. J. Psychiatry* **139,** 1196–1198.

[35] B. Martin, D. J. Harvey, and W. D. M. Paton (1977) Biotransformation of cannabidiol in mice. Identification of new acid metabolites. *Drug Metab. Dispos.* **5,** 259–267.

[36] J. R. Bailey, H. C. Cunny, M. G. Paule, and W. Slikker, Jr. (1987) Fetal disposition of Δ^9-tetrahydrocannabinol (THC) during late pregnancy in the Rhesus monkey. *Toxicol. Appl. Pharmacol.* **90,** 315–321.

[37] A. H. Conney (1967) Pharmacological implications of microsomal enzyme induction. *Pharmacol. Rev.* **19,** 317–366.

[38] J. R. Gillette, D. C. Davis, and H. A. Sasame (1972) Cytochrome P-450 and its role in drug metabolism. *Annu. Rev. Pharmacol.* **12,** 57–84.

[39] A. Y. H. Lu and S. B. West (1980) Multiplicity of mammalian microsomal cytochromes P-450. *Pharmacol. Rev.* **31,** 277–294.

[40] D. W. Nebert, D. R. Nelson, M. Adesnik, M. J. Coon, R. W. Estabrook, F. J. Gonzalez, F. P. Guengerich, I. C. Gunsalus, E. F. Johnson, B. Kemper, W. Levin, I. R. Phillips, R. Sato, and M. R. Waterman (1989) The P450 superfamily: Updated listing of all genes and recommended nomenclature for the chromosomal loci. *DNA* **8,** 1–13.

[41] D. E. Ryan, P. E. Thomas, L. M. Reik, and W. Levin (1982) Purification, characterization and regulation of five rat hepatic microsomal cytochrome P-450 isoenzymes. *Xenobiotica* **12,** 727–744.

[42] F. P. Guengerich, G. A. Dannon, S. T. Wright, M. V. Martin, and L. S. Kaminsky (1982) Purification and characterization of rat liver microsomal cytochrome P-450: Electrophoretic, spectral, catalytic and immunochemical properties and inducibility of eight isozymes isolated from rats treated with phenobarbital or β-napthoflavone. *Biochemistry* **21,** 6019–6030.

[43] D. J. Waxman and C. Walsh (1982) Phenobarbital-induced rat liver cytochrome P-450: Purification of two closely related isozymic forms. *J. Biol. Chem.* **258,** 11937–11947.

[44] R. Masuda-Mikawa, Y. Fujii-Kuriyama, M. Negishi, and Y. Tashiro (1979) Purification and partial characterization of hepatic microsomal P-450's from phenobarbital and 3-methylcholanthrene-treated rats. *J. Biochem.* **86,** 1383–1394.

[45] N. A. Elshourbagy and P. S. Guzelian (1980) Separation, purification and characterization of a novel form of hepatic cytochrome P-450 from rats treated with pregnenolone-16α-carbonitrile. *J. Biol. Chem.* **255,** 1279–1285.

[46] S. A. Wrighton, P. Maurel, E. G. Schuetz, P. B. Watkins, B. Young, and P. S. Guzelian (1985) Identification of the cytochrome P-450 induced by macrolide antibiotics in rat liver as the glucocorticoid responsive cytochrome P-450p. *Biochemistry* **24,** 2171–2178.

[47] D. E. Ryan, L. Ramanathan, S. Iida, R. E. Thomas, M. Haniu, J. E. Shively, C. S. Lieber, and W. Levin (1985) Characterization of a major form of rat hepatic microsomal cytochrome P-450 induced by isoniazid. *J. Biol. Chem.* **260,** 6385–6393.

[48] J. M. Lasker, J. Raucy, S. Kubota, B. P. Bloswick, M. Black, and C. S. Lieber (1987) Purification and characterization of human liver cytochrome P-450-ALC. *Biochem. Biophys. Res. Commun.* **148,** 232–238.

[49] S. Loewe (1944) Studies on the pharmacology of marihuana, in *The Marihuana Problems in the City of New York* by the Mayor's Committee on Marihuana. Jaques Cattell, Lancaster, PA, pp. 149–212.

[50] J. V. Dingell, K. W. Miller, E. C. Heath, and H. A. Klausner (1973) The intracellular localization of Δ^9-tetrahydrocannabinol in liver and its effects on drug metabolism in vitro. *Biochem. Pharmacol.* **22,** 949–958.

[51] G. M. Cohen, D. W. Peterson, and G. J. Mannering (1971) Interactions of Δ^9-tetrahydrocannabinol with the hepatic microsomal drug metabolizing system. *Life Sci.* **10,** 1207–1215.

[52] D. Kupfer, I. Jansson, and S. Orrenius (1972) Spectral interactions of marihuana constituents (cannabinoids) with rat liver microsomal monooxygenase system. *Chem. Biol. Interact.* **5,** 201–206.

[53] A. J. Siemans, H. Kalant, J. M. Khanna, J. Marshman, and G. Ho (1974) Effect of cannabis on pentobarbital-induced sleeping time and pentobarbital metabolism in the rat. *Biochem. Pharmacol.* **23,** 477–488.

[54] W. D. M. Paton and R. G. Pertwee (1972) Effect of cannabis and certain of its constituents on pentobarbitone sleeping time and phenazone metabolism. *Br. J. Pharmacol.* **44,** 250–261.

[55] B. B. Coldwell, K. Bailey, C. J. Paul, and G. Anderson (1974) Interaction of cannabinoids with pentobarbital in rats. *Toxicol. Appl. Pharmacol.* **29,** 59–69.

[56] H. K. Borys, G. B. Ingall, and R. Karler (1979) Development of tolerance to the prolongation of hexobarbitone sleeping time caused by cannabidiol. *Br. J. Pharmacol.* **67,** 93–101.

[57] L. M. Bornheim, H. K. Borys, and R. Karler (1981) Effect of cannabidiol on cytochrome P-450 and hexobarbital sleep time. *Biochem. Pharmacol.* **30,** 503–507.

[58] K. Hamajima, K. Watanabe, S. Narimatsu, Y. Tateoka, I. Yamamoto, and H. Yoshimura (1983) Sex difference in the effects of Δ^9-tetrahydrocannabinol and cannabidiol on pentobarbital-induced sleeping time and hepatic microsomal drug metabolizing enzyme systems in mice. *Yakugaku Zasshi* **103,** 1289–1297.

[59] K. Bailey and P. Toft (1973) Difference spectra of rat hepatic microsomes induced by cannabinoids and related compounds. *Biochem. Pharmacol.* **22,** 2780–2783.

[60] K. Watanabe, K. Hamajima, S. Narimatsu, I. Yamamoto, and H. Yoshimura (1986) Effects of two cannabinoids on hepatic microsomal cytochrome P-450. *J. Pharmacobiodyn.* **9,** 39–45.

[61] L. M. Bornheim, and M. A. Correia (1987) Cannabidiol: Effect on hepatic cytochrome P-450 isozymes. *The Pharmacologist* **29,** 76.

[62] L. M. Bornheim and M. A. Correia (1989) Effect of cannabidiol on cytochrome P-450 isozymes. *Biochem. Pharmacol.* **38,** 2789–2794.

[63] L. M. Bornheim and M. A. Correia (1990) Selective inactivation of mouse liver cytochrome P-450IIIA by cannabidiol. *Mol. Pharmacol.* **38,** 319–326.

[64] K. A. Hostetler, S. A. Wrighton, P. Kremers, and P. S. Guzelian (1987) Immunochemical evidence for multiple steroid-inducible hepatic cytochromes P-450 in the rat. *Biochem. J.* **245,** 27–33.

[65] P. E. Graves, L. S. Kaminsky, and J. Halpert (1987) Evidence for functional and structural multiplicity of pregnenolone-16α-carbonitrile-inducible cytochrome P-450 isozymes in rat liver microsomes. *Biochemistry* **26**, 3887–3894.

[66] H. K. Borys and R. Karler (1979) Cannabidiol and Δ^9-tetrahydrocannabinol metabolism. *Biochem. Pharmacol.* **28**, 1553–1559.

[67] R. Karler, P. Sangdee, S. A. Turkanis, and H. K. Borys (1979) The pharmacokinetic fate of cannabidiol and its relationship to barbiturate sleep time. *Biochem. Pharmacol.* **28**, 777–784.

[68] R. D. Sofia and H. Barry III (1970) Depressant effect of Δ^1-tetrahydrocannabinol enhanced by inhibition of its metabolism. *Eur. J. Pharmacol.* **13**, 134–137.

[69] S. Burstein and D. Kupfer (1971) Hydroxylation of *trans*-Δ^1-tetrahydrocannabinol by hepatic microsomal oxygenase. *Ann. NY Acad. Sci.* **191**, 61–67.

[70] E. W. Gill and G. Jones (1972) Brain levels of Δ^1-tetrahydrocannabinol and its metabolites in mice — correlation with behavior, and the effect of the metabolic inhibitors SKF 525-A and piperonyl butoxide. *Biochem. Pharmacol.* **21**, 2237–2248.

[71] H. D. Christensen, R. I. Freudenthal, J. T. Gidley, R. Rosenfeld, G. Boegli, L. Testino, D. R. Brine, C. G. Pitt, and M. E. Wall (1971) Activity of Δ^8- and Δ^9-tetrahydrocannabinol and related compounds in the mouse. *Science* **172**, 165–167.

[72] R. Mechoulam (1970) Marijuana chemistry. *Science* **168**, 1159–1166.

[73] G. Jones and R. G. Pertwee (1972) A metabolic interaction in vivo between cannabidiol and Δ^1-tetrahydrocannabinol. *Brit. J. Pharmacol.* **45**, 375–377.

[74a] L. M. Bornheim and M. A. Correia (1990) Effects of cannabidiol on mouse hepatic cannabinoid metabolism. *FASEB J.* **4**, A1973.

[74b] L. M. Bornheim and M. A. Correia (1991) Purification and characterization of the major hepatic cannabinoid hydroxylase in the mouse: A member of the cytochrome P-450 IIC subfamily. *Mol. Pharmacol.*, submitted.

[75] K. Watanabe, M. Arai, S. Narimatsu, I. Yamamoto, and H. Yoshimura (1986) Effect of repeated administration of 11-hydroxy-Δ^8-tetrahydrocannabinol, an active metabolite of Δ^8-tetrahydrocannabinol, on the hepatic microsomal drug-metabolizing enzyme system of mice. *Biochem. Pharmacol.* **35**, 1861–1865.

[76] B. Mantilla-Plata and R. D. Harbison (1976) Influence of alteration of tetrahydrocannabinol metabolism on tetrahydrocannabinol-induced teratogenesis, in *The Pharmacology of Marijuana*. M. C. Braude and S. Szare, eds. Raven, New York, pp. 733–742.

[77] T. Bino, A. Chari-Bitron, and A. Shakar (1972) Biochemical effects and morphological changes in rat liver mitochondria exposed to Δ^1-tetrahydrocannabinol. *Biochem. Biophys. Acta* **288**, 195–202.

[78] M. K. Poddar, K. C. Bhattocharya, and J. J. Ghosh (1974) Potentiating effect of cannabidiol on Δ^9-tetrahydrocannabinol-induced changes in hepatic enzymes. *Biochem. Pharmacol.* **23**, 758–759.

[79] M. El-Sourogy, A. Y. Malek, H. H. Ibrahim, A. Farag, and A. El-Shihy (1966) The effect of *cannabis indica* on carbohydrate metabolism in rabbits. *J. Egypt. Med. Assoc.* **49**, 626–628.

[80] C. M. Soni and M. L. Gupta (1978) Effect of cannabis (bhang) extract on blood glucose and liver glycogen in albino rats. *Indian J. Physiol. Pharmacol.* **22**, 152–154.

[81] A. Pasquale (de), G. Costa, and A. Trovato (1978) The influence of cannabis on glucoregulation. *Bull. Narc.* **30**, 33–41.

[82] C. J. Hillard, A. S. Bloom, and M. D. Houslay (1986) Effects of Δ^9-tetrahydrocannabinol on glucagon receptor coupling to adenylate cyclase in rat liver plasma membranes. *Biochem. Pharmacol.* **35**, 2797–2803.

[83] A. C. Howlett, M. Ross Johnson, L. S. Melvin, and G. M. Milne (1987) Nonclassical cannabinoid analgetics inhibit adenylate cyclase: Development of a cannabinoid receptor model. *Mol. Pharmacol.* **33**, 297–302.

[84] M. Herkenham, A. B. Lynn, M. D. Little, M. Ross Johnson, L. S. Melvin, B. R. DeCosta, and K. C. Rice (1990) Cannabinoid receptor localization in brain. *Proc. Natl. Acad. Sci. USA* **87**, 1932–1936.

[85] N. L. Benowitz, T. Nguyen, R. T. Jones, R. I. Herning, and J. Bachman (1980) Metabolic and psychophysiologic studies of cannabidiol-hexobarbital interaction. *Clin. Pharmacol. Ther.* **28**, 115–120.

[86] S. Agurell, S. Carlsson, J. E. Lindgren, A. Ohlsson, H. Gillespie, and L. Hollister (1981) Interactions of Δ^1-tetrahydrocannabinol with cannabinol and cannabidiol following oral administration in man. Assay of cannabinol and cannabidiol by mass fragmentography. *Experientia* **37**, 1090–1092.

[87] C. A. Hunt, R. T. Jones, R. I. Herning, and J. Bachman (1981) Evidence that cannabidiol does not significantly alter the pharmacokinetics of tetrahydrocannabinol in man. *J. Pharmacokin. Biopharm.* **9**, 245–260.

[88] I. G. Karniol, I. Shirakawa, N. Kasinski, A. Pfeferman, and E. A. Carlini (1974) Cannabidiol interferes with the effects of delta-9-tetrahydrocannabinol in man. *Eur. J. Pharmacol.* **28**, 172–177.

[89] W. S. Dalton, R. Martz, L. Lemberger, B. E. Rodda, and B. Forney (1976) Influence of cannabidiol on delta-9-tetrahydrocannabinol effects. *Clin. Pharmacol. Ther.* **19**, 300–309.

[90] A. W. Zuardi, I. Shirakawa, E. Finkelfarb, and I. G. Karniol (1982) Action of cannabidiol on the anxiety and other effects produced by delta-9-THC in normal subjects. *Psychopharmacology* **76**, 245–250.

[91] W. S. Dalton, R. Martz, B. E. Rodda, L. Lemberger, and R. B. Forney (1976) Influence of cannabidiol on secobarbital effects and plasma kinetics. *Clin. Pharmacol. Ther.* **20**, 695–700.

[92] H. R. Prasanna, K. D. Nakamura, S. F. Ali, M. H. Lu, W. Slikker, Jr., and R. W. Hart (1989) Altered hepatic microsomal function and elevated protooncogene expression as residual effects in rats exposed to delta-9-tetrahydrocannabinol. *Biochem. Biophys. Res. Commun.* **160,** 217–221.

[93] N. Sethi, P. K. Agnihotri, and S. Srivastava (1989) Aminopyrine-*N*-demethylase activity of rat liver after administration of crude cannabis extract. *Indian J. Med. Res.* **90,** 36–38.

[94] E. L. Abel, S. E. Tan, and M. Subramanian (1987) Effects of Δ^9-tetrahydrocannabinol, phenobarbital, and their combination on pregnancy and offspring in rats. *Teratology* **36,** 193–198.

[95] E. L. Abel (1985) Alcohol enhancement of marihuana-induced fetotoxicity. *Teratology* **31,** 35–40.

[96] S. L. Corson (1986) Effects of Δ^9-THC, the principal psychoactive component of marijuana, during pregnancy in the Rhesus monkey. *J. Reprod. Med.* **31,** 1071–1081.

[97] D. E. McMillian, L. S. Harris, R. F. Turk, and J. S. Kennedy (1970) Development of marked behavioral tolerance to 1-Δ^9-tetrahydrocannabinol (Δ^9-THC) and cross tolerance to 1-Δ^8-tetrahydrocannabinol (Δ^8-THC) in the pigeon. *Pharmacologist* **12,** 258.

[98] V. P. Dixit (1981) Effects of cannabis sativa extract on testicular function of presbytis entellus entellus. *Planta Med.* **41,** 288–294.

[99] L. Lemberger, N. R. Tamarkin, J. Axelrod, and I. J. Kopin (1971) Delta-9-tetrahydrocannabinol: Metabolism and disposition in long-term marihuana smokers. *Science* **173,** 72–74.

[100] N. L. Benowitz and R. T. Jones (1977) Prolonged delta-9-tetrahydrocannabinol. Effects of sympathomimetic amines and autonomic blockades. *Clin. Pharmacol. Ther.* **21,** 336–342.

[101] C. A. Hunt and R. T. Jones (1980) Tolerance and disposition of tetrahydrocannabinol in man. *J. Pharmacol. Exp. Ther.* **215,** 35–44.

[102] M. C. Kew, I. Bersohn, and S. Siew (1969) Possible hepatotoxicity of cannabis. *Lancet* **1,** 578,579.

[103] J. S. Hochman and N. Q. Brill (1971) Chronic marihuana usage and liver function. *Lancet* **2,** 818,819.

[104] F. S. Tennant, M. Preble, T. J. Prendergast, and P. Ventry (1971) Medical manifestations associated with hashish. *J. Am. Med. Assoc.* **216,** 1965–1969.

[105] W. J. Coggins, E. W. Swenson, W. W. Dawson, A. Fernandez-Salas, J. Hernandez-Bolanos, C. F. Jiminez-Antillon, J. R. Solano, R. Vinocour, and F. Faerron-Valdez (1976) Health status of chronic heavy cannabis users. *Ann. NY Acad. Sci.* **282,** 148–161.

[106] S. Cohn, P. J. Lessin, P. M. Hahn, and E. D. Tyrell (1976) A 94-day cannabis study, in *Pharmacology of Marijuana*, vol. 2. M. C. Braude and S. Szara, eds. Raven, New York, pp. 621–626.

[107] E. K. Cruickshank (1976) Physical assessment of 30 chronic cannabis users and 30 matched controls. *Ann. NY Acad. Sci.* **282,** 162–167.

[108] J. A. Farrow, J. M. Rees, and B. S. Worthington-Roberts (1987) Health, developmental, and nutritional status of adolescent alcohol and marijuana abusers. *Pediatrics* **79,** 218–223.

[109] A. Mellors (1974) Lysosomal damage by cannabinoids: A mechanism for hepatoxicity and reduced cellular immunity. *Fed. Proc.* **33,** 1386.

[110] C. M. Shapiro, A. R. Orlina, P. J. Unger, M. Telfer, and A. A. Billings (1975) Marihuana induced antibody response and laboratory correlates. *Clin. Res.* **23,** 488A.

In Vivo Microscopy
of the Effects of Ethanol
on the Liver

Robert S. McCuskey

Introduction

In vivo microscopic studies of the mammalian liver, to date, have been restricted principally to studies of rats and mice, although a few studies have been reported using hamsters, guinea pigs, and rabbits.[1] Nevertheless, these studies have provided valuable information concerning the liver, particularly its microvascular compartment. The latter is composed of portal and central venules, hepatic arterioles and sinusoids, as well as associated neural elements that may modulate or modify vascular mechanisms controlled locally or by hormones. This system is responsible for regulating everything that enters and leaves the sinusoids where the exchange processes occur between the blood and the hepatic parenchymal cells. Since the microcirculation is dynamic, it is best studied using in vivo microscopic methods, which permit the rate, duration, magnitude, and direction of dynamic events to be directly visualized, evaluated, quantified, and recorded continuously in life. Surprisingly, however, only a limited number of in vivo microscopic studies have been reported on the basic hepatic microcirculatory response to alcohol.[2–5]

Following the ingestion of alcohol, significant alterations occur in host defense mechanisms including depressed reticuloendothelial (RES) function as well as altered immune, lymphocyte, granulocyte, and platelet functions. These increase the host's susceptibility to infection.[6–8] Ethanol ingestion produces increased hepatic oxygen consumption, fatty liver, hepatomegaly, hepatocellular damage, and, with prolonged consumption, hepatitis, fibrogenesis, and cirrhosis may result. Alterations in hepatic blood flow accompany these responses. Acutely administered ethanol increases hepatic blood flow.[9,10] The acute vasodilatory effect of ethanol is not thought to be a result of vascular actions of metabolites of ethanol, acetalaldehyde, or acetate,[11–14] but is suggested to be a result of adenosine.[14] The potential role of vasoactive mediators released from Kupffer cells, however, has not been evaluated.

Kupffer cells are one of the cellular compoments of the sinusoids in the liver and are a major part of the RES. Several studies have demonstrated that Kupffer cell function is affected by alcohol in both experimental animals and man. Clearance of microaggregated albumin and endotoxin is depressed in rats following both acute and chronic administration of alcohol.[15–17] Acute human alcoholics with no evidence of liver disease also have a depressed RES that returns to normal several days following alcohol withdrawal.[18] Furthermore, patients also have been reported to have a depressed RES as evidenced by reduced clearance of microaggregated albumin;[19] and, another group lacked a concentration gradient of immune complexes between portal and hepatic veins.[20] Finally, elevated levels of systemic, circulating endotoxin have been reported in humans intoxicated with alcohol[21] and during alcoholic liver disease[17,21,22] suggesting spillover of gut-derived endotoxin no longer being cleared by alcohol-depressed hepatic Kupffer cells. As a result, Kupffer cell dysfunction and endotoxin have been implicated in the etiology of alcoholic liver disease.[16,17,22] This concept is further supported by recent animal studies which demonstrated that, in the presence of alcohol, normally innocuous doses of endotoxin become toxic and result in severe liver damage.[23] Hypoxia, such as reported for centrilobular hepatocytes in rats acutely dosed with ethanol,[3,5] also potentiates the hepatotoxicity of endotoxin.[24]

Endotoxins, lipopolysaccharides of the cell walls of gram-negative bacteria, have manifold toxic and, in low concentrations, beneficial effects.[25–28] Kupffer cells are the principal site for the removal of circulating endotoxins from the blood.[29–33] Following the endocytosis of endotoxin, a variety of toxic and beneficial mediators are released from Kupffer cells, as well as other macrophages. Among the mediators produced are tumor necrosis factor (TNF), interleukin-1 (IL-1), eicosanoids, and reactive free radicals. These are thought to participate in the host response to endotoxin (reviewed in ref. 31). Although high concentrations of endotoxins, such as are found during gram-negative sepsis, usually precipitate a toxic response including hepatic microvascular and parenchymal dysfunction, low levels of gut-derived endotoxin such as normally found in the portal blood, may contribube to nonspecific resistance by modulating Kupffer cell activity (reviewed in ref. 31). Unfortunately, little is known about the role of these substances in mediating blood vessel and cellular injury in the liver during health as well as in the presence of alcohol and/or infection.

At the microcirculatory level, limited knowledge exists about alcohol-induced alterations in the hepatic microvasculature, how such alterations are exacerbated in the presence of endotoxemia and/or infection, and the role played by Kupffer cells in these processes. The few published in vivo microscopic studies report that acute, oral administration of ethanol to rats increases both portal and hepatic arterial blood flow resulting in an average net increase in the velocity of erythrocyte flow through the sinusoids.[2–5] The increased flow in the sinusoids, however, was heterogeneous, with some sinusoids exhibiting dramatic increases in cellular velocity, whereas others had little or no increase and some a decrease. As a result, some centrivenular areas became hypoxic while others exhibited an increase in oxygenation.[2–5] There are no reports of in vivo microscopic examination of livers in animal chronically ingesting ethanol.

Owing to this lack of knowledge concerning the microvascular pathophysiology induced in the liver by acute and chronic alcohol alone or in the presence of endotoxin and/or infection, we initiated studies to elucidate the hepatic microvascular responses, including Kupffer cell function, during these conditions. This chapter summerizes our methodology for high resolution in vivo microscopy of the liver and the observed dynamic responses of hepatic microvasculature to acute intragastric ethanol administration in mice alone or in combination with endotoxin.

In Vivo Microscopic Methods

Basic Methods

The basic methods that have been used to study the living liver with the light microscope include examination of surgically exposed organs in situ or as isolated, perfused preparations.[34] Each method has advantages as well as limitations.

Microscopic study of surgically exposed organs in situ usually permits high resolution examination of the microvasculature with its supplying vessels and nerve supplies intact. However, these preparations are subject to movements induced by the heart, respiratory, and gastrointestinal systems, which, at times, can preclude critical microscopic study of the liver. Another limitation is the requirement to use anesthesia, which limits the duration of the study to relatively short periods of time (2–12 h). In spite of these limitations, the use of such methods has resulted in a better understanding of the structure and function of the microvasculature in the liver under a variety of experimental conditions. Although most such studies have been of the intact liver *in situ*, the isolated, perfused liver[35] also is a suitable candidate for high resolution in vivo microscopy. Such preparations are not subject to induced movements and permit critical control of blood pressure and flow. However, they usually are of very short duration since structural and functional deterioration frequently becomes evident after 1–2 h.

The livers of a variety of small laboratory animals, including rats, mice, hamsters, rabbits, and guinea pigs, can be studied by light microscopy using transillumination of relatively thin (3–5 mm) areas of the organ. Thicker areas of the organs in these species as well as the thicker livers of larger animals such as cats, dogs, and monkeys can be examined only by epi-illumination. It should be noted, however, that the resolution obtainable using epi-illumination usually is inferior to that realized with transillumination.[34]

Transillumination Methods

Two basic methods of transillumination have been used for light microscopy of the spleen. These include the use of quartz, glass, or plastic light rods or fiber optic light guides, which generally are not focusable; alternatively, a focusable condenser contained on a modified compound microscope is used. Although the first method permits microscopic examination of the organ in its normal anatomical position, examination at high magnifications with good resolution rarely is possible. As a result, most in vivo microscopic studies of the microvasculature of the liver during the past 30 yrs have used a modified compound trinocular microscope.[1,31,34]

The compound trinocular microscope normally is equipped for both trans- as well as epi-illumination of the organ to be studied. After the animal is anesthetized, the liver is exteriorized through a left subcostal incision and positioned over a window of optical grade mica or glass in a specially designed tray mounted on the microscope stage. The tray has provision for the drainage of irrigating fluids, and the window overlies a long working distance condenser. The liver is covered with a piece of Saran or Mylar film, which sometimes is cemented to a moveable U-shaped metal or plastic frame. The Saran or Mylar holds the organ in position and limits movement induced by the heart, respiration, and intestines, yet it is flexible enough to avoid compression of the underlying hepatic microvasculature. In addition, the plastic film helps to maintain homeostasis by limiting exposure of the surface of the organ to the external environment. Homeostasis is further insured by constant suffusion of the organ with Ringer's solution, which is maintained at body temperature by proportional regulating heaters electronically clamped to rectal temperature. Once the organ is exteriorized and positioned on the window overlying the substage condenser, it is transilluminated with selected wavelengths of monochromatic light between 400 and 800 nm obtained by placing a monochromater in the light-path between a broad spectrum xenon lamp and the substage condenser. The microscopic images of the microvasculature and its surrounding tissue are secured at magnifications up to 1500× using both dry and water immersion objectives. The resulting optical images are either studied and photographed directly or are televised through a projection ocular (1.6–5.0×). A silicon or intensified silicon (SIT or ISIT) vidicon camera is used depending on the sensitivity and resolution required as well as the wavelenghts of light to be imaged. The resulting video images are either video taped or recorded on motion picture film using a camera whose motor is synchronized with the framing rate of the video system.

The use of specific wavelengths of monochromatic light enhance definition of cellular detail through the selective absorption or transmission of these wavelengths by specific tissue and cellular components. When such monochromatic, microscopic images are televised, the contrast between tissue and cellular components can be enhanced further by readjustments of the brightness and contrast controls on the video monitor. Thus, the images of a particular structure(s) can be enhanced or supressed depending on the wavelength of light selected and the adjustments of the television system. For example, the use of wavelengths of light that are selectively absorbed by hemoglobin contained in the circulating erythrocytes aids in the study of patterns of blood flow or the overall morphological organization of a microvascular bed in the organ, particularly at low or moderate magnifications. However, for studying the highly vascular liver at high magnifications, it is useful to transilluminate the organ at wavelengths of light between 575 and 750 nm to eliminate the absorption of light by the hemoglobin contained in the numerous erythrocytes flowing in the microvasculature. This not only increases the amount of light transmitted through the liver, but it also enhances the definition of the endothelium and other cellular components. When such images are televised using a silicon vidicon having a peak spectral response between 600 and 800 nm, the following usually can be observed: differentiation of the microvasculature into portal and central venules, hepatic arterioles, and sinusoids; patterns of blood flow in these vessels; the shape and deformation of individual blood cells; differentiation of the endothelium of most vessels; identification of most cells contiguous with the microvasculature; and some cytoplasmic and nuclear detail. Under optimal conditions, the measured resolution is 0.3–0.5 µm when using 80–100× water immersion objectives.

Epi-Illumination Methods

In addition to transillumination, the liver can be epi-illuminated through the objective lens using appropriate optics. As indicated earlier, the resolution obtained using this method of illumination is considerably less than that obtained by transillumination. However, epi-illumination is particularly useful for studying the patterns and distribution of fluorescent probes of microvascular and cellular function. Potential uses of fluorescent probes include the study the phagocytic and endocytotic properties of Kupffer cells under a variety of conditions, the transport of material from the sinusoid into parenchymal cells, differences in the patterns between cellular and plasma flow, and entrapment of labeled leukocytes and tumor cells, and so on.[1,34–41] For intensely fluorescing materials, epi- and transillumination can be combined to provide improved definition of the cellular localization of a variety of fluorescent probes. Alternatively, weakly fluorescing probes may first be imaged and recorded by epi-illumination and their localization subsequently identified by transillumination. In many cases, the use of intensified (SIT or ISIT) video cameras coupled with digitial image processing and/or filtered techniques are necessary to obtain images of reasonable quality and for extraction of the desired information, especially if this information is to be quantified. Such techniques are just beginning to be used in studying the microvasculature of organs by in vivo microscopy.

In Vivo Microscopic Studies of the Effects of Ethanol on the Liver

Initial experiments using endotoxin-sensitive NMRI mice dosed intragastrically with 1 g/kg ethanol demonstrated a 31% increase in the numbers of phagocytic Kupffer cells/microscopic field 1 h after ethanol ingestion. However, 5 g/kg intragastric ethanol resulted in a 19% reduction in phagocytic Kupffer cells.[42] In contrast, 5 g/kg ethanol elicited a 30% increase in the number of phagocytic Kupffer cells in endotoxin nonresponding C_3H/HeJ mice.[42] Subsequently, more extensive experiments were conducted to better define the hepatic microvascular responses to different doses of ethanol and relate these to blood ethanol levels in C57Bl/6 mice.

Ethanol doses of 1 gm/kg of body wt in C57Bl/6 mice produced systemic blood ethanol levels of 0.1% 30 min after dosing. Portal levels were not significantly higher than levels in systemic blood; by 3 h no detectible blood ethanol was found. In contrast, ethanol doses of 4 g/kg of body wt resulted in blood levels of 0.35% by 30 min, these levels were still evident at 3 h but had dropped to 0.1% by 6 h. Only modest changes in transaminases were detected even at the highest doses (5 g/kg of body wt) of acute ethanol administration with these values remaining in the normal range.[43,44]

Based on these results, the hepatic microvascular responses to a single acute low (1 g/kg of body wt) and high dose (4 g/kg of body wt) of intragastric ethanol was studied in more detail by high resolution in vivo microscopy at 30 min and 3 h after dosing.[43,45] Similar examinations were made of control animals dosed with isocaloric sucrose in water. The high dose of ethanol (4 g/kg) elicited hepatocellular damage as evidenced by the formation of vacuoles and/or swollen organelles, endothelial cellular swelling, and transient plugging of sinusoidal blood flow by leukocytes. Following challenge with a standardized iv dose of 1.0 μm latex particles, there appeared to be less uptake by Kupffer cells although the number of phagocytic cells was not significantly different from controls. Although the low dose of ethanol (1 g/kg) elicited considerably less change in the microcirculation, it did elicit a 63% enhancement of phagocytosis of latex particles by Kupffer cells.[43,45–47] The number of phagocytic Kupffer cells also increased, particularly by 3 h when the blood ethanol level had returned to undetectable levels. Further evidence of Kupffer cell activation was provided by a 128% increase in the clearance rate of a bolus injection of endotoxin from the blood of the animals treated with 1 g/kg ethanol.[46,47] Kupffer cells are the principal site for such clearance.[30,33]

These studies demonstrated that an acute single dose of ethanol differentially affects the hepatic microvascular system, including Kupffer cell phagocytic function, in a dose dependent manner. That ethanol affects Kupffer cell function is evident from enhanced phagocytic activity elicited by low doses of ethanol and the lack of effect or suppression of phagocytosis with high doses. Since the latter responses were not seen in endotoxin nonresponsive mice where enhanced phagocytosis was observed instead, the effects of ethanol on phagocytic activity appear to depend on the state of Kupffer cell activation, which is low in C_3H/HeJ mice.[37,38] Differential, dose dependent effects on Kupffer cell phagocytic function also are elicited by both endotoxin and TNFα,[31,36–41] suggesting a possible role for these substances in the responses to ethanol.

Many of the microvascular events, e.g., endothelial cellular swelling, leukocyte adhesion, and plugging of sinusoids, also mimic responses elicited by injection of endotoxin and tumor necrosis factor alpha (TNFα), as well as sepsis.[31,36–41] Since endotoxin was not detected in the plasma of mice acutely treated with ethanol and all of these events were eliminated when anti-mouse TNF was administered prior to ethanol,[45–47] TNF released from Kupffer cells is strongly suggested to be responsible for the intravascular events elicited by ethanol. Further evidence is provided by the observation that ethanol failed to elicit leukocyte adhesion to the endothelium of C_3H/HeJ mice whose Kupffer cells and other macrophages do not produce TNF. It should be noted, however, that leukocyte adhesion can be elicited in these mice by the administration of exogenous TNF.[40] Taken together, these data support the reported involvement of TNF in the hepatic response of macrophages to ethanol.[48,49]

Acknowledgments

These studies were supported by NIAAA Specialized Alcohol Research Center Grant, IP50AA 08037, a grant from the Arizona Disease Control Research Commission, and the A. V. Humboldt Stiftung (US Senior Scientist Prize to RSM).

References

[1] R. S. McCuskey (1988) Hepatic microcirculation, in *Sinusoids in Human Liver: Health and Disease.* P. Bioulac-Sage and C. Balabaud, eds. Kupffer Cell Foundation, Leiden, pp. 151–164.

[2] N. Sato, H. Eguchi, Y. Takei, T. Hijioka, S. Tsuji, T. Matsuura, N. Hayashi, S. Kawano, T. Kamada (1987) Microcirculatory aspects for the mechanism of alcoholic liver disease-sinusoidal blood flow and oxygenation at periportal regions of hepatic lobules in rats, in M. Tsuchiya, M. Asano, Y. Mishama, and M. Oda, eds. *Microcirculation — An Update,* vol. 2. Excerpta Med, Amsterdam, pp. 345–348.

[3] N. Sato, T. Matsumura, S. Kawano, and T. Kamada (1987) Hepatic microcirculation and hepatic cellular-metabolism, in *Microcirculation — An Update,* vol. 2. M. Tsuchiya, M. Asano, Y. Mishama, and M. Oda, eds. Excerpta Med, Amsterdam, pp. 345–348.

[4] H. Eguchi, N. Sato, M. Minamiyama, T. Matsumura, S. Kawano, and T. Kamada (1987) Heterogeneous response in hepatic sinusoidal blood flow to acute ethanol ingestion in rats. *Alcohol Alcohol.* **Suppl. 1,** 519–521.

[5] N. Sato, S. Kawano, T. Matsumura, H. Yoshihara, T. Hijioka, H. Eguchi, T. Matsunaga, et al. (1988) Abnormal heterogenic distribution of hepatic sinusoidal blood flow and oxygenation after acute ethanol consumption in rats: Direct evidence for pericentral hypoxemia, in *Biomedical and Social Aspects of Alcohol and Alcoholism.* K. Kuriyama, A. Takada, and H. Ishii, eds. Elsevier Science, Tokyo, pp. 775–778.

[6] H. G. Adams and C. Jordan (1984) Infections in the alcoholic. *Med. Clin. NA* **68,** 179–200.

[7] D. B. Louria (1963) Susceptibility to infection during experimental alcohol intoxication. *Trans. Assoc. Am. Physicians* **76,** 102–112.

[8] J. P. Nolan (1965) Alcohol as a factor in the illness of university service patients. *Am. J. Med. Sci.* **249,** 135–142.

[9] H. Castenfors, E. Hultman, and B. Josephson (1960) Effect of intravenous infusions of ethyl alcohol on estimated hepatic blood flow in man. *J. Clin. Invest.* **39,** 776–781.

[10] S. Shaw, E. A. Heller, and H. S. Friedman (1977) Increased hepatic oxygenation following ethanol administration in the baboon. *Proc. Soc. Exp. Biol. Med.* **156,** 509–513.

[11] B. M. Altura and B. T. Altura (1982) Microvascular and vascular smooth muscle actions of ethanol, acetaldehyde, and acetate. *Fed. Proc.* **41,** 2447–2451.

[12] B. M. Altura and A. Gebrewold (1981) Failure of acetaldehyde or acetate to mimic the splanchnic arteriolar or venular dilator actions of ethanol: Direct in situ studies on the microcirculation. *Br. J. Pharmacol.* **73,** 580–582.

[13] F. J. Carmichael, V. Saldivia, Y. Israel, and H. Orrega (1986) Does acetaldehyde (ACT) mediate the ethanol (E) induced increase in liver blood flow? *Hepatology* **6**, 1125.

[14] F. J. Carmichael, V. Saldivia, Y. Israel, and H. Orrega (1987) Effect of acetate on splanchnic hemodynamics. *Hepatology* **7**, 1061.

[15] M. V. Ali and J. P. Nolan (1967) Alcohol induced depression of reticuloendothelial function in the rat. *J. Lab. Clin. Med.* **70**, 295–301.

[16] J. P. Nolan, A. Leiborwitz, and A. L. Vladutiu (1980) Influence of alcohol on Kupffer cell function and possible significance in liver injury, in *The Reticuloendothelial System and the Pathogenesis of Liver Disease.* H. Liehr and M. Grun, eds. Elsevier/North Holland, Amsterdam, pp. 125–136.

[17] J. P. Nolan and D. S. Camara (1982) Endotoxin, sinusoidal cells, and liver injury. *Prog. Liver Dis.* **7**, 361–376.

[18] Y. K. Liu (1979) Phagocytic capacity of reticuloendothelial system in alcoholics. *J. Reticuloendothel. Soc.* **25**, 605–613.

[19] W. G. E. Cooksley, L. W. Powell, and J. W. Halliday (1973) Reticuloendothelial phagocytic function in human liver disease and its relationship to haemolysis. *Br. J. Haematol.* **25**, 147–152.

[20] R. L. Kaufman, J. C. Hoefs, and F. P. Quismorio, Jr. (1982) Immune complexes in the portal and systemic circulation of patients with alcoholic liver disease. *Clin. Immunol. Immunopathol.* **22**, 44–54.

[21] C. Bode, V. Kugler, and J. C. Bode (1987) Endotoxemia in patients with alcoholic and nonalcoholic cirrhosis and in subjects with no evidence of chronic liver disease following acute alcohol excess. *J. Hepatol.* **4**, 814.

[22] H. Liehr (1983) Endotoxins and alcoholic hepatitis, in *Clinical Hepatology.* G. Cosmos and H. Thaler, eds. Springer Verlag, Berlin, pp. 336–339.

[23] B. S. Bhagwandeen, M. Apte, L. Manwarring, and J. Dickeson (1987) Endotoxin induced hepatic necrosis in rats on an alcohol diet. *J. Pathol.* **152**, 47–53.

[24] Y. Shibayama (1987) Enhanced hepatotoxicity of endotoxin by hypoxia. *Pathol. Res. Pract.* **182**, 390–395.

[25] D. Schlessinger, ed. (1980) *Endogenous Mediators in Host Responses to Bacterial Endotoxin, Microbiology–1980.* American Society of Microbiology, Washington.

[26] E. Szentivanyi, A. Nowotny, and H. Friedman, eds. (1986) *Immunobiology and Immunopharmacology of Bacterial Endotoxins.* Plenum, New York.

[27] B. Urbaschek, ed. (1987) Perspectives on Bacterial Pathogenesis and Host Defense. *Rev. Infect. Dis.* **9 (Suppl. 5)**, S431–659.

[28] A. Nowotny, ed. (1983) *Beneficial Effects of Endotoxins.* Plenum, New York.

[29] R. V. Mairer and R. Ulevitch (1981) The response of isolated rabbit hepatic macrophages (H-MO) to lipopolysaccharide (LPS). *Circ. Shock* **8**, 165–181.

[30] J. C. Mathison and R. Ulevitch (1979) The clearance, tissue distribution and

cellular localization of intravenously injected lipopolysaccharide in rabbits. *J. Immunol.* **123,** 2133–2143.

[31] R. S. McCuskey, P. A. McCuskey, R. Urbaschek, and B. Urbaschek (1987) Kupffer cell function in host defense. *Rev. Infect. Dis.* **9(Suppl. 5),** S616–619.

[32] R. S. Munford (1978) Endotoxins and the liver. *Gastroenterology* **75,** 532–535.

[33] D. J. Ruiter, J. van den Maulen, A. Brouwer, M. J. R. Hummel, B. J. Mauer, J. C. M. von den Ploeg, and E. Wisse (1981) Uptake by liver cells of endotoxin following its intravenous injection. *Lab. Invest.* **45,** 38–45.

[34] R. S. McCuskey (1986) Microscopic methods for studying the microvasculature of internal organs, in *Physical Techniques in Biology and Medicine Microvascular Technology.* C. H. Baker and W. F. Nastuk, eds. Academic, New York, pp. 247–264.

[35] R. J. Stock, E. V. Cilento, and R. S. McCuskey (1989) A quantitative in vivo study different molecular weight FITC-dextrans in the hepatic microcirculation. *Hepatology* **9,** 75–82.

[36] R. S. McCuskey (1988) Hepatic microcirculation in disease, in *Sinusoids in Human Liver: Health and Disease.* P. Bioulac-Sage and C. Balabaud, eds. Kupffer Cell Foundation, Leiden, pp. 315–322.

[37] R. S. McCuskey, R. Urbaschek, P. A. McCuskey, N. Sacco, W. Stauber, C. A. Pinkstaff, and B. Urbaschek (1982) Studies of Kupffer cells in mice sensitized or tolerant to endotoxin, in *Sinusoidal Liver Cells.* D. L. Knook and E. Wisse, eds. Elsevier/North Holland, Amsterdam, pp. 387–392.

[38] R. S. McCuskey, R. Urbaschek, P. A. McCuskey, N. Sacco, W. T. Stauber, C. A. Pinkstaff, and B. Urbaschek (1984) Deficient hepatic phagocytosis and lysosomal enzymes in the low endotoxin-responder, C_3H/HeJ mouse. *J. Leukocyte Biol.* **36,** 591–600.

[39] R. S. McCuskey, R. Urbaschek, P. A. McCuskey, and B. Urbaschek (1983) *In vivo* microscopic observations of the responses of Kupffer cells and the hepatic microcirculation to Mycobacterium bovis BCG alone and in combination with endotoxin. *Infect. Immunol.* **42,** 362–367.

[40] R. S. McCuskey, R. Urbaschek, P. A. McCuskey, and B. Urbaschek (1989) Hepatic microvascular responses to tumor necrosis factor, in *Cells of the Hepatic Sinusoid,* vol. II. E. Wisse, D. L. Knook, and K. Decker, eds. Kupffer Cell Foundation, Leiden, pp. 272–276.

[41] R. S. McCuskey (1986) Hepatic microvascular dysfunction during sepsis and endotoxemia, in *Cytoprotection and Cytobiology,* vol. 3. M. Tsuchiya, ed. Excerpta Medica, Amsterdam, pp. 3–17.

[42] R. S. McCuskey, P. A. McCuskey, H. Eguchi, E. G. Crichton, R. Urbaschek, and B. Urbaschek (1990) In vivo microscopy of the liver following acute administration of ethanol, in *Alcohol, Immunosuppression and AIDS.* A. Pawlowski, D. Siminary, and R. Watson, eds. A. Liss, New York, pp. 341–350.

[43] H. Eguchi, P. A. McCuskey, and R. S. McCuskey (1991) Kupffer cell activity and hepatic microvascular events after acute ethanol ingestion in mice. *Hepatology* **13,** 751–757.

[44] H. Eguchi, P. A. McCuskey, and R. S. McCuskey (1990) Microvascular responses in the liver to ethanol. *FASEB J.* **4,** A1250.

[45] H. Eguchi, P. A. McCuskey, P. Scuderi, and R. S. McCuskey (in press) TNFα plays a role in hepatic microvascular events following acute ethanol ingestion in $C_{57}Bl/6$ mice, in *Cells of the Hepatic Sinusoid,* vol. III. E. Wisse, D. L. Knook, and R. S. McCuskey, eds. Kupffer Cell Foundation, Leiden.

[46] R. S. McCuskey (in press) Responses of the hepatic sinusoid lining and microcirculation to combinations of endotoxin, cytokines and ethanol, in *Cells of the Hepatic Sinusoid,* vol. III. E. Wisse, D. L. Knook, and R. S. McCuskey, eds. Kupffer Cell Foundation, Leiden.

[47] R. S. McCuskey, H. Eguchi, P. A. McCuskey, R. Urbaschek, and B. Urbaschek (in press) Some effects of ethanol on Kupffer cell function and host defense mechanisms in the liver, in *Proceedings of the International Congress of Mucosal Immunology.* M. Tsuchiya, ed. Elsevier, Tokyo.

[48] C. J. McClain and D. A. Cohen (1989) Increased tumor necrosis factor production by monocytes in alcoholic hepatitis. *Hepatology* **9,** 349–351.

[49] D. L. Thiele (1989) Tumor necrosis factor, the acute phase response and the pathogenesis of alcoholic liver disease. *Hepatology* **9,** 497–499.

Interrelationships Between the Brain and the Liver

David H. Van Thiel and Ralph E. Tarter

Introduction

For years it has been known that individuals with subclinical portal systemic encephalopathy manifest features that are common to a number of psychiatric problems. These include euphoria, depression, mental slowing, inappropriate affect, and disturbances of behavior as well as sleep. It is not surprising, therefore, that patients with advanced liver disease having low-grade unrecognized, or subclinical portal systemic, encephalopathy are, on occasion, inappropriately admitted to psychiatric facilities.[1-4] Among the most frequent psychiatric diagnosis assigned to such individuals are anxiety reaction, psychotic depression and hysteria.[5] Moreover, patients with subclinical hepatic encephalopathy have mistakenly been diagnosed as having psychomotor epilepsy, a frontal-lobe tumor, narcolepsy, Parkinson's disease, multiple sclerosis, or cerebral arteriosclerosis.[3-5]

Traditionally, portal systemic encephalopathy has been graded into four categories, based on the findings of a clinical examination.[6] If no abnormality consistent with clinical encephalopathy is present, a grade of 0 is

From: *Drug and Alcohol Abuse Reviews, Vol. 2: Liver Pathology and Alcohol*
Ed: R. R. Watson ©1991 The Humana Press Inc.

assigned. It is important to note, however, that cerebral dysfunction frequently can be demonstrated in such individuals when sophisticated neuropsychological tests are utilized to identify the presence of a subclinical encephalopathy. A grade of 1 is assigned if the individual exhibits a shortened attention span, is unable to perform simple mental operations efficiently, and has symptoms of anxiety. A grade of 2 is assigned if the individual demonstrates apathy, time disorientation, inappropriate behavior, and personality changes. Progression into the next stage of severity, identified as grade 3 encephalopathy, occurs with the emergence of features of semistupor, somnolence, confusion, and spatial disorientation. The final stage, stage 4, or true coma, occurs when the patient is unresponsive.

In a variety of different studies, psychological tests of cognitive capacity have been shown to be sensitive measures for detecting cerebral dysfunction (the presence of an encephalopathy) that is not otherwise clinically demonstrable. Such testing procedures have been shown to be particularly valuable in detecting subclinical encephalopathy in individuals with chronic liver disease. Elsass, Lund, and Ranek[7] compared eight cirrhotics who had undergone a portacaval shunt with eight cirrhotic individuals who had not undergone such a procedure, in order to get evidence of hepatic encephalopathy. They demonstrated that the shunted group was more impaired than was the nonshunted group on four of seven tests of cognitive functioning that were administered. The differences between groups were most apparent on tests that assessed visuospatial capacity, but were also evident on tests of verbal memory. In another investigation comparing alcoholic individuals with and without cirrhosis, Gilberstadt et al.[8] obtained evidence for visuospatial deficits in the former group from abnormal scores on the WAIS performance subtest and the trailmaking test, a writing-speed and reaction-time test. Overall, 50% of the cirrhotic subjects that were examined exhibited some impairment on at least one test and obtained a nonverbal IQ that was, on average, 10 points lower than that of the noncirrhotic subjects studied. When five commonly assessed measures of liver injury were compared between these two groups of alcoholic individuals, the serum levels of albumin, γ-globulin, the prothrombin time, ICG retention time at 20 min and blood ammonia levels were able to account for 23–56% of the variance in performance abnormalities exhibited in the cognitive tests utilized in this investigation. However, the best predictor of neuropsychological test performance was the serum albumin level.

More recently, controlling for the untoward effects of alcohol abuse, Tarter et al. compared a group of 30 biopsy-proved nonalcoholic patients with cirrhosis to a group of patients with Crohn's disease and without liver disease.[9] The latter disease group was selected as a control for this study because it controls for the effects of chronic illness as a contributing factor to the measured cognitive performance being assessed. Moreover, the physicians caring for such patients and the major medical therapy (glucocorticoids) utilized to treat individuals with Crohn's disease are the same as those used to treat individuals with cirrhosis. The results of this study demonstrated that individuals with cirrhosis demonstrate deficits on tests that measure visuospatial praxis and perceptual motor capacity. In contrast, intellectual ability, assessed by the Peabody picture vocabulary tests and Raven's progressive matrices, as well as language and memory and memory capacity, were normal in the cirrhotic subjects who were studied.

Individuals with different types of liver disease have been compared on a battery of neuropsychological tests to determine if the cerebral dysfunction present in such individuals varies according to the type of liver disease.[10] Indeed, the cognitive impairments identified were found to vary according to the pathogenesis of the liver disease. Thus, the nature and the severity of the neuropsychological abnormalities present in individuals with liver disease appear to vary as a function of the pathogenesis of the liver disease and, presumably, also of the specific pathophysiologic mechanisms responsible for the liver disease.

Specifically, three different groups of cirrhotic subjects were studied. The first consisted of individuals with postnecrotic cirrhosis (viral and autoimmune liver disease); the second consisted of individuals with advanced cholestatic liver disease (primary biliary cirrhosis and primary sclerosing cholangitis); and the third consisted of individuals with alcohol-induced liver disease.[10] All the subjects studied had, at the time of study, a clinical rating of either 0 or 1 for the degree of encephalopathy that they manifested utilizing the criteria of Parsons-Smith et al.[6] A comprehensive battery of neuropsychological tests was administered to each subject. Each of the individual tests comprised in the test battery previously had been shown to be a sensitive measure for detecting and quantitating cerebral dysfunction. Language, attention, hearing, memory, visuospatial abstracting, and psychomotor processes were evaluated.

The cognitive impairments detected were not the same across all study groups. A progression of impairments was found from those with cholestatic liver disease to those with hepatocellular liver disease and finally to those with Laennec's (alcohol-induced) cirrhosis.[10] The percentage of tests outside the normal range was 20% for individuals with cholestatic liver disease, 32% for those with postnecrotic cirrhosis and 37% for those with Laennec's cirrhosis. Utilizing chi-square analysis, it could be demonstrated that individuals with alcoholic cirrhosis and with postnecrotic cirrhosis performed statistically more poorly than did a group of control individuals with Crohn's disease (a group with a chronic gastrointestinal disease, whose medications and physicians were as to those of the cirrhotic patients, but who were without demonstrable liver disease). It is of some interest to note that the deficits detected were not present for all the cognitive processes assessed in any of the three different groups of patients with liver disease. Specifically, none of the liver-disease groups differed from the Crohn's-disease control group on tests evaluating language, indicating that their communication capabilities were unaffected by the presence of liver disease. However, the three liver-disease groups were clearly distinguishable from the chronic Crohn's-disease control group on several cognitive measures. Specifically, individuals with both Laennec's cirrhosis and postnecrotic cirrhosis and, to a lesser degree, individuals with cholestatic liver disease, were found to be impaired on tests assessing attention and concentration. None of the three liver-disease groups differed from each other on the tests assessing these particular functions. This suggests that the deficits found in attention and concentration in these subjects represent deficits specific to liver disease, rather than deficits that are pathophysiologically specific. On tests of cognitive capacity, however, differences among the three different liver-disease groups were identifiable. Specifically, on tests of perceptual motor capacity, the alcoholic individuals with cirrhosis scored less well than did those with cholestatic liver disease, but comparably to those with postnecrotic cirrhosis. On tests evaluating learning and memory, individuals with cholestatic liver disease were found to be less impaired than were individuals with alcoholic cirrhosis.

The reasons underlying these group differences remain unclear, but appear to be related to the differing pathophysiologic consequences of the primary liver disease characterizing each group.[4,10] Thus it appears quite plausible that distinctive biochemical and metabolic disturbances associated with either cholestatic or hepatocellular liver disease selectlvely cause specific neuropsycholocigal dysfunctions. Presumably because individuals with Laennec's cirrhosis demonstrate the effects of liver disease *per se* as well as the neurotoxic effects of alcohol, the severity of cerebral impairment present in this group was greatest.[10–12]

In another study using neuropsychological tests that measure visuopractic capacity, visual scanning, and perceptual motor speed, it was found that individuals with chronic nonalcoholic cirrhosis were impaired compared to individuals with a chronic medical illness.[9] Specifically, when 30 individuals with chronic nonalcoholic cirrhosis were compared to 10 patients with Crohn's disease, the individuals with nonalcoholic cirrhosis performed less well on the symbol digit modalities test, a measure of speed of visual scanning and of repetitive motor responding. The subjects with cirrhosis also had more difficulty assembling blocks into various spatial configurations than did the controls. In addition, they performed less well than controls on the Purdue pegboard, a test of perceptual motor speed. Moreover, they required more time than the controls to complete the trailmaking test and the tactual performance test. Although no differences in recalling the shapes of the blocks was noted, individuals with cirrhosis were less able to remember the location of the figures on the board than were the controls. In contrast to the difference in time required to complete the perceptual motor speed tests, simple motor speed tests were performed at the same rate by individuals with cirrhosis and those with Crohn's disease.

When the psychiatric status of the cirrhotic individuals was evaluated using the Minnesota Multiphasic Personality Inventory (MMPI), they did not exhibit any more disturbances than did individuals with Crohn's disease.[9] This finding indicates that the neuropsychological deficits recognized in cirrhotic individuals cannot be a consequence of their being more emotionally disturbed than the controls. In fact, on a 16-factor personality questionnaire, individuals with Crohn's disease reported more disturbances than did individuals with cirrhosis.[9] However, utilizing the sickness impact profile, individuals with nonalcoholic cirrhosis report more disturbances in sleep and rest, body care and movement, and recreation and pastimes, and experience more physical dysfunction than do controls with Crohn's disease.[9]

Because computed tomography (CT) scanning provides the opportunity for in vivo examination of the brain for structural abnormalities that can be clinically identified, and because quantitation of the relative position and distances between identifiable cerebral nuclei and the size and volume of the ventricles, and of the presence of cortical sucal widening can be accomplished, this modality provides unique information about the morphology of the brain that is not otherwise detectable. Thus, a formal CT scan study of the brain of individuals with stable cirrhosis has been performed recently.[13]

Specifically, 49 nonalcoholic cirrhotic individuals, 20 of whom had hepatocellular disease (either postnecrotic cirrhosis or autoimmune chronic active hepatitis) were compared with 29 patients with advanced cholastatic disease (either primary biliary cirrhosis or sclerosing cholangitis). The CT scans were performed in a standard manner using a GE 9800 scanner; serial scans were obtained at 10-mm intervals through the entire head on a plane parallel to that of the planum sphenodale. During the scanning procedure, diatriazoate megulamine iodinated contrast medium was administered intravenously to all of the subjects studied. Moreover, for each variable assessed, three independent measurements were obtained and a mean score was computed.

Even more recently, alcoholics with cirrhosis have been compared to nonalcoholics with cirrhosis in terms of their performance on a panel of neuropsychological test procedures to determine whether prior alcohol abuse adversely affects the neuropsychological test performance beyond that effect attributable to the presence of a subclinical hepatic encephalopathy associated with stable cirrhosis.[12] In this study, 24 individuals with Laennec's cirrhosis were compared to 26 subjects with postnecrotic cirrhosis. The group of alcoholics with cirrhosis had a mean age of 41 yr and an educational level of 13.5 yr on average. The mean estimated WAIS IQ was 107 for the alcoholics; those with postnecrotic cirrhosis had a mean age of 44 yr, 14.9 yr of formal education, and an estimated WAIS IQ of 110. The results obtained by both of these groups were compared to those of a group of 18 community-dwelling normal men, recruited by advertisement, who had a mean age of 39 yr, an educational level of 14 yr and a WAIS IQ of 112. Specifically, a battery of 18 neuropsychological test procedures was utilized, and the three groups were compared using one-way analysis of covariance. Significant group effects were found for the trailmaking test (both parts A and B), symbol digit, digit span forward, Benton vision retention test, Brown-Peterson memory test, Stroop test, and grooved pegboard (dominant hand).

The results were evaluated further using a set of orthogonal constructs comparing the control group vs the liver-disease groups and the alcoholic cirrhotic group vs the nonalcoholic cirrhotic group.[12] In all cases, the normal controls differed from the combined liver disease groups ($p < 0.05$). The alcoholic and nonalcoholic cirrhotic groups differed significantly only on part B of the trailmaking test ($p < 0.05$). Thus, the neuropsychological test performance of alcoholics with cirrhosis was found to be essentially equivalent to that of nonalcoholics with cirrhosis. This finding clearly documents that individuals with cirrhosis and those with coexisting alcoholism performed similarly on a battery of neuropsychological tests. Thus it appears as if the presence of liver disease, more than the problem of alcoholism, determines the neuropsychological deficits found in cirrhotic alcoholics.[12] It is noteworthy that a gradation of impairments between the groups was evident on certain tasks. Although not reaching statistical significance, the results of three different tests suggested that certain cognitive processes may be more impaired in alcoholics, implicating an independent effect of alcohol abuse on test performance. Nonetheless, it appears that the presence of advanced liver disease is more important than alcoholism in determining the overall neuropsychological deficits found in cirrhotic alcoholics. In this regard, it is interesting to note that recent studies of medically intact alcoholics have failed to reveal any substantial impairment on neuropsychological test performance.[14,15] The demonstration that liver disease underlies a large portion of the cerebral dysfunction found in alcoholics has important ramifications for alcohol treatment programs.[16]

In a recent clinical investigation, an attempt was made to determine whether routinely obtained measures of hepatic injury correlated to or accounted for the latency scores obtained using event-related evoked potentials in cirrhotic individuals who were not overtly encephalopathic.[17] Fifty-eight nonalcoholic cirrhotic individuals were studied. Each had cirrhosis proved by liver biopsy. In addition, a panel of five routine measures of hepatic injury or function was obtained on each. These included measures of serum albumin, serum globulin, prothrombin time, fasting blood ammonia, and ICG retention at 20 min. Each subject underwent a visual evoked-potential examination, brain stem auditory evoked-potential recording, and median nerve somatosensory evoked-potential recordings. All of the evoked-potential recordings obtained were in the normal–mildly-abnormal range when control values obtained in neurologically intact individuals were used for the comparisons. When univariate correlations between the hepatic injury measures and the evoked-potential latency scores were obtained, no association among the various variables was evident. When multiple-linear-regression analysis was undertaken, however, it was found that the ICG retention correlated to the latency in the visual and brain stem auditory evoked-potential responses, indicating that this measure of hepatic injury, in the absence of overt, clinically evident hepatic encephalopathy, is a sensitive biochemical measure of subtle neurophysiologic disturbance as detected by visual and auditory evoked-response latency recording.

In an additional study, similar evoked-potential recordings were obtained in 116 individuals with advanced liver disease.[18] The same biochemical measures of hepatic injury and function were related to the short-latency evoked potentials and were found to correlate only poorly to the presence of subclinical neuropsychologically demonstratable hepatic encephalopathy. Prior studies had shown that individuals with nonalcoholic cirrhosis, who did not otherwise demonstrate evidence of hepatic encephalopathy, perform abnormally on neuropsychological tests.[9] These findings have been interpreted to reflect the presence of a subclinical form of hepatic encephalopathy in those with cirrhosis.

Other studies have shown that biochemical measures of hepatic injury can, to some extent, predict performance on certain neuropsychological tests.[11] However, the interpretation of these latter studies is difficult, since both the type of patients and test measures utilized have varied, and multivariate procedures have not been used. To address this issue, 79 patients with advanced liver disease, either primary biliary cirrhosis or postnecrotic cirrhosis, were investigated, employing both univariate and multivariate statistical procedures to determine which of five measures of hepatic injury or function thay are in common use reflect the presence of subclinical hepatic encephalopathy as detected by a battery of neuropsychological tests.[19] None of the patients studied in this investigation had a current or lifetime history of psychiatric illness, nor was there a history of alcohol or other substance abuse, neurologic injury, or other complicating medical disorder that might confound the results obtained on the neuropsychological test procedures. The study population had a mean age of 43 yr and spanned the socioeconomic spectrum, with the typical subject being a member of the middle class and having 14 yr of formal education. Importantly, the neuropsychological and biochemical measures obtained were collected within a 72-hr time-period. The five tests evaluating hepatic function consisted of the serum albumin level, the serum γ-globulin level, the prothrombin time, ICG retention at 20 min, and the fasting blood ammonia level. Twelve separate indices of neuropsychological performance were assessed. These included tests evaluating visuospatial and psychomotor processes, functions known to be abnormal in subjects with subclinical hepatic encephalopathy. The administration of the test battery required only 30–40 min and was conducted in a single session. Subjects with liver disease performed on the border line between normal and mildly impaired individuals on most of the neuropsychological tests utilized. More severe hepatic injury was found to be associated with greater neuropsychological test performance impairment. The serum albumin level correlated to five of the 12 neuropsychological test variables; the prothrombin time correlated to four. The γ-globulin level, the ammonia level, and ICG retention at 20 min each correlated with only one test variable. A stepwise multiple-regression analysis revealed that the prediction of an impaired neuropsychological test performance was substantially enhanced when all five variables were included in the analysis. Significant correlations were obtained for nine of the 12 neuropsychological measures, indicating that liver-injury status predicts a substantial amount of the test-score variance on a wide variety of neuropsychological performance measures. The serum albumin was the most powerful predictor. Of the nine significant correlations, it entered the regression equation first on five, and second for two. The prothrombin time was the second-most-important predictor of an encephalopathic process and entered the regression equation first for two neuropsychological variables and second for five others. Considering the multifactorial pathogenesis of subclinical portal systemic encephalopathy, the good physical condition of the subjects studied, and the absence of overt neurologic disease, it is remarkable that these five routine tests of hepatic injury could account for such a substantial proportion of the variance observed on the various neuropsychological tests used to assess cerebral dysfunction.[19] Especially interesting was the observation that the fasting serum ammonia level was the poorest predictor of an encephalopathic process. The serum ammonia level has been considered for decades to be the primary cerebral toxic agent in hepatic encephalopathy. Nonetheless, the serum ammonia level did not identify the presence of a subclinical encephalopathy in the cirrhotic individuals studied or even contribute a significant amount of variance on the test measures of identified cerebral dysfunction. Together, the serum albumin and the prothrombin time provided the most powerful estimate of an encephalopathic process. Clearly, any encephalopathic process occurring as a consequence of advanced liver disease has a multifactorial basis, and, although the albumin level and prothrombin time may account for a large portion of the variance observed on neuropsychological measures, they alone are not responsible for the cognitive deficits present in individuals with subclinical hepatic encephalopathy. It should be emphasized that, in aggregate, the five biochemical measures utilized explained <30% of the total variance observed for the measured neuropsychological test performance. This finding underscores the complexity of the metabolic factors responsible for hepatic encephalopathy, but also suggests that the encephalopathic process, as measured by neuropsychological tests, may be attributable to factors other than those that assess liver injury.[19] Tarter and Alterman,[20] have concluded that the cognitive deficits observed in alcoholics are multifactorial in origin and are not attributable to alcohol neurotoxicity only, but also reflect a disruption of other organ systems that affect cerebral functioning.

The relationship between alcohol-induced liver disease and cognitive dysfunction in alcoholics has only recently been examined in any detail. In one study, the magnitude of the cerebral atrophy present in alcoholics, as determined by computed tomography was found to vary with the severity of their liver disease.[21] In two other studies, the electroencephalographic abnormalities present in alcoholic individuals were found to be more pronounced in those with cirrhosis than in those without cirrhosis.[22,23] Despite these findings, it must be noted that, in general, alcoholic and nonalcoholic individuals with cirrhosis perform similarly on various cognitive tests. Based on these findings, at least two independent groups of investigators have concluded that cirrhosis more than alcohol abuse, is responsible for the cognitive impairments present in alcoholics with liver disease.[24,25] To assess this observation in greater detail, 15 alcoholics with biopsy-confirmed cirrhosis and a mean age of 44 yr completed a neuropsychological test battery during which time a panel of biochemical measures assessing hepatic function, including serum values for aspartate transaminase (SGOT), alanine transaminase (SGPT), alkaline phosphatase, total bilirubin, albumin, globulin, prothrombin time, fasting blood ammonia, and ICG retention at 20 min were determined.[11] Significant correlations between these biochemical measures of liver function and cognitive-performance measures were obtained. The degree of abnormality of the alanine transaminase level correlated significantly to four of the cognitive variables, whereas the prothrombin time and fasting blood ammonia level each correlated to three. The aspartate transaminase level, alkaline phosphatase, and ICG retention at 20 min each correlated with two cognitive-test measures. The bilirubin, albumin, and γ-globulin levels each correlated to only one. All but four of the correlations were circumscribed to visuospatial and memory processes, suggesting an association between these particular capacities and the severity of the liver disease present. This study suggests that biochemical measures of hepatic dysfunction can account for a significant amount of the variance observed in cognitive test performance scores obtained by individuals with alcohol-associated cirrhosis.

Similar results have been reported by Gilberstadt et al.[8] It is noteworthy that the correlations in the Gilberstadt study were also most prevalent on tests evaluating visuospatial and memory processes. These are precisely the types of tests on which alcoholics most frequently have been demonstrated to perform poorly. Moreover, the magnitude of the correlations were rather substantial, accounting for 23–56% of the test variance. From these findings, it would appear that neuropsychological deficits commonly reported in alcoholics may be mediated as a consequence of hepatic dysfunction and are not a consequence of alcohol neurotoxicity *per se*.[11,24]

In vivo, the gross appearance of the brains of individuals with cirrhosis has been shown to demonstrate evidence for both cerebral edema and cortical atrophy.[13,26] In addition, correlations between individual CT variables and an individual's performance on a neuropsychological test battery have been reported. Subjects in this study underwent a battery of neuropsychological tests including standardized measures of intelligence, language, attention, memory, visuospatial, and psychomotor capacities. Although not overtly encephalopathic, the patients with advanced liver disease exhibited quantifiable CT scan abnormalities. Specifically, when the sulci-width scores of the subjects with liver disease were compared to those of published norms, it was clear that the individuals with liver disease manifested cerebral atrophy confined to the anterior cortical regions. In contrast to these findings of atrophy in the frontal areas, the nonfrontal sulci of these same patients were similar to those of normal individuals. However, when compared to published norms, individuals with chronic liver disease have been shown to have identifiable morphological abnormalities consisting of indices that include the bicaudate diameter, the bicaudate index, the maximum width of the third ventricle, and the cella media distance. Not all of the CT measurements that were assessed revealed abnormalities, however. The maximum distance between the anterior horns of the lateral ventricles as well as the widths of the inner and the outer skulls, were similar in cirrhotics and the normal controls. When comparisons were made between the CT-scan appearance of the brain of patients with hepatocellular disease and those with cholestatic disease, no significant differences between the two groups could be identified.

Because several of the psychometric tests utilized in the neuropsychological test battery utilized by Tarter et al. measure the same, or similar, aspects of psychological functioning, a factor analysis of the data was performed.[13] The derived factor scores for each subject were then correlated to the individual's CT scores. Whereas univariate correlations illustrated that cerebral morphologic status was associated with an individual's performance on a given test, multivariate analysis demonstrated the degree to which each of the various CT parameters assessed were associated with empirically derived categories of cerebral dysfunction defined by mutually exclusive domains of neuropsychological test performance. All of the psychometric tests utilized in this investigation could be aggregated into three psychological categories.[13] Factor 1, which accounted for 62.8% of the total pooled variance, received its highest loadings from tests measuring psychomotor efficiency. Factor 2, which accounted for 24.7% of the total variance, received its highest loadings from tests of learning capacity. Factor 3, which accounted for only 12.5% of the total variance, received its highest loading from tests measuring perceptual motor coordination. When the factor scores obtained for each subject were related to the various CT scan variables assessed, widening of frontal sulci correlated significantly to factor-1-comprising tests that measure attention, spatial capacity, expressive language fluency, and response-sequencing ability. These processes are known to be subserved primarily by frontal regions of the cerebrum; thus it is not particularly surprising that the identified anterior cerebral atrophy was associated with poor performance on tests assessing these functions. The distance between the tips of the anterior horns of the lateral ventricles correlated to factors 1 and 2, and the bicaudate diameter and bicaudate index were found to correlate to all three factors. The maximum width of the third ventricle correlated only to factors 1 and 3. The outer skull diameter was associated with abnormalities in learning and memory capacity. Overall psychomotor efficiency correlated to five independent CT variables, learning capacity correlated to four and measures of perceptual motor coordination correlated to three.

The finding that gross cerebral morphologic abnormalities exist and can be recognized in patients with nonalcoholic cirrhosis has significant implications. First, they indicate that, despite a normal appearance on a clinical neurologic examination, quantifiable neuroanatomical abnormalities can be identified on CT scans in individuals with nonalcoholic cirrhosis. Second, the absence of overt clinical neuropsychiatric manifestations by these subjects suggests that there must be an anatomic basis for the subclinical manifestations of hepatic encephalopathy identified in these subjects. It remains to be determined whether any pharmacologic, dietary, or surgical intervention available for the treatment of chronic hepatic encephalopathy can either eliminate or ameliorate the anatomic abnormalitites identified. Such would be expected if the CT scan and neuropsychological disturbances identified actually were a consequence of a subclinical portasystemic encephalopathy and had a metabolic causation.

This important study documented in vivo evidence of cerebral morphologic abnormalities in patients with advanced chronic liver disease in individuals who did not exhibit overt clinical signs or symptoms of hepatic encephalopathy.[26] The changes from normal appeared to reflect the combined presence of cerebral atrophy and edema. Additionally, several CT indices could be correlated to the magnitude of the subclinical encephalopathy identified in the subjects studied using a battery of psychometric tests. Thus, these data suggest rather strongly that subclinical hepatic encephalopathy is not a neuropsychiatric disease characterized by a metabolic dysfunction alone, but also involves identifiable and quantitatable cerebral morphologic abnormalities. Moreover, these data provide an explanation for the impaired neuropsychological capacities found in patients with chronic liver disease who do not manifest clinical evidence of encephalopathy. Finally, it is especially noteworthy that the serum ammonia level, the biochemical factor commonly thought to be the principal cerebral toxic agent responsible for hepatic encephalopathy, was the least powerful chemical predictor of any of the CT scan abnormalities detected in the subjects studied.[26]

The most recent innovative and radical treatment for portal systemic encephalopathy is orthotopic liver transplantation.[27] This surgical procedure is offered principally to individuals with advanced chronic liver disease who are no longer responsive to standard forms of medical therapy.[28,29] The effect of hepatic transplantation on portal systemic encephalopathy is not, as yet, entirely clear. However, in one small cadre of patients, no cognitive deficits were found in liver-transplant recipients when they were studied, on average, 1 yr after their transplant surgery.[27]

Specifically, in a recent study, the results of neuropsychological testing in 10 individuals surviving orthotopic liver transplantation were compared with those of 10 medical controls with established, but stable, Crohn's disease.[27] The two groups did not differ from each other on measures of verbal and nonverbal intelligence. However, the transplant patients performed significantly better than the patients with Crohn's disease at learning associations on a 10-item list of word pairs. Accuracy of recall of the word-pair associations tested 30 min later was the same for both groups. On two perceptual motor tests, the transplant recipients performed significantly better than the control patients with Crohn's disease. The transplant recipients exhibited faster finger-tapping speed than the controls and also performed better on tests of perceptual motor speed. In contrast, the two groups did not differ in either attention or concentration capacities. Specifically, the transplant recipients could repeat strings of digits (in both a forward and backward sequence), recite the alphabet, perform serial additions, and count backwards as competently and as rapidly as the controls. Similarly, no differences between the two groups were evident on the star-drawing test, another assessment of perceptual motor performance. Moreover, the transplant recipients performed as well as the controls in terms of the time it took to draw a star within a 1/4-in. boundary. The number of errors committed in performing the task was also comparable. In addition, no group differences were observed in the ability to sequentially match symbols with numbers.

Tests of spatial organization also failed to discriminate between posttransplant survivors and individuals with Crohn's disease. Specifically, no differences were noted in their ability to copy patterns with blocks or in their ability, when blindfolded, to place geometric blocks in a form board.

Language capacities assessed by a subtest of the Boston Diagnostic Aphasic Examination were almost identical in the two groups.[27] Confrontation naming, requiring the naming of common objects, and responsive naming, involving answering a variety of questions, were also similar. Fluency or speed of verbal output did not differ between the two groups. Finally, comprehension as measured by the token test, was the same for both groups.

The MMPI profiles of surviving transplant recipients and controls revealed a significant difference only on the hypochondriasis scale. Interestingly, scores of the patients with Crohn's disease were in the more pathologic direction compared to scores of those surviving a liver transplant.[27] The profiles of transplant recipients on the 16 personality-profile tests showed that they did not differ from the Crohn's disease controls on any of the personality scales. Finally, utilizing the sickness-impact profile, none of the scales discriminated between the transplant survivors and the controls with Crohn's disease. These data indicate that patients who survive orthotopic liver transplantation are not impaired on measures of neuropsychological capacity when compared either with a medical-disease control group of stable individuals with Crohn's disease or with population norms. On measures of psychiatric status and social functioning, they performed as well as individuals with Crohn's disease. However, when contrasted with values obtained by a normative population, the transplant recipients presented a profile of moderate anxiety, somatic distress, and concern.[27] Moreover, routines of everyday living were somewhat disrupted, as evidenced by the finding that their condition negatively affected sleep and rest, eating and appetite, and work capacity and recreation. Impairments of >20% were observed in each of these scales, on which a score at or near 0 would be a normal value. Thus, a generally good, but not normal, neuropsychiatric outcome for liver-transplant recipients was documented.[27]

Recent studies have demonstrated that vitamin E deficiency is prevalent in patients with chronic liver disease and that the magnitude of the measured vitamin E deficiency correlates directly to the severity of measured visuomotor deficits.[30] These investigations indicate that nutritional correlates of hepatic injury can account for a substantial proportion of the variance observed on certain neuropsychological test scores obtained by cirrhotics. This implies further that vitamin E deficiency rather than hepatic encephalopathy *per se* is the basis for at least some of the neuropsychological dysfunction present in cirrhotic individuals with latent portal systemic encephalopathy. Vitamin E deficiency is known to produce neurological dysfunction; thus, its contribution to the neurologic dysfunction of individuals with cirrhosis is not entirely unexpected.[30,31]

The preceding is a brief overview of the current status of brain–liver interactions as seen in individuals with alcoholism, alcoholic liver disease, other forms of liver disease, and before and after liver transplantation. Much has been learned in the last decade about the effect of nonneurologic organ dysfunction on brain performance. Much remains to be learned. It is anticipated that the results herein reported will hasten the development of this new and evolving information and help to put it into perspective both for neurobehavioralists and for hepatologists, surgeons, and others who care for individuals with liver disease.

Acknowledgments

This work was supported by grants NIAAA32556 and NIDDK06601.

References

[1] L. Havens and C. Child (1955) Recurrent psychosis associated with liver disease and elevated blood ammonia. *N. Engl. J. Med.* **252,** 756–759.

[2] C. Leevy (1982) Exploring the brain liver relationship. *Mod. Med.* **42,** 17–22.

[3] W. Summerskill, L. Davidson, S. Sherlock, and R. Steiner (1956) The neuropsychiatric syndrome associated with hepatic cirrhosis and an extensive portal collateral circulation. *Q. J. Med.* **25,** 245–266.

[4] R. E. Tarter, K. L. Edwards, and D. H. Van Thiel (1988) Neuropsychological dysfunction due to liver disease, in *Medical Neuropsychology.* R. E. Tarter, D. H. Van Thiel, and K. L. Edwards, eds. Plenum, New York, pp. 75–97.

[5] S. Sherlock, W. Summerskill, L. White, and E. Pheur (1954) Portal systemic encephalopathy: Neurological complications of liver disease. *Lancet* **2,** 453–457.

[6] B. Parsons-Smith, W. Summerskill, A. Dawson, and S. Sherlock (1957) The electroencephalograph in liver disease. *Lancet* **2,** 867–871.

[7] P. Elsass, Y. Lund, and L. Ranek (1978) Encephalopathy in patients with cirrhosis of the liver: A neuropsychological study. *Scand. J. Gastroenterol.* **13,** 241–247.

[8] S. J. Gilberstadt, H. Gilberstadt, L. Zieve, B. Bregel, R. O. Collier, Jr., and C. J. McClain (1980) Psychomotor performance defects in cirrhotic patients without overt encephalopathy. *Arch. Intern. Med.* **140,** 519–521.

[9] R. E. Tarter, A. M. Hegedus, D. H. Van Thiel, R. R. Schade, J. S. Gavaler, and T. E. Starzl (1984) Non alcoholic cirrhosis associated with neuropsychological dysfunction in the absence of overt evidence of hepatic encephalopathy. *Gastroenterology* **86,** 1421–1427.

[10] R. E. Tarter, A. M. Hegedus, D. H. Van Thiel, N. Edwards, and R. R. Schade (1987) Neurobehavioral correlates of cholestatic and hepatocellular disease: Differentiation according to disease specific characteristics and severity of the identified cerebral dysfunction. *Int. J. Neurosci.* **32,** 901–910.

[11] R. E. Tarter, A. M. Hegedus, D. H. Van Thiel, J. S. Gavaler, and R. R. Schade (1986) Hepatic dysfunction and neuropsychological test performance in alcoholics with cirrhosis. *J. Stud. Alcohol* **47,** 74–77.

[12] R. E. Tarter, D. H. Van Thiel, A. M. Arria, J. Carra, and H. Moss (1988) Impact of cirrhosis on the neuropsychological test performance of cirrhosis. *Alcohol. Clin. Exp. Res.* **12,** 619–621.

[13] P. Bernthal, A. Hays, R. E. Tarter, D. H. Van Thiel, J. Lecky, and A. Hegedus (1987) Cerebral CT scan abnormalities in cholestatic and hepatocellular disease and their relationship to neuropsychological test performance. *Hepatology* **7,** 107–114.

[14] I. Grant, K. Adams, and R. Reed (1984) Aging, abstinence and medical risk

factors in the prediction of neuropsychological deficits among chronic alcoholics. *Arch. Gen. Psychiatry* **41,** 710–718.

[15] K. Adams and L. Grant (1986) Influence of premorbid risk factors on neuropsychological performance in alcoholics. *J. Clin. Exp. Neuropsychol.* **8,** 362–370.

[16] C. McClain, T. Potter, J. Kromhout, and L. Zieve (1984) The effect of lactulose on psychomotor performance tests in alcoholic cirrhotics without overt encephalopathy. *J. Clin. Gastroenterol.* **6,** 325–329.

[17] R. E. Tarter, R. Sclabassi, S. L. Sandford, A. L. Hays, J. P. Carra, and D. H. Van Thiel (1987) Relationship between head injury status and event related potentias. *Clin. Electroencephalogr.* **18,** 15–19.

[18] S. L. Sandford, R. E. Tarter, R. Sclabassi, and D. H. Van Thiel (1987) Sensory information processing in patients with non alcoholic cirrhosis. *J. Neurol. Sci.* **80,** 269–276.

[19] R. E. Tarter, S. L. Sandford, A. L. Hays, J. P. Carra, and D. H. Van Thiel (1989) Hepatic injury correlates with neuropsychological impairment. *Int. J. Neurosci.* **44,** 75–82.

[20] R. E. Tarter and A. I. Alterman (1984) Neuropsychological deficits in alcoholics: Etiological considerations. *J. Stud. Alcohol* **45,** 1–9.

[21] W. Acker, C. J. Aps, S. K. Majunder, G. K. Shaw, and A. D. Thomson (1982) The relationship between brain and liver damage in chronic alcoholic patients. *J. Neurol. Neuropsychol. Psychol.* **45,** 984–987.

[22] T. Kardel and B. Stigsby (1975) Period amplitude analysis of the electroencephalogram correlated with liver function in patients with cirrhosis of the liver. *Electroencephalogr. Clin. Neurophysiol.* **38,** 605–609.

[23] T. Kardel, P. Zander-Olsen, B. Stigsby, and K. Tonneson (1972) Hepatic encephalopathy evaluated by automatic period analysis of the electroencephalogram during lactulose treatment. *Acta Med. Scand.* **192,** 493–498.

[24] R. E. Tarter, A. M. Hegedus, J. S. Gavaler, R. R. Schade, D. H. Van Thiel, and T. E. Starzl (1983) Cognitive and psychiatric impairments associated with alcoholic and non-alcoholic cirrhosis. *Hepatology* **3,** 830.

[25] S. Rehnstrom, G. Sinert, J. A. Hansson, G. Johnson, and J. Vang (1977) Chronic hepatic encephalopathy: A psychometrical study. *Scand. J. Gastroenterol.* **12,** 305–311.

[26] R. E. Tarter, A. L. Hays, S. S. Sandford, and D. H. Van Thiel (1986) Cerebral morphological abnormalities associated with non-alcoholic cirrhosis. *Lancet* **2,** 893–895.

[27] R. E. Tarter, D. H. Van Thiel, A. M. Hegedus, R. R. Schade, J. S. Gavaler, and T. E. Starzl (1984) Neuropsychiatric status after liver transplantation. *J. Lab. Clin. Med.* **103,** 776–782.

[28] T. E. Starzl, A. J. Demetris, and D. H. Van Thiel (1989) Medical progress: Liver transplantation (Part I) *N. Engl. J. Med.* **321,** 1014–1022.

[29] T. E. Starzl, A. J. Demetris, and D. H. Van Thiel (1989) Medical progress: Liver transplantation (Part II) *N. Engl. J. Med.* **321,** 1092–1099.

[30] A. M. Arria, R. E. Tarter, V. S. Warty, J. L. Renner, and D. H. Van Thiel. Prevalence and treatment of vitamin E deficiency in adults with chronic liver disease: Preliminary results from a clinical trial of alpha tocopherol (Submitted).

[31] A. M. Arria, R. E. Tarter, V. Warty, and D. H. Van Thiel (1990) Vitamin E deficiency and psychomotor dysfunction in adults with primary biliary cirrhosis. *Am. J. Clin. Nutr.* **52,** 383–390.

Morphine and Liver Damage

Louis Shuster

Introduction

Recurring reports of a high incidence of liver dysfunction in narcotic addicts have led several investigators to examine the possibility that narcotic drugs, such as heroin and morphine, may be hepatotoxic. The overwhelming consensus is that most of the liver damage encountered among narcotic addicts is attributable to viral hepatitis contracted by the use of dirty needles. This conclusion is supported by the lack of hepatotoxicity in federal-prisoner patients who were injected with large amounts of sterile morphine under controlled conditions.[1] There is also no evidence of increased hepatotoxicity in addicts maintained on oral methadone.[2] Conversely, there is a correlation between the duration of exposure to hypodermic equipment and the cumulative incidence of liver disease.[3]

Initial attempts to develop an animal model of morphine-induced liver damage used rhesus monkeys. The results were negative.[4] However, subsequent work with rats and mice has yielded clearcut evidence that narcotics can produce liver damage. The intriguing aspect of this phenomenon is that, according to various investigators, as many as six different mechanisms may be involved. This review presents the evidence for and against the postulated mechanisms in the light of what is known about other drugs that are unequivocally hepatotoxic.

From: *Drug and Alcohol Abuse Reviews, Vol. 2: Liver Pathology and Alcohol*
Ed: R. R. Watson ©1991 The Humana Press Inc.

Narcotic-Induced
Liver Damage in Rats and Mice

Enzyme Changes and Histology in Rats

Axelrod[5] observed that chronic administration of morphine to rats decreased the ability of a liver fraction containing microsomes and soluble proteins to carry out the *N*-demethylation of morphine to formaldehyde. He postulated that the morphine-induced inactivation of morphine-metabolizing enzymes might serve as a model for changes in narcotic receptors, leading to the development of narcotic tolerance in the central nervous system.[6] Similar observations were made by other workers, who found that the decrease in metabolism was not specific to morphine, but could also be seen with other drugs metabolized by the mixed-function oxidase system, such as hexobarbital.[7–9] The main reason for the decline in enzyme activity is a decrease in the amount of cytochrome P-450 in the endoplasmic reticulum.[9]

Gurantz and Correia[10] found that the acute injection into rats of a single high dose of morphine (45–50mg/kg ip) produced a loss of cytochrome P-450 as soon as 1 h after injection. This loss could be attributed to dissociation of the heme moiety and was followed by a three- to fourfold increase in microsomal heme oxidase activity. Morphine-injected rats also displayed evidence of hepatotoxicity in the form of two- to threefold increases in the activity of SGOT and SGPT. This change was prevented by the simultaneous injection of the narcotic antagonist naloxone.

The initial impression was that these morphine-induced changes were limited to adult male rats. Kato et al.[11] found that morphine pretreatment did not decrease the hydroxylation of hexobarbital in female rats, or in mice and rabbits of either sex. Even in male rats there was no change in aniline hydroxylation, an activity that, unlike hexobarbital hydroxylation, is not controlled by androgens. There was an interesting parallel between morphine treatment and adrenalectomy. Both treatments produced similar decreases in hexobarbital hydroxylation, but only in male rats.[9,11] Thus, morphine administration seemed to decrease specifically only that form of cytochrome P-450 that is controlled by androgens in adult rats. Among other treatments that specifically decrease this form of cytochrome P-450 are hypoxia, ACTH, formaldehyde, thyroxine, and repeated injection of epinephrine in oil.[8]

Changes in Liver Function in Mice

The sc injection of morphine into mice, in doses ranging from 5 to 40 mg/kg, inhibits the hepatic clearance of both sulfobromophthalein, a dye that is conjugated to a glucuronide, and indocyanine green, a dye that is not conjugated. This inhibition is counteracted by naloxone. The involvement of a morphine metabolite appears unlikely, because methadone, which is metabolized by a different pathway from morphine, produces the same effect. Cannulation experiments indicate that the effect of morphine is not attributable to biliary spasm.[12] Hurwitz[13] had previously shown that morphine inhibition of the clearance of phenol red in mice was mainly attributable to a decrease in the apparent volume of distribution, rather than a lower rate of elimination. The relationship of these findings to narcotic-induced liver damage is still unclear.

Liver Damage in Mice

The broadening of the scope of morphine-induced hepatotoxicity resulted from a chance observation made with male ICR mice. Thureson-Klein et al.[14] were studying the brains of mice that had been implanted with pellets of morphine base. They observed that these animals had pale, fatty livers. Examination of liver sections by electron microscopy revealed a marked accumulation of lipid droplets and degranulation of the rough endoplasmic reticulum. The total extractable lipid content increased by 100%. Similar changes were produced by the injection of morphine, 40 mg/kg, every 8 h.

The same group of workers later showed that the implantation of morphine pellets in mice produced a twofold increase in SGPT and SGOT, which could be prevented by concurrent repeated injection of naloxone. Transaminase levels were increased about 50% by a single subcutaneous injection of morphine sulfate, 40 mg/kg. The same increase could be produced by injecting 20 µg of morphine sulfate by the intraventricular route. Elevation of transaminases after pellet implantation could be prevented completely by prior hypophysectomy or, to a lesser extent, by adrenalectomy. These results suggested that morphine may be affecting the liver indirectly, by acting on narcotic receptors in the central nervous system to activate the pituitary-adrenal axis.[15]

Further evidence for the role of narcotic receptors was provided by Needham et al.[16] By using a different strain of mice and increasing the dose of morphine to 100 mg/kg, they obtained eightfold increases in SGOT at 16–18 h after intraperitoneal injection. There was a correlation with narcotic potency. Levorphanol was hepatotoxic, but dextrorphan was not, and hydromorphone was more potent than morphine. Naloxone prevented liver damage when injected before morphine or up to 30 min afterward. Naloxone injected 60 min after morphine was ineffective. This observation suggests that the initial damage takes place within the first hour after morphine administration. Another indication that narcotic receptors play an important role was the observation that hydromorphone did not produce liver damage in mice that had been made tolerant to hydromorphone. Intracerebral injections of either morphine or the opioid peptide D-[Ala^2]-met-enkephalinamide elevated SGOT levels three- to fourfold.[16]

Figure 1 shows dose-related increases in SGOT after intracerebral injections of the enkephalin analog FK-3324 (tyr-D-ala-gly-mephe-met-(O)ol). A strain of mice, CXBK, that has fewer narcotic receptors in the brain than C57Bl/6 mice,[17] also showed considerably less liver damage from morphine.[16]

A possible role for β-adrenergic receptors was indicated by the observation that morphine hepatotoxicity was partially blocked by pretreatment with reserpine or by propranolol, a β-blocker, but not by the α-blocker dibenzyline.[16]

In contrast to the findings in rats, liver damage from morphine was more pronounced in female C57Bl/6B By mice than in males. There was no sex difference in B$_6$AF$_1$/J hybrids, and in Balb/cBy mice, the males were more sensitive.[16]

Needham et al. also investigated the possible role of morphine metabolism in hepatotoxicity. Normorphine, the product of *N*-demethylation of morphine, was not hepatotoxic at a dose of 50 mg/kg. Pretreatment with phenobarbital, an inducer of cytochrome P-450, did not potentiate liver damage from morphine. Chloramphenicol, an inhibitor of mixed-function oxidases, provided partial protection. SKF 525-A, another potent inhibitor, did not protect at all. On the other hand, the latter compound was by itself hepatotoxic at a dose of 50 mg/kg[16] However, SKF 525-A has some narcotic activity that is partially reversed by naloxone[18] and it has been reported to cause liver damage in dogs.[19]

Liver damage from morphine and hydromorphone, as indicated by both SGOT levels and staining of liver sections for fat, was considerably

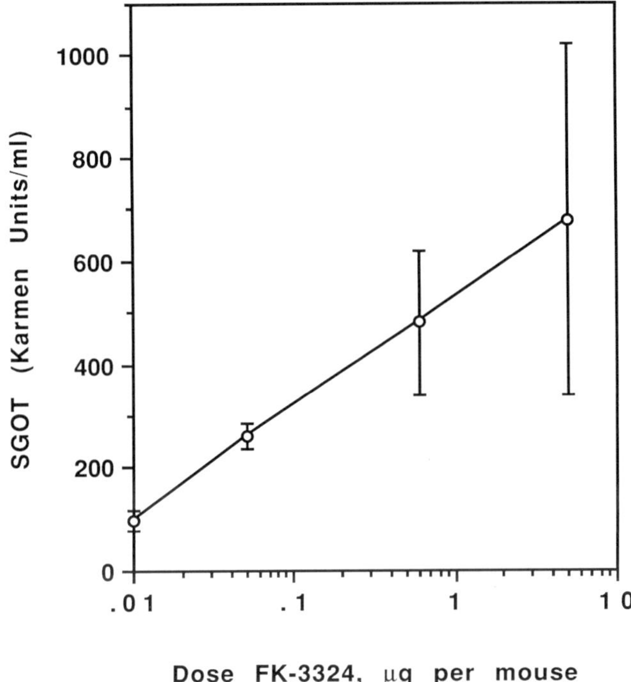

Dose FK-3324, μg per mouse

Fig. 1. Effect of intracerebral injection of the enkephalin analog FK-3324 on SGOT levels. B_6AF_1/J male mice were injected intraventricularly with 10 μL of the drug dissolved in 0.15M NaCl. They were bled for determination of SGOT 18 h later. The SGOT level in saline-injected mice was 73 Karmen U/mL. Each value is the mean ± SEM for 3–6 mice.

more pronounced in mice kept on pine shavings than in mice kept on corn-cob bedding.[16] The effect of exposure to pine bedding reached a maximum at 10 d, and was reversible (Fig. 2). Exposure to pine bedding is known to induce drug-metabolizing enzymes, and can potentiate markedly the hepatotoxicity of cocaine by stimulating its conversion to an active metabolite.[20]

In summary, the experiments of Needham et al.[16] suggest that, although central narcotic receptors play a key role in liver damage from morphine in mice, there may also be a component involving morphine metabolism in the liver. They did not observe an appreciable decrease in the hepatic

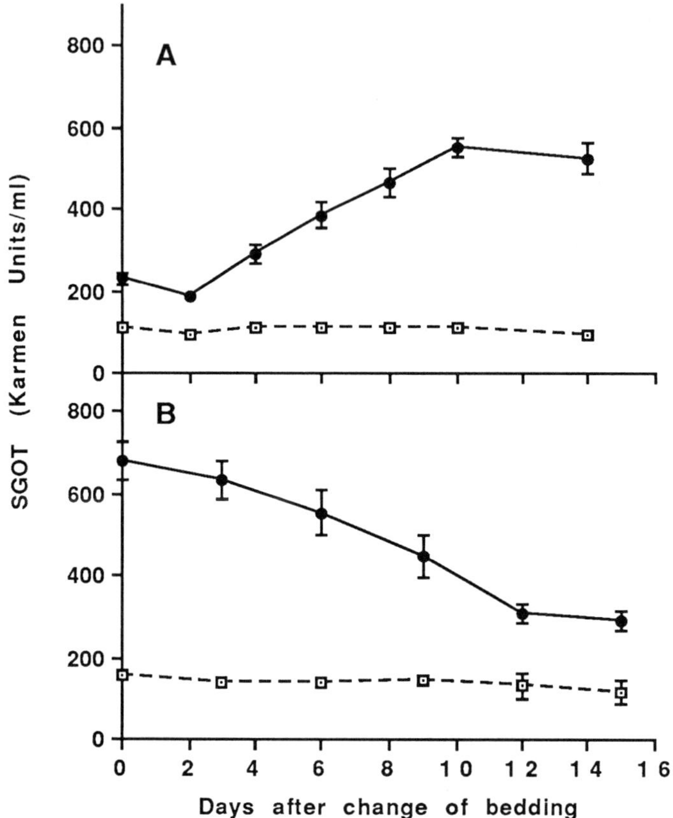

Fig. 2. Effect of changing bedding on the hepatotoxicity of morphine. C57Bl/ 6By male mice were kept on either pine or corn-cob bedding for 2 wk, then switched on day 0. At various times after the changeover different groups were injected ip with morphine sulfate, 100 mg/kg, and bled 18 h later for the determination of SGOT. Each point represents the mean value for 5 mice ± SEM: **(A)** changed from corncob bedding to pine shavings. **(B)** changed from pine shavings to corn-cob bedding. Dotted lines represent values for saline-injected controls.

cytochrome P-450 levels in mice injected with morphine. The following sections of this review deal with the mechanisms involved in liver damage from morphine. In the male rat, morphine metabolism appears to be of primary importance; in the mouse, the role of central narcotic receptors is more pronounced.

Metabolism of Morphine to Active Intermediates

Changes in Liver Glutathione Levels

The metabolic activation of hepatotoxins such as carbon tetrachloride and acetaminophen is believed to lead to the formation of free radicals that react with protein and with nucleophiles, such as glutathione. These reactions can be detected as covalent binding of hepatotoxin to cellular proteins and as a decrease in the concentration of reduced glutathione in the liver. In the case of acetaminophen, it has been postulated that a decrease of >80% in the concentration of glutathione in the liver leaves cells unprotected against free-radical oxidants such as peroxides and superoxide, that are produced in the course of normal metabolism. Oxidation of unsaturated fatty acids in cellular membranes and the release of lysosomal enzymes causes necrosis.[21]

It was therefore intriguing that two groups of workers found that high doses of morphine and other narcotics lowered hepatic glutathione levels at the same time that they produced elevation of serum transaminase activities in mice and rats.[22,23] The changes produced by morphine, SKF 525-A, L-α-acetylmethadol, and propoxyphene were diminished or prevented by pretreatment with the narcotic antagonist naltrexone. However, it was not clear whether naltrexone was acting centrally, to block narcotic receptors, or peripherally, to inhibit morphine metabolism.[22]

Pretreatment of rats with the cytochrome-P-450 inducer phenobarbital potentiated the effect of morphine on serum transaminase levels, but did not affect the change in liver glutathione, and 3-methylcholanthrene, which induces cytochrome P-448, was without effect.[23]

Metabolic Formation of a Glutathione Adduct

The incubation of tritiated dihydromorphine with rat liver microsomes and NADPH led to covalent labeling of soluble and microsomal proteins. Labeling was inhibited by carbon monoxide, by naloxone, and by glutathione. Activation of morphine via *N*-demethylation followed by *N*-hydroxylation was ruled out by the finding that normorphine and ethylmorphine (which is *N*-demethylated more readily than morphine) were much less hepatotoxic than morphine.[23]

An adduct of tritiated morphine and glutathione was isolated from enzyme incubation mixtures and identified by proton NMR and mass spectrometry as 10-α-S-glutathionyl-morphine.[24] This structure was confirmed by additional studies on an adduct of activated morphine with *N*-acetyl-cysteine.[25] The postulated metabolism of morphine to an active species that can react with both glutathione and proteins in illustrated in Fig. 3. The nature of the activation at the C-10 benzylic carbon has not yet been defined.

Morphinone as an Active Metabolite of Morphine

An entirely different metabolic activation step for converting morphine to a hepatotoxic metabolite has been proposed by Nagamatsu et al.[26,27] They argue that morphine is oxidized at position 6 by a cytosolic dehydrogenase to morphinone, which can bind covalently to the sulfhydryl groups of both glutathione and proteins (Fig. 4). The LD_{50} of morphinone in mice was about 50 mg/kg, that is, one-tenth that of morphine. Pretreatment with 1 g/kg of either glutathione or cysteine protected mice against a lethal dose of morphinone (80 mg/kg), but not against morphine (700 mg/kg). Morphinone (30 mg/kg) produced a greater decrease in liver glutathione than the same dose of morphine or dihydromorphine. In vitro, morphinone, but not morphine, reacted rapidly with both glutathione and cysteine to cause the disappearance of free sulfhydryl groups.[26] This reaction is typical of α, β-unsaturated ketones. Nagamatsu et al.[27] also isolated a morphinone–cysteine conjugate from proteolytic digests of liver protein from mice that had been injected with morphine.

Morphine-6-dehydrogenase was purified from guinea pig liver cytosol by Yamano et al.[28] Both NAD and NADP served as cofactors. The enzyme oxidized morphine, nalorphine, normorphine, codeine, and ethylmorphine, but was inactive with dihydromorphine, and only slightly active with dihydrocodeine. At pH 7.4 the activity of the enzyme was only one-fifth that at pH 9.1 or 9.7. However, morphinone was identified as a metabolite of morphine in guinea pig bile and urine, showing that it is formed under physiological conditions.

An interesting feature of morphine-6-dehydrogenase is that the same enzyme also functions to reduce naloxone to 6-α-naloxol.[29] For this reaction, either NADH or NADPH can serve as a cofactor. The pH optimum for naloxone reduction is 6.2–6.8. The enzyme has the general properties of a ketone reductase.[30] In addition to naloxone, the enzyme also reduces

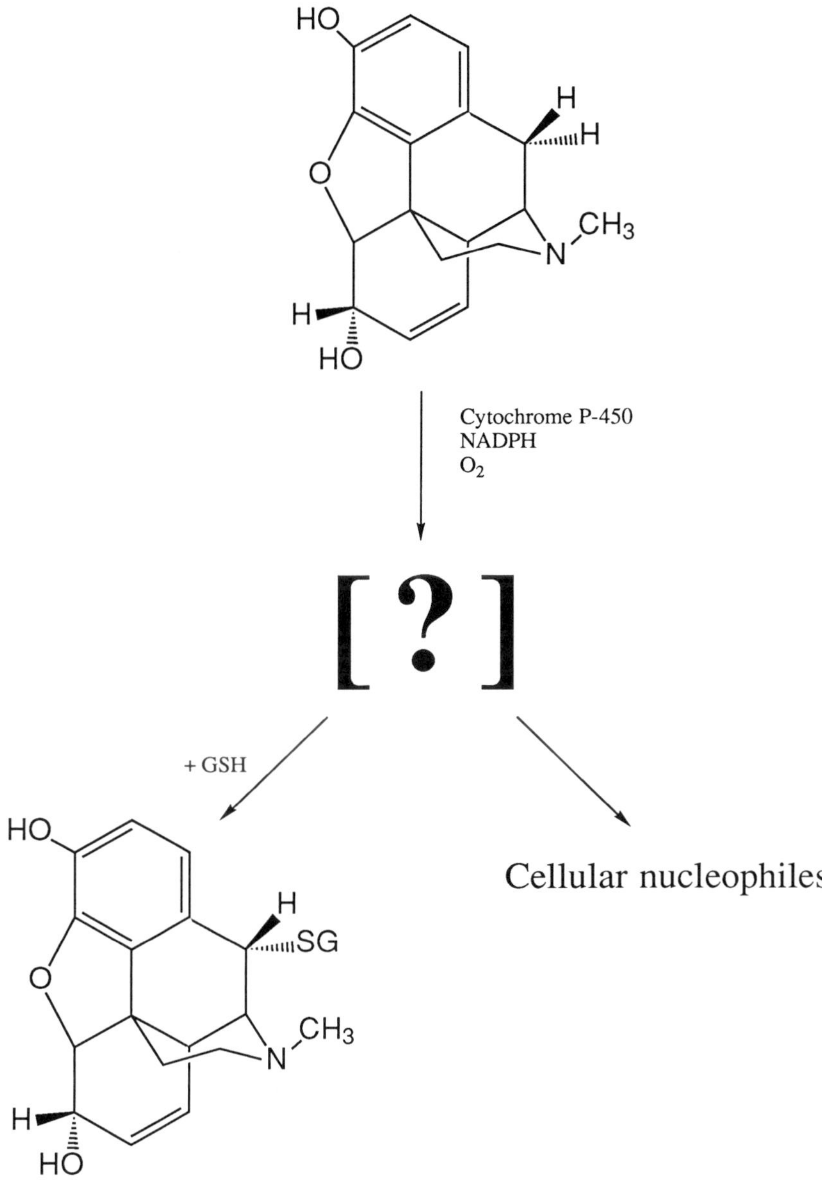

Fig. 3. Metabolism of morphine to an intermediate activated at C-10. This reaction scheme is based on Correia et al.[24]

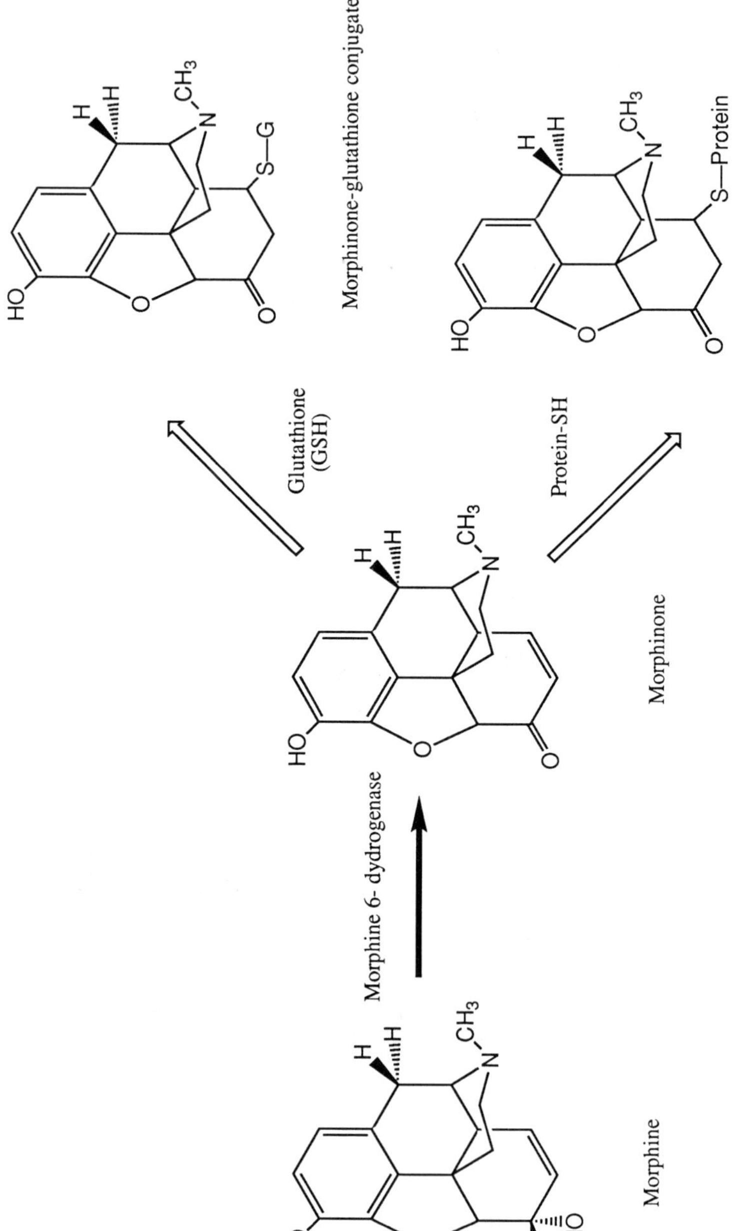

Fig. 4. Activation of morphine by morphine-6-dehydrogenase to morphinone. This reaction scheme is based on Nagamatsu et al.[27]

naltrexone, morphinone, and oxycodeine. Dihydromorphinone and dihydro-codeinone are poor substrates, and other aliphatic and aromatic ketones were not reduced. The enzyme appears to be specific for the oxidation and reduction of position 6 of morphine analogs with an unsaturated bond at C-7,8 and/or a C-14 hydroxyl group.

The addition of morphine to isolated rat hepatocytes at a concentration of 0.25 m*M* produced a 75% decrease in glutathione levels within 2 h.[31] This change was accompanied by a 20% decrease in viability. The same concentration of morphinone produced a complete loss of both glutathione and viability, as measured by the leakage of lactate dehydrogenase. The loss of glutathione in cells incubated with morphine was matched by the formation of a morphinone–glutathione conjugate. Naloxone prevented the formation of this conjugate and protected the cells against the toxic effects of morphine. Dihydromorphinone and normorphine produced only minor decreases in either glutathione levels or cell viability.

In vivo experiments carried out in rats showed that naloxone prevented the decrease in liver glutathione and increases in serum transaminases following morphine injections, but had no effect on the changes produced by morphinone. This finding suggests that naloxone protection against the hepatotoxicity of morphine is attributable to the inhibition of the formation of morphinone.[31]

Codeinone as an Active Metabolite of Codeine

Nagamatsu et al.[32] have also described the metabolism of codeine by 9000-g supernatant fractions of rat and guinea pig liver homogenates. The rat liver preparation produced codeinone, morphine, and norcodeine in the presence of NAD, but only the latter two metabolites in the presence of NADP. The guinea pig liver preparation made considerably less codeinone with NADP than with NAD. The acute toxicity of codeinone in mice was 30 times greater than that of codeine. Nagamatsu et al.[32] also postulated that codeinone could undergo further reduction of the 7,8-unsaturated bond to yield hydrocodeine, which could be reduced to 6-hydrocodol by morphine-6-dehydrogenase. Subcutaneous injection of codeine (100 mg/kg) and codeinone (5 mg/kg) into mice produced a 10% decrease in hepatic glutathione levels. The simultaneous injection of naloxone (10 mg/kg) prevented the decline after codeine, but not after codeinone. The injection of 10 mg/kg codeinone produced death from convulsions within 2 h. This death was prevented by glutathione or cysteine (500 mg/kg), but not by naloxone (50 mg/kg). Naloxone did protect against the lethal effect of 200 mg/kg codeine. The finding that death from codeinone was prevented by injecting 50 mg/kg phenobarbital suggests that the main toxicity of codeinone is attributable to its action as a convulsant, rather than to depletion of glutathione and liver damage.[33]

The interpretation of codeine hepatotoxicity is complicated by results obtained with isolated rat hepatocytes.[34] Hepatocytes exposed to codeine concentrations of $0.25M$ or higher for 1 h or more displayed leakage of LDH and a decline in GSH levels. There was no change in the content of NADPH or cytochrome P-450. The toxicity of codeine was not affected by pretreatment of the rats with phenobarbital, even though this treatment increased the level of cytochrome P-450. On the other hand, addition of the mixed-function oxidase inhibitor metyrapone at a concentration of 1.0 mM largely prevented the toxic effects of 0.5 mM codeine. The addition of methimazole, an inhibitor of FAD-containing monoxygenase, potentiated damage from codeine. Ellington and Rosen conclude that a cytochrome P-450-mediated pathway is responsible for the conversion of codeine to hepatotoxic intermediates.[34]

Comparison of Postulated Metabolic Pathways

The characteristics of the two pathways for metabolic activation of morphine are summarized in Table 1. The evidence supporting the morphinone pathway seems considerably stronger than that for C-10 oxidation. The morphinone intermediate has been identified, as has the specific enzyme that makes it. The toxicity of morphinone has been investigated, as has its reaction with both glutathione and proteins. The intermediate postulated by Correia et al.[24] remains unidentified. One way to reconcile the apparent conflict is to suggest that the C-10 product may be formed from morphinone. However, morphine dehydrogenase is a cytosolic enzyme, and the C-10 product can be formed from morphine by isolated microsomes. Another major difficulty is the hepatotoxicity and depletion of glutathione produced by dihydromorphine, hydromorphone, and levorphenol. None of these compounds has a 7,8 double bond that could be oxidized to an α, β-unsaturated ketone.

Table 1
Comparison of Metabolic Pathways for Activation of Morphine

	Nagamatsu et al.[27] Yamano et al.[28]	Correia et al.[23,24]
Species	Rat, guinea pig	Rat
Enzyme	Morphine-6-dehydrogenase	Cytochrome P-450
Cellular location	Cytoplasm	Smooth endoplasmic reticulum
Cofactors	NAD, NADP	NADPH
Optimal pH	9.1–9.7	7.4
Metabolic product	Morphinone (-α-unsaturated ketone)	Unknown
Substrate specificity	Morphine analog unsaturated at C-7,8 and/or having OH at C-14	(–)-3-Hydroxy-*N*-methyl morphinan
Product of metabolite with glutathione	8-S-Glutathionyl morphinone	10-α-S-glutathione morphine
Product of metabolite with proteins	8-S-Cysteinyl morphinone	10-α-S-cysteinyl morphine adduct

A serious problem with all theories that attribute the hepatotoxicity of morphine to metabolic activation is the wealth of evidence implicating narcotic receptors in the CNS. It is possible to demonstrate hepatotoxic effects from small amounts of narcotics injected directly into the brain. Furthermore, opioid peptides, which are not susceptible to any of the metabolic transformations described above, can also produce liver damage when injected into the brain.

Central Actions Related to Hepatotoxicity

Evidence for the Role of Narcotic Receptors

As described in the section on "Enzyme Changes and Histology in Rats," it is possible to produce fatty liver damage and elevation of serum transaminases in mice by injecting narcotic drugs or opioid peptides directly into the brain. Hepatotoxicity from narcotics injected peripherally is reduced or absent in narcotic-tolerant mice or in animals with a genetic deficiency of mu receptors in the brain.

Centrally-Mediated Changes
in Hepatic Glutathione

James et al.[22] reported that several narcotics lowered hepatic glutathione and increased SGPT levels when administered to mice orally or by ip injection. They concluded that the two effects were unrelated. Subsequent studies by this group have concentrated on the role of central narcotic receptors in lowering hepatic glutathione. The maximal decrease following intracerebroventricular injections of narcotic drugs was about 30%.

The effect of an intracerebroventricular (icv) injection of 100 μg of morphine was completely blocked when 100 μg of naltrexone was given by the same route.[35] Centrally administered naltrexone also prevented glutathione depletion after ip administration of morphine.[36] When a number of selective narcotic agonists were tested, only those that stimulate mu or delta receptors were capable of lowering hepatic glutathione.[35] The depression of hepatic glutathione cannot be attributed to morphine-induced hypoxia or hypothermia, nor does it result from intracellular oxidation of GSH to GSSG.[37]

Evidence for a Role
of Central Adrenergic Receptors

Pretreatment of mice with yohimbine or prazocin partially prevents the depletion of hepatic glutathione after icv morphine. Adrenalectomy completely prevents depletion, and this change is reversed by the injection of hydrocortisone. Peripheral autonomic blockers (i.e., propranolol, atropine, and hexamethonium) or destruction of peripheral adrenergic terminals with 6-hydroxydopamine are ineffective. Roberts et al. concluded that central adrenergic receptors may play a role in lowering hepatic glutathione.[38] James et al.[39] had previously demonstrated that epinephrine administered subcutaneously can lower hepatic glutathione levels, and morphine is known to cause the release of epinephrine from the adrenal medulla.[40] Epinephrine injected subcutaneously into mice produces a dose-related increase in serum transaminase levels (Table 2).[41] The question arises whether epinephrine released from the adrenals by central actions of morphine can

Table 2
Epinephrine-Induced Liver Damage in Mice

Epinephrine dose, mg/kg	Number surviving	SGOT Karmen U/mL ± SEM
1	6/6	195 ± 35
2	6/6	453 ± 90
5	6/6	2114 ± 858
7.5	10/17	6015 ± 1512
10	3/8	25529 ± 14739

[a]B_6AF_1/J male mice, kept on pine shavings, were injected sc with epinephrine dissolved in 0.15M NaCl and emulsified with olive oil. They were bled from the tail 18 h later, and SGOT was assayed according to Shuster et al.[54]

then act on central adrenergic receptors to lower hepatic concentrations of glutathione.

The results of Roberts et al.[38] suggest that the role of the adrenals in the glutathione-lowering action of morphine relates to the presence of glucocorticoids rather than to epinephrine. It should be borne in mind that the 25% decrease in hepatic glutathione produced by morphine in these experiments is unlikely to be responsible for liver damage. An overnight fast will produce a 50% decrease in hepatic glutathione in mice.[42]

A similar situation has been described for other drugs that produce liver damage following metabolic activation. The hepatotoxicity of cocaine in phenobarbital-induced mice is blocked by phentolamine and yohimbine. The effect of adrenergic blockers on the glutathione-lowering action of cocaine was considerably less than that on serum transaminase levels.[43]

A role for peripheral adrenergic receptors in the liver cannot be ruled out. For instance, phenylephrine and epinephrine cause the efflux of glutathione from the isolated perfused rat liver. This effect is blocked by the alpha antagonist prazocin.[44]

Changes in Lipid Metabolism

One peripheral adrenergic mechanism that could contribute to fatty necrosis is a change in lipid metabolism. Activation of hormone-sensitive lipase could release free fatty acids that can be transported to the liver where they can give rise to lipid peroxides. At 12 h after the implantation of a subcutaneous pellet of morphine base into mice there is a sixfold increase in the triglyceride content of the liver, and a 90% decrease in the activity of oleyl CoA: 1-ocyl-GPC-acyltransferase activity.[45] Another change in lipid metabolism, reported by Lamb and Dewey,[46] is a doubling of microsomal phosphatidate phosphohydrolase activity, which can also lead to increased triglyceride synthesis. This change has been encountered after exposure to other hepatotoxins as well as to ACTH.[47] Naloxone, which blocks the ACTH-releasing action of morphine,[48] also prevents the rise in phosphatidate phosphohydrolase after morphine.[46]

Although some of the lipolytic activity of morphine in vivo could be attributed to the release of epinephrine from the adrenal glands, there is also evidence for direct stimulation of lipases in vitro. Various narcotics increased the activity of a lipase from the mold *Rhizopus arrihizus*. The most potent was etorphine, which produced 38% stimulation at a concentration of 50 n*M*. Levorphanol was about 86 times more potent than its nonnarcotic enantiomer dextrophan. Higher concentrations of all the opiates tested were inhibitory.[49]

Thus, there are several mechanisms by which morphine could stimulate lipolysis of peripheral triglycerides and synthesis of hepatic lipids. Some of these mechanisms are also encountered in other situations that produce a fatty liver, such as partial hepatectomy, a carbohydrate-rich diet, and exposure to ethanol. The mechanism in these cases appears to involve glucocorticoid stimulation of protein synthesis leading to increased activity of phosphatidate phosphohydrolase. Perfusion of isolated rat liver with cortisol produces a threefold increase in activity of this enzyme, and the increase is prevented by actinomycin D.[50]

Interactions Between
Narcotics and Other Drugs

Synergism with Other Hepatotoxins

Morphine potentiates the hepatotoxic effects of cocaine and acetaminophen in mice.[22] An example of synergism between cocaine and hydromorphone is shown in Table 3. Synergism implies that two different mechanisms may be involved. James et al.[22] have suggested that potentiation by morphine results from a 25% decrease in hepatic glutathione levels. An effect of morphine metabolites seems to be ruled out by the finding of

Table 3
Effect of Epinephrine and Adrenalectomy
on Narcotic-Induced Liver Damage

Treatment	n	SGOT Karmen U/mL $\pm$ SEM
Hydromorphone, 50 mg/kg+ sham operation	4	739 ± 69
Hydromorphone, 50 mg/kg+ adrenex	6	322 ± 69
Morphine, 50 mg/kg	4	138 ± 14
Morphine, 50 mg/kg + epinephrine, 1 mg/kg	6	555 ± 120

[a]Male B_6AF_1/J male mice, kept on pine shavings, were injected ip with hydromorphone or morphine dissolved in $0.15M$ NaCl, and sc with epinephrine in NaCl emulsified with olive oil.

Adrenalectomy was carried out under pentobarbital anesthesia. The mice were given 0.9% NaCl in their drinking water and tested 7–10 d after surgery.

marked synergism between intracerebral morphine and systemic cocaine or acetaminophen.[36]

Effect on the Metabolism of Other Drugs

The subcutaneous implantation of pellets of morphine base into rats produces significant decreases in the cytochrome P-450 and phospholipid content of liver microsomes, and decreased activity of NADPH-Cytochrome c reductase and glucose-6-phosphatase. Although these changes may simply reflect damage to the endoplasmic reticulum, they also lead to a marked decrease in the rate of mixed-function oxidase activity. For example, there is a 70% decrease in the activity of *p*-chloro-*N*-methylaniline demethylase.[51] This finding is an extension of the original observation that morphine treatment decreases the activity of morphine-*N*-demethylase.[5] Morphine-induced changes in the metabolism of aniline and hexobarbital have also been reported.[9,11]

It is important to point out that all these effects of morphine on microsomal drug metabolism seem to be specific to adult male rats. They have not been demonstrated in mice.[9,11] Regulation of microsomal drug metabolism in male rats involves interactions among male sex hormones, the adrenal glands, and the hypothalamic–pituitary axis. It is unlikely that morphine is decreasing effective androgen levels, because simultaneous administration of testosterone does not antagonize the morphine-induced depression of drug metabolism.[9]

Possible Interactions with Ethanol

It would not be surprising if morphine could potentiate fatty liver damage from ethanol just as it acts synergistically with other hepatotoxins. If the oxidation of morphine to morphinone or to another reactive intermediate plays an important role, one could speculate on interactions with pyridine nucleotide coenzymes. The coenzyme for the oxidation of ethanol by alcohol dehydrogenase is NAD. Metabolism of ethanol, by increasing levels of NADH and NADPH, leads to increases in the biosynthesis of lipids. Conversion of NAD to NADH should decrease the activity of morphine-6-dehydrogenase, which requires either NAD or NADP. If this enzyme is responsible for activation of morphine to a hepatotoxic intermediate, then ethanol might decrease liver damage from morphine. On the other hand, chronic ethanol can induce the mixed-function oxidase system by increasing the synthesis of cytochrome P-450IIE.[52] It would be helpful to know which subfamily of cytochrome P-450 might play a role in the metabolic activation of morphine to hepatotoxic intermediates.

Questions to be Resolved

Even in experimental animals, the picture of morphine-induced liver damage that has emerged to date is fragmentary and confused. It is difficult to correlate results from rats, where there is good evidence of metabolic activation and mechanism-based destruction of cytochrome P-450, to those from mice, where narcotic receptors in the CNS appear to play an important role. Several puzzling aspects of liver damage from narcotics in mice are still unexplained. One is the pronounced effect of age, as illustrated in Fig. 5. The increased sensitivity between the ages of 8 and 24 wk cannot be attributed to differences in the activity of hepatic mixed-function oxidases. Lauterburg et al.[53] have reported a marked age-related decline in the rate of turnover of hepatic glutathione, but no change in glutathione concentration, in rats. They suggest that this change may be responsible for age-related increases in sensitivity to hepatotoxins such as acetaminophen.

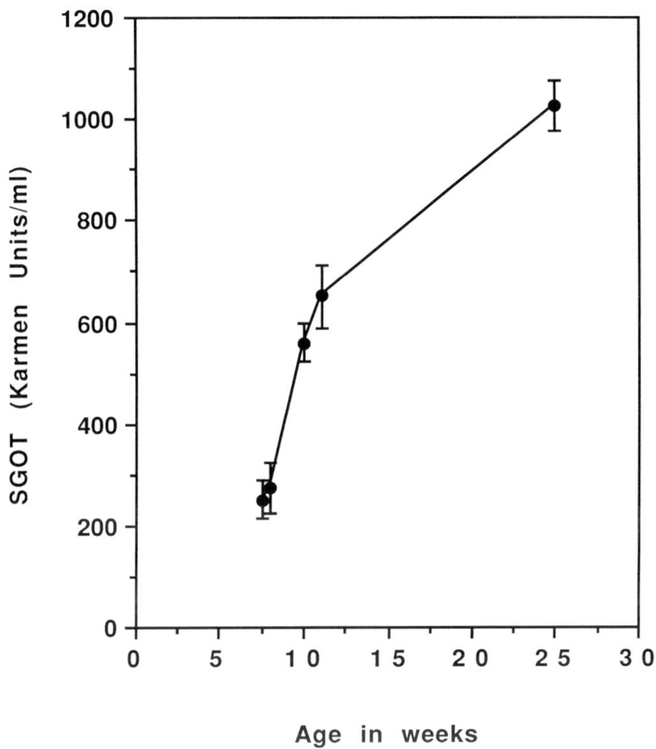

Fig. 5. Narcotic-induced liver damage in mice of different ages. Male B_6AF_1/J mice kept on pine bedding were bled 18 h after the injection of hydromorphone · HCl, 50 mg/kg ip. Each value is the mean ± SEM for 5 mice.

We have also found that pretreatment of mice with a single dose of morphine — one that by itself does not produce liver damage — protects against the hepatotoxicity of a subsequent dose of hydromorphone given as long as 2 wk later (Fig. 6). By this time any slight analgesic tolerance that could have been caused by the initial dose would certainly have worn off.

These questions are not likely to be amenable to experiments with simpler systems, such as perfused livers or cultured hepatocytes. Not enough attention has been paid to species and strain differences. Eventually it may prove fruitful to look more closely at human subjects who have received

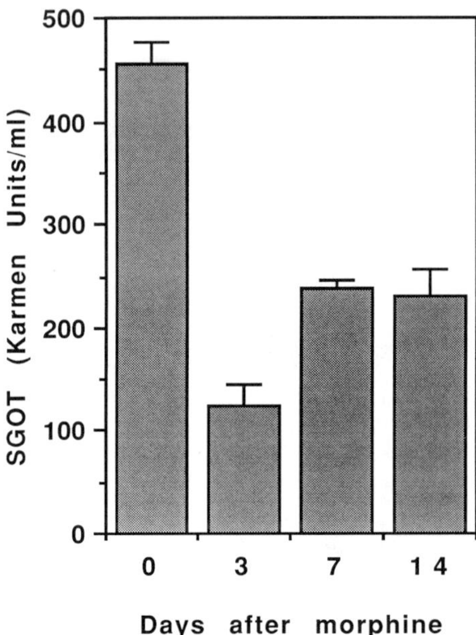

Fig. 6. Effect of pretreatment with morphine on subsequent liver damage from hydromorphone. Male B_6AF_1/J mice were given a single injection of morphine sulfate, 25 mg/kg ip. At various times after this treatment different groups were injected with hydromorphone, 50 mg/kg, and bled 18 h later for determination of SGOT. Each bar represents the mean value for 5 mice ± SEM. The mice were 10 wk old at the beginning of the experiment.

very large doses of narcotic drugs under controlled conditions—for example, surgery patients who are injected intravenously with several hundred milligrams of morphine for general anesthesia.

Acknowledgments

Some of the experiments described here were supported by Grant #DA-01885 from the National Institute on Drug Abuse. I am grateful to James Powers for technical assistance and to Sandoz Pharmaceuticals Corporation for providing compound FK-3324.

References

[1] C. W. Gorodetzky, J. D. Sapira, D. R. Jasinski, and W. R. Martin (1968) Liver disease in narcotic addicts. I. The role of the drug. *Clin. Pharmacol. Ther.* **9,** 720–724.

[2] M. J. Kreek, L. Dodes, S. Kane, J. Knobler, and R. Martin (1972) Long-term methadone maintenance therapy: Effects liver function. *Ann. Intern. Med.* **77(4),** 598–602.

[3] J. D. Sapira, D. R. Jasinski, and C. W. Gorodetzky (1968) Liver disease in narcotic addicts. II. The role of the needle. *Clin. Pharmacol. Ther.* **9,** 725–739.

[4] F. P. Brooks, G. A. Deneau, H. P. Potter, Jr., J. G. Reinhold, and R. F. Norris (1963) Liver function tests in morphine-addicted and in nonaddicted rhesus monkeys. *Gastroenterology* **44,** 287–290.

[5] J. Axelrod (1956) Possible mechanism of tolerance to narcotic drugs. *Science* **24,** 263–264.

[6] J. Cochin and J. Axelrod (1959) Biochemical and pharmacological changes in the rat following chronic administration of morphine, nalorphine and normorphine. *J. Pharmacol.* **125,** 105–110.

[7] D. H. Clouet and M. Ratner (1964) The effect of altering liver microsomal *N*-demethylase activity on the development of tolerance to morphine in rats. *J. Pharmacol. Exp. Ther.* **144,** 362–372.

[8] R. Kato and J. R. Gillette (1965) Sex differences in the effects of abnormal physiological states on the metabolism of drugs by rat liver microsomes. *J. Pharmacol. Exp. Ther.* **150,** 285–291.

[9] N. E. Sladek, M. D. Chaplin, and G. J. Mannering (1974) Sex-dependent differences in drug metabolism in the rat. IV. Effect of morphine administration. *Drug Metab. Dispos.* **2,** 293–300.

[10] D. Gurantz and M. A. Correia (1981) Morphine-mediated effects on rat hepatic heme and cytochrome P-450 in vivo. *Biochem. Pharmacol.* **30,** 1529–1536.

[11] R. Kato, K. I. Onoda, and A. Takanaka (1971) Species differences in the effect of morphine administration or adrenalectomy on the substrate interactions with cytochrome P–450 and drug oxidations by liver microsomes. *Biochem. Pharmacol.* **20,** 1093–1089.

[12] A. Hurwitz, H. R. Fischer, J. D. Innis, S. Ronsse, and Z. Ben-Zvi (1985) Opioid effects on hepatic disposition of dyes in mice. *J. Pharmacol. Exp. Ther.* **232,** 617–623.

[13] A. Hurwitz (1981) Narcotic effects on phenol red disposition in mice. *J. Pharmacol. Exp. Ther.* 216, 90–94.

[14] A. Thureson-Klein, J. W. Yang, and I. K. Ho (1978) Lipid accumulation in mouse hepatocytes after morphine exposure. *Experientia* **34,** 773–774.

[15] Y. H. Chang and I. K. Ho (1979) Effects of acute and continuous morphine administration on serum glutamate-oxalacetate transaminase and glutamate-pyruvate transaminase activities in the mouse. *Biochem. Pharmacol.* **28,** 1373–1377.

[16] W. P. Needham, L. Shuster, G. C. Kanel, and M. L. Thompson (1981) Liver damage from narcotics in mice. *Toxicol. Appl. Pharmacol.* **58,** 157–170.

[17] A. Baran, L. Shuster, B. E. Eleftheriou, and D. W. Bailey (1975) Opiate receptors in mice: Genetic differences. *Life Sci.* **17,** 633–640.

[18] T. Lehman and G. R. Petersen (1978) Naloxone — reversible analgesic action of SKF–525A in mice. *Psychopharmacol.* **59,** 305–308.

[19] E. C. Dick, S. M. Greenberg, J. F. Herndon, M. Jones, and E. J. Van Loon (1960) Hypocholesteremic effects of 2–diethylaminoethyl 2, 2–diphenylvalyrate (SKF–525A) in the dog. *Proc. Soc. Exp. Biol. Med.* **104,** 523–526.

[20] M. L. Thompson, L. Shuster, and K. Shaw (1979) Cocaine-induced hepatic necrosis in mice. The role of cocaine metabolism. *Biochem. Pharmacol.* **28,** 2389–2395.

[21] A. R. Boobis, D. J. Fawthrop, and D. S. Davies (1989) Mechanisms of cell death. *Trends Pharmacol. Sci.* **10,** 275–280.

[22] R. C. James, D. R. Goodman, and R. D. Harbison (1982) Hepatic glutathione and hepatotoxicity: Changes induced by selected narcotics. *J. Pharmacol. Exp. Ther.* **221,** 708– 714.

[23] M. A. Correia, J. S. Wong, and E. Soliven (1984) Morphine metabolism revisited: I. Metabolic activation of morphine to a reactive species in rats. *Chem. Biol. Interact.* **49,** 255–268.

[24] M. A. Correia, G. Krowech, P. Caldera-Munoz, S. L. Yee, K. Straub, and N. Castagnoli (1984) Morphine metabolism revisited. II. Isolation and chemical characterization of a glutathionylmorphine adduct from rat liver microsomal preparations. *Chem. Biol. Interact.* **51,** 13–24.

[25] G. Krowech, P. S. Caldera-Munoz, K. Straub, N. Castagnoli, and M. A. Correia (1986) Morphine metabolism revisited. III. Confirmation of a novel metabolic pathway. *Chem. Biol. Interact.* **58,** 29–40.

[26] K. Nagamatsu, Y. Kido, T. Terao, T. Ishida, and S. Toki (1982) Protective effect of sulfhydryl compounds on acute toxicity of morphinone. *Life Sci.* **30,** 1121–1127.

[27] K. Nagamatsu, Y. Kido, T. Terao, T. Ishida, and S. Toki (1983) Studies on the mechanism of covalent binding of morphine metabolites to proteins in mouse. *Drug Metab. Dispos.* **11(3),** 190–194.

[28] S. Yamano, E. Kageura, T. Ishida, and S. Toki (1985) Purification and characterization of guinea pig liver morphine 6-dehydrogenase. *J. Biol. Chem.* **260,** 5259–5264.

[29] S. Yamano, F. Nishida, and S. Toki (1986) Guinea-pig liver morphine 6-dehydrogenase as a naloxone reductase. *Biochem. Pharmacol.* **35(23),** 4321–4326.

[30] R. L. Felsted and N. R. Bachur (1980) Mammalian carbonyl reductases. *Drug Metab. Rev.* **11**, 1–60.

[31] K. Nagamatsu, Y. Ohno, H. Ikebuchi, A. Takahashi, T. Terao, and A. Takanaka (1986) Morphine metabolism in isolated rat hepatocytes and its implications for hepatotoxicity. *Biochem. Pharmacol.* **35**, 3543–3548.

[32] K. Nagamatsu, T. Terao, and S. Toki (1985) In vitro formation of codeinone from codeine by rat or guinea pig liver homogenate and its acute toxicity in mice. *Biochem. Pharmacol.* **34**, 3143–3146.

[33] K. Nagamatsu, K. Inoue, T. Terao, and S. Toki (1986) Effects of glutathione and phenobarbital on the toxicity of codeinone. *Biochem. Pharmacol.* **35**, 1675–1678.

[34] S. P. Ellington and G. M. Rosen (1987) Codeine-mediated hepatotoxicity in isolated rat hepatocytes. *Toxicol. Appl. Pharmacol.* **90**, 156–165.

[35] R. C. James, W. D. Wessinger, S. M. Roberts, G. C. Millner, and M. G. Paule (1988) Centrally mediated opioid induced depression of hepatic glutathione: Effects of intracerebroventricular administration of mu, kappa, sigma and delta agonists. *Toxicology* **51**, 267–279.

[36] N. P. Skoulis, R. C. James, R. D. Harbison, and S. M. Roberts (1989) Depression of hepatic glutathione by opioid analgesic drugs in mice. *Toxicol. Appl. Pharmacol.* **99**, 139–147.

[37] N. P. Skoulis, R. C. James, R. D. Harbison, and S. M. Roberts (1989) Perturbation of glutathione by a central action of morphine. *Toxicology* **57**, 287–302.

[38] S. M. Roberts, N. P. Skoulis, and R. C. James (1987) A centrally-mediated effect of morphine to diminish hepatocellular glutathione. *Biochem. Pharmacol.* **36**, 3001–3005.

[39] R. C. James, S. M. Roberts, and R. D. Harbison (1983) The perturbation of hepatic glutathione by α_2 adrenergic agonists. *Fundam. Appl. Toxicol.* **3**, 303–308.

[40] M. Vassalle (1961) Role of catecholamine release in morphine hyperglycemia. *Am. J. Physiol.* **200**, 530–534.

[41] L. Shuster, C. A. Garhart, J. Powers, Y. Grunfeld, and G. Kanel (1988) Hepatotoxicity of Cocaine, in *Mechanisms of Cocaine Abuse and Toxicity.* NIDA Research Monograph 88. D. Clouet, K. Asghar, R. Brown, eds. National Institute on Drug Abuse, Rockville, MD, pp. 250–275.

[42] R. R. Brooks and S. F. Pong (1981) Effects of fasting, body weight, methycellulose, and carboxymethycellulose on hepatic glutathione levels in mice and hamsters. *Biochem. Pharmacol.* **30**, 589–594.

[43] R. C. James, M. A. Schiefer, S. M. Roberts, and R. D. Harbison (1987) Antagonism of cocaine-induced hepatotoxicity by the alpha adrenergic antagonists phentolamine and yohimbine. *J. Pharmacol. Exp. Ther.* **242**, 726–732.

[44] H. Sies and P. Graf (1985) Hepatic thiol and glutathione efflux under the influence of vasopressin, phenylephrine and adrenaline. *Biochem. J.* **226**, 545–549.

[45] G. Y. Sun, D. W. Hallett, and I. K. Ho (1978) Effect of morphine on hepatic lipid metabolism. *Biochem. Pharmacol.* **27**, 1779–1782.

[46] R. G. Lamb and W. L. Dewey (1981) Effect of morphine exposure on mouse liver triglyceride formation. *J. Pharmacol. Exp. Ther.* **216**, 496–499.

[47] H. P. Glenny and D. N. Brindley (1978) The effects of cortisol, corticotropin and thyroxine on the synthesis of glycerolipids and on the phosphatidate phosphohydrolase activity in rat liver. *Biochem. J.* **176**, 777–784.

[48] J. P. Heybach and J. Vernikos (1981) Naloxone inhibits and morphine potentiates the adrenal steroidogenic response to ACTH. *Eur. J. Pharmacol.* **75**, 1–6.

[49] P. D. Kelly and J. R. Traynor (1981) Effects of narcotic analgesics on lipase activity in vitro. *Br. J. Pharmacol.* **73**, 301P–302P.

[50] M. A. Lehtonen, M. J. Savolainen, and I. E. Hassinen (1979) Hormonal regulation of hepatic soluble phosphatidate phosphohydrolase. Induction by cortisol in vivo and in isolated perfused rat liver. *FEBS Lett.* **99**, 162–166.

[51] V. Amzel and T. A. Van Der Hoeven (1979) Morphine-induced depression of the hepatic microsomal drug-metabolizing enzyme—effect on the lipid component. *Biochem. Pharmacol.* **29**, 658–661.

[52] M. J. Coon and D. R. Koop (1987) Alcohol-inducible cytochrome P-450 (P-450 ALC). *Arch. Toxicol.* **60**, 16–21.

[53] B. H. Lauterburg, Y. Vaishnav, W. G. Stillwell, and J. R. Mitchell (1980) The effects of age and glutathione depletion on hepatic glutathione turnover in vivo determined by acetaminophen probe analysis. *J. Pharmacol. Exp. Ther.* **213**, 54–58.

[54] L. Shuster, A. Bates, and C. A. Hirsch (1978) A sensitive radiochemical assay for serum glutamic-oxaloacetic transaminase. *Anal. Biochem.* **86**, 648–654.

Index